To See with a Better Eye

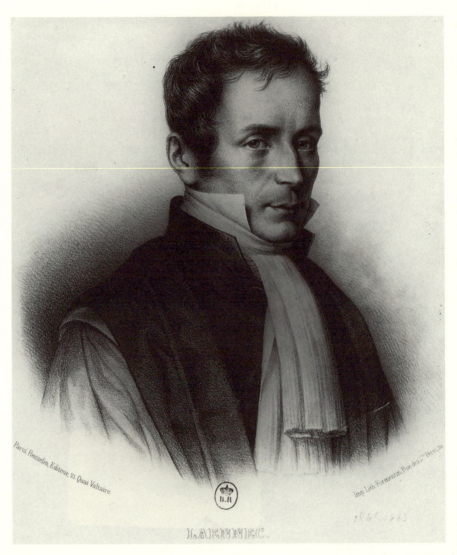

LAENNEC.

Frontispiece. Laennec in academic robes, after the engraving by Ambroise Tardieu for Panckoucke's *Biographie médicale*, ca. 1823–1824. Laennec's cousin, Christophe, did not think that this portrait resembled its subject, because he was not wearing his glasses. Photograph: Roger-Viollet, Paris.

To See with a Better Eye

A LIFE OF R.T.H. LAENNEC

• *JACALYN DUFFIN* •

PRINCETON UNIVERSITY PRESS

PRINCETON, NEW JERSEY

Library of Congress Cataloging-in-Publication Data

Duffin, Jacalyn
To see with a better eye :
A life of R. T. H. Laennec / Jacalyn Duffin.
p. cm.
Includes bibliographical references and index.
ISBN 0-691-03708-6 (cloth: alk. paper)
1. Laennec, R. T. H. (René Théophile Hyacinthe), 1781–1826.
2. Physicians—France—Biography. I. Title.
R507.L25D84 1998
610'92—dc21
[B]   97-19779 CIP

This book has been composed in Galliard

Princeton University Press books are printed on acid-free paper, and meet the guidelines
for permanence and durability of the Committee on Production Guidelines for Book
Longevity of the Council on Library Resources

http://pup.princeton.edu

Printed in the United States of America

1 3 5 7 9 10 8 6 4 2

• FOR ROBERT DAVID WOLFE •

He is the greatest physician who is the most profound in thought, as he will see, with a better eye, the nicest phenomena of life and predict more remotely the kind of disease which threatens an individual.

—*Corvisart [1806], 19*

Medicine is not a new science.

—*Hippocrates*, Ancient Medicine, *cited by Laennec 1804h, epigraph*

• CONTENTS •

LIST OF ILLUSTRATIONS — xi

LIST OF TABLES — xiii

ACKNOWLEDGMENTS — xv

INTRODUCTION — 3

PART ONE: PATHOLOGY: ANATOMY, PHYSIOLOGY,
AND THE BODY POLITIC — 9

CHAPTER ONE
Youth and Revolution — 11

CHAPTER TWO
Student in the Paris School — 24

CHAPTER THREE
Research and Academic Aspirations — 54

CHAPTER FOUR
Clinical Practice, Clinical Physiology — 77

CHAPTER FIVE
The Restoration: Politics, Hospitals, and Patients — 102

PART TWO: AUSCULTATION — 119

CHAPTER SIX
The Discovery — 121

CHAPTER SEVEN
The Treatise on Mediate Auscultation: The Lungs — 151

CHAPTER EIGHT
The Treatise on Mediate Auscultation: The Heart and
Clinical Reasoning — 174

PART THREE: DISEASE — 207

CHAPTER NINE
Reception and Impact of Auscultation: Reviews, Diagnoses,
and Broussais — 209

CHAPTER TEN
Return to Paris: Elite Practice and Professor in the Clinic — 240

CHAPTER ELEVEN
At the Collège de France: The Second Unpublished Book | 259

CHAPTER TWELVE
Between the Quick and the Dead: Pathology, Physiology,
and Clinical Medicine | 286

APPENDIX A
A Note on Sources: Scientific Papers and Correspondence | 305

APPENDIX B
Laennec's Finances | 311

APPENDIX C
Patients in the Two Editions of the *Traité de l'auscultation* | 314

APPENDIX D
Laennec's Network: A Glossary of Frequently Cited Names | 324

APPENDIX E
The Family of R. T. H. Laennec | 328

LIST OF ABBREVIATIONS | 329

NOTES | 333

*BIBLIOGRAPHY OF R. T. H. LAENNEC: PUBLICATIONS, REVIEWS,
AND OTHER PROFESSIONAL ACTIVITIES* | 397

BIBLIOGRAPHY | 407

INDEX | 437

Frontispiece: Laennec in academic robes, after engraving by
    Ambroise Tardieu, ca. 1823   ii
1.1. Laennec's birthplace   12
1.2. Portrait of Laennec's uncle, Guillaume Laennec   14
1.3. Théophile-Anne-Françoise Laennec, la petite tante de Miniac   20
2.1. Jean-Nicolas Corvisart des Marets   26
2.2. Jean-Noël Hallé   31
2.3. Case history of wigmaker, Antoine Michel, "cadet Rousseau."   34
2.4. Gaspard-Laurent Bayle   39
2.5. *The Death of Bichat*   41
2.6. "I am a doctor since yesterday," letter, 1804   52
3.1. Detail of Laennec's drawings of his new "genre" of worm,
    acephalocysts   57
3.2. Laennec's unpublished treatise on pathological anatomy,
    1804–1808   66
3.3. Chapter on cirrhosis from Laennec's unpublished treatise on
    pathological anatomy   72
4.1. The chateau at Couvrelles near Soissons   81
4.2. Laennec, the Dubois portrait   86
4.3. Laennec's patient, René de Chateaubriand   88
4.4. Laennec's patient, Céleste Buisson de la Vigne, Madame de
    Chateaubriand   89
4.5. Laennec's clerical friend Pierre-Vincent Dombideau de
    Crouseilhes, Bishop of Quimper   95
6.1. Laennec listening at a wooden beam, from film by Maurice
    Cloche, 1949   123
6.2. Laennec "Memoire sur l'auscultation," 23 February 1818   128
6.3. Laennec's stethoscope of 1819   130
6.4. Laennec practicing direct auscultation on a patient at the
    Necker hospital   135
6.5. Views of pulmonary emphysema, 1819   144
6.6. Case history of Marie-Magdeleine Grigy, February 1818   146
7.1. First edition of Laennec's treatise on mediate auscultation,
    August 1819   153
7.2. Stages in the life history of the tubercle, 1819   159
7.3. Man cured of chronic pleurisy with retraction of the chest   161
8.1. So-called portrait of Laennec, labeled and signed by
    J. J. Ansiaux   175
8.2. Laennec's Latin essay on angina pectoris, December 1810   195
9.1. An early image of mediate auscultation   212

9.2. The manor of Kerlouarnec, at Ploaré   220
9.3. Laennec's drawing of a door, ca. 1820   221
9.4. The marsh known as Palud de Cosquer, near the town of
      Pont l'Abbé   222
9.5. Presumed self-portrait of Laennec, as the "hermit"
      of Kerlouarnec   223
9.6. F. J. V. Broussais   226
9.7. Schematic representation of the pathophysiology of
      Broussais and Laennec   228
10.1. Laennec's patient, the Duchesse de Berry   242
10.2. Caricature of Laennec at Bordeaux, 1824   255
10.3. Letter from Laennec announcing his marriage,
       2 December 1824   257
11.1. Sketch of Laennec by C. J. B. Williams, 1825   262
11.2. Laennec's opening address at the Collège de France,
       December 1822   264
11.3. "Existence of vital principle," undated manuscript in
       the hand of Laennec   265
11.4. Mériadec Laennec, the young cousin   281
11.5. Laennec's tomb, Ploaré   284
11.6. Plaster cast of the cranium of Laennec, made in 1934   285
12.1. Bronze statue of Laennec erected in the town square
       of Quimper in 1868   292

Table 2.1. Laennec in the Paris School, 1801–1804   30
Table 3.1. Laennec's Classification of Intestinal Parasites,
   1804–1826   56
Table 3.2. Laennec's Classification of Anatomical Lesions,
   1804–1826   62
Table 3.3. Laennec's Treatise of Pathological Anatomy, ca.
   1803–1808: Structure and Cases   71
Table 5.1. Hospital Movement at Necker Hospital during
   Laennec's Presence, 1816–1819   109
Table 5.2. Hospital Movement at Necker Hospital during
   Laennec's Presence, 1821–1822   109
Table 5.3. Occupations of Six Hundred Forty-Six Patients in
   Laennec's Hospital Records (Necker and Charité Hospitals,
   1816–1826)   113
Table 6.1. Theses of Laennec's Students and Other Associates,
   1818–1823   148
Table 7.1. Clinical Records Pertaining to Puerile Respiration
   and Asthma   172
Table 8.1. Laennec's Classification of Organic Lesions of the
   Heart, 1822–1826   181
Table 8.2. Laennec's Criteria for Diagnosis of Cardiac Hyper-
   trophy and Dilatation   190
Table 8.3. Diagnoses of Heart Disease in the *Traité de l'ausculta-
   tion* and the Manuscripts   198
Table 8.4. Correlation of Auscultatory Evidence with Pathology
   and Physiology: Clinical Examples   203
Table 9.1. Admission Diagnoses of Patients Who Died in Necker
   Hospital, 1816–1823   214
Table 9.2. Comparison of Admission and Postmortem Diagnoses
   for Patients Who Died in the Necker Hospital, 1822 and 1823   215
Table 9.3. Diagnosis of Heart Disease at Admission among Patients
   Who Died in the Necker Hospital during Laennec's Presence,
   1816–1823   216
Table 9.4. Final Diagnosis of Heart Disease in Patients Who Died
   in the Charité Hospital during Laennec's Presence, 1823–1826 217
Table 10.1. Hospital Movement at the Charité Hospital,
   1823–1826   246
Table B.1. An Estimation of Laennec's Changing Financial
   Situation, 1804–1826   311

Table B.2.　Laennec's Wills and Estate　　　　　　　　　　313
Table C.1.　Complete Case Histories in the *Traité de l'auscultation médiate*, 1819 and 1826　　　　　　　　　　316
Table C.2.　Brief Case Histories First Used in the *Traité de l'auscultation médiate*, 1819　　　　　　　　　　317
Table C.3.　Brief Case Histories First Used in the *Traité de l'auscultation médiate*, 1826　　　　　　　　　　320

• *A C K N O W L E D G M E N T S* •

MIRKO DRAZEN GRMEK welcomed me as his student in November 1982, suggested Laennec as a dissertation topic, patiently tolerated the first historical research of a clinician, responded to my writing with alacrity and constructive criticism, and, in the end, became my friend. His unfailing support has been an ingenious blend of prodding and reticence—an inspiration in itself. Toby Gelfand supervised my postdoctoral fellowship in Ottawa where I was able to expand the work begun in France. He gently counseled me through the rough passages in my North American debut, while his enthusiasm for and knowledge of French medicine was the basis of our friendship and a stimulus to my work.

The families of Laennec "descendants" were warmly receptive to my study of their illustrious ancestor, readily opening their homes and their archives to a Canadian intruder. I thank M. Hervé and Mme Bernadette de Miniac of Rennes; the family of Bertrand Laennec in Lyons, especially M. François Laennec and Dr. Eric and Mme Laurence Laennec; M. Yves and Mme Lorraine Laennec of Paris; M. François Puget of Quimper; M. Rousselot and the Chéguillaume family of Nantes. Many others in France also willingly donated their help: they include M. André Halna du Frétay, the owner of Kerlouarnec, who greeted my endeavour with a hearty welcome, Dr. Paul Clouard of Quimper, and Dr. J. P. Kernéis and Dr. Charles Dubois, both of Nantes. I also thank Professor Jackie Pigeaud of the Université de Nantes for his permission to consult the Laennec papers and for the many excellent evenings that we spent, together with Alfrida Pigeaud, "laennecisant." My friends François and Martine Gallouin of Vitry-sur-Seine eagerly solved problems of every imaginable sort with dazzling energy and speed.

Many archivists and librarians facilitated my work. It is a pleasant duty to acknowledge the courtesy and cheerful efficiency of Laure Teulade, Sonia Bosc and their predecessor, Nelly Galkowski, of the Musée Laennec in Nantes. I also am grateful for the help of Agnès Marcetteau of the Nantes Médiathèque; municipal archivist Hervé Glorinnec and archivist of the évêché Jean-Louis Le Floch, both in Quimper; Robert Bonfils and his colleagues at the Archives des Jéuites in Vanves, the friendly archivists at the Archives of the Assistance Publique and of the Collège de France in Paris. Janine Samion-Contet, B. Molitor, and their associates made my visits to the Bibliothèque Interuniversitaire de Médecine successful and pleasant, while the many kindnesses of Monique Chapuis, Jacqueline Chapuis, Michelle Lenoir, her predecessors, and their colleagues of the Académie de Médecine of Paris, have allowed me to think of their magnificent library as home away from home for many years.

I have benefited from the treasures of several excellent libraries in North America and Britain and am honored to mention the names of people who thoughtfully directed me to materials that I might otherwise have overlooked: they are Toby Appel, Mike Barfoot, Lois Black, Elaine Challacombe, Jon Erlen, Tom Horrocks, Wayne Lebel, Paul Kligfield, Ed Morman, Ellen Nagle, Phil Teigen, Dorothy Whitcomb, and Barbara Williams. The staff of the Bracken Library at Queen's University quickly retrieved rare items from distant libraries on many occasions.

I am deeply indebted to those who took the time to read and criticize earlier drafts of the entire manuscript: they are Ann La Berge, Olga Kits, Paul Potter, R. D. Wolfe, John Harley Warner, Cherrilyn Yalin, and an anonymous reader for Princeton University Press. Guenter Risse, Leonard Wilson, and the late Dr. Miguel Chiong kindly commented on specific chapters, and their keen observations came to influence other portions of the writing. I have enjoyed opportunities to speak about Laennec to a number of medical and historical audiences in France and in North America, from San Francisco to St. John's Newfoundland and from Mexico City to Winnipeg—the questions that emerged from these contacts shaped the final product. Several scholars engaged with my work in diverse ways; for their special favors recognition belongs to Maria Teresa Andrès, Françoise Blateau, K. Codell Carter, Dale Dotten, Bruce Fye, Peter Galbraith, Caroline Hannaway, Joel D. Howell, James Leith, Otto Marx, Russell C. Maulitz, Terrie Romano, the late Roselyne Rey, the late Jacques Roger, Ana Cecilia de Romo, Charles Rosenberg, Joan Sherwood, Mark E. Silverman, William Summers, Dora B. Weiner, and George Weisz.

Danielle Gourevitch, Rodopi Press and the editors of the *Bulletin of the History of Medicine,* the *Canadian Bulletin of Medical History, Canadian Medical Association Journal, Medical History, History and Philosophy of Life Sciences,* the *Journal of the History of Medicine and Allied Sciences, Transactions and Studies of the College of Physicians of Philadelphia,* as well as the organizers of conferences and editors of cited volumes gave permission to use of material published earlier. At Princeton University Press, Emily Wilkinson, Kevin Downing, and Madeleine Adams treated my concerns with remarkable consideration, tact, and speed, while Teresa Carson's meticulous copy editing brought both clarity and moral support.

I acknowledge with thanks the vital funding of the Hannah Institute for the History of Medicine, which, for twelve years, has been the source of the material conditions of my employment, as well as provider of a special grant to facilitate travel in France. Dr. Duncan Sinclair, most unusual of deans, read my work, was excited by its potential, and supported the sabbatical year that gave me the liberty to finally complete the research and writing. I am grateful to him and to Queen's University for this privilege.

Since their infancy, my now grown children, Jessica and Joshua, have put up with too many, long conversations about stethoscopy and French politics.

But they always encouraged me with their curiosity and skepticism, and they willingly participated in the final journey to tie up loose ends, sharing in the joyful rediscovery of Laennec's family, his Breton world, and especially his "swamp." This book is dedicated to my husband, Robert David Wolfe, because of the conceptual, practical, psychological, and editorial sustenance that he infused into its production, because he believed in my becoming an historian, and because he took us to live in France.

To See with a Better Eye

Biography is considered by more than one modern

historian to be a weed whose proliferation in the fields of

history is deadly for the advancement of true knowledge.

—*G. de Bertier de Sauvigny 1948, vii*

THE LIFE of R. T. H. Laennec (1781–1826) spanned the French Revolution, the first Empire, and the Restoration. Through sickness, war, and poverty, he studied medicine, practiced his Catholic faith even when it was banned, tended his patients, dissected their cadavers, and taught his students. A prominent clinician, he waged a bitter polemic with one of the most popular doctors in Paris, conducted physiological experiments, and wrote three books on pathology, diagnosis, and disease, only the second of which was published. In his spare moments, he cultivated letters, played music, hunted, hiked, and danced. He also developed the technique of mediate auscultation and invented the stethoscope, both of which were described in the two editions of his published book (1819 and 1826). When he died at age forty-five, Laennec was one of the most famous doctors in Europe, but the laudatory memory of his work is a truncated and twisted version of what he had tried to say.

Laennec is venerated for auscultation and for his piety. In the purple prose of physicians, he has become the "founder of modern medicine"; the "crowning glory" of the Paris school; a medical "prince," a "messiah," the "greatest clinician" of France, of the nineteenth century, of modern medicine, and of all time; his invention has been compared to that of Gutenberg, while he has been called "a sort of medical Newton or Galileo," "the French Sydenham," and "the French Hippocrates."[1] For Catholic physicians in France, his name is synonymous with an accord between medicine, health, and ethics, while in his native Brittany, his life has become the mystical stuff of legends.[2] The centenary of his death and the bicentenary of his birth were both marked by lavish ceremonies attended by the most distinguished physicians and politicians of France.[3]

Faced with the enormous jumble of hyperbole, legend, and fact, it might be reasonable to ask why we need yet another book about this man. I have three answers. First, Laennec's work has not been examined for more than three-quarters of a century. Distortions and inconsistencies in existing accounts have been suspected for some time, but they are inadvertently perpetuated by the inadequacies of earlier histories and by the nature of the secondary literature on nineteenth-century medicine. The numerous Laennec biographies—almost all of which are based on the careful but undeniably hagiographic study of Alfred Rouxeau (1854–1926)[4]—contain errors of fact and omission. These mistakes have been picked up and replicated by other scholars, and even novelists, poets, and filmmakers who have found inspiration in a romantic life lived in romantic times.[5] The glory that covers Laennec's name conceals the man almost as effectively as do the novels and the Breton myths.

Second, examination of a single life through dramatic political and medical changes can offer new perspectives on a process previously studied through institutions, disciplines, and groups. Scholars compartmentalize history into artificial though useful divisions defined by topic or period. For early nineteenth-century France, we have studies of the Revolution, the First Empire, and the Restoration; for its medicine, we have a rich literature about hospitals, practitioners, patients, pathology, physiology, and other sciences. Biography reminds us that individual lives transit these units and allows us to test, sometimes even disrupt, the neat definitions of their boundaries. Laennec was deeply engaged with the political turmoil of his time, and he participated actively in all aspects of the intellectual endeavor of the medical community in which he worked.

Third, none of the Laennec biographies incorporates the insights of the last four decades of scholarly work on the social history of early nineteenth-century French medicine.[6] Only a handful of these excellent new contributions—notably those on pathology—mention him at all, and he is curiously absent from the rest, despite his lofty stature in medical circles. Perhaps recent scholars hesitate to mention Laennec because they are understandably wary of the vast, untapped collection of his manuscripts and of the laudatory, even reverential nature of literature about him. In short, my task has been to put Laennec back into the history of French medicine and to put the new social history of nineteenth-century medicine into the story of Laennec.

The primary sources for this study are Laennec's scientific papers and his correspondence (see Appendix A). I have also used the indirect testimony of his patients, the published and unpublished cases, including the illnesses of his friends, his family, and himself. The patient records are the "laboratory notebooks" of his research; each encounter was an experiment that tested his ideas about pathology, diagnosis, therapy, and disease. A case record is a complex text. Usually written by a student over a period of time, it contained three principal ingredients: first, a translation of the patient's own account of illness; second, a report of repeated examinations of the patient's body in life and, often, also in death—a process that changed dramatically in Laennec's time; and third, an interpretation of the combined meaning of the first two. I am interested in how these texts testify to Laennec's research and how, in turn, they were shaped by the very discoveries that they document. Who were the patients? Did the doctor's analysis of their problems differ from his assessment of trouble in his friends, his family, his society, and himself? How did the case histories contribute to his understanding of disease? The potential of auscultation was revealed through a retelling of these tales in a fashion that satisfied the ambient desire to connect altered structure with disturbed function. Doctors' stories were forever changed by Laennec's invention.[7]

I have also examined Laennec's private life, not only for its admittedly diverting elements, but for two other reasons. First, the details of his private life and his political views cannot be separated from his professional life, his medical achievements, or the evolution of his scientific ideas. In fact, there is a remarkable consistency between his perception of personal and social well-being and his holistic theory of disease. Second, some of these events have never been fully told, especially the family lawsuits and the dismissal of his uncle in the White Terror.

My work is divided into three parts, each corresponding to one of Laennec's three books. Part One centers on the formation of his ideas about the new science of pathological anatomy. As a medical student, Laennec began to write a treatise on this subject and its potential for explaining the sites and etiology of disease. But his education, early research, and clinical practice also demonstrated the limitations of pathological anatomy and brought him to recognize a clinical pathophysiology that went beyond structural change. His blatant royalism during the Bourbon Restoration gave him an appointment in the hospital that was to become the proving ground for stethoscopic research. The early years discussed in Part One set the intellectual stage for his discovery and development of mediate auscultation.

Part Two focuses on the production and content of the *Treatise on Mediate Auscultation*, the only one of his three books to appear in print. I use the published and manuscript case histories to reconstruct the process of discovery of mediate auscultation as a series of breakthroughs leading to Laennec's invention of the stethoscope, his elaboration of signs of internal organic change, his fashioning of neologisms to describe them, and his identification of new organic lesions. Gradually, he came to appreciate the power of his invention not only in its well-known applications to anatomical medicine, but also in a lesser-known realm of physiology and pathophysiology of the lungs and heart. An analysis of Laennec's clinical reasoning in the construction of diagnostic signs reveals the psychological and epistemological priorities that governed an early nineteenth-century physician's use of evidence. The criteria he imposed on this ensemble of inductive evidence expressed the probability-based, decision-making orientation of one whose existence straddled the sensualist philosophy of the late eighteenth century, when a high value was placed on accurate observation, and the dawn of positivist thought, when medicine purported to eschew theories about cause and began the self-conscious project to link clinical signs to numbers. Laennec's semiology reveals a personal dialogue with these emerging ideals.

Part Three focuses on disease, the topic of Laennec's intended four-volume treatise based on his lessons at the Collège de France. I reexamine his relationship with his rival, François-Joseph-Victor Broussais (1772–1838), purveyor of "physiological medicine," and I demonstrate that their polemic revolved around a fundamental agreement about the primacy of function over structure in the study of disease—an agreement that was hampered by the inadequacies of a new vocabulary. Following the publication of his treatise, Laennec became preoccupied with rebutting critics who, like Broussais, complained that his discovery did nothing for therapeutics, and he conducted little-known experiments to test Hippocratic concepts, auscultation, and drugs. For his lectures, he built a synthetic theory of disease that incorporated pathological anatomy as well as compensating for its limitations; he addressed all diseases, including those that, he thought, would never be explained by anatomical change. I believe that the tenets of this theory, which he thought of as "eclectic," were perceived as an unwelcome, even paradoxical form of vitalism and that this perception has played a role in the historiographic distortion of his ideas.

Patient records were my methodological focus, because I wanted to explore the process of Laennec's discovery and the meaning of auscultation of heart and lung in his practice. My research confirms what others have already observed: auscultation was indeed both a product of and an impetus for the new anatomical medicine; and the stethoscope had a prompt and significant impact on diagnostic practice and on the naming and concepts of disease. I also show that Laennec had been guided by his teacher Jean-Nicolas Corvisart des Marets (1755–1821), his friend Gaspard-Laurent Bayle (1774–1816), and several other colleagues who had come close to listening to the chest, although he did not always credit them. Whether or not he was personally responsible for the early nineteenth-century mutation in "gaze," his life began as the process started and ended when it was in full sway. He was actively involved in the doubly semiotic process of developing a new discourse—to define clinical signs and to label disease, by weighing the advantages and limitations of new ideas, old words, neologisms, and signs. He and his colleagues were conscious that they lived in revolutionary times, and this awareness created a competitive atmosphere and sparked a number of miniature priority disputes, which can be characterized as jostling over "discoveries" that have long since been disregarded.

Some of my findings were unexpected. Not only did the illness histories of Laennec's private life and clinical practice bring him to discover a method of revealing internal organic change, they also emphasized his growing conviction that pathological anatomy could not explain all diseases, nor could it account for their causes. These histories provided what he construed to be evidence of the physiological influence of psyche upon soma. He conceived of his stethoscope, his clinical practice, and his disease theory in physiological terms. Influenced by Matthieu-François-Régis Buisson (1776–1804), the

cousin of M. F. Xavier Bichat (1771–1802), Laennec first spoke of auscultation as a physiological process as early as 1802. He conducted what he believed to be physiological experiments until the year of his death. He never
relinquished a basic psychosomatism that made his medical theory of disease
coherent with his personal experience of illness and death in his patients,
family, and friends. In a parallel way, he embraced a physiological philosophy
of social and political life that corresponded to the ideas of Félicité de
Lamennais (1782–1854), René de Chateaubriand (1768–1848), and Louis
G. A. de Bonald (1754–1840), to whom he had been led again by Buisson
and other devout friends in the Congrégation coterie.

Laennec's views on physiology drove me to the secondary literature on
early nineteenth-century physiology, where I was startled to discover that he
could not be found. Histories of pathological anatomy never fail to recognize him, but those of physiology ignore him. In some ways, the imbalance
is created by historians' anachronistic compartmentalization: in the early
nineteenth century, neither discipline had yet been fully separated from
clinical medicine. Laennec's absence may also have been due to his lack of
credibility among contemporary physiologists whose enmity he had earned
with his political and religious conservatism. His unpopularity in these well-
circumscribed circles poses an interesting problem for the historian. It has
usually been explained as the result of his conservative sympathies, the long-
standing polemic with Broussais, the extraordinary manner of his appointment to the Collège de France, and his shady involvement in the royalist
coup of the Faculty. But, as Erwin Ackerknecht observed, other conservative,
Catholic doctors did not evoke the same personal and professional hostility.[8]
Furthermore, these old religious and political disagreements do not explain
why he does not appear in histories of physiology, if he practiced physiology.
Stephen Jacyna made a similar observation about the relative absence from
histories of medicine of Laennec's contemporary, François Magendie
(1783–1855), who is well examined in histories of physiology; he too found
parallels between Restoration physiology and its philosophy.[9] I do not dispute the importance of the social factors in determining the reception of
Laennec's "eclectic" theories—indeed they probably alerted his critics—
however, the hostility emerged from an intellectual reaction to his physiology. I find that Laennec's invisibility as a physiological investigator is the
result of suppression and distortion of his thought by rivals, enemies, and
family during his life and in the years immediately after his death. George
Weisz has shown convincingly how the ambitions of pathologists entered
into the later construction of his posthumous reputation.[10] His reputation
was also shaped by views of physiology, pathology, and clinical medicine, and
their relationship to perceptions of vitalism that have characterized different
periods in the two centuries that separate us from him.

Laennec was an excellent observer, a brilliant scholar, an inspired thinker,
and an artist, but he could also be proud, selfish, occasionally vindictive, and

his finely honed sense of justice and his conservatism in both politics and medicine were certainly not to everyone's taste, then or now. If he emerges less saintlike from my study than from those of my predecessors, I hope that he will seem more human and no less worthy of examination as an intriguing representative of his time, a vigorous if challenging specimen in the formal garden of its history.

PART ONE

Pathology: Anatomy, Physiology, and the Body Politic

A book is like a voyage that takes us out of the circle
of our habits and our way of seeing.

—*A. von Haller, 1757, cited by Laennec,*
Traité d'anatomie pathologique, *ca. 1804–1808*

Youth and Revolution

I often feel a touch of melancholy when I think that
these times, so stormy for the State, have been for me
the happiest of my life.

—Laennec to his father, 4 September 1798

THE EARLY LIFE OF R. T. H. Laennec, like that of most French people of the late eighteenth century, was marked by war, suffering, illness, and loss, but his trauma was alleviated by optimism and the frivolity of youth. Motherless at five, sent to the army at fourteen, seriously ill at seventeen, he was a dedicated student, talented in music, and not a little vain. The dramatic political changes of the Revolution, First Empire, and Restoration marked him deeply and influenced the course of his career. The romantic story of his life has been told many times; twentieth-century biographers—myself included—are indebted to Alfred Rouxeau, the Breton physiology professor whose hagiographic account was based on a thousand family letters that he located and transcribed (see Appendix A).[1]

Laennec was born on 17 February 1781 at the inland port of Quimper near the western tip of Brittany. He was the first child of Théophile-Marie Laennec (1747–1836) and Michelle-Gabrielle-Félicité Guesdon (1754–1786), who became parents ten months after their marriage. Both families had respectable roots in the regions of Finistère: the child's paternal grandfather and great-grandfathers on both sides had been mayors of Quimper.[2] Maternal grandparents claimed distant relationship to the writer Elie Fréron (1718–1776) and the poet François de Malherbe (1555–1628); the father's ancestors included several generations of lawyers.

The Laennec family lived at the mother's birthplace, which they shared with her father until his death on 10 October 1781 (fig. 1.1). Their home stood on the quay overlooking the confluence of the Steir and Odet Rivers opposite a park; it was demolished in the twentieth century.[3] The old man left the house to his daughter and his position as bailiff in the municipal bureaucracy to her husband.

Laennec's father, Théophile-Marie, was the eldest of the five children born to lawyer Michel Laennec (1714–1782) who lived at the manor of Kerlouarnec (Place of the Foxes) near Douarnenez twenty kilometers northwest of Quimper. Like his father, Théophile-Marie became a lawyer, and in

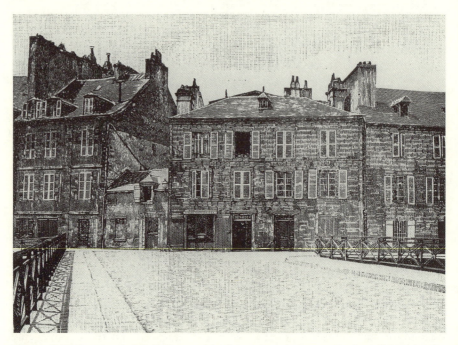

Figure 1.1. Laennec's birthplace, with the open window, was demolished in the twentieth century, but the house to the left was still standing in 1995. A monument now marks the site. Image discovered by Guermonprez and published in Rouxeau [1912], 14. Photograph: Queen's Medical Photography Services.

1781 he held positions as king's counselor and officer of the Admiralty of Quimper. By the 1790s he was unhappily situated as a magistrate in the civil court at the town of Quimperlé. Intelligent, but unreliable, selfish, and sometimes deceitful, he thought that he belonged in Paris and that he deserved the indulgence of others to help him pursue his destiny. His passions were plotting, rhyming, gossip, and writing prose. The unsettled times and his capricious nature resulted in ever-precarious employment, and he contracted many debts. For four years after his father died on 31 October 1782, Théophile-Marie prevented his three living siblings from receiving any benefit from the estate. The beautiful property of Kerlouarnec he kept for himself, but it slid into the serious decline from which his physician son would later try to retrieve it. Laennec *père* seems to have blown with whatever political breeze passed his way hoping with each change to find a comfortable niche in the new order. In the Terror, he tried to ingratiate himself with the revolutionary tribunals; once it became possible to restore confiscated fortunes, he became the champion of émigrés; in the early Empire, he published an ode to Napoleon; and he cheered with his son at the return of the King in 1814.[4]

Little is known of the infancy of the Laennec children. A brother, Michel (Michaud), was born 14 July 1782, and a sister, Marie-Anne, in 1785. A single reference to a *nourrice* (wet nurse) in one of the father's letters led Rouxeau to conclude that the future doctor, always called Théophile by his family, spent a year away from the home in the care of a Breton-speaking wet nurse. Laennec's mother died on 15 November 1786, two days after giving birth to a baby girl whose first breath had also been her last.[5] Most historians have attributed the mother's death to tuberculosis, and some have blamed her for unwittingly infecting her famous son, but the evidence pointing to the mother's tuberculosis is slim: she died young, as did her brothers and her sons; and her physician brother-in-law once described her as "frail."[6] More likely, she succumbed to childbed fever or another complication resulting from her delivery two days before. Rouxeau refused to accept the tuberculosis hypothesis for the mother's death, because of Laennec's much later surprise at learning of phthisis (tuberculosis) in his family.[7]

The widowed Théophile-Marie was considered incapable of caring for his three living children. The little girl was taken by his wife's sister, Madame de la Potterie, and in January 1787, the two boys were sent to live with the father's youngest brother, abbé Michel Laennec (1750–1801), doctor of the Sorbonne and priest of the small parish of Elliant, sixteen kilometers east of Quimper. There they began their studies and learned catechism, but at the end of a year, the abbé left to become canon at the larger community of Tréguier on the north coast of Brittany. By March 1788, the children were sent back to their father in Quimper. The priest-uncle and the father both appealed to their middle brother, Guillaume-François Laennec (1748–1822), physician at Nantes. Guillaume found the request "bizarre," but he agreed to care for the "orphans." Rouxeau tells us that the little boys sailed into the port of Nantes on 15 May 1788. France was on the verge of its long and bloody Revolution, and more than nine years would pass before either child saw his father again.[8]

Guillaume Laennec became a second father to his nephews (fig. 1.2). Born at Kerlouarnec, he had left Finistère to study medicine in Paris, Montpellier, and London. While in Paris from 1769 to 1772, Guillaume frequented the home of Elie Fréron, writer and critic of Voltaire, and he was an eager student of the private anatomy lessons of the surgeons Raphaël Bienvenu Sabatier (1732–1811) and Antoine Petit (1722–1794). But he had difficulty paying for the expensive Parisian cadavers, which could not be obtained from the cemeteries as they had been in Brittany. In 1773, he completed his degree in Montpellier where he followed the classes of Paul-Joseph Barthez (1734–1806). After a few months in London, he practiced first in Quimper, then as a temporary medical officer in the navy at Brest, before settling on marriage and a career in Nantes.[9]

A well-documented family legend testifies to the legalistic fighting spirit of this medical descendant of a long line of jurists. Upon his engagement to the youthful Désirée de Gennes de Matignon in 1781, Guillaume was required by his future father-in-law to leave Quimper for a larger town befitting his bride from Rennes, the capital of Brittany. Guillaume thought it wise to

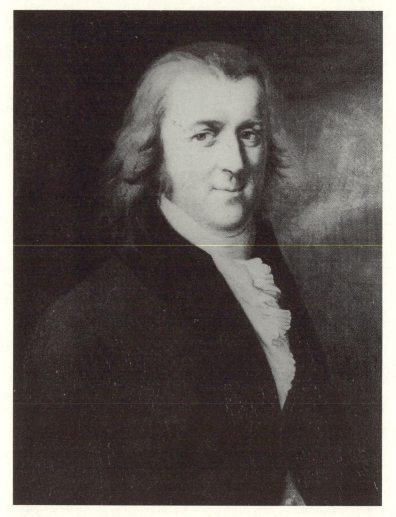

Figure 1.2. Portrait of Laennec's uncle, Guillaume Laennec, physician at Nantes, by Descarins, 1793. Original belongs to the family of Bertrand Laennec of Lyons. Source: Photograph of the copy in Musée Laennec, Nantes. Photographer: M. Certain.

avoid the city of his in-laws and instead chose Nantes where six of twelve doctors had recently died. Despite the apparent need for doctors, jealous physicians in the medical faculty had influenced municipal authorities to deny privileges to Guillaume and his fellow Montpellier graduate, surgeon Pierre-François Blin (1756–1834); the newcomers could undertake thirty-nine months of supplemental training, write five examinations, and pay twenty-four hundred livres in fees. At first Guillaume complied and passed three of the five examinations, but he became impatient following his marriage in July 1783, and tried to renegotiate the terms of his situation. After four unsuccessful attempts at finding a compromise, he adopted the creative strategy of suing the University. Representing himself and relying on a 1707 law, he argued for more than two years through nine hearings in the parliament at Rennes and finally won his case and that of Blin in 1785.[10]

Guillaume's success galvanized the attention of his fellow citizens; a few months later the faculties of law, letters, and theology (but not medicine) elected him *Procureur général* of the University. In that capacity, he brought six new doctors to Nantes and, three years later, controlled seven of eleven votes in the medical faculty. In March 1788, he was elected Rector of the University. Guillaume was not a man to inspire feelings of indifference; either he was loved or he was hated. More denunciations and bitterly won triumphs lay ahead.

The young Laennec and his brother arrived in Nantes shortly after Guillaume's election as Rector. They joined their cousin, four-year-old Christophe, but Guillaume's family soon grew to include three more sons and a daughter. The earliest known autograph of the future doctor is his nine-year old signature on the baptismal record of his cousin, Ambroise, born in February 1790.[11] The Laennecs of Nantes lived in a grand building in the Place Bouffay, near a (now vanished) branch of the Loire. Several servants worked under the watchful and economically shrewd eye of Guillaume's mother-in-law, Madame de Gennes, who had moved from Rennes after her husband's death. She was said to have been more fond of young Théophile than she was of any of her own grandchildren. Well into his late adolescence, the boy entrusted her and her daughter with the management of his meager resources and his wardrobe.[12]

Nantes suffered greatly during the Revolution. Guillaume Laennec was relatively comfortable, but his old enemies and the political instability compelled him to be vigilant. The privileges of a physician and an administrator were suspect, contact with aristocracy was dangerous, and connection to a priest could be fatal. In contrast to his older brother, Guillaume's political sympathies were more closely guarded, and his religious sentiments leaned toward the skeptical, although he once described himself "a bit Jansenist."[13] Years earlier at the festivities surrounding the marriage of the Dauphin (soon to be Louis XVI) to fourteen-year-old Marie Antoinette, he had been dismayed to witness the trampling of dozens of Parisians; to his father, Guillaume deplored the unnecessary, royal extravagance and complained that the money spent on fireworks could have funded several courses in obstetrics.[14] Guillaume may have welcomed the democratization of some structures following the meetings of the Estates General, but he was cynical about the benefits of the Convention. In the 1790s, he was named to several regional committees, only to resign or be removed. Papers testify to his willingness to provide certificates that would exempt fellow citizens from extreme privation or restore their lost property; others describe him as a "demagogue" and enemy of the Revolution.[15]

Shortly after the execution of Louis XVI on 21 January 1793, a counter-revolutionary war exploded in the Vendée, southeast of Brittany. The uprising was the result of dissatisfaction with the economic situation and had been triggered by reaction to a massive conscription effort for the wars with the Rhineland, the Netherlands, and Austria. The counterrevolutionaries, or *Chouans*, were a mixture of peasants, Catholics, royalists, and smugglers, with backing from foreign opportunists.[16] The Terror in Brittany was dominated by an effort to put down these uprisings. Instability and outright violence continued at intervals with more or less vigor until mid-1800.

In March 1793, a guillotine was erected in Place Bouffay in front of the Laennec home, and over the following three months, some fifty people were executed. An enthusiastic crowd was expected to fill the windows overlooking the square. To spare his family from this gruesome obligation, Guillaume Laennec moved to a newer dwelling a short distance away in Place de l'Egalité (now Place Royale) at the end of June 1793.[17] Earlier that same year, when the property of the clergy was confiscated, he had acquired the large country house at Petit Port north of town on the border of the bucolic valley of the Cens. There the children could seek refuge for longer periods of time when the wars were quiescent.[18]

In October 1793, Jean-Baptiste Carrier (1756–1794) was sent to quell the uprisings in the west as the representative on mission of the Convention government. He emptied the prisons, rounded up "brigands," encouraged pillaging and the rape of women and children, and ruthlessly shot or guillotined hundreds. For a quicker and less costly method of execution, he drowned countless, bound prisoners in a series of *noyades*, which entailed scuttling crowded barges in the Loire. Guillaume's son, Christophe, recalled a frightening night when Carrier came to the family home for food and drink and was angered when Madame de Gennes voiced her opposition to his agenda. As punishment, her physician son-in-law was sentenced to six weeks of hospital arrest at the Hôtel Dieu (renamed the Temple de l'Humanité).[19] According to other sources, Guillaume's "arrest" may have had nothing to do with his mother-in-law's indiscretion and he was confined to the hospital with five other doctors because of the overwhelming medical need.[20] By early February 1794, Carrier had been recalled. The mortality under his three-month reign of terror in Nantes is unknown, but the carnage is considered to have been the highest in France with estimates ranging from four to twenty thousand deaths.[21]

In late 1794, Guillaume Laennec traveled to Paris as an accuser of Carrier. The trial focused on the unauthorized executions and his responsibility for deaths of children and women, some of whom had been pregnant. In his deposition, Guillaume described Carrier's "republican marriages": a boy and a girl—or an old man and an old woman—were stripped, tied together, and thrown in the river. He wrote to his wife of the arrest of the "monster" and his trial: "Nantes has her revenge!"[22] Carrier was executed on 16 December 1794. While in the capital, Guillaume lobbied successfully for a commission as a military physician and for support of the fragile botanical garden, which had been the mainstay of hospital remedies until the troubles caused it to be expropriated and neglected.[23] Two years later he appealed for the right to reestablish formal medical training in Nantes, but the faculty would not be resurrected until 1808.[24]

Throughout these turbulent times, the nephews attended school: first in the preparatory courses of the Institution Tardivel; then at the Collège de l'Oratoire. Schools and their curricula were reorganized as a result of the revolutionary mistrust of the priest instructors; however, "religion" persisted as a subject, joined with *logique morale* and "development of the rights of man."[25] The earliest surviving record of Laennec's schooling is from the summer of 1792, when he was listed as one of seventeen students in the *quatrième* class.[26] The boys appear to have excelled in their studies of rhetoric, ancient languages, Latin, natural history, drawing, literature, mathematics, physics, and chemistry.[27] In their spare hours, they played games and music and learned to swim and hunt with their younger cousins. Théophile enjoyed additional lessons in flute, drawing, and dance, and he kept a rock collection, which his uncle referred to as his personal "quarry," relating it to the boy's initial desire to study engineering.[28] At the age of seventeen, after visiting a political café, Laennec revealed himself to be a supporter of the Republic, fascinated by the effect of the government's suppression of newspapers, which, he said, had left "a profound and deep chagrin that enveloped all the thoughts [of journalists and their friends] and even penetrated their discourse." And he pondered the irony of his situation: "I often feel a touch of melancholy when I think that these times, so stormy for the State, have been for me the happiest of my life."[29]

The family suffered financial stress and the loss of their only daughter, Emerance, who died at the age of twenty months. Guillaume mourned for his pretty baby girl, "conceived in the dark days of the Terror, carried in the convulsive anguish of fear, nursed by a mother who was fed rotten beans and crusts"; the child was yet "another victim of the Revolution," he said, and the painful memory of her death would go with him to the grave.[30] The bereaved mother suffered for a long time, and her despair was aggravated by a miscarriage a few months later.[31]

Laennec's other uncle, the abbé Michel Laennec, had refused to swear allegiance to Civil Constitution of the Clergy (12 July 1790)—legislation that sought to make priests salaried servants of the state. He left his parish at Tréguier and went to live by the baths of St. Julien in Paris near the Sorbonne, where he could attend to his poor health. In the summer of 1792, he decided to follow the advice of a doctor and seek a cure in Bath, England; before leaving, he obtained a passport to certify that he had not fled or been deported. He took the English waters and set out to return by way of Jersey in October, but the carefully prepared documents were rejected by the authorities. The ailing abbé spent the remainder of his life in Germany, Scotland, and London waiting for permission to reenter France. He opened a plea for help with a veiled reference to the revolutionary hatred of religion that might prevent his letter from being transmitted to his siblings because their very names proclaimed a love of God.[32] Guillaume tried to send money to Jersey, but, as he later told it, traces of his benevolence nearly cost him his head, and he had to burn the letters from his clerical brother to avoid suspicion. The abbé uncle, who had baptized the future doctor and been his first teacher, died in March 1800 in Southampton when the coach carrying him tipped over and he was crushed "under the full weight of a large Englishman."[33] A few years later, however, a Breton physician told Laennec that his priest-uncle had suffered from phthisis.[34]

Théophile-Marie seems to have provided no assistance to his exiled brother, although he thought he had found himself a fortune. In February 1794, he married Geneviève Agnès Julie Urvoy St. Bedan, widow of the rich émigré, Joseph-Etienne André Lehec, who had died eight months before. Laennec *père* gloated over his new wealth to family and friends, and promised to reunite his children at the home in Quimper as soon as the court battle over his wife's inheritance was settled in Saint Brieuc.[35] The following year, the new stepmother sent the boys gifts of 500 and 300 livres with a promise of more just to "get acquainted"; however, her largesse ended with the initial gift.[36] In 1795, Théophile-Marie lost his job as magistrate at Quimperlé, either because he was now the relative of an émigré, or because he was absent pursuing the restoration of his wife's fortune. He was soon reinstated, but was continually petitioning for new positions in other cities, or making his family do so on his behalf. The lawsuits over the Lehec estate dragged on for more than twenty years.[37]

In order to amplify the older nephew's meager resources, uncle Guillaume decided to use his influence to place Théophile as a medical aide in the revolutionary army. In September 1795, at the age of fourteen, Laennec enlisted as a surgeon third class; he was not always paid for his duties, but patients were not lacking. He later claimed a total of thirty-four months of service: sixteen months in the Armée Côte de Brest, from 6 Vendémiaire An IV to 30 Nivôse An V (29 September 1795 to 19 January 1797), and eighteen months in the military hospitals and ambulance of the Armée de l'Ouest, from 1 Vendemiaire An VIII to 1 Germinal An IX (23 September 1799 to 22 March 1801).[38] Wartime Nantes was served by two hospitals with a combined capacity of more than four thousand beds: the civil hospital in the former Hôtel Dieu and the military hospice, which occupied six different clerical buildings, including convents, seminaries, and schools.

Early experience in the army was something that an entire generation of French physicians came to share, and it has been observed that military upbringing probably served to define a medical cohort socially.[39] By the age of sixteen, young Laennec was thoroughly committed to a future in medicine. A certificate, signed by his commanding officer in support of his second tour of duty, testified to his skills and the appreciation of patients and superiors during his first tour of duty.[40] He had already learned to dissect the human body, and when he went back to school, he continued to read medical books: Philippe Pinel (1745–1826) on diseases, Antoine-François Fourcroy (1755–1809) on chemistry, and an unidentified Platner.[41] He reported to his father that he was the only student in his class studying Greek, which he already considered to be important for understanding ancient medical texts; he hoped (in vain) to learn English, too.[42] The uncle was pleased with the lad and praised the "compendium," which he had written after reading Pinel's *Nosographie* "for the first time." He said, "I knew right away that he would be an excellent physician because he had found the *optima methodus studendi*." And he cited Voltaire, "any man who seeks to learn by reading a book without a pen in hand, will never learn well."[43]

Most letters to Laennec *père* during this period contain requests for money from the boys or from their uncle on their behalf. Théophile-Marie occasionally sent small amounts that did not satisfy their needs; more often he made promises that he failed to keep. In April 1796, he called Michaud home to Quimper, but Théophile waited in Nantes and dreamed of going to Paris to complete his education. In a peculiar gesture of support, the father sent his overworked brother the documents necessary to sue the Van Berchem family for a debt owed to his second wife's dead grandmother. The money derived from a successful case could be used for Théophile. To everyone's surprise, Van Berchem paid a small portion of the debt before his death; the widow paid another, but she also died soon after. Four years later, and despite his brother's repeated urgings to keep suing the Van Berchem estate, Guillaume rejected further action as a waste of time.[44]

Finally in the summer of 1797, young Laennec was sent the funds to visit his father for the first time in a decade. Full of enthusiasm, he took the next available ship, but unfavorable winds led to a long delay in the town of Paimboeuf not far from Nantes. He reached Quimper in early July, where finally he met his new stepmother and renewed acquaintance with his brother Michaud, sister Marie-Anne, and his young paternal aunt, Théophile-Anne-Françoise, only three years his senior (fig. 1.3). But he was disappointed to discover that his father was in St. Brieuc on the north coast of Brittany still pursuing his wife's fortune. In letter after letter, he begged his *cher papa* to return; but there were no replies.[45]

After almost two months of waiting, Laennec set out on foot to find his father at St. Brieuc more than one hundred kilometers away across the Armorican plateau. He walked by the slate quarries in Chateaulin and the mines at Poullaouen and Huelgoat so that he could add some new specimens to his geological collection.[46] Little is known of what happened at the reunion, but it is clear father and son found pleasure in each other's company and possibly also in the recognition of a common lively intelligence and a sensitivity for wit and rhyme. Few historians have commented on the marked similarities in the family's epistolic prose—the transports of joy or anger at personal injustices that characterize the writing of Laennec, his father, and his uncle. Together father and son composed a poem satirizing the submission of law to

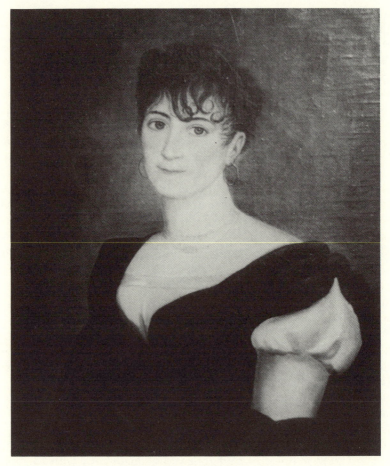

Figure 1.3. Théophile-Anne-Françoise Laennec, la petite tante de Miniac. Favorite and confidante of her nephews, she married Armand de Miniac mayor of the town of Lannion in 1800. Anonymous portrait belonging to the de Miniac family. Photograph: M. Hervé de Miniac of Rennes.

commerce, and they went with their architect friend, Mathurin Crucy, to visit the navy installations in Brest.[47]

Laennec walked the 225 kilometers back to Nantes from Quimper in four and a half days. When his trunk arrived, he found his clothes in tatters because the package containing his precious rock collection had fallen open. To the uncle's mild alarm, the boy, who already tended to expensive taste in clothing, now had more effete demands: he needed a private dancing master and insisted that his attire measure up to the fashion of the day. "The arts are the balm of life," his father told him; young Laennec concurred, and he poured his energies into finding a position for his father on the tribunal in Nantes so that both families could live together.[48]

The bloom did not last long. By late November, Laennec was wondering why his father and stepmother failed to send the promised amounts to bolster his shabby wardrobe; more seriously, he began to think he would not have sufficient resources to attend school.[49] Guillaume had not deprived Théophile of any serious request, especially when it came to his studies. But he despaired of his brother ever taking charge of the expenses generated by the clothing, food, and education of his offspring. With his own family still growing, both he and his nephew were conscious that it was time that the father began to contribute more. From the summer of 1797, he warned his brother that plans must be made for Théophile's study in Paris.[50]

As the promised Lehec fortune failed to materialize, Théophile-Marie's second marriage became somewhat less than happy. He took to hiding his letters and his person from his spouse, and he tried to pass his responsibilities on to others.[51] His daughter, Marie-Anne, was already showing signs of the strange character that led some to think her mad; she was packed off to live with "two old ladies" who would teach her manners. His younger sister, Théophile-Anne-Françoise, may have chosen marriage with Armand de Miniac, jurist and future mayor of Lannion, in order to escape her sister-in-law and to avoid the veil; as the "little aunt" de Miniac, she remained the fond confidante of her nephews.[52]

In May of 1798, seventeen-year-old Laennec fell ill with the first in a life-long series of illnesses: night sweats, chest pain, nosebleeds, and a high fever, which continued unabated for three weeks. Concerned for his "naturally delicate" nephew, Guillaume summoned his colleague, Le Meignen (1731–1803), whose remedies caused the boy to pass a large intestinal worm. Convalescing over eight days at Petit Port under the diligent care of his aunt and *maman* de Gennes, the patient blithely wrote to his father, "I narrowly escaped the arms of Death."[53]

The following summer, Laennec went northwest again to visit his father at St. Brieuc. He had been instructed to extract an unequivocal commitment of financial support for study in Paris, but the entreaties did not bear fruit. Instead, the father proposed to keep his son with him and out of school until spring. Guillaume was outraged, "consumed by chagrin," he said. "What the devil do you expect him to do in Saint-Brieuc?" he demanded. "To keep him till spring, is to lose him!"[54] With his coffers still empty, Laennec once more trekked back to Nantes, whence he cheerfully reported that he had encountered neither "*Chouans* nor '*chats-huants.*' "[55] But he had been lucky, because the war was escalating again.

Two weeks later, in a dense fog on the night of 19–20 October 1799, Nantes was attacked by counterrevolutionaries, estimated at twelve hundred to four thousand strong. Shooting erupted in the square below the Laennec family home, and Christophe awoke his older cousin, who took his gun and disappeared into the night. When he had not returned by morning, Christophe and his grandmother searched for his body among the dead. Two days later, Laennec told his father that he had been among the fifty citizens who fired at a column of three hundred brigands advancing on the home of the *Payeur général*. The rebels retreated, leaving seven dead in the street and at least twenty other bodies floating in the Loire; fifty people were wounded and carried to the military hospice for care. Fixated on his studies, despite the skirmishes in the streets, Laennec concluded the letter with a reminder for the long-promised money for his education.[56] Two days later, the attack was renewed and rebuffed again.

Sometime in the same autumn, Laennec was sent to Petit Port to fetch sacks of grain, but a band of outlaws stole his mare and his cargo, although they did him no harm. According to his cousin, the theft caused embarrassment more than fear, since the events were broadcast about the town by the drawing instructor at whose home he had sought refuge.[57]

Efforts to bring the Vendean war to a close were renewed in the wake of Napoleon Bonaparte's coup d'état of 18 Brumaire An VIII (10 November 1799). Laennec had applied for readmission to the military service hoping for promotion and the associated raise in pay.[58] He had reenlisted in the fall of 1799, and in late January 1800 left for Vannes in the Morbihan Gulf with the ambulance corps of the republican *Armée de l'ouest*. Under General Brune, the army had just brought about a decisive victory over Georges Cadoudal and his *Chouans* before Laennec's arrival, but he was there when the treaty was signed on 2 February 1800.[59] Laennec's victorious month at the front seems to have been slow. He spent his free time "on his knees" in his duty room composing his lengthy poem, *La guerre des Vénètes*. The "heroi-comic" epic was a thinly disguised parody about the adventures of one Docteur Cennéal (Laennec, spelled backwards) and his medical comrades whose delight and amazement at finding themselves still alive at the end of a bloody war was the theme of the final stanza.[60] Laennec's sister was said to have enjoyed reciting the epic and his father was so pleased that he made plans for its publication.[61] Laennec was released from active duty on 28 February 1800, and to his great relief was back in Nantes four days later.[62]

The year 1800 was a difficult one for the future doctor. He had accomplished all he could in Nantes, and although he continued working at the military hospice, he knew that it would soon be closed.[63] His aunt Désirée had been chronically ill, following her miscarriage and a painful operation for mastitis; his uncle was hinting at finding him a wife.[64] It was time to move on. One day at dinner in late August, he read a letter from his father, turned ghastly pale, excused himself quietly, and went to his room. The uncle found his nephew crying and so "shaken" that he feared for his life: "You have put death in the heart of your son," Guillaume accused his brother, whose newest crime had been the decision to send Michaud to Paris, leaving the older son behind. "He needs only two or three years in Paris," the uncle continued, "the first money you find . . . should be for him."[65]

Furious with this turn of events, Guillaume and his nephew began to campaign for an equal opportunity.[66] Either by shame or by a true change in fortune, the father suddenly turned *volte face* and chastened his son: "You have so little memory. You forget the extent of my resources in this region—resources that have just swelled with the inheritance from my poor [brother] abbé Laennec, and the forthcoming logging at Kerlouarnec. . . . Tell me quickly the hour and the day that your uncle would like you to leave."[67] This strange reply was encouraging, but Michaud reported from Paris that the funds, which he had been instructed to send, were tied up in bonds and could not be liberated until peace. Guillaume accused Michaud of hoarding the money for himself and his brother of lying; Théophile's jealousy could scarcely be hidden.[68]

The father suggested that Michaud pawn a diamond worth fifteen hundred livres, but no one, including the "old Jew Isaac," would offer more than a derisory price for the jewel.[69] The uncle threatened to send his moping nephew back to Quimper, but finally the father came through. Guillaume expressed his thanks and relief to his brother, with a description of the emotional leave-taking: he was in bed with a cold when his nephew came to say good-bye with promises to be frugal and "tears in his eyes." Traveling halfway by carriage and the rest on foot, Laennec left Nantes for Paris on 20 April 1801.[70]

Laennec had experienced the Revolution as both citizen and soldier, and of his first twenty years, he had spent seven in the study and practice of medicine. The firsthand experience of the effects of war and misery became a lens for his subsequent clinical encounters. A true son of Théophile-Marie, he loved music, poetry, and languages, and he felt more Breton than French. He prided himself on excellence in everything he attempted, and was eager for Paris, expecting both to learn and to make contributions at its new school of medicine.

Student in the Paris School

Anatomy, though so carefully cultivated, has yet not
supplied medicine with any really important observations.
One may scrupulously examine a corpse, yet the necessities
on which life depends escape one. . . . Anatomy may cure a
sword wound, but will prove powerless when the invisible
dart of a particular miasma has penetrated beneath our skin.
Between surgery and medicine lies an infinite gap
which nothing can fill.

—*Louis Sebastien Mercier [1788], 97*

In the natural sciences, when observation and experiment
have gathered facts, destroyed or rectified old ideas, it
becomes necessary to create new classifications which link
the elements of the newly acquired knowledge and
distribute them in a methodical order.

—*Laennec 1802f, 169*

THE ECOLE DE SANTÉ: ANATOMY AND DISEASE CONCEPTS

Laennec's destination was the seven-year-old medical school in Paris, where
he would spend three years as a student and many more as a devoted alum-
nus. He already had gathered clinical experience in Brittany, but his exposure
to professional leaders in the capital sharpened his learning and honed his
skills as a participant in a newly created medical culture. There he was influenced intellectually and spiritually, and he became known as a brilliant but
single-minded young man with an aptitude for the new science of pathological anatomy and a penchant for preserving the past.

In December 1794, the medical school of Paris had reopened after a five-
year hiatus caused by the revolutionary abolition of faculties and professional

academies. Restructured on a plan devised by the chemist, A. F. Fourcroy, it briefly bore the new name "Ecole de Santé," a name chosen to reflect an emphasis on health and its maintenance rather than disease and its repair. Eighteen of the twenty-seven professors were new recruits, twelve of whom had been members of the College of Surgery or its associated Ecole Pratique de Dissection. Most were liberal-leaning supporters of the Revolution who had been entertained in the salons of the *Idéologues,* where they were exposed to sensualist philosophy and converted to hospital reform and the goals of public health. In this cradle of positivistic medicine, they claimed to value Hippocrates above Galen, observation above theorizing, material fact above ephemeral idea, and numerical evidence over anecdote; causes could be respected, but not known. Their philosophical spokesman was Pierre-Jean-George Cabanis (1757–1808), who was eventually appointed historian of medicine in the new school.[1]

The stature of surgery in the new school was soon enhanced by Napoleon, who relied on the skills and inventions of military surgeons to keep his army fighting. Among those elevated to Baron in the aristocracy of the First Empire, were surgeons Dominique-Jean Larrey (1766–1842) and René-Nicolas Desgenettes (1762–1837), and Bonaparte's personal physician, Jean-Nicolas Corvisart des Marets (fig. 2.1). These men seem to have had little trouble reconciling their acquired nobility with their recent revolutionary sympathies. The transfer of political power to surgery was an additional boost to its rising credibility in academic institutions and in medical epistemology. In keeping with postrevolutionary ideals, instruction was revised to promote practical, rather than theoretical medicine, through anatomical dissection, clinical experience, and a melding of surgical and medical skills. Symbolically the Ecole de Santé occupied a magnificent new building that had been intended to house the Académie de Chirurgie, abolished in 1793.[2]

The definition of disease and its relationship to the body was part of the main research agenda in the medical schools of early nineteenth-century Europe, especially Paris. The hospital was the principal site of investigation (the "laboratory"), each patient an experiment, and the findings were discussed in journals and at societies, virtually all of which were reconstructed following the Revolution.[3] Here it is essential to distinguish between "illness," which is the subjective experience of individual suffering, and "disease," which is a historically contingent and constructed idea about illness.[4] Embedded in disease concepts are ideas about the perceived nature of the illness and sometimes also about its cause and/or rational treatment. In Laennec's lifetime, disease concepts changed from constructs based on patients' subjective symptoms or feelings, described in the patient's history, to concepts based on specific changes in the patient's body, detected objectively through physical examination. Pathological anatomy and experimental physiology both grew out of this preoccupation with the definition of disease, but they had yet to be institutionalized as distinct academic disciplines.

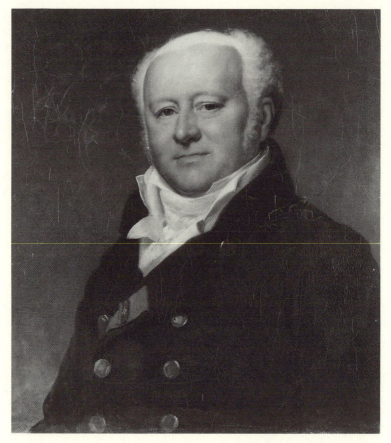

Figure 2.1. Jean-Nicolas Corvisart des Marets, by François Gerard. Professor of clinical medicine, Napoleon's personal physician and Laennec's teacher at the Charité hospital, Corvisart practiced and disseminated Auenbrugger's diagnostic technique of percussion. Source: Musée de Versailles. Photograph: Réunion des Musées Nationaux de France.

Michel Foucault described a fundamental change that occurred in the structure of medical knowledge: using only printed works published in France, he contended that the disease models we still use today were "born" in early nineteenth-century Paris. He studied the "discourse," or specialized language, as a disciplinary vehicle for ideas; the term, medical "gaze," borrowed from Corvisart, refers to the new way in which doctors would conceptualize disease: "the paradoxical ability to *hear a language* as soon as it *perceives a spectacle*."[5] With their new "gaze," doctors learned how to see the disease that may lie beyond the patient's senses. Critics of modern medicine portray this change in medical knowledge as the first step in a downward spiral that compartmentalized medical practice and reduced patients to powerless dependents, obligated to their physicians for knowledge about their own conditions. Some historians have pointed to precursors for educational practices and the accompanying epistemological shifts in schools operating elsewhere and earlier in eighteenth-century Europe.[6] Nevertheless, the postrevolutionary Paris school institutionalized the changes on a grand scale, and whether or not the trend originated in France, it was Laennec's future work on auscultation that would consolidate it and revolutionize how diseases are constructed and how doctors and patients relate to each other through diagnosis.

In the late eighteenth century, diseases were classified on the basis of symptoms, that is, the subjective feelings of sickness experienced by patients and "examined" by doctors through interview and observation. A "disease," then, was an idea assembled from a constellation of subjective symptoms that depended on their type, sequence, severity, and rhythm. Nosologists (or those who studied diseases) sorted diseases into Classes, Orders, Genera, and Species; some systems included more than two thousand types of diseases as did that of the Montpellier professor François Boissier de Sauvages (1706–1767). This "symptomatic" or "botanical" method was not unlike that applied to the study of plants and animals, and among the eighteenth-century nosologists can be found Carolus Linnaeus (1707–1778) and Erasmus Darwin (1731–1802), grandfather of Charles. In Edinburgh, William Cullen (1712–1790) compared various nosological systems and constructed one of his own. While in Paris, Philippe Pinel adapted and revised yet another disease classification, the massive *Nosographie philosophique* that Laennec had begun to read in Brittany.[7]

In order to learn about diseases, eighteenth-century medical students were required to memorize nosological classifications. When confronted with a patient having a certain combination of symptoms evolving in a certain sequence, astute observers would be able to apply a name to the patient's condition, or impose a diagnosis. Armed with the name of the disease, they could recall or research the correct treatment to alleviate the symptoms. To make a diagnosis, the patient's history—the subjective account of the illness—was of paramount importance. Physical signs—derived from the pulse, touching, and observation of skin and excreta—were contributory, but of lesser importance. In the eighteenth century, a physical disease was not an anatomical object, it was a physiological event; for its recognition, the patient was the final arbiter. A person could not be sick without feeling sick.

Anatomical information about the patient was mostly irrelevant to diagnosis, though not uninteresting. The physical examination was relatively cursory and of secondary importance to the history. Doctors would notice the patient's general appearance, the temperature of the skin to touch, changes in the face, hair, and nails. Those in England might count the pulse, whereas those in France would simply feel and describe it qualitatively. Surgeons sometimes palpated (felt) the abdomen for tumors or masses, but in the days before anesthesia and antisepsis, their routine work was limited to the treatment of wounds and procedures on the appendages of the body: arms, legs, breasts, genitalia. Operations on the thorax and abdomen had been performed since antiquity; notoriously dangerous, however, they were confined to the draining of abscesses and were undertaken with great trepidation, only in dire circumstances.[8]

Anatomy was not ignored by medical teachers and students. Since the early sixteenth century, some, such as Antonio Benivieni (1443–1502), had turned their attention to the study of abnormal or pathological anatomy. Several great compendia of changes in the internal organs had been published, including those of Théophile Bonet (1620–1689) and Giovanni Battista Morgagni (1682–1771).[9] In the eighteenth century, dissection rose to such prominence that, as Barbara Stafford has said, it became a "paradigm for any forced, artful, contrived, and violent study of depths" and a metaphor for "investigative method."[10] In 1772, the Collège de France created a chair of human anatomy from one of its three chairs of medicine, occupied by Antoine Portal (1742–1832) until its abolition in 1832. Private courses in dissection, like those that had been attended by Guillaume Laennec, were popular in the provinces as well as in Paris, where, as Dora Weiner has shown, amphitheaters were located within a strategically short distance of the morgue of the Hôtel Dieu hospital.[11] But anatomy was not formally taught in the Paris medical school until after the Revolution.

In 1794, François Chaussier (1746–1828) was brought from Dijon to fill the new chair of anatomy and physiology. His position was supported by a department of anatomical studies (*travaux anatomiques*) with a *chef* and six prosectors, a system that had been carried over from the assimilated Ecole Pratique. The 1798 revision of laws pertaining to anatomical subjects meant that three hundred cadavers were provided for approximately one-tenth to one-quarter of the total medical student body of twelve hundred.[12] In 1801, Guillaume Dupuytren (1777–1835) was appointed *chef* of anatomical studies, and two years later he would found the Société Anatomique. A chair in pathological or abnormal anatomy was still three and a half decades away and would be Dupuytren's legacy to his faculty. In Laennec's student days, pathological anatomy was, as he called it, an "entirely new science."[13]

Anatomy, of both normal and pathological subjects, may have been respected as a scientific discipline even before it was formally integrated into the medical curriculum; however, its application to the clinical setting was not clear, and it could not be integrated epistemologically with the nosological disease concepts. Doctors were skeptical of the use of anatomy for three quite justifiable and equally powerful reasons. First, the organic changes observed in cadavers might be the products of death itself, not of a prior disease process. Second, the organic changes might eventually be proven to be associated with diseases rather than with death, but they could not be detected inside a body until the patient was already dead. Third, "signs" embedded in the patients history or some yet to be invented physical technique might lead a doctor to the knowledge of the internal changes before the patient became a cadaver, but the anatomical changes could not be repaired. Each of these reasons was sufficient to constitute what could be called an "epistemological obstacle."[14] No doctor—and for the aforementioned reasons, not even a surgeon—could hope to treat internal anatomy; doctors treated diseases. And diseases were about function and perceptions of function: pains, fevers, rashes, swelling, the coughing of blood, and the loss of weight, movement, speech, or consciousness. Treatment should aim to relieve these symptoms; it could not hope to repair alterations to the internal organs.

In the early days of the Paris school, doctors struggled with the problem of how to integrate the older disease concepts with the information generated by centuries of dissection. Semiology, or study of the clinical signs that could guide a doctor to the diagnosis or the prognosis of a patient's condition, was an important aspect of medical knowledge; new books were being written on the subject in an attempt to bridge the gap between anatomy and nosology.[15] Pinel tried to bring anatomy into his *Nosographie*, a favorite example being his use of the observations of Johann Georg Roederer (1726–1763) and Karl Gottlieb Wagler (1731–1778), who found that autopsies of the Göttingen citizens, who had died in a 1762 epidemic of "mucous fever," usually revealed inflammation of the digestive tract. Pinel's use of their observation seems to have stimulated great interest in Roederer and Wagler, prompting the two French translations, which appeared within a few months of each other, and resulting in the work of P. A. Prost (d. 1832) on gastric fevers—works that would be reviewed by the young Laennec.[16]

By 1800, young experts in anatomy and pathological anatomy became critics of nosology. They claimed that, unlike plants and animals, diseases were not beings and should not be classified in the same way. Diseases were disorders in function; they were physiological and anatomical. These students turned the sensualistic philosophy of their school back on its instructors to argue that diseases should be classified only on the basis of changes that could be seen, felt, tasted, smelled, and heard by the doctor—changes that could be detected by an objective observation, independent of the patient's subjective account. Alterations that were amenable to this kind of perception were those of the internal organs.

Laennec immediately became a participant in the process of integrating anatomy and symptomatology, a process that had only begun as he arrived in Paris. Some of his successors leaned toward the total subjugation of the patient's symptoms to a new, anatomical imperative. At first, he leaned in the same direction, but eventually, he favored a combination of anatomy and nosology to explain disease.

TABLE 2.1
Laennec in the Paris School, 1801–1804

Term/Course	*Professor*
Messidor An IX (June–July 1801)	
Surgery (private course)	Boyer
12 Floréal An IX (2 May 1801): first registration	
Medical Physics and Hygiene	Hallé and Desgenettes
Matiera Medica	Peyrilhe
Internal Pathology	Pinel and Bourdier
6 Frimaire An X (27 Nov 1801): second registration	
Anatomy and Physics	Chaussier and Duméril
Chemistry and Pharmacy	Fourcroy and Deyeux
Internal medicine clinic	Corvisart and Leroux
Messidor An X (June–July 1802): third registration	
Physics and Hygiene	Hallé and Desgenettes
Internal Pathology	Pinel and Bourdier
Botany	Richard
Legal Medicine, History of Medicine	Leclerc and Cabanis
4 Frimaire An XI (25 Nov 1802): fourth registration	
No courses indicated in register	
Admitted to the Ecole Pratique de Dissection by examination	
16 Fructidor An XI (3 Sep 1803)	
Prizes: First prize in Surgery	
First prize in Medicine (shared)	
4 Pluviôse An XII (25 Jan 1804)	
Petition "Au citoyens professeurs"	
22 Prairial An XII (11 June 1804)	
Defense of thesis	

Sources: Laennec, MS petition, "Au citoyens professeurs," Demandes d'inscription, AN AJ 16 / 886 and ML, photograph; Laennec letters to his father and uncle from 20 Messidor An IX (9 July 1801) to 16 Fructidor An XI (3 Sep 1803), MS de Miniac, nos. 31, 32, 35, 43, 44, transcribed in Bouvier 1980, 193–97, 226–28 and Crochet 1982, 26, 27–30; Secretary of the Faculty of Medicine to Rouxeau, 1910, cited in Bouvier 1980, 192, 199, 213–14, 228.

LAENNEC IN PARIS

Laennec arrived in the capital at the end of April 1801. He moved into his brother's small apartment in the labyrinthine network of narrow streets in the old Latin quarter. By early May, he was introduced to the Breton enclave and had enrolled in the medical school. There he would study medicine, surgery, and anatomy, participate in the resurrection of academic societies, immerse himself in the teachings and the philosophy of the leaders of the new school, and fall under the spell of their outspoken young critics (see table 2.1).

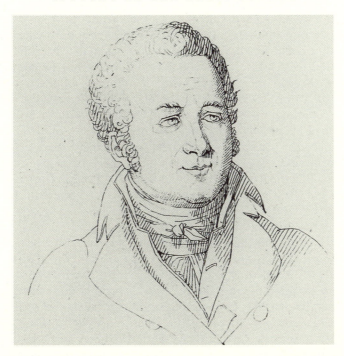

Figure 2.2. Jean-Noël Hallé, professor of hygiene and Laennec's lifelong mentor. Engraved by Frany after a portrait by Gounod, in *Biog. NC.* Photograph: Queen's Medical Photography Services.

The organization of the school was still evolving; its curriculum, examinations, and licensing requirements would not be resolved until the "laws of Ventôse and Germinal An XI" (March 1803).[17] Jean-Noël Hallé (1754–1822) was among Laennec's first professors and became his lifelong admirer and patron (fig. 2.2). The artistic son of a painter and a survivor of the old Faculty, Hallé was tolerated by the new order, despite his "royalist" leanings that had led him to plead openly but unsuccessfully for the life of Antoine-Laurent Lavoisier (1743–1794). Since 1794, Hallé had been a popular teacher in the chair of "medical physics and hygiene"; he liked to trace the history of ideas and expounded on a concept of well-being that integrated the psychic with the physical. As a hygienist, he was selected by the Institute to report on the discovery of vaccination by Edward Jenner (1749–1823), and he was immediately convinced of its value. In 1805, he would be named *médecin ordinaire* to the imperial court, but a falling out with Napoleon meant that he made few visits to the Tuileries. In the same year, he took over the Collège de France chair of practical medicine, vacated by a busy Corvisart who was preoccupied with the onerous tasks of *premier médecin* to the self-proclaimed Emperor. At the Collège de France, Hallé devoted a series of lectures to Hippocrates; he held the position for seventeen years until his death, when he would be replaced by his favorite disciple, Laennec.[18]

Three months after Théophile's arrival, the Laennec brothers were almost out of money, one semester in Paris had cost as much as a year anywhere else. The diamond could not be sold, and the restaurateur who provided their meals wanted to be paid. They began a tradition of borrowing from each other, from Breton friends, and from the mothers of friends, Mme de Laubrière and Mme de Varennes. Théophile could not afford the nine francs a month to continue the private lessons of the surgeon Alexis Boyer (1757–1833); he had been obliged to spend twenty-five francs on five volumes of chemistry in order to keep up with classes, and he had been sick several times. The first enthusiasm may have faded, but he had become acquainted with the booksellers along the banks of the Seine, and he had begun working on Latin and Greek, which, he claimed, were "essential" for success in his medical examinations.[19] The revolutionary distaste for classical languages notwithstanding, it was customary for medical students to be examined partly in Latin; they closed their theses with classical aphorisms, on which they were prepared to answer questions. In the first year and a half, their father contributed 450 francs to his sons, only about one-third of what they had spent; Guillaume gave them the rest and berated his brother for his negligence.[20]

In the middle of 1801, Laennec began his clinical studies with Corvisart at the school's *clinique interne* in the Charité hospital (called "l'Hospice de l'Unité" during the revolutionary period); there, an exclusive Société d'Instruction Médicale had just opened to extol the virtues and methods of bedside teaching.[21] Like Hallé, Corvisart was a survivor of the old faculty; unlike Hallé however, he had little use for the medical classics, and supported the idea of translating the few, truly useful, old books from Latin into the vernacular. While reading the *Aphorisms* of Maximilian Stoll (1742–1788) in preparation for his lessons at the Collège de France, he had stumbled across a reference to percussion, a method for examining a patient's chest that he had never before encountered.[22] Research led him to the little-known Latin book on the technique, published by Leopold Auenbrugger (1722–1809) in 1761 and already translated into French by Rozière de la Chassagne in 1770.[23]

Percussion, or tapping on the chest with the ends of the fingers, yields a resonant sound when the underlying parts of the lungs are healthy and filled with air, or a dull sound when they are abnormally filled with fluid, pus, or tumor. Auenbrugger was the son of an innkeeper and had seen his father use the same method to measure the level of wine or beer in a cask. His acoustic sensibilities extended to music, and he also penned the libretto for Antonio Salieri's opera, *Der Rauchfangkehrer* (*The Chimneysweep*), first performed in 1781. But Auenbrugger's ingenious contribution to medical semiology was ignored, for the same reasons that practitioners had been ambivalent about anatomy. Diseases of the chest were not known by names that related to anatomical structures; they were known by names for disordered functions, the symptoms suffered by the patient: fever, difficulty breathing, cough, wheezing, spitting blood, pain, and palpitations.

Corvisart immediately began to test Auenbrugger's percussion in his clinical practice at the Charité hospital, where he insisted that every death be investigated by an autopsy. To the amazement of colleagues and students, he was able to predict the postmortem findings long before the patient died. His rounds were well attended and his *ouvertures* became a sort of public declaration of the accuracy of his clinical acumen. He spoke of "tact" and "gaze" (or glance, "*coup d'oeil*") of a good clinician, schooled in both the science and art of medicine: special senses that would lead him to "see with a better eye" and to predict "the kind of disease which threatens an individual." His students imputed large doses of these qualities to their teacher. Heart disease became his special interest, because it often appeared as a surprise finding at autopsy. Using percussion, Corvisart could tell which hearts would be enlarged; and using palpation, or gentle application of his hand to the front of the patient's chest, he could sometimes distinguish a *frémissement cataire*, a catlike purring or "thrill," which he said indicated alteration of the valves inside the heart. The clinical link that Corvisart could establish between the state of the organs inside his still-living patients and their symptoms was unprecedented.[24]

As Laennec joined the service, Corvisart was deep in his research on clinical examination and percussion in preparation for two new books: a treatise on heart disease and a translation and commentary of Auenbrugger's *Inventum novum*. His private duties as physician to the First Consul waxed greatly, slowing the work so that the books did not appear until 1806 and 1808, respectively. With Boyer and Jean-Jacques Leroux des Tillets (1749–1832), Corvisart also edited the monthly *Journal de médecine, chirurgie, et pharmacie*, which began in Vendémiaire An IX (September–October 1800). Corvisart's *Journal de médecine* reported on the clinical discoveries of the Paris school—especially those of his hospital—reviewed recent literature, and provided the *constitutions médicales*, which were detailed tables of meteorological observations related to the health of the population.

Corvisart appears to have amplified his clinical teaching in the Hippocratic style of Stoll, by having students collect his aphorisms—"if-and-then" sentences that usually conveyed a clinical condition and its associated meaning as diagnostic, prognostic, or therapeutic signs. Laennec and at least one other student, François-Victor Mérat de Vaumartoise (1780–1851), recorded Corvisart's aphorisms. The majority of the 135 aphorisms in Laennec's manuscript pertained to the diseases of the heart or lung, and included allusions to percussion (nos. 6, 11), precordial thrill (no. 42), jugular veins (nos. 54, 55, 56), chemical changes of sputum (no. 44, 53), and the difficulty of recognizing the causes of disease (no. 43). Corvisart taught the inventor of the stethoscope that "the palpitations of the heart are sometimes so intense that the sound of the heart can be heard beating against the chest wall" (no. 8).[25] Laennec annotated these pearls of wisdom with references to cases he had seen in the *clinique interne* between spring 1801 and spring 1802.[26]

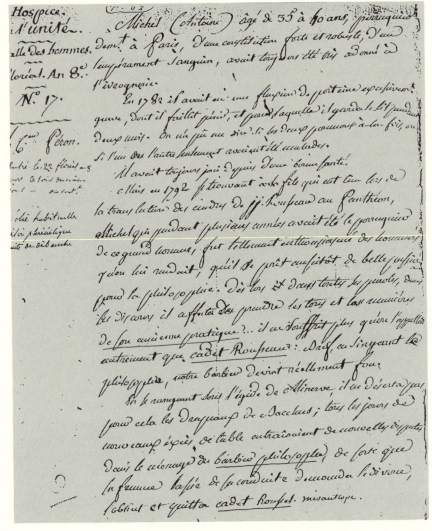

Figure 2.3. Title page of the case history of wigmaker, Antoine Michel, nicknamed "*cadet Rousseau, misantrope*" [*sic*], 22 Floréal An VIII (12 May 1800). Some historians have identified this document as Laennec's first clinical history, but the date, location, and handwriting are incompatible with that assertion. Nevertheless, it was kept with his papers, its style resembled his, and it exemplified his special interest in fatal diseases that left no organic lesions. Source: Musée Laennec, MS Cl. 8 [I], f. 1–3.

Aside from their value as medical documents, clinical records were stories told as evidence for new ideas about anatomy and disease. A manuscript at the Musée Laennec, written in an unknown hand, described the history of a man who died a year before Laennec's arrival in Paris; it seems to have been a cautionary tale against the possibility of finding the cause of disease in the organs of the cadaver (fig. 2.3). The history concerned the final illness of forty-year-old Antoine Michel, former wigmaker to Jean-Jacques Rousseau and overly fond of drink. In 1794, Michel was so overcome with emotion during the ceremony to transport Rousseau's remains to the Panthéon that he developed a passion for philosophy and went mad. "But," the author continued, "in placing himself under the protection of Minerva, he did not abandon Bacchus, and with each successive day, more excesses of the table brought new disputes into the home of the barber-philosopher." The man's wife sought and obtained a divorce from "*cadet Rousseau*, misanthrope," as he was now nicknamed. He was admitted to the Hospice de l'Unité on 22 Floréal An VIII (11 May 1800) in a state of agitation, but Corvisart's pre-scription of a large phlebotomy from his foot was to no avail, and he died that night. The autopsy revealed nothing to explain the man's demise. The writer concluded with a question: "Could the patient have died from this sort of attack of *acute mania*?"[27] The rich blend of classical references, ironic humor, and erudite curiosity was exactly the kind of prose that Laennec and his father admired so much, but the presence of this possibly fictitious docu-ment among his papers has yet to be explained. Some historians have identi-fied it as Laennec's first clinical history, but the date, location, and handwrit-ing are incompatible with that assertion. It may have served as a model for the records Laennec would write as a member of the Société d'Instruction Médicale. The final question would haunt his entire career. Could a person die without a significant anatomical change? Many of Laennec's colleagues would come to believe that the answer had to be "no," but he was always sure that the answer was "yes."

Toward the end of his first year in Paris, Laennec wrote the history of a twenty-two-year-old man who had first been admitted in September 1801 and died in March 1802. Before the autopsy, Corvisart reviewed the patient's clinical history, which had included pronounced pulsations in the jugular veins, and he percussed the chest of the cadaver. He predicted that the au-topsy would reveal pleural effusions, an enlarged heart with a dilated right ventricle, and lesions in the left side of the heart where he expected to find the primary cause of the illness. Corvisart was right; in addition to the changes he had specified, an ossified mitral valve was found in the left heart. Leroux was satisfied with the student's report of yet another anatomoclinical success worthy of his colleague's reputation; without telling the author, the editor made some abbreviations and alterations and published the case in the *Journal de médecine*.[28]

Laennec was angered by the manner in which his first article had appeared in print, the resulting clash of literary styles, and the lack of originality. "It cannot contribute anything to the progress of the art, given the scant details and absence of anything new," he complained to his father. He vowed not to show his next project to the professors until he had decided that it was ready for press. It would be a long presentation and analysis of six case histories of patients who had died of a new condition that the twenty-one-year-old student called "peritonitis," or inflammation ("-itis") of the peritoneum, the membrane lining the abdomen and its organs. Laennec said that he had been "contemplating" the peritonitis article for nearly a year and was working "alone."[29]

The idea of peritonitis was a direct extrapolation of the tissue-based pathology that seems to have originated with John C. Smyth (1741–1821) in England and permeated the teaching of Pinel and Bichat.[30] Tissue theory held that a range of pathological changes could characterize various types of tissues, independent of the organs in which they were found. Inflammation of the serous wrappings of the abdomen was a tissue concept worthy of Bichat himself; indeed, he had even collected some examples of the condition. When the student thought that his work was complete, he showed it to Leroux, who again found the essay "so much to his taste" that he wanted to appropriate it for Corvisart and himself, naming the real author only as "editor." After "several arguments," Laennec would consent only to a change in title to indicate that the case histories had been, "collected under the eyes of professors Corvisart and J. J. Leroux." Even this concession annoyed him, because "neither one nor the other had ever been involved"; he admitted, however, "it was in their hospital that I collected the cases," and "otherwise, Leroux is quite a good man."[31]

Laennec's article described the illnesses and detailed autopsy findings in six patients: five males ranging in age from seven to sixty years; and a thirty-two-year-old woman, Anne G., who died of fever following a delivery and an attack of fainting brought on by her "aberrant" husband's declaration that he was "leaving her forever." The article filled more than a hundred pages in two consecutive issues of the *Journal de médecine* late in the summer of 1802.[32] Generally considered to be the first description of peritonitis as a separate clinical entity, it brought the student-author immediate acclaim.

Dupuytren, whom Laennec described as "one of the leading anatomists of Paris," invited him to use his *laboratoire* for research. An unidentified member of the Société Médicale d'Emulation, possibly Dupuytren or Hallé, presented a summary of the peritonitis article and recommended its author be invited to join. Laennec hoped that his father could send money for clothes befitting the future invitation, but begged him not to brag about the "little" triumphs: "It is a very bad practice here in Paris to make a lot over one success, it will almost always be an obstacle to ever achieving a second."[33] Laennec had not bothered to apply to the elite Ecole Pratique de Dissection, but Leroux now insisted that he place himself in a position to compete for the prizes that it had recently inherited from the defunct

Académie de Chirurgie. In the fall of 1802, he passed the examination of the "school-within-the-school" and was admitted to a more senior level than the one that he had requested.[34]

Laennec was influenced by the clinics of Corvisart, but he did not like his teacher. At first, he appeared to enjoy proximity to the political action and reported to his father on inside information about Bonaparte's health.[35] Soon, however, the sentiments cooled, compromised perhaps by the close brush with plagiarism. In answer to one of his father's requests to use his connections to find him a position in Paris, Laennec wrote a credible but less than attractive description of his professor: "I know only M. Corvisart who is too lazy to write any book, although he is the *coryphée* of practical medicine; who does not want to see patients because it bothers him; who would hold it against me if I would speak to him of business; who would not open a letter or throw it on the fire, if one were to disturb him with such matters. His character pleases me so little that I have scarcely sought to know him better. In Paris, almost all the learned men of letters and of science are the same."[36] Laennec continued to see Corvisart professionally and socially for a long time, but by 1806 he still felt incapable of asking a favor of the man who had invited him "a hundred times to dine at his home."[37]

Two Theses of 1802: New Definitions for Pathology and Physiology

In 1802, two important theses were defended in the Paris school by charismatic older students: Gaspard-Laurent Bayle and Matthieu-François-Régis Buisson. Laennec was caught up in the energy of these brilliant reactionaries, whose dissertations broadly encompassed a programmatic statement for the remainder of his life. Both Bayle and Buisson criticized the dominant political ideas of their professors, and both were preoccupied with the classification systems of emerging disciplines. Bayle's thesis was devoted to pathological anatomy and its relationship to classification of disease; Buisson's, to the classification of physiological functions. The influence of Bayle on Laennec is well known; that of Buisson has been ignored. Between their two examinations came the death of Bichat, an event that had a direct effect on the reception of the second thesis.

Bayle and Laennec were close and, despite the seven-year difference in age, parallels in their early lives favored their friendship. They came from opposite corners of France and from different social circumstances to live side by side in the same street, rue du Jardinet, but like most of their peers, they began medical training as apprentice surgeons in the military. Their bond was strengthened by love of poetry, languages, art, music, and by regional patriotism. From Bayle, whom he called his "intimate friend," the previously indifferent Laennec was lead to a deep attachment to Catholicism, and to his political conservatism.[38]

Bayle was born at Le Vernet in the Alps of Provence in southern France and set out to become a priest (fig. 2.4). In 1792, after two years in a seminary, he was ready to take holy orders, but abruptly abandoned religious studies because he feared that he would never be "perfect" enough for clerical duties. He read Voltaire, Diderot, and Helvetius and turned from religion to law and politics. Chosen to serve as a counterrevolutionary voice on his departmental council, he received Paris exiles more warmly than his alarmed parents deemed wise; they sent him off to Montpellier. There he became disillusioned with politics and law, and entered medical school. Three years later, he was a surgical aide in the army and found God once again, through J. J. Rousseau, the patristic writings, and the Bible. In 1798, Bayle went to Paris to study with Corvisart and, by 1801, he had been recognized for academic excellence and was serving as an assistant in anatomical work and as a clinician in an unofficial capacity at the Charité hospital.[39]

Bayle was artistic, analytical, and passionate. He had a fondness for entomology and skill in classifying. As a child, he collected insects and, when confronted with an unfamiliar species, invented his own taxonomy. He also wrote poetry, but upon becoming a medical student, he burned all his poems because their very existence, "begging improvement," tormented him so much that he could neither work nor sleep.[40] He studied and spoke Provençal, cultivated classical languages, and preferred to read ancient medical texts in Greek. Once he had rediscovered his spiritual way, he openly practiced his Catholicism during revolutionary atheism. These traits display a reactionary turn of character and remarkable individual strength. To pursue "dead languages," to favor royalism, and to cultivate religion in the iconoclastic times of the Revolution and the early Empire were activities certain to draw notice, if not court disaster. Even in his medical epistemology, Bayle displayed a curious mixture of conservatism and originality.

Bayle's thesis attacked Pinel's classification of disease, by constructing nosology and practical medicine as two different, but related approaches to the same problem.[41] Nosology, or the observation of symptoms of diseases, was useful to both the theoretical "*médecins observateurs*" (nosologists) and the clinical "*médecins pratiques*" (like Bayle). But, Bayle said, the variety of individual suffering was infinite, and the number of different diseases should be finite. Therein lay the problem of an approach to diseases based only on the symptoms: there would be too many different types of disease to be practicable, a "*labyrinthe inextricable*." Instead, he proposed a classification of disease built on the organic lesion. The "*médecin pratique*" was able to sort out the useful "*symptômes constans*"—that is, those that were reflections of quality not of degree—from the confusing "*symptômes variables*" of the individual case by the exercise of the "delicate tact" and "admirable gaze," described by Corvisart. Bayle closed his thesis with a presentation of nine clinical cases of "gangrenous pustules" that he had collected in Provence.

Perhaps to soften anticipated hostility, Bayle used terms of respect when criticizing the nosologists, and he admitted to some reservations about the

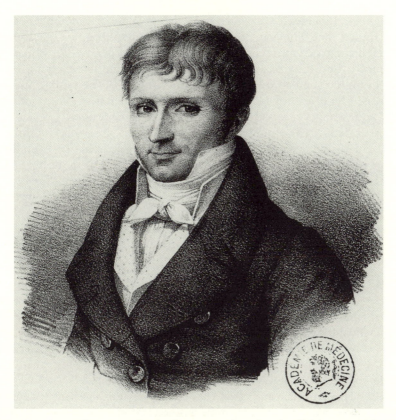

Figure 2.4. Gaspard-Laurent Bayle. Laennec's friend and collaborator. Lithograph by Didion, Académie Nationale de Médecine. Source: Académie Nationale de Médecine.

universal applicability of pathological anatomy to medical practice. Tremendous advances in pathological anatomy had occurred in the previous century, he said, but because the state of physical diagnosis was still limited, the relevance of findings in the dead to the living patient was sometimes obscure. After all, a clinician could know a disease only by its symptoms; therefore, Bayle maintained, the work of the nosologists must not be ignored, even though it ought to become a supplement to pathological anatomy. Patients suffered from diseases, not from organic lesions; diseases were alterations of function, not ensembles of symptoms, and not organic changes. Acknowledging the long held mistrust of anatomy, he agreed that the doctor's task was to relieve the symptoms; no one could hope to alter an organic change even if it could be proved to be part of the illness and/or it could be diagnosed before death.

Bayle defended his thesis on 4 Ventôse An X (23 February 1802). Laennec was one of two friends who kept a shorthand record of the proceedings and the examiners included Corvisart and Pinel.[42] With considerable audacity, Bayle argued that Pinel's method resulted in hair-splitting distinctions that hampered the true comprehension of the nature of disease. Pinel may have recognized the utility of localizing the disease to an ailing organ, but, in Bayle's opinion, he had overstated the importance of the symptom for the diagnosis. The disease should be recognized by qualitative "constant symptoms" and, whenever possible, by associated organic lesions.

Exasperated by the young upstart, Pinel said that he would be throwing away useful distinctions, if he ignored nosology. Bayle tried to explain that he did not reject the value of the observed differences, but he doubted their utility as a means of distinguishing separate diseases. The example of confluent versus discrete smallpox was inspired by the case reports of gangrenous pustules. In Pinel's view, these were two different diseases, because the patients with the former type were beyond medical help and would invariably die, whereas those with the latter stood a chance of recovery. Bayle said that they were different intensities along a continuum of a single disease; any further distinction was not useful.

Pinel: You have shown clearly that the path of the naturalists and that of the nosologists are not the same. . . . In general, classifications are intended to help the memory, to make distinctions between cases, and why do you not want me to make two species [of disease] when it could save the life of a patient?

Bayle: I see no application for differences in intensity . . .

Pinel: They are different species! The distinction is too important; it's not for our amusement that we make distinctions between diseases. . . . Why would you want to confuse them?

Bayle: I am not confusing anything, we differ [Pinel interrupted twice] . . . I beg you to let me give my reasons because you must judge me according to my experiences.

Pinel: True, true . . .[43]

And so it continued. Pinel seemed to appreciate the objections, but he had difficulty admitting that his system of classification was not useful; clumsy as it was, it was the best available and sometimes it worked. Nevertheless, Bayle was granted his degree.

A few months later, on 21 July 1802, the school was shocked to learn of the death of Bichat (fig. 2.5). Originally from Lyons, protégé of Pierre Joseph Desault (1738–1795) and later of his widow, the thirty-year-old physician had been energetically conducting research in pathological anatomy and physiology, although his exact place in the school had been never been formalized.[44] Historians have long tried to perceive a personal connection between Laennec and Bichat, and some have imagined that the young Breton joined the long, almost "penitential" procession of mourners.[45] Plausible though these conjectures may be, there is no evidence that Laennec ever studied with Bichat, even less that he was an admirer. On the contrary,

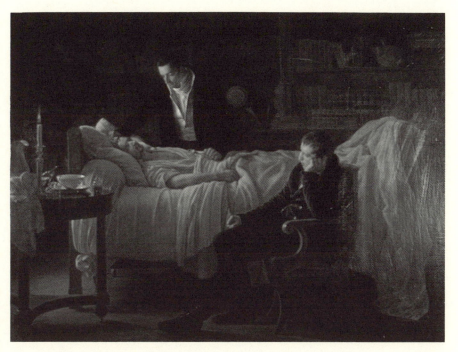

Figure 2.5. *The Death of Bichat,* painting by Louis Hersent, salon of 1817, bequest to the Faculté de Médecine de Paris by Pierre Petroz in 1891. Source: Association des Amis du Musée d'Histoire de la Médecine de l'Université René Descartes.

he joined in criticisms of Bichat's *Recherches physiologiques,* all the while paying obligatory lip service to the tragic loss of young genius that quickly became pro forma in the Paris school. The only firm link that can be established between Laennec and Bichat is through the latter's first cousin and critic, Régis Buisson, whose thesis defense took place a scant six weeks after Bichat's death.

Buisson, like Bichat, was also from Lyons, and, like Bayle and Laennec, he had served in the republican armies.[46] As part of his medical training, he collected autopsy results for Bichat at the Hôtel Dieu, using a rigorous format that corresponded to his cousin's theoretical views on pathological anatomy. He also helped to write the *Recherches physiologiques* and edited at least one of the five volumes of his cousin's *Anatomie descriptive,* published posthumously, with a biography of his deceased cousin.[47] An outstanding student, Buisson had shared a prize in the public examinations of 1801, but his profound religious sentiments were said to pervade, if not pervert, his thinking: in trying to integrate his spirituality with his physiology, Buisson was said to have claimed that he could "prove anatomically" that childbirth would have been painless if only "our grandmother Eve" had not sinned.[48] Buisson abhorred the materialistic skepticism of his chosen profession. He deployed medical metaphor to describe medical materialism as a "deadly epidemic" of a "contagious" and "fatal disease" that had afflicted "almost all" those who practiced and taught medicine in Paris.[49] In reaction, he joined five other devout medical students to found the Congrégation, which held its first clandestine meeting on 2 February 1801 at the home of the Jesuit priest, Jean-Baptiste Bourdier Delpuits (b. 1736). Buisson was elected the first prefect.[50]

For his thesis, Buisson conducted a three-hundred-page critique of the materialism in Bichat's *Recherches physiologiques*, and he proposed a new classification of physiology.[51] Influenced by Louis G. A. de Bonald, his own spiritualism, and the Jesuit uncle to whom he would dedicate the work, he "rejected" Bichat's divisions between "*vie organique*" and "*vie animale*." These artificial terms "sinned by an intrinsic vice" in that they were not mutually exclusive and not "perfectly natural."[52] Bichat seemed to forget Bonald's idea that man was "an intelligence served by organs," he said, and human consciousness and emotions affected all physiological domains be they "animal" or "organic."[53] To know if a denomination is well chosen, one must ask first, what is it that one wishes to express; second, if the word truly expresses that thought; and third, if there is not already an underlying meaning fixed in the minds of society.[54] But even the "savages" of Lithuania, Aveyron, and Canada do not deserve Bichat's epithets of animal and organic life; they have language, laws and religion—imperfect perhaps—but far beyond those of animals.[55] He recognized the ancient divisions of functions in human organisms, such as vision, speech, hearing, locomotion, and absorption, and conceived of an "active" and "passive" component to each, emphasizing that both components could be influenced by mind and emotion. For example, passive hearing was "audition"; active hearing was "auscultation."[56]

Buisson defended his long and controversial thesis on 7 September 1802. In response to a request from the Protestant theologian Pierre Picot (1745–1822) of Geneva, he gave his version of the conditions leading up to and surrounding the defense. He claimed to be proud that his opinions caused him to be among the first in his school to have been labeled an "imbecile," a "maniac par excellence," and a member of a "fanatic party"; he found it ironic that the professors had been obliged to give public recompense to "imbeciles" at the end of each year. His defense was the first occasion in the short history of the new medical school that anyone had tried to uphold ideas that were "diametrically opposed to materialism."[57] In anticipation of a lively dispute, more than five hundred young people assembled, some anxious for his success, others hoping for his defeat. All, including the candidate, were surprised by the respectful tone of the professors, only one of whom made "specious objections." His success and the spontaneous applause showed that audience and professors alike were satisfied with his performance.[58]

One month later, Laennec published a guardedly admiring eleven-page review of Buisson's thesis in Corvisart's *Journal de médecine*. He rehearsed the basic divisions of Buisson's physiological classification and recognized its debt to Bonald, the "modern physocologist" [sic]. The critique of Bichat might appear "singular," he said, "even misplaced in the eyes of those who were not aware of the bond between the author and the illustrious physiologist"; however, he reminded the readers that the thesis was well underway *before* "death ravaged physiology of one of its brightest lights." In other words, Bichat had been aware of the criticism. On the "intrinsic merit" of Buisson's thesis, Laennec pretended to "abstain," except to say it was notable for "clarity, purity of style, and the order and method that governed it."

More significantly, the future inventor of the stethoscope described Buisson's concepts of the passive and active components of the human hearing and voice in the following way:

He distinguishes two sorts of hearing, the passive or *audition*, the active or *auscultation*, a division based on equally exact observations, and on which is based the difference between the words, *to hear* and *to listen*.

Moving on to the examination of the voice, he distinguishes three types: the voice strictly speaking, song, and the spoken word. He asks this question, "Do humans have a specific voice [*voix propre*] like most animals?" . . . After developing some interesting rapports based on a study of children . . . he concludes by saying: "there are two sorts of voice in man, a *native voice* that he loses after infancy, and a *natural voice* that *society alone* gives him for the rest of his life."[59]

As defined by Buisson, then, auscultation was an active physiological process that engaged both the mind and hearing of the listener. The voice, one of the first and most important objects of Laennec's future stethoscopic research, was also a physiological process, invested with intrinsic and extrinsic elements reflecting the mind and the biology of its owner. Not only did Buisson's thesis herald the discovery of auscultation, which supposedly took place some fifteen years later, but it also pointed to the essentially *physiological* framework on which, I will show, the technique would be conceived and developed, by furnishing a vocabulary to convey it.

The following year, Laennec reviewed his "friend" Buisson's edition of Bichat's posthumous *Anatomie descriptive*. He made reference to his own discovery of the liver membrane and complained of various "defects," including differences in style and the disproportionate attention given to certain matters at the expense of others; however, he acknowledged that the book would become a classic, to be read with pleasure like the works of Boyer.[60] Buisson in turn published a review of Laennec's thesis, which will be examined below, but a few weeks later he was dead, possibly of an infected wound sustained during an autopsy.[61] His name would never again appear in Laennec's printed or manuscript work, and it has all but vanished from historical view.[62] Woe betide those who criticize Bichat.

THE CONGRÉGATION: A POLITICAL AND RELIGIOUS CONVERSION

Buisson's influence on his fellow students was considerable in both the short and long terms. He brought Bayle into the Congrégation on 25 July 1802 (four days after Bichat's death). On the following 23 March, Laennec, too, had enrolled and was quickly filled with the political and religious sentiments of his new-found friends.[63] He had been a proud republican soldier, but now he was openly royalist. In the correspondence, references to the religious conversion are scant, except for a letter to his father in late February 1803 which seems to credit Delpuits and either Bayle or Buisson: "I have turned to Him who alone can give real happiness, and your son is entirely back in the bosom of religion. I owe this good fortune to the counsel and advice of two men, each as talented as he is virtuous. The first is the most educated to have ever graduated from the Paris school; the other is one of the last children of the Company of Jesus, which possibly was destroyed only because it was one of the most invincible obstacles to the establishment of philosophy."[64]

In the Congrégation, Bayle and Laennec made lifelong friends: the medical students, Louis-Aimé Fizeau (1776–1864), Simon-Gabriel Bruté de Remur, Charles Savary des Brulons (d. 1814); the clerics, Antoine-Jerome-Paul Tesseyre (d. 1818) and Hyacinthe-Louis de Quélen (1778–1839), the future archbishop of Paris; the former aristocrats and royalists who would reclaim power after the Restoration of the throne, including the nobleman Mathieu-Jean-Félicité, Duc de Montmorency (1767–1826), who had hidden during the Terror at the home of Germaine Necker Mme de Staël (1766–1817). Bayle died too soon to profit from his acquaintance with aristocrats and clerics, but these contacts would serve Laennec well after the Restoration.

The meetings of the Congrégation opened with a mass, followed by an essay read by Delpuits or by one of the members, and a general discussion. Numbers grew so quickly that by 1803 the group had to be divided into two sections, each with its own vice-prefect; Laennec was chosen as vice-prefect of the second group in 1807, and it was likely in that capacity that he read his undated reflections on "*Ego sum via, veritas, et vita*" (I am the way, the truth, and the life).[65] Like members of a counterrevolutionary salon, they sometimes gathered informally in the homes of ladies, such as Mlle Delavau, who lived in the rue Dominque d'Enfer near the Jardin de Luxembourg and whom the guests called "*ma tante*." Her brother, Guy Delavau (1788–1874), became a member in 1807, prefect in 1817, and prefect of police in 1821.[66] The evenings may have embraced lighter amusements that included the poems of Buisson satirizing the free-thinking Chaussier and other medical professors for their atheism, anticlericalism, and pretentious use of big words, or possibly also Laennec's "*Cantique sur la fausse philosophie*" ("Canticle on False Philosophy").[67] Mlle Delavau appeared in Laennec's papers as a reliable witness to the mix of superstition and religion that had character-ized the seances of the mesmerizer Charles Deslon (1750–1786).[68]

Laennec's newfound royalism led him to reject Bonaparte and the promise of the First Empire. In the summer of 1804, he was shocked to learn that his father had privately published a twelve-page pamphlet, "Homage of a Father, or my Votes for Napoleon Bonaparte," expressing his enthusiastic support in Latin, French, and Breton. His son was filled with "profound pain," and advised him to destroy the dangerous pamphlet, or withhold it until he had considered three questions that seemed to echo Buisson: "First, what were you trying to do? Second, what ought you to avoid? And finally third, what is your goal?"[69] The father revised his pamphlet, but still the son did not approve.[70]

Between 1801 and 1804, Laennec watched as Napoleon proclaimed the Concordats and relegitimized the association between church and state. As a manifestation of the renewed relations, Pope Pius VII came from Rome to preside over the imperial coronation on 2 December 1804, during which Bonaparte unexpectedly seized the crown from the pontiff and placed it on his own head. Laennec complained that the excitement had caused a tempo-rary increase in the cost of clothing, and on the day of the coronation, he kept to his room. His uncle Guillaume thought his decision stemmed from the prudence that he had learned from the thieves who had entered his dwelling to steal money and part of his flute.[71] More likely, it was a form of political protest.

The Pope stayed in Paris for a few more weeks and, according to a fairly reliable source, Laennec was among those members of the Congrégation who were presented to Pius VII in a nearby chapel following mass at Saint Sulpice on 18 December 1804. The Pope's pleasure at meeting "talented" students from "different branches of science and the arts," was reported in the newspapers, and he was quoted as having said, "Nothing has been more agreeable than [hearing] the religious sentiments expressed by these young people."[72] A descendant of one of Laennec's fellows, told how His Holiness smiled and said, "*medicus pius res miranda* [a pious doctor is a thing of wonder]."[73]

Ironic as it may seem from this distance, there was an elitist, almost daring, antiestablishment cachet about the "student culture" of the Congrégation; members were known to cultivate a heady mix of "forbidden" topics: reli-gion, royalism, and scientific truth. Their opposition to the physiological classifications and the perceived "materialism" of Bichat mirrored their op-position to political ideals of postrevolutionary France. J. V. Pickstone has argued that Bichat's popularity among many students of the Directory and Empire may have been due to the resonance of his physiological ideas with their political goals.[74] Not all students were admirers, however; and tending to support Pickstone's argument, the Congrégation opponents of Bichat also saw themselves as the enemies of the Revolution. They prided them-selves on being the intellectual cream of the school, and their academic success lent credibility to the medical and political disagreements with professors. Their distinctions included Fizeau's first prize in An X (1801–2) and his successful defense of a thesis on fever.[75] Some members of the Congrégation may have been motivated by the prospect of regaining lost fortunes and titles, but others, like Buisson, Bayle, and Laennec, had once been revolutionary soldiers and willing republicans. They viewed their participation as a reasoned choice—"physiologically active" to use a Buissonian turn of phrase—based on their superior understanding of lived experience. If the best and brightest of the Paris school opposed the faculty to recognize *Dieu et le Roi*, then there was hope for the future. And when that future finally came, they seized opportunities to move from the covert to the powerful, confident in the absolute wisdom of their righteous vision and making full use of the network of social connections established in their youth.[76]

STUDENT-AUTHOR/STUDENT-TEACHER

Laennec's achievements more than measured up to the high standards of the Congrégation. While still a student, he wrote articles on his discoveries in anatomy and pathology: on visceral membranes; on a bursa in the shoulder; on how to demonstrate the internal arachnoid membrane; on how to determine whether a throat slit by a razor is the result of murder or suicide. And with Bayle, he published another observation on heart disease: the case of a twenty-two-year-old shoemaker, in whom the postmortem finding of valvular disease had been predicted antemortem on the basis of the pulse alone, because the man was considered to be "too sick" for examination by percussion and palpation.[77] This report was similar to Laennec's first article on a heart patient, the one that he thought had been unoriginal. Why the second essay was published is not known; however, in contrast to the first, this case tends to suggest that Corvisart's special technique of percussion was not always needed to come to an accurate anatomical diagnosis.

Modesty was not a feature of Laennec's early writing, although sometimes he attributed his small anatomical discoveries to "chance."[78] His essay on the best method to demonstrate visceral membranes of the abdominal organs was published as a letter to "Citoyen Dupuytren," in whose laboratory he and Bayle were working. He was formally respectful, perhaps a bit flattering, but he did not minimize the gloating triumph of his claim to having made an original observation supported by a thorough review of the literature: "In no author have I found any trace of a more precise indication of the visceral membranes."[79] It was his most important work to date, he announced to his literary father, but he also confessed that the style was inelegant because he had rushed to print fearing that "those to whom [he] had spoken would publish it as their own, as so often happens here."[80] Similarly, his essay on the demonstration of the internal arachnoid began with an elogious summary of Bichat's observations on the cerebral membranes; however, the technique, which had been "impossible" for Bichat, was "very easy" for Laennec.[81] Even in his early book reviews, he sometimes managed to find a way to bring his own achievements to the fore.[82] Such talent and confidence in a student was a force to be reckoned with.

By the end of February 1803, Laennec had confided in his father that he was collaborating with another "anatomist" (probably Bayle) on Dupuytren's treatise of pathological anatomy, but the project had to be kept secret. In May, he began to speak of giving his own private course in pathological anatomy the following winter, partly because he was desperate for the money needed to sustain a serious bid for the newly resurrected school prizes. At least one Parisian solicited his help as a medical ghostwriter. The different dates and descriptions suggest that there may have been two men: in the passage of March 1803, the would-be author was described as a "very rich man" whose "book would have little to do with medicine";[83] a year later, he was a "professeur de l'Ecole," a "savant who does not write his books alone."[84] Laennec abandoned the idea by October 1804, complaining that he had received only half of what he was owed for his labors in the project. Perhaps one of the unnamed men was Corvisart, whose book on the heart was eventually compiled by his former student, C. E. Horeau.

The examinations of the summer of 1803 justified the high value that Laennec placed on his own abilities. He spent five of the six hours of the combined examination in medicine and chemistry on the medical question, leaving only one hour to reply to the question in chemistry. For the practical examination in surgery, he was asked to disarticulate the arm of a cadaver at the shoulder with Dupuytren as assistant. He told his uncle that, as he left the room, he had overheard his examiner, Antoine Dubois (1756–1839), remark to Dupuytren: "*ce coup de bistouri, charmant!*"[85] Laennec went on to explain that Dubois had been "speaking of the stroke by which I cut the tendons of the supraspinatus, infraspinatus, small round, and biceps, and the capsule of the joint at the same time as I was rotating the arm below and inside so that the head of the humerus rolled under the blade of the instrument and came out the moment the incision was complete." He was sure that he would stand first in surgery and medicine, and he expected to be a runner-up in chemistry and pharmacy and in anatomy and physiology.

Laennec did not achieve the two anticipated positions as runner-up, but he took first prize in surgery out of fifteen competitors, and he shared the first prize in medicine with the runner-up, Billerey, out of the dozen who wrote.[86] He was ecstatic about being the only student to win two awards, his family and housemates with him. Letters flew between Paris and Brittany describing the examinations, the borrowed suit of clothes, the lavish prizes, the "brilliant" ceremony, the dinner at the home of Fourcroy, now director of public education, with the physician minister of the interior, Jean-Antoine Chaptal (1756–1832), and the special moments in conversation with these great men. Later, he was vexed to learn that his *cher papa* had made and circulated thirty copies of his letter announcing the success; but father and uncle had to be forgiven for their joy and pride. Just the year before Michaud had taken all the prizes at the Ecole des Quatre Nations and had already found himself a good job in Beauvais at the prefecture of the department of the Oise. Soon the long, expensive studies of the orphan pair would draw to a close, and Théophile would also find a position worthy of his achievements. A professorship is what he wanted and now had reason to expect. He told his father about the beautiful instruments for surgical amputation that he had won: "deluxe cutlery," which for him were only "objects for show because I will never do surgery unless in an emergency when there is no one else." The academic labors were already beginning to pay off: Pinel was "friendly," Hallé "charmed," and Leroux, who foresaw an academic future for him in Paris, had already proposed that he work as a paid editor for the *Journal de médecine*.[87] The thesis and the final examinations remained.

The final year of Laennec's medical studies was a curious mixture of the very new and the very old. With Bayle, he was an original member of the Société Anatomique, which held its first meeting on 12 Frimaire An XII (3 December 1803). The president was the founder, Dupuytren, who, although he had yet to defend a thesis, had just taken up a surgical position at the Hôtel Dieu hospital (in 1802 or 1803, reports differ). Laennec had assisted Dupuytren in his research and anatomy classes in the spring of 1803, and developed his own ideas about how to organize, teach, and publish the "entirely new science" of pathological anatomy.

Courses on dissection and normal anatomy as it applied to surgery were numerous, but courses on abnormal or pathological anatomy were relatively rare. The secretive experiences with Bayle in working on the textbook of Dupuytren, the latter's chronic inability to publish, and the brief flirtation with ghostwriting may also have led Laennec to the conclusion that he would never derive any benefit from his discoveries if he did not develop them for himself. He announced his private course in pathological anatomy in the fall of 1803. The precocious pedagogic adventure was taken as an affront by Dupuytren, whose well-known personal ambition and paranoid suspicions may have begun to rub off on his young associate; soon they would be openly engaged in verbal combat (see chap. 3).[88]

Laennec's course opened for the first of its three cycles on 14 Frimaire An XII (6 December 1803), two days after the first meeting of the Société Anatomique. "No one has ever embarked on a teaching career under such fortunate auspices," he told his father; some people might give him trouble because he had not yet graduated, but he was sure he could "smooth over these little difficulties," since so many students were begging him to start. He expected an audience of one hundred and an income of 600 francs; however, by the end of the first month he realized that lecturing to the "good number" who turned up might enhance his reputation, but would do nothing for his finances.[89] A description of Théophile's two-hour "inaugural" lecture was handed down, and possibly embellished, through generations of descendants: at first hesitant, then increasingly confident, the twenty-two-year-old instructor spoke like a "great master" with a "quantity of expressions that were rare even in Paris"; he ended to thunderous applause.[90] The location of the classes and the source of cadavers are unknown. In the third year, his audience dwindled to only six students, who were taught in Laennec's apartment.[91]

While teaching his first course, Laennec abandoned Dupuytren to work with Bayle on their own treatise of pathological anatomy.[92] The extensive notes that he wrote in preparation for the course and for the book, as well as those taken by a student who was in attendance during 1803–1804, show that the lessons and the textbook were developed in parallel.[93] Both sets of papers follow an order that reflected Laennec's classification of anatomical lesions, a conceptual invention which he proudly viewed as yet another personal discovery and to which he would adhere, with only minor modifications, for the rest of his life (see table 3.2). References to the contributions of members of the Paris school including Bichat, Dupuytren, Bayle, and himself, were numerous; those to English writers were few, but Laennec did not neglect the work of Morgagni and the ancients, including Galen, Aristotle, and Hippocrates.

LAENNEC'S THESIS ON HIPPOCRATES

Hippocrates was much talked about by doctors in the late eighteenth and early nineteenth centuries, and their uses of the ancient texts have been an object of study.[94] Laennec had originally planned to write his thesis on the "new science," and it is not clear why he decided to concentrate on ancient medicine instead. In the competitive style of his friends, he may have been provoked by another student who was preparing a thesis on doubts about the existence of Hippocrates; perhaps, he was goaded by Corvisart's skepticism over the value of ancient medicine, while Hallé's interest in history may have served as a model.[95] Laennec's Hippocrates would be new and different. Not only would he be elucidated through respectable philological method, worthy of an erudite member of the Congrégation, but the so-called new ideas, which Paris professors flattered themselves in having invented, would be shown to have originated long before with the "Father of Medicine." Laennec's unorthodox thesis claimed that Hippocrates, who, as far as anyone can tell had never performed an human autopsy in his hypothetical life, could be read as a positivistic advocate of pathological anatomy, a venerable critic of Pinel's nosology, and a hoary partisan of the twin theses of Bayle and Buisson.[96]

A study of Hippocrates afforded two other advantages: it might cool the warming tension between Laennec and his rival Dupuytren by deflecting attention away from pathological anatomy; and it could also improve his qualifications for an academic plum: the chair of Hippocratic medicine and rare diseases. Founded in 1794, the chair was held by the dean of the school,

Michel Thouret (1748–1810), but the occupant had yet to give a single lecture and, in fact, never would. In late January 1804, Laennec sought permission to sit his doctoral examinations two years early on the basis of his service as a surgical aide; by mid-February, the professors had given their consent, provided he pay the fees for the two years from which he would be exempt.[97] He began what he mistakenly hoped would be a final campaign on the paternal purse for books and clothes, explaining that he could save time if he bought books instead of using the library and that he had been passed over for a minor position because of his shabby attire.[98]

Laennec's thesis has attracted the attention of historians and philologists alike, not only because it offered the enchanting example of one "great man" looking at another, but because it contained an unusual interpretation of Hippocratic texts that has been described as an "uneasy reconciliation" of ancient wisdom with the new Paris medicine.[99] Laennec said that he hoped that a physician who understood Greek would eventually conduct a synthetic analysis of Hippocratic anatomy, physiology, nosology, semiotics, and therapeutics in both surgery and practical medicine. Since "particular circumstances" gave him "only a few days" to devote to his thesis, he would confine himself to "the doctrine of Hippocrates" as it applied to practical medicine.[100]

In Laennec's thesis, "doctrine," or theory, was distinguished from "method" as the ensemble of "systematic" ideas about diseases; it was the most evanescent part of medical knowledge. Disease systems or concepts were used for facilitating the understanding of a vast collection of facts; for example, diseases could be studied according to their causes, their symptoms, their organic lesions, or their treatments. Method followed; it was the recognition of disease and the application of rational or empirical therapy to that disease. The texts of Hippocrates were pleasing to the modern reader because they seemed to contain many "facts" and little doctrine, and he claimed that most doctors adhered to the method, but only a few understood the doctrine that he was about to elucidate.

In Hippocrates, according to Laennec, doctrine could be reduced to the following systematic idea: "among the symptoms presented by a disease, there are those that are specific and characterize the disease [*symptômes propres*]; there are others which can be found in any disease [*symptômes communs*]." Common symptoms were nonspecific, the "epiphenomena" of sickness, and a result of intensity not of quality; they might have a bearing on prognosis, but they had nothing to do with categories of disease. Fever and crises were good examples of "common symptoms." Laennec's approach mirrored the semantics of Bayle: his *symptôme propre* was the equivalent of Bayle's *symptôme constans;* the examples concerning degrees of intensity were almost identical to those of Bayle in their intent to undermine the nosological categories of Pinel.

When Laennec's Hippocrates chose to speak of nosology, he displayed the "healthiest" points of view. Hippocrates "wanted to base the distinction between diseases on the nature of organic lesions that they caused in the animal economy; and this basis, when it exists (because there are diseases that leave no trace of their existence) is certainly the most solid that one could choose."[101] The parenthetical remark clearly recognized the existence of cases like *cadet Rousseau*. He continued: doctors stop at a study of epiphenomena, because they are obliged to treat the symptoms; only a few diseases can be cured by specifics (e.g., syphilis) or by destroying the cause (e.g., surgical diseases). Symptomatic treatment can be effective if it is directed to the main symptom, but it can be abused if the doctor focuses on the secondary symptom (*symptôme du symptôme*).

Prognosis was more important to Hippocrates than was diagnosis, and it sometimes seemed to Laennec that diagnostic signs had actually been "pruned" from the ancient writings. With flagrant disregard for epistemological relativism, Laennec fretted over Hippocrates's apparent ignorance of the "internal organic diseases." He came up with the anachronistic suggestion that the Old Man of Cos must have followed the advice, now ascribed to Bichat, and "opened a few cadavers"—he simply did not open enough.[102] But when Hippocrates spoke of different fevers, Laennec said, he was not designating the diagnostic categories understood by the nosologists; he was giving merely adjectival descriptions of the epiphenomena of illness. The types of fevers recognized by modern writers could be reduced to five; examples of all five types could be found in the works of Hippocrates, but they were not separate diseases. As Bayle had argued two years earlier, he accused the nosologists of being distracted by perceptible differences in intensity, which had been recognized by Hippocrates two thousand years before. In trying to make different diseases of these categories, the nosologists fell victim to a habit of systematization, a habit that the Father of Medicine had been able to resist.

Laennec examined the role of inflammation in different tissues as a source of fevers, especially in the mucous membranes as described by Roederer and Wagler and cited by Pinel. But he refused to construct different diseases out of the fevers that accompanied each of these different anatomical lesions, just as he rejected distinctions based on symptoms. He concluded with an unconventional idea, which was difficult for his colleagues to accept, but which he would retain till the end of his life (all the while attributing it to Hippocrates): there is only one type of fever, or at most two. In support of this idea, he cited the 1802 theses of two men: his friend from the Congrégation, Fizeau, and his future enemy, François-Joseph-Victor Broussais (1772–1838).[103]

Laennec wrote his thesis quickly, because he was preoccupied by his work in pathological anatomy, his teaching, and the final examinations; in compensation for its brevity, he hoped it would be "provocative" (*piquant*).[104] As a philosophical disquisition on the problem of nosology and its relationship to ancient texts, it belonged with the critical essays of Bayle, Buisson, and Fizeau. The epigraph was a passage from *Ancient Medicine*, a cautionary tale

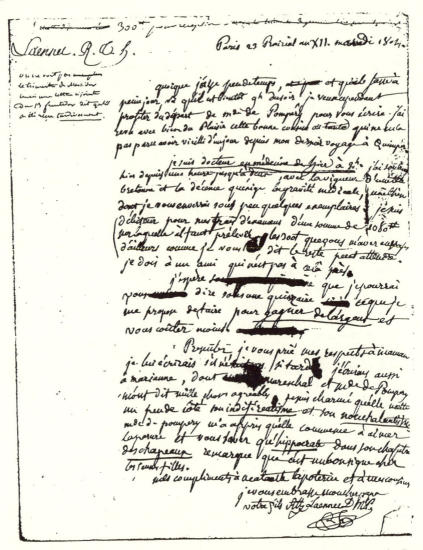

Figure 2.6. "I am a doctor since yesterday," begins the second paragraph. Letter announcing the successful thesis examination, and signed with the new credentials D[oct.] M[ed.] P[aris.] Laennec to his father, 23 Prairial An XII (12 June 1804). Source: MS de Miniac, no. 61. By permission of M. Hervé de Miniac, Rennes. Photograph: Queen's Medical Photography Services from photocopy.

for the new Paris school and a refrain for his own existence: "Medicine is not a new science. . . . But anyone who, casting aside and rejecting all these means, attempts to conduct research in any other way or after another fashion, and asserts that he has found out anything, is and has been the victim of deception."[105]

Laennec's father insisted that the thesis be dedicated to Chaptal and provided some fawning copy. His son ignored the suggestion and chose his uncle instead: "I owe him this small token of gratitude for all his generosity."[106] Historians have claimed that because Laennec's thesis was published, it was an epoch-making event; however, it is difficult to find evidence to confirm this statement. Many contemporary theses were published. Laennec simply made an advantageous arrangement with Didot for two hundred copies of the thesis, on the promise of his forthcoming treatise of pathological anatomy, which he had been told might be sold for two thousand livres. The professors seem to have been little disturbed by their energetic student chastising them for being less original than they had thought. Perhaps they were bored with the snobbish attacks from the Congrégation coterie. The examination committee was supposed to consist of Baudeloque, Boyer, Chaussier, Corvisart, Deyeux, and Bourdier as president; however, Corvisart did not appear, and Baudeloque, Chaussier, and Deyeux sent as their replacements Sue, Pinel, and Thillaye.[107] The defense lasted an hour on 22 Prairial An XII (11 June 1804), and the size of the audience is unknown. "I am a doctor since two o'clock yesterday," Laennec told his father: he had argued "with the vigor of a Breton head and the decency required for medical gravity" (fig. 2.6). More than one thousand livres were still needed for the unpaid fees, but he hoped to be able to announce how he would be earning his living within the next two weeks.[108]

Buisson's review of the thesis was guarded. He said,

> One would have to be very rigorous to find that the opinion, which M. Laennec allows himself to hold, is bold or rash. This opinion is based far less on the authority of Hippocrates than it is on present-day observation, but what better route than observation to discover the true and false in medical theory? Is a true theory anything other than the ensemble of consequences necessarily deduced from observed facts? . . . Everything here boils down to a dispute over words . . . Diagnostic and prognostic signs are necessarily linked; and while it is useful to separate them to appreciate their retrospective importance, it is impossible to separate them absolutely either in study or in practice.[109]

Laennec's reaction to this dismissive review by the leader of the Catholic scholars is unknown; perhaps he did not respond because the influential Buisson was soon dead. And in spite of the review, the young graduate was confident: his prizes, his publications, his reputation as a researcher in a new field, his mastery of the central debates over the nature of disease, his classical erudition, and his proven ability to teach convinced him that he would be offered the first available position in the Paris school.

Research and Academic Aspirations

If medicine has lost something with the destruction of
the old companies known under the names of Faculties
and Colleges, it has in a certain way made amends for
the loss with the advantages for the advancement of
science offered by the new organization of studies
[in pathological anatomy].

—Laennec 1805h, 158

LAENNEC would remain dependent on his father's less than generous largesse for four more years, and his confident expectation of a position in the
Paris school would not be filled for more than a decade. His student awards
and his publications were impressive, but they could not overcome the requirements of political acceptability. Academic security would come only
after 1815 and the Restoration, through the connections he had established
in his youth. In the months immediately following his thesis defense, he
could not imagine the long wait that lay ahead.

This chapter traces Laennec's early career as an independent researcher
and active contributor within the postrevolutionary medical societies of
Paris. He continued to pour his energies into the less lucrative research of a
future professor, cultivating members of scholarly societies, styling himself as
an erudite medical pundit, and sparring with Dupuytren. He devised a new
classification of anatomical lesions, but his treatise on pathological anatomy
progressed slowly. By 1811, he came to the disappointing realization that an
official position might never come his way. In the interval, he had established
a clientele that distracted him from his original academic goals into the role
of a busy clinician serving a peculiar subset of Paris society. His practice will
be the topic of the next chapter.

SCHOLARLY SOCIETIES AND JOURNALS

Laennec's research activities continued through Corvisart's *Journal de médecine*, which he served as editor, contributor, and reviewer until late 1808,
and through the Société de l'Ecole de Médecine, which would always be his
most important intellectual outlet. The Société de l'Ecole was founded by

permission of the minister of the interior as compensation for the defunct Société Royale de Médecine, the archives of which it had inherited, and the Académie Royale de Chirurgie. Members were paid two francs and fifty centimes for their participation at weekly meetings.[1] Essay contributions by members or correspondents were read, and small committees were charged with assessing the research and reporting back to the assembly on its value. The proceedings and a subset of the original papers with the evaluators' reports were published in the society's *Bulletin*. The Société de l'Ecole dissolved when Louis XVIII created the Académie Royale de Médecine in 1820. Its papers were left to the new Académie and are now held within the archives of its descendant, the Académie Nationale de Médecine.[2]

As part of the admission process in early 1804, Laennec spoke to the Société de l'Ecole about his research on parasites. Bayle had already presented a statistically rich description of the clinical and organic changes in phthisis.[3] Their election to the Société was soon ratified by ministerial approval, and they attended their first meeting as adjunct members on 30 August 1804. Laennec had been recruited with fifteen others as part of a drive to enlarge and rejuvenate the aging membership.[4] As he told his father, the society would now be in a position to fulfill its assigned role of "preserving and increasing medical science in France"; after he had "aged a little" in his new position, he would send a "small purse" of his earnings to his stepmother for her games of Boston. Wary of his father's unfailing capacity to embarrass him, he said "remember that this title should not be written as part of an address."[5] The father failed to follow the advice, and the son soon stopped sending his good news. Laennec *père* then began asking for word of his son from his brother and various other spies.[6]

Between 1804 and 1811, Laennec was one of the most active members of the Société de l'Ecole: his name appeared in the proceedings as frequently as any other, including Dupuytren and the physiologist Julien-Jean-César Legallois (1770–1814). Here, he presented his discoveries in pathological anatomy, developed his reputation as a parasitologist, and collaborated on small committees with established luminaries—such as his professors Chaussier, Larrey, Pinel, André-Marie-Constant Duméril (1774–1860), Baron Georges Cuvier (1769–1832), and Pierre-François Percy (1754–1825)—to evaluate the work of future luminaries, including J. E. D. Esquirol (1772–1840), J. M. G. Itard (1774–1838), and L. L. Rostan (1790–1866). Here also, he would describe his early research in auscultation.

Laennec's first contribution to the Société de l'Ecole was a lengthy analysis and classification of vesicular worms, read as part of his candidacy on 16 February 1804. He had been contemplating the project long before he had graduated, perhaps even since the days in Brittany when he had passed a large worm at the end of his serious illness in 1798. By March 1806, he told his father that the *Mémoire sur les vers vésiculaires* (Essay on Vesicular Worms), promised for more than two years, was finally being printed and would fill almost two hundred pages and be illustrated with four engravings based on his own drawings. Initially, he had hoped to sell the work for twenty-five

TABLE 3.1
Laennec's Classification of Intestinal Parasites, 1804–1826

Family ("famille")	*Type* ("genre")	*Sort* ("sorte")
Helminthes (roundworms)	*Ascarides*	*A. lombricoides*
		A. vermicularis
	Tricephalus	
	Filiairia	
	Hamularia	
	Crinon	
Agastres (flatworms)	*Taenia*	*T. solium*
		T. lata
		T. visceralis (rejected 1806)
	Polystoma pinguila	
	Hexathyridium venaria	
	Distoma r. fasciola	
	Distoma hepaticum	
	Distomus intersectus ("discovered" 1807, rejected 1826)	
Vesiculaire (vesicular worms)	*Cysticercus*	*C. finnu*
		C. fibreuses
		C. de fischer
		C. dicystus (1805)
	Polycephali	
	Ditrachyerus	
	Acephalocystides (hydatids) (Laennec's type)	*A. ovoidea* (1804)
		A. granulosa (1804)
		A. surculigera (1804)
		A. cystifiri (1822)
		A. étranglé (1822)
		A. ansa (1822)
		A. applati (1822)

Sources: Laennec, 1812a; Collège de France, lessons 24–27, 1822–1823, BIUM, MS 2186 (IV) f. 96r–106v; Laennec 1807a; *Traité* 1826, 1:275–276.

louis (Fr 600), but he began to despair of seeing its completion. The *Mémoire* was printed slowly over four months in 1806 and was not released until 1812.[7]

Laennec devoted ten pages of the long essay on vesicular worms to reviewing the history of parasitology from the ancient writers, Aretaeus of Cappadocia (first century A.D.) and Galen (second century A.D.), to his own time. He presented an outline of his classification, which consisted of four types: three were already recognized; the fourth, "*Acephalocystides*," was his own creation, previous examples of which, he said, had been confused with other varieties or labeled as "hydatids" (see table 3.1). Citing the contributions

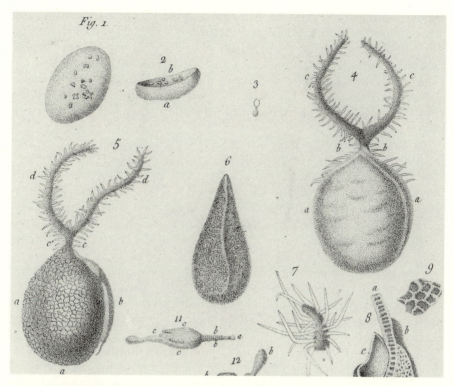

Figure 3.1. Detail from figures engraved from Laennec's drawings of his new "genre" of worm, acephalocysts. The worm, ditrachyceros, is shown in its natural size (Fig. 3) and as seen under the microscope (Figs. 4, 5). Source: Laennec 1812a, plate 4 detail. Wangensteen Historical Library of Biology and Medicine, University of Minnesota. Photograph: D. Van Slyke.

and assistance of Dupuytren, Antoine Dubois (1756–1837), Pierre Lassus (d. 1807), Percy and other Paris physicians, he elaborated on the description of each of the four types ending with a long section justifying the advent of his new fourth type and discussing the related diseases and their treatment (fig. 3.1).

During his years with the Société, Laennec would make a dozen reports and presentations on human parasites, of which at least three concerned previously unknown species, and one a recognized species that he claimed should be nonexistent.[8] With Larrey, he also reported on a case of elephantiasis, but they did not recognize the parasitic cause.[9] Just as Bayle was known to have a fondness for insects, Laennec became the resident worm specialist. By 1822, he had added four more "sorts" to his group of "acephalocysts," one or two of which might constitute separate species.[10] The Académie de Médecine possesses Laennec's hand-colored drawing of an incomplete and still unidentified "worm" sent by the surgeon Chartier of Lorris (Loiret) to

Duméril, professor at both the Museum and the Faculty of Medicine, and president of the Société de l'Ecole.[11] According to Huard and Théodoridès, who published a reproduction of Laennec's drawing, the "worm" is now thought to have been a "pseudo-worm" or a piece of intestinal tissue.[12] Laennec later retracted his "discovery" of *distomus intersectus*, saying that it was an "error committed in my youth" when he saw a new type of parasite "in the larva of a fly that happened to fall into the chamber pot" of one of his patients.[13]

To study parasites, Laennec owned and used a microscope, which he may also have applied to the study of anatomical lesions.[14] Much has been made of the mistrust of the microscope prior to 1820. Bichat, Dupuytren, and by inference Laennec, are said to have opposed it. Historians explain the mistrust by pointing to the unreliability of the instrument prior to the development of compound achromatic lenses in the 1830s.[15] But Laennec referred to microscopy several times throughout his career. His reservations about its limits in pathological anatomy are discussed in chapter 11.

Laennec viewed parasites as "living foreign bodies"—a subset of anatomical lesions—but in pursuing the investigation of other species, he also hoped to carry his work beyond the realm of medicine into the wider domain of the natural sciences. For the *Journal* and the Société, he reviewed manuscripts and publications on zoological topics, and in 1809 he was named with L. J. S. Thillaye (1776–1860) to attend and report on meetings of the Institut de France, within which resided the successor to the old Académie des Sciences.[16]

The special interest in living organisms and their classification brought the young graduate to the attention of Cuvier, who was already well established in the academic and political world of Paris. In November 1804, they reported favorably on the incomplete essay, "Considerations on the Natural History of the Worms of Man," by the medical doctor, Fortassin (d. 1804), whose sudden death had curtailed his investigations and whose autopsy became another anatomical case in the *Journal de médecine*.[17] Cuvier and Laennec held similar views on politics and science, and would be colleagues at the Collège de France, where Cuvier held the chair of natural history from 1800 to 1832. Like Laennec, he leaned to the right, supported religion, abhorred social disorder, and adopted an all embracing vision of physiology.[18]

Many book reviews in Corvisart's *Journal* were written by Laennec, who signed with a variety of different initials, which he clarified in a letter to his father.[19] In this capacity, his specialties were pathological anatomy, nosology, parasitology, and philology, including ancient authors and translations in general. With minor variations, his reviews usually followed a formula: survey of the history and literature of the topic; summary of the contents of the work under review; where necessary, an appreciation of the quality of translation; and, finally, a brief assessment of the merits of the work.

Laennec's character can be sensed on reading his reviews: bright, quick, sarcastic, often arch, and confidently erudite. A mocking humor bubbled to the surface, especially when he was compelled to defend the honor of his native Brittany. Thus, after correcting some matters of grammar and etymology, he responded to his former professor, Pierre Lassus, who had described Quimper as "dirty and sad" and plagued with "endemic" scabies: "Although I think M. Lassus's observation is inaccurate, I will not dwell upon whether or not Quimper is dirty and sad. I know that one should not argue about matters of taste . . . But that my compatriots are affected with endemic scabies, I will deny. . . . There is proportionately more scabies in Paris than in any place in Lower Brittany, even in Quimper-Corentin."[20]

Laennec made fun of the medical "discoveries" of an author "who forgets he is a dentist" and dared to suggest that Bichat died of the previously unappreciated disease of "cachexia": "What, *messieurs!*" he asked his readers, "Are you indifferent to a theory that could be among the most useful to your profession?"[21] He reveled in elaborate word play and referred again to Quimper in reviewing a vitalistic essay reminiscent of Paracelsus.[22] In reviews of translations, he could be caustic: for example, he once wrote that the pleasing aspects of a work owed more to Hippocrates than to the translator, who might have done better "if he had a real talent for translating." [23] He devoted the first twenty pages of his review of J. L. F. Terr's poem, "Hygea, or the Art of Being Well," to a rollicking survey of poetic literature pertaining to health and medicine with seventy-eight references; and he closed with a stinging remark: "If there were no other poems except 'Hygea' and 'The Art of Blowing One's Nose,' then [Terr] would certainly deserve the 'Palm of Poetry.' "[24]

The arrogance of Laennec's student publications softened, but he rarely missed an opportunity to remind readers of his own abilities and contributions to medical science. In marveling over the mini-industry in translating works from Latin to the vernacular, he lamented the passing of a common language for the dissemination of research.[25] The special interest in translating Roederer and Wagler's treatise on mucous fever had been prompted by Pinel, whose treatise, he said, few physicians had actually read.[26] A review of one such translation allowed him to refer to the anti-Pinelian idea, articulated in his own dissertation, that there was only one type of fever.[27] Similarly, he used a review of Duméril to promote his own classification of parasites and another of Bichat to recall his discovery of the visceral membranes.[28]

Laennec was not above adopting a moralizing tone to harp on his pet peeves: excessive haste to publish and the creation of neologisms—ironically the very "sins" that he did or would commit himself. The author who had no talent for translating was chided for not hesitating, according to the advice of Horace: "*Nonumque prematur in annum.*"[29] In complaining of the "negligence" and "inaccuracy" he found in Prost's reductionist work on lesions in the gastrointestinal tract, he said: "One is never pressed to have a scientific work appear, especially if one proposes to give it the pompous title of *Medicine Enlightened by the Opening of Bodies.*" This disapproval extended to a scathing criticism of Prost's simplistic pathological anatomy and later of his systematic therapeutics on bleeding as a therapy for mental illness.[30] These attacks were an early declaration of his position in the later dispute with Broussais.

Laennec pontificated on neologisms too: "One must never make a new word, unless one has a new thing to express."[31] But even new ideas need not spawn neologism, and he congratulated Paul-Joseph Barthez (1734–1806) for having presented "many new ideas without creating new words." Barthez's style may sometimes be difficult, he said, but his ideas were not, and his work demonstrated that those who cultivate science should not neglect letters.[32] Old and new words were of concern to others, too, including his teacher Leroux, who joined in a self-conscious appreciation of the contemporary program to redefine and reclassify disease.[33] Their writings and the criticisms of Buisson may have led Laennec to adopt a conservative stance on the issue.

In his capacity as journalist, Laennec was called upon to review the work of well-placed professors of France and other countries. Former teachers and superiors could not be blamed if at times they found their protégé to be a bit insufferable. His review of an article by Garnier, first surgeon to the king of Westphalia, ended with the promise that he "did not intend to attack a man to whom surgery owes so much," a pronouncement considerably weakened by the modifying platitude: "*errare humanum est.*"[34] The 1806 *Mémoires* of the elite Société d'Emulation, of which he was not a member, were "perhaps inferior," he said, to the previous collections, and he criticized their style.[35] But when Laennec, future inventor of the stethoscope, reviewed Corvisart's translation of Auenbrugger on percussion, the Emperor's doctor got off with only a light rebuke for his anticlassicism. Corvisart had "entirely rejected the doctrine of the ancients," said Laennec, and he hinted that the "motives" for doing so had been political rather than clinical. His former teacher should remember that Hippocrates had described the succussion sound first and that the ancient doctrine of critical days had yet to be proven wrong. Nevertheless, Corvisart deserved the high esteem of his former students, he wrote, because his "rare tact," "perspicacity," and "continuing observations" allowed him to make "astonishingly certain diagnoses" of the mysterious "thoracic viscera . . . enclosed in a sort of osseous cage."[36]

Laennec had expected six hundred francs a year from his collaboration on Corvisart's *Journal*, but he was rarely paid the full amount, and sometimes he was not paid at all.[37] Reviewing books limited his time for research, but he managed to publish a few of his own essays, articles, and reports for the Société de l'Ecole. Among these can be found an unusual and possibly original case of compression of the thoracic duct by an aortic aneurysm;[38] the presentation of the new pathological lesion common to several different organs, which he called "melanosis";[39] and a detailed analysis of the doctrine of Franz-Joseph Gall (1758–1828).[40]

The last-named publication was a lengthy three-part assessment of the system of Gall as described by four French language works on the topic.

Gall's ideas, like those of the Scottish physician John Brown (1735–1788), the German physician Franz-Anton Mesmer (1734–1815), and Prost, were not to be trusted, said Laennec; reductionist theories were "seductive" because they promised to "facilitate the work" needed to learn a science. His special interest in Gall seems to have stemmed from its popularity, its originality as an exercise in classification of the metaphysical "organs," and the criticisms made by others of its intrinsic materialism. He concluded that Gall's theory might have detrimental effects on society if the courts were to recognize the concept of involuntary homicide. He also wondered how one could conceive of a God, if one accepted the idea of a *don fatal.* But he did not think that Gall could be labeled a "materialist," because he neither attacked nor excluded the "spirituality of the soul." These comments suggest that Laennec may have been inspired to conduct the analysis for a meeting of the Congrégation. Later, he welcomed the publication of yet another work on the doctrine of skull, "one of which Dr. Gall could not complain," since it was "the most methodical and complete" that had ever been published on craniomancy, "whatever one might think" of the practice.[41] Disapproval of a theory did not obviate knowing about it.

Similarly, when Brown's work appeared in French, Laennec said that his "friend" R. J. Bertin (1757–1827) had rendered a great service in translating and incidentally improving upon the "barbaric" Latin of Brown, because the system that tilted against "pretended errors that have never existed" could now be understood in order to be combated and refuted.[42] Refutation loomed large in his immediate and distant future.

PATHOLOGICAL ANATOMY AND THE DISPUTE WITH DUPUYTREN

The most important of Laennec's many articles that appeared in the few years following his graduation was his "Note on Pathological Anatomy," read at the Société de l'Ecole on 28 December 1804 and published in early 1805.[43] The reasons for its importance are twofold: first, it heralded and summarized the structure of his unpublished treatise on pathological anatomy; second, it was itself a "discovery"—a declaration of a classification, a not-to-be-trusted-but-inevitably-necessary theory, a systematic approach to the new science. Laennec tried to move beyond the regional- and organ-based approach of Bonet and Morgagni, and beyond the tissue-systems approach of Bichat, all of whom tended to follow an order dictated by the method of dissection. Laennec would build a classification of organic lesions that incorporated and respected the results of his predecessors.[44] With little modification, he would use the same classification in 1812 and again in 1822. He would eventually construct part, but definitely not all, of his conception of disease on this basis of this theory (see table 3.2).

The jewel in the crown of the classification was the idea of "accidental production," a term he had coined to account for tissues that he thought of

TABLE 3.2
Laennec's Classification of Anatomical Lesions, 1804–1826

Alteration	Type	Examples
Nutrition	Hypertrophy	
	Atrophy	
Form and position	Luxations	
	Hernias	
Texture	Dissolution	
	Accumulation/extravasation of fluid	
	Inflammation and sequelae (transferred here 1812)	
	Accidental productions:	Analogous
		Ossifications
		Fibrous tissue
		Serous membranes
		Erectile tissue
		Vascular tissue
		Lymphatic tissue
		Hairy tissue
		Horny tissue
		Fatty tissue
		Transformations
		Nonanalogous
		Tubercles
		Inflammation (only 1804)
		Degenerations (only 1804)
	(After 1804 the items below each form a separate type)	
	Scirrhus	
	Colloid	
	Gelatinous/gumma	
	Squamous	
	Encephaloid	
	Melanosis	
	Cirrhosis	
	Sclerosis	

Sources: Laennec, "Note sur l'anatomie pathologique," 1804; "Anatomie pathologique," 1812; "Traité d'anatomie pathologique," 1804–1808, BIUM, MS 2186 (III a,b,c) and ML, MS Cl. 7 lot a; Lessons at the Collège de France, 1822–1826, BIUM, MS 2186 (IV) and ML, MS Cl. 2 lot a (A) and (B).

as newly arisen without obvious cause. He subdivided the group into "analo-gous" productions (comprised of tissues found in the healthy body) and "nonanalogous" productions (comprised of extraordinary tissue). The class loosely corresponds to the current term, "neoplasm" (meaning new forma-tion or growth), which is equally without implications concerning physio-logical origin; and the subdivisions, to "benign" and "malignant." In the subgroup of nonanalogous accidental productions, Laennec situated the "tubercle" together with cirrhosis, sclerosis, inflammation, and what are now thought of as various types of cancer, *encephaloïdes*, *melanoses*, and *squirrhe*. The advantage of the category came from the ingenious manner in which it neatly separated pathological anatomy from pathological physiology: "acci-dental production" implied nothing about the process by which lesions formed; it simply described them.

Understanding this category is essential to understanding Laennec's pa-thology, both to appreciate the competitive atmosphere surrounding the cutting-edge research, and to comprehend his later disputes with Broussais. For Laennec, all organic lesions arose from physiological processes; inflam-mation was a structural entity, separate from all other pathological lesions, tubercles and cancers included. His pride in the creation of this classification was evident, and he claimed priority in a footnote heavy with irony. It pleased him, he said, to see that Dupuytren had also recommended the same classifi-cation in an article published in the previous issue of the *Bulletin de la Société de l'Ecole*; "this conformity in the way of seeing things seems to me to argue in favor of the classification." But, he "could prove" that it was his idea, that he had presented it first, and that it had formed the basis of his teaching early in An XII (1803–1804).[45]

Dupuytren responded to the footnoted insinuation by immediately accus-ing Laennec of plagiarism. If the classification and the concept of accidental productions had been stolen, Laennec, not Dupuytren, was the culprit. He claimed that he had taught the classification in his classes of An X (1801–1802), which Laennec had attended and for which he had written a letter of thanks. He had continued using it the following year when Laennec, Fizeau, and Bayle were his assistants. His priority was proven in that he had pub-lished a month before Laennec. Referring to Laennec's criticisms of Bichat (and perhaps obliquely to Buisson's, too), Dupuytren said that there had been a "motive" that everyone would recognize in Laennec's apparent "af-fection" for the dead genius—this from Dupuytren who, on hearing about the tragic end of Bichat, is said to have exclaimed, "Now I can finally breathe!"[46]

Laennec replied. He did not doubt the influence of teachers: long before Dupuytren, there had been his instructors in Nantes. Indeed, he had been present for the course in An X, which is how he knew that Dupuytren had never presented such a classification. Underlining inconsistencies in his op-ponent's argument, he gave the sequence of events from his perspective, supporting not only his claim to priority, but also the suggestion that Dupuytren had stolen from the former student. He demanded a public opening of Dupuytren's course notes, now in the hands of Hallé, and said that he would not speak on the subject again, even if attacked.[47] This response clarified the unarticulated reasons why he had stopped working with Dupuytren and had rushed his article to press.

Dupuytren counterattacked, and the editors of the *Journal* invoked closure on the ugly dispute; their periodical would not become a forum for polemic between valued colleagues.[48] Maulitz has shown that there may have been differences in their approaches to the new sciences, the one pragmatic, the other theoretical.[49] Laennec's biographers have used the debate to highlight the clarity, wisdom, restraint, and justification of his arguments; however, they fail to point out that the first printed accusation had been made by Laennec, whether or not he had been the injured party. He had already shown himself to be utterly unwilling to have his creations expropriated, and he would never shrink from a fight.

In the end, it was a dubious honor that the two men had contested; the concept of "accidental production" was soon challenged, then forgotten. As early as 1826, vigorous objections arose to the category because it was thought to incorporate too many different changes. Imbued with a "physiological" orientation, contemporaries complained that it revealed nothing about the origin of lesions, the very advantage that had made it seem useful to its originator(s?).[50] By the late century, Laennec was said to have been "dazzled" (Trousseau) by his "erroneous theory" (Hanot).[51] Laennec always distinguished between classifications pertaining to pathology and those pertaining to physiology, but his expertise in the former did not preclude an interest in the latter; an understanding of both was essential for a comprehensive approach to disease.

In the wake of the public dispute, Laennec continued to serve as vice-president of the Société Anatomique with Dupuytren at the helm, but their enmity eventually poisoned what had been a flourishing enterprise. Within a year of its founding in December 1803, the Société Anatomique had grown from seventy members to nearly two hundred, and applications had to be limited to those with an inside advocate. In the first three and a half years, more than 356 lectures had been read at the weekly meetings. In September 1805, a few months after the quarrel with Laennec, Dupuytren stepped down as president; three others shared the task over the next eighteen months, but a malaise crept over the group. From mid-1806, sessions were held infrequently and irregularly; the original six rules, which had sufficed for nearly three years, were increased to twenty in October, and to forty by the next July. On 5 August 1807, Laennec became president of the Société Anatomique. It seems to have been a sort of coup d'état, a last ditch attempt to rescue the society. The minutes show that he reviewed the principal goals: the study of anatomy, physiology, and pathological anatomy. A "few abuses" had taken place, he said, but from that moment on, he proposed that priority be given to "facts and questions" of anatomy and physiology.[52] Perhaps he was referring to the actions of Dupuytren, who was known to have marshaled students into the service of his treatise of pathological anatomy by having them collect pathological lesions from all cadavers dissected in the Ecole Pratique.

At the opening session of the following year on 29 December 1808, Laennec gave another speech, the manuscript of which has been preserved. There had been a "longer than usual interruption" of five months brought on by "particular circumstances," he said, and he repeated the purposes of the Société. It was not a scholarly venue for the presentation of original discoveries and the advancement of careers; it was, as it had always been, a company of students and physicians who wanted to perfect their skills in anatomical science. Sessions should center on the presentation of a clinical history followed by the autopsy findings. A subject did not have to be a complete novelty in order to be worthy of presentation and discussion. The works of Morgagni, Walter, and Bichat were "closed books for anyone who had not seen enough to have learned how to read them . . . To open cadavers, observe, repeat observations, and communicate them to colleagues was the only way to grasp pathological anatomy." This "new science could bring a precision and certainty to diagnosis that can sometimes astonish those doctors who find it more convenient to mistrust anatomy than to study it." He hoped many students would join.[53] Immediately following this speech, and as if to support the principles enunciated, François Magendie (1783–1855) presented an eye, in which the retina had been converted into a fibrous membrane, and he supervised a student in practicing an operation for cataract on a cadaver.[54]

But Laennec had seized command of a sinking ship. During the sessions that followed, attendance dwindled, meetings were held only twice a month, and the society dissolved on 20 April 1809. Dupuytren appears to have already abandoned the group and may have been making students aware that an association with Laennec might jeopardize one with himself. Laennec would attempt a revival in 1814, but with little success, and the Société Anatomique lay dormant until its reconstitution by Jean Cruveilhier (1791–1874) in January 1826; at that time, both Laennec and Dupuytren were invited to be honorary presidents.[55]

TREATISE OF PATHOLOGICAL ANATOMY: THE FIRST UNPUBLISHED BOOK

Laennec seems to have stopped teaching his course on pathological anatomy after its third round in 1805–1806, but the treatise continued to grow with an expected completion date of late 1806 (fig. 3.2). He and Bayle worked together and shared clinical cases related to their special interests. For example, as Bayle compiled his mémoire on swelling of the glottis, Laennec donated the 1805 case of unsuccessful laryngotomy on the medical student

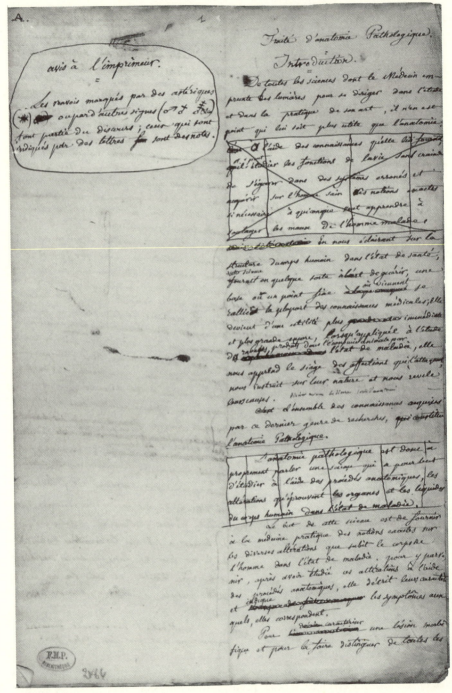

Figure 3.2. Title page of Laennec's unpublished treatise on pathological anatomy, 1804–1808. In the upper left, the author wrote instructions for the printer. Source: BIUM, MS 2186 (IIIa), 1r. Photograph: Bibliothèque Interuniversitaire de Médecine, Paris.

Signiolle, who died crying "in a choked voice that the [surgical] opening was not wide enough."[56] By June 1805, he told his father that the first volume of his own projected two-volume treatise was almost complete, but he still needed financial support: "It's a terrible thing, the novitiate of a scientific career."[57] He was referring not only to the lack of money, but to the atmosphere of his work, the agony of the dying patients, the minute attention to detail, the revolting stench of their bodies that had begun to putrefy long before they had died, especially in the summer when dissection classes had closed but research continued. "I live among the dead and the dying," he told his cousin, and he described the "scenes of death" that made up what he and his colleagues often called the "painful career" (*carrière pénible*).[58]

Dissecting brought the mortal danger of accidental finger-prick. In August 1804, Laennec explained to his father, "I am writing with my middle and ring fingers, since my index is bound up and covered with a cataplasm due to a scalpel stick." Eventually he would have "seven or eight personal experiences" with autopsy injuries, including the famous inoculation of a tubercle "sometime around 1806"; however, he reassured his father who had fretted about the danger, "no one cares about precautions more than I."[59] The father was encouraging. "Hurry up slowly," he said, "remember it is a basic book for medicine and for your reputation; but hurry . . . remember Dupuytren is there . . . and if he publishes before you do, he will accuse you of having stolen his work again."[60]

Part of Laennec's incomplete treatise of pathological anatomy has been preserved; it is the first of his two unpublished books.[61] Some have contended that it would have been the first French language treatise on pathological anatomy, predating those of Cruveilhier and Gabriel Andral (1797–1876), in 1816 and 1829 respectively.[62] But Laennec had no such illusions. He cited Xavier Bichat's *Anatomie générale* (An X [1801–1802]), which he "always assumed that [his] readers had read," because it was "one of the foundations of pathological anatomy."[63] Among his precursors, he also wrote of Portal's five-volume treatise, based on his Collège de France lessons, and of the collection of autopsies published by J. F. Lobstein of Strasbourg, which he had reviewed for the *Journal* in September 1805. But the lengthy article by Félix Vicq d'Azyr (1748–1794) for the *Encyclopédie méthodique* was "merely a compilation, lacking method, often lacking taste, and in every respect unworthy of the author's reputation, which otherwise was so well deserved." Laennec also mentioned at least two French translations of works that he recognized as having emerged from the tradition of Bonet and Morgagni: Portal's translation of the "mediocre" histories of Joseph Lieutaud; and a French translation of Matthew Baillie's *Morbid Anatomy*. But Morgagni's *De Sedibus* was the touchstone; it was better, he thought, than the four hundred autopsies in Albrecht von Haller's treatise, in which excellent observations had been marred by theoretical preoccupations.[64]

Laennec thought that the rise of pathological anatomy was perhaps one of the few benefits of the Revolution, and he said so, in his review of Lobstein, with the statement used as an epigraph at the beginning of this chapter.[65] His treatise opened with a philosophical preface that reflected his political and religious conservatism and contained some familiar criticisms of the tenets of the Paris school. Nature was "nothing more than the ensemble of connections (*rapports*) established by the Creator between Beings." Science, was "the ensemble of knowledge derived from comparison and methodical re-union of facts." "Positive facts," were important, of course; "consequences always flow from them." But science was "not simply the accumulation of facts, as some tried to pretend"; it always included a system to link the facts, "a methodical knowledge of principles." Laennec did not share the opinion of those who saw reasoning as a heresy, who would reject any form of classi-fication, who claimed to rely solely on quantity (numbers), who denied all physical truths unless they derived from the senses alone. He used the exam-ple of William Harvey's experiments to show that observations made on li-gated vessels did not, in themselves, constitute the theory of circulation; the theory came only when the observations were united with a form of reason-ing, deduction. To refuse to admit to the participation of mental operations in science was not "philosophical" it was merely "stupid." Although he did not say so, it was also anti-Buisson. Laennec's criticisms of the pretensions of early positivism bear a striking resemblance to those made more than a cen-tury later when positivism held full sway.[66]

In keeping with these ideals, his own book was not intended as a compen-dium and would not provide examples of every lesion (as it seems Dupuytren may have been trying to do). He was concerned more with approach and method and would give case observations, simply as a guide for future re-search. On the other hand, he would endeavor to provide references to orig-inal discoveries, because "there is nothing more interesting for researchers than the course of their own science."[67]

Having criticized the new positivistic trends of the Paris school, Laennec then praised and partly espoused them, by recalling the basic premises of Bayle's thesis. The purpose of the science of pathological anatomy was "to furnish practical medicine with exact notions about the diverse alterations that affected the human body in a state of disease," using the procedures of anatomy and clinical medicine. Nosology encompassed all that could be known about diseases; it could be examined from five perspectives: (1) the causes; (2) the organic alterations; (3) the disturbance in function; (4) the symptoms and their course; (5) the treatment. The last two perspectives al-ready formed the sciences of semiology and therapeutics. Therefore, three approaches remained to amplify nosology: etiological, anatomical, and symptomatic. Of these three, the anatomical method must be preferred because it alone relied on positive, objective, and observable facts. Since an-tiquity, the best understood diseases were those, like pneumonia, that were named and identified by their organic changes.

The etiological and symptomatic methods should not be "banished," Laennec said, but they should remain only as supplementary, because they were too theoretical, too variable, or too subjective to be verified. He criticized nosological nomenclatures like Pinel's, which were based on symptoms: "What uncertainty . . . reigns in distinctions and denominations of diseases for which the names are drawn from the nature of symptoms! Has anyone ever been able to assign a precise distinction between the soporific disorders, such as coma, cataphora, and coma-vigil? Has one ever been able to identify the precise point that separates asthma from dyspnea, orthopnea, and angina of the chest?"[68]

Pathological anatomy sometimes had recourse to chemistry, especially when it came to identifying aspects of altered parts. He cited the effects of heating an enlarged liver and of immersing a "white degeneration" in acid to determine if it was albuminous or fatty. Although pathological anatomy contributed to nosology, pathological chemistry would contribute less to nosology and more to etiology and therapeutics; it should be developed as its own discipline to the advantage of medicine. Nevertheless, pathological anatomy ought not to be concerned only with solids, but also with body liquids: their quantity and quality, such as the chemical composition of saliva, urine, bile, and blood.[69]

Knowledge of physiology and normal anatomy were essential for a good pathologist. Through physiology the clinician would learn that in addition to solids and liquids the body contains a nervous influence, a "vital principle," that could also be altered to constitute a cause of organic change. If a person suffered from shortness of breath and no signs could be found of heart disease, phthisis, or any other disease of the chest organs, then one must conclude that the disease was due to a "lesion of the vital principle," a real disease that could not be elucidated by dissection.[70] The altered vital principle could make a person sick, but it could also heal: Laennec said that miraculous cures of serious organic disorders may have been effected through the same mechanism. He then reviewed the history of pathological anatomy, taking up again the thorny questions of whether or not the Egyptians, Hippocrates, and Aristotle had performed human autopsies. He closed the preface by situating his work as a new approach to an old discipline.[71] This conception of the physiological cause and nature of disease would be elaborated in his later work on auscultation and disease.

Laennec's letters suggest that he worked with Bayle, but the introduction was written in the first person singular, an unusual choice in French even for a solitary author. He may have continued to revise the introduction long after Bayle's death, since he still spoke of completing the treatise after 1819.[72] In any case, the ideas expressed in the unpublished treatise bear a strong resemblance to Bayle's, especially those about pathological anatomy and the physiological "vital lesion."[73] Some historians have quite reasonably suggested that they originated with Bayle: debunking Laennec's contributions to the pathological anatomy of tuberculosis, Roselyne Rey asked, "What was left for Laennec to find that could not already be found in Bayle?"[74] But Laennec rolled priority back further, to Abraham Kaau Boerhaave (d. 1758) and Hippocrates.[75]

Prominent in Laennec's teaching notes, but not in the treatise, was a discussion of what he described as the four-part method of doing pathological anatomy: dissecting a cadaver, judging among the findings, writing reports, and preparing specimens. For the order of dissection, Laennec preferred Morgagni's method (head, thorax, abdomen) over Bichat's (start with the body region indicated by the symptoms). In judging the significant from the insignificant, he reminded his students that a knowledge of general anatomy—normal structure, color, and texture—was essential. The pathological anatomist must also understand how to distinguish between the physiological effects of three modes of death (brain, heart, lung). This observation was "not the discovery of Bichat," as many claimed, but had been recognized "with clarity" since at least the time of Galen. Reports should follow a rigorous order in simple language, from the general to the specific, and the attentive student must never use a word that he does not completely comprehend. He gave a brief summary of the advantages and disadvantages of various substances used in preparing specimens for demonstration and preservation.[76]

After the introduction, the treatise proceeded in chapters devoted to various types of lesions, beginning with alterations in texture and working through the rest of his classification. Each chapter followed a specific order: general description, with references to the original observations. The extant material covers only the "analogous" and some of the "nonanalogous" accidental productions. Laennec believed himself to be the discoverer of four new types in the latter category: melanosis, cirrhosis, encephaloid matter, and sclerosis.[77] They were supported by cases from his earliest experiences in Nantes or Paris, several of which had been collected during summer research. The anatomical "discoveries" were "made" by the recognition of unusual findings, and "confirmed" by failure to find previous references to similar lesions in the literature (see table 3.3).

In time, Laennec managed to publish most of what he considered to be his discoveries; only his "discovery" of "sclerosis" seems not to have appeared in print. An essay on melanosis was read at the Société de l'Ecole in January 1806, and excerpts were published in the *Bulletin*. The chapter on "encephaloid" or "cerebriform (medullary)" cancer, which now appears to correspond roughly to "adenocarcinoma," was revised and published an 1815 volume of *Dictionnaire des sciences médicales*.[78] The chapter on cirrhosis received international attention.

Laennec's cirrhosis was an accidental production, which he mistakenly believed that he had been first to recognize; it had been described earlier by English writers.[79] He did, however, coin the name for the lesion, a derivative of the Greek word χιρρός meaning "tawny colored," which refers to the characteristic color of a cirrhotic liver (fig. 3.3). His prototypical observation was the history of Françoise Cuvi, a thirty-nine-year-old servant who had died at the Cochin hospital in the summer of 1804.[80] Drinking habits were not mentioned in her case or any other case diagnosed cirrhosis by Laennec,

TABLE 3.3

Laennec's Treatise of Pathological Anatomy, ca. 1803–1808: Structure and Cases

Analogous accidental productions
  Ossification
    Case: male, Bataille, Charité, summer 1803, BIUM, MS 2186 (IIIa), f. 42r
  Cartilages
    Case: female, a lady, patient of Dr. G. Laennec, Nantes, ML, Cl. 7a, 2r
  Fibrous
    Case: female, 48 yr, Charité, summer 1802, ML, Cl. 7a, f. 14–18
    Case: male, Charité, patient of Bayle, ML, Cl. 7a, f. 26r–v
  Serous membranes
    Case: female, 26 yr, actress, ML, Cl. 7a, f. 48r–v
    Case: female, Chevalier, summer 1803, ML, Cl. 7a, 51–53
  Mucous membranes
    Case: male, summer 1803, ML, Cl. 7a, f. 69–70
  Synovial membranes
    Case: male, elderly, Charité, winter 1803–1804, ML, Cl. 7a, f. 73v
  Cellular membranes (adhesions)
    Case: female, 37 yr, Cochin, autumn 1803, ML, Cl. 7a, f. 97
  Horny tissue
  Hairy tissue
  Tissues with analogies to the above
Nonanalogous accidental productions
  I. Melanosis
    Case: male, Hasenfrat, tailor, Charité, summer 1803, ML, Cl. 7a, f. 132–135
  II. Tawny degenerations, cirrhosis
    Case: female, Cuvi, 39 yr, servant, summer 1804, ML, Cl. 7a, f. 143v
  III. Encephaloides
    Case: male, 35 yr, mason, Charité, spring 1804, ML, Cl. 7a, f. 153r
    Case: female, Filiault, 40 yr, Cochin, summer year?, ML, Cl. 7a, f. 160r–v
    Case: male, 72 yr, saddler, Cochin, summer 1804, ML, Cl. 7a, f. 165r–v

Source: Laennec, "Traité d'anatomie pathologique," ca. 1804–1808, BIUM, MS 2168 (III, a,b,c) and ML, MS Cl. 7 lot a.

including that of Jean Edmé, which he would publish in his 1819 treatise.[81] This chapter was later published in French, in both France and England, and Laennec's former student Robert Carswell (1793–1857) gave pride of place to his special interest in the condition in his atlas of pathological anatomy.[82] In English, Laennec's name has been affixed eponymically to alcoholic liver cirrhosis, but in France his etymological interest in liver disease is virtually unknown. The result is a strange pattern of veneration: a French chest physician is remembered by anglophones for a lesion of the liver that had already been described in Britain. Not only was greater attention given to Laennec's cirrhosis in English literature, but in France, his connection to cirrhosis was suppressed through a concerted effort to combat his "theoretical" and "systematic" ideas, among which could be included the concept

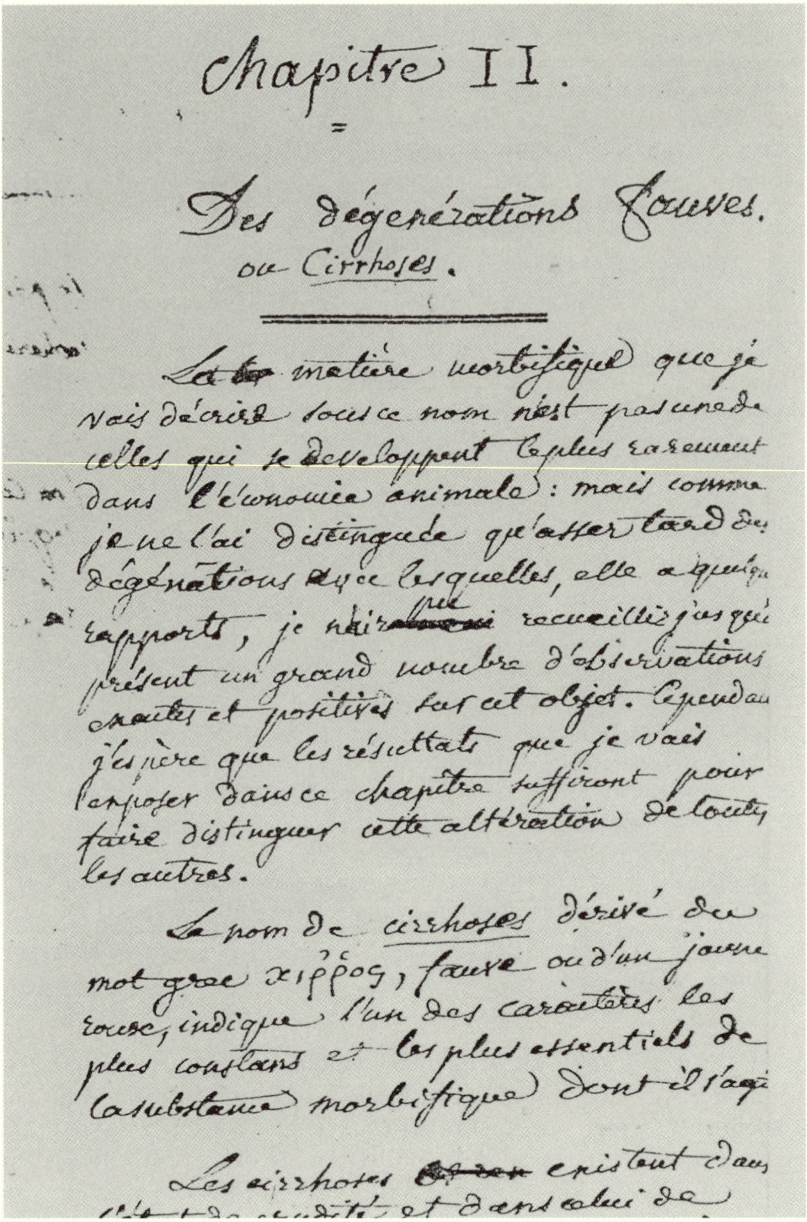

Chapitre II.

Des dégénérations rousses.
ou Cirrhoses.

La matière morbifique que je vais décrire sous ce nom n'est pas une de celles qui se developpent le plus rarement dans l'économie animale: mais comme je ne l'ai distinguée qu'assez tard des dégénérations avec lesquelles elle a quelques rapports, je n'ai pu recueillir jusqu'à présent un grand nombre d'observations exactes et positives sur cet objet. Cependant j'espère que les résultats que je vais exposer dans ce chapitre suffiront pour faire distinguer cette altération de toutes les autres.

Le nom de cirrhoses dérivé du mot grec κιρρος, fauve ou d'un jaune roux, indique l'un des caractères les plus constans et les plus essentiels de la substance morbifique dont il s'agit.

Les cirrhoses existent dans

Figure 3.3. First page of Laennec's chapter on cirrhosis from his unpublished treatise on pathological anatomy (detail). His derivation of the word "cirrhosis" from Greek is explained in the second paragraph. Laennec's name was eponymically affixed to alcoholic liver cirrhosis after this manuscript chapter was published in Britain. Source: Musée Laennec, MS Cl. 7, Cahier VV, f. 140r. Photograph: Queen's Medical Photography Services from ML photocopy.

of "accidental production."[83] When the movement crushed the general theory, it also eradicated the specific example. Only J. M. Charcot (1825–1893), participating in the late-century surge of nationalistic sentiment, tried to revive French interest in Laennec's role in cirrhosis; unaware of the chapter on cirrhosis, however, he set eponym-hunters on the wrong track by citing the case of Edmé.[84]

The manuscript treatise contains nothing on the other categories of nutrition, form, and position, and there is a significant absence of material on tubercles or inflammation. Laennec's early thoughts about these conditions, however, can be derived from the more complete notes for his course, from the student notebook, and from those copied (and presumably revised) by his cousin, Mériadec, for a posthumous edition of the treatise that never appeared. The ideas about tubercles and inflammation are discussed in chapters 7 and 12.[85]

THE CHAIR OF HIPPOCRATIC MEDICINE AND RARE DISEASES

When a professor died, a domino effect worked its way down through the ranks from the vacated position, as young scholars vied for new opportunities. Dupuytren's career made leaps forward with the deaths of the anatomist, Honoré Fragonard (1732–1799) and of the surgeon, Sabatier, but not without considerable lobbying in the intervals, lobbying that extended to his mother's writing directly to Napoleon.[86] After the death of the surgeon Lassus in early 1807, Laennec's hopes for an academic appointment were raised. Expecting that Dupuytren would become professor of surgery, he prepared to fill the resulting vacancy as chief of anatomical studies. But this time, Dupuytren was passed over, and the thwarted Laennec pretended not to have wanted the position anyway, because it would interfere with his clinical practice.[87]

Michel Thouret died on 19 June 1810, having given no lectures during the fifteen years he held the chair of Hippocratic medicine and rare diseases. No position could be better suited for Laennec, but at first he thought that the chair would be abolished. To his surprise, the *Grand maître* of the University allowed it to continue, and a competition was announced. Laennec expressed his reasons for hope to his uncle: he could claim to be an expert in new and rare diseases through his accomplishments in pathological anatomy; as for ancient medicine, his thesis had been on Hippocrates and he had been studying ancient texts for three years. He was prepared, he said, for a test in which he might be expected to translate a Hippocratic text from Greek without the help of a dictionary.[88] Laennec's knowledge of the classics was evident to all who read the reviews in Corvisart's *Journal*, where he did not hesitate to cite ancient writers, argue over etymology, or criticize a translation.[89] The monetary security would be welcome, but he was also committed to the possibility of reviving the long neglected teaching.

Laennec's manuscripts contain four sets of papers that may be products of his preparation for the anticipated competition: parts of a Latin essay on angina pectoris and three collections concerning ancient authors. The Latin essay on angina was read at the Société de l'Ecole in December 1810 and is discussed in chapter 8, but the timing of his decision to speak in Latin suggests that it was part of his bid for the vacated chair. The first collection, entitled *Cours sur la doctrine d'Hippocrate*, consists of forty pages of fragments, ideas and citations, including an analysis of the first five cases of the treatise, *Epidemics I*, in response to the writings of Henry Cope, who had tried to prove the utility of Hippocratic signs. It may represent the plan of the first course he hoped to teach in 1811.[90]

The second collection is a French translation of a Greek-Latin edition of the first three books of Aretaeus, *The Causes and Signs of the Acute and Chronic Diseases*.[91] The writings of Aretaeus are considered to be among the earliest medical texts that relate disease to anatomic change, and the particular selection reflects a preoccupation with physical signs of disease. In a passage on syncope with signs of a heart ailment—Laennec translated a line as "the beats of the heart change into palpitations."[92] This passage led the medical classicist Francis Adams (1796–1861) to think that Aretaeus had anticipated cardiac auscultation, and he claimed that Laennec's admiration for Aretaeus and Hippocrates derived from similarities in their diagnostic approach.[93] Laennec would return to Aretaeus and other ancient authors in his lessons at the Collège de France and in his 1826 discussion of phthisis.[94]

The third collection is an incomplete French translation from the Latin books of Caelius Aurelianus (fifth century A.D.) *On Acute and Chronic Diseases*, itself a translation from the lost Greek text of Soranus of Ephesus (first to second century A.D.).[95] Caelius Aurelianus and Soranus were members of the "Methodist school" of physicians who linked diseases to the textural state of tissues. According to Fernand Robert, Laennec used the presence of "Methodist" ideas as evidence that a text was not Hippocratic.[96] Again, the choice of text may have been significant, because of its preoccupation with fevers and the nosological problems they posed. Fevers were difficult to reconcile with the anatomoclinical method, as Bayle and Fizeau, among others, had already shown. Foucault suggested that it was the problem of fever that led the Société d'Emulation to announce its 1809 essay competition on responses to the question, "What are the diseases that can be considered specifically as organic?"[97] Perhaps it was the additional challenge of this question, in conjunction with the job competition, that prompted Laennec to reconcile his own ideas concerning fever, first expressed in his thesis, with those in the ancient texts—a reconciliation that would culminate in his 1821 essay, "Fevers according to the Doctrine of Hippocrates and the Findings of Pathological Anatomy."[98]

After a year of deliberations, however, the Faculty decided to abolish the chair late in the summer of 1811. Some historians have contended that, given an opportunity, Laennec would have obtained the position easily. But he had serious opposition from the chevalier François-Christophe-Florimond de Mercy (1775–1849), who had already obtained permission from Thouret to open a private course in Greek medicine and had been lobbying the Faculty with letters and presentations of his work. De Mercy enjoyed the protection of Chaussier, the professor of anatomy and physiology and a noted hellenist, and a decade later after the Restoration, he was still striving to persuade the faculty to revive the chair.[99] His translations have been criticized by Emile Littré (1801–1881) and by Charles Daremberg (1817–1872),[100] but at least one of his editions enjoyed the approval of a commission of the Société de l'Ecole de Médecine, comprised of Chaussier, Hallé, and Laennec. They examined his *Conspectus Febrium*, in which he tried to elucidate the problem of fever by applying modern diagnostics to the ancient clinical histories in the Hippocratic treatises, *Epidemics I* and *III*. So impressed was Laennec with the initiative that he recommended de Mercy for corresponding membership in the Société.[101] A single remark in a letter suggests that they may have been friends.[102]

The energetic pursuit of the chair of Hippocratic medicine left Laennec with a collection of citations in Greek and Latin on a wide variety of topics including semiology, therapeutics, nosology, and specific diseases with references to at least thirty-five different ancient authors. Hippocrates was cited more frequently than all other authors with the exception of Morgagni.[103] Laennec's preoccupation with an ancient-modern dialogue has been noticed by Jackie Pigeaud, who described Laennec's Hippocrates as having been philologically "open with blurred contours," and by Ackerknecht, who said that it had become "almost impossible to develop the proper empathy for Laennec's faith in an eternal science of medicine, immutable and known in most of its aspects."[104] Laennec sought more than a benediction for his style of observation; he wanted to inform his research into the fundamental questions of nosology with ancient clinical experience, reexamined in the light of pathological anatomy. This goal is exemplified by his admiration for the works of de Mercy, Cope, Jean-François Aubry (d. 1795), John Barker (1708–1748), and Anne-Charles Lorry (1726–1783).[105]

With the abolition of Thouret's chair in 1811, Laennec relinquished all aspirations for an official place in academic medicine. He had virtually abandoned the *Journal* by 1808, and the Société Anatomique had died under his leadership. The pace of his discoveries and communications slowed, although he continued to attend the meetings of the Société de l'Ecole and, prompted by several friends, he was dragged out of relative retirement to contribute to an ambitious new *Dictionnaire des sciences médicales*. For this project, a team of writers produced sixty volumes of state-of-the-art definitions between 1812 and 1822. They were whipped along by Charles-Louis-Fleury Panckoucke (1780–1844), whom Laennec jokingly described an "evil spirit" and "son of the man who had been ruined by the *Encyclopédie*." He predicted that the work would consume all his free time and bankrupt the publisher; however, his contributions derived entirely from his earlier writings in dissection and parasitology.[106] It is a measure of Laennec's reputation that he was selected over Dupuytren or other academic contenders to write the entry on pathological anatomy, a recapitulation of the 1804 article that had so angered his rival.

Laennec had established himself as an expert in the new science of pathological anatomy, conscious of both its potential and its limitations. This accomplishment was the tedious but essential groundwork—the preparation of his mind—for his future discovery and the direction in which he would choose to apply it. But Laennec was not well, and pathological anatomy was an all-consuming science, he said, befitting only the energies of healthy young men with few obligations.[107] In abandoning what seemed to be a hopeless academic pursuit, he could enjoy the healthier activities of hunting and hiking. Secure in the quality of his achievements and confident in his knowledge of both past and future trends in medicine, he decided to devote himself to his clinical practice, which had been growing steadily since 1805 and might finally bring an end to the ongoing financial difficulties. His experience as a clinician would consolidate his belief in the limitations of pathological anatomy and underscore the importance of physiology in disease.

Clinical Practice, Clinical Physiology

The present age can be seen as an epoch distinguished
for physiology.

—*Laennec on Buisson, 1802f, 169*

For every illness, the patient has his story [or romance].

—*Veron, 1853–1855,* 1:120

OVER THE COURSE of his career, Laennec worked in private practice, in public hospitals, in teaching clinics, and as a volunteer in both urban and rural
environments. As a result, most of the contemporary "styles" of medical
practice, as described by Jacques Léonard, from the country doctor to the
grand patron, can be found in the career of this one physician.[1] His own
health was precarious, but he discovered the restorative benefits of regular
exercise, physical rest, and psychic diversion. Personal illness and the stories
of his patients reminded him that pathological anatomy could not explain all
diseases. These experiences brought him face to face with a clinical physiology that recognized the influence of the psyche on the soma. He extended
this realization from individuals to the collective, believing that the health of
the body politic was a function of the mind politic. Just as the characteristics
of certain diseases have been shown to affect the explanations constructed to
account for them, the tales of sickness and recovery in himself, in others, and
in society, shaped and were consistent with the grand theory about all diseases that he would elaborate at the end of his life.[2]

PATIENTS IN THE FAMILY: THE PSYCHIC CURE

Laennec did not set out to become a clinician, but his practice grew steadily
while he conducted his early research and publishing; he relished the atten-
tions of a certain political and religious subset of society, and after 1808,
patients were his main source of income (see Appendix B). His postgraduate
existence was well documented in the letters of his cousins, Christophe
(1785–1858), Ambroise (1790–1839), Mériadec (1797–1873), and Em-

manuel (1802–1879), the sons of Guillaume Laennec. One after another they came to Paris to complete their education and live with or near Laennec: Christophe and Emmanuel studied law; Ambroise and Mériadec chose medicine. Laennec was eager to accommodate them, viewing it as an opportunity to contribute to the debt that he "would never be able to repay."[3] Their letters reminding Guillaume of their monetary needs incidentally describe Laennec's evolution from scholar to practitioner.

Guillaume was more reliable in his financial support than his brother or his own father had been: when Ambroise complained that he had not provided enough for Mériadec, the father responded that his sons were right "to scold" and increased the pension.[4] But he, too, had difficulty in sustaining the Parisian studies of four young men. In 1808, new laws concerning the Imperial University of France allowed the reopening of the long-closed faculty of medicine at Nantes. Guillaume was restored to his professorship and began teaching medical therapeutics. The detailed notes of his revived course in *materia medica* covered many authors and a wide variety of therapies including botanicals, metals, electricity, and galvanism.[5] The academic change eased his financial situation, and Laennec made sure that a brief notice describing the "easy and brilliant elocution" of his uncle's inaugural speech appeared in Paris.[6]

Only three years younger, Christophe was like a second brother to Laennec and would always be his closest confidant. He came to Paris in early 1804, just before his cousin's graduation, and witnessed his transformation from a scholar, immersed in teaching and research, to a busy practitioner with an illustrious clientele.[7] He helped his cousin move next door to the slightly larger apartment that had been vacated by Bayle, who had found a position at the Charité hospital and married Louise-Sophie Moutard-Martin, the sister of a medical colleague, in the summer of 1805.[8] With four rooms, moldings, and two mirrors, the second-floor apartment at 3 rue du Jardinet had a touch of class; Laennec made it his home for almost fifteen years.[9]

At the beginning of his stay, Christophe was impressed by Théophile's insouciance in living so near the financial edge and his facility in borrowing, talents keenly honed from years of insecurity. In a letter to his mother, he wrote that, despite "apparent disorder," his cousin had "quite a bit of finesse in the affair" of borrowing, which he does "admirably" and "with great science." When he had money, he would pay off the debts that "cried out the most loudly"; smaller ones did not trouble him.[10] The talent was turned on the observer, who was obliged to reach into his own pockets to pay the rent when the one father had reneged on his financial duty while the other had not.[11]

Laennec's first patients failed to enhance his coffers because they came from his family and included himself. When the cousins or his brother were sick, he gave them free, often unasked for advice; he also treated his stepmother through the mail at her request.[12] The cousins resented the medicines and thought that their doctor-relative was too much given to dosing and bleeding himself.[13] The whole family worried about his younger brother, Michaud.

Laennec maintained only a loose affiliation with Michaud, who had been working at the prefecture in Beauvais eighty kilometers north of Paris since early 1803. Physically alike, small and uncommonly gaunt, they seem to have had remarkably dissimilar personalities; yet, they bore each other a distant respect. Laennec described his brother as a man "who knew the price of money" and whose "defect" was to "push exactitude and orderliness to the point of rigor so that his desire to proceed correctly in affairs, made him seem hard in words."[14] Concerned as he was about Michaud's health, the young physician agonized more over his brother's cynicism and indifference to religion. He begged their father to inspire in Michaud a return toward faith: "The poor boy has great need of it," but "above all do not let him know that it comes from me for fear that he will be defiant."[15]

Michaud coughed blood in late January 1805 at the end of a long "cold." Laennec instructed him by letter, but did not trust the patient to follow his orders. When he received no news, he and Christophe assumed that the illness had resolved, but a mutual friend warned them of Michaud's deterioration. Laennec extracted money from his father for a visit to Beauvais; however, he seems to have had little actual inclination to see his sick brother and kept postponing the trip. Finally, Michaud came to Paris for a few days in August 1805 to work on a grammar textbook for the teachers in his department. Christophe reported that Michaud was even more sickly than his brother, and he refused to rest. Since Laennec had now seen Michaud, he decided that the journey to Beauvais was no longer necessary. Instead, he would spend the money on a vacation in the interests of his own health, professing mild regret that his brother would not join him.[16]

Laennec is known as one of the great invalids of tuberculosis history; at least two biographies have framed his existence as an example of the power of *spes phthisica* (the hopeful temperament of the consumptive).[17] References to his frail health were frequent in the letters; however, the exact nature of the various ailments that plagued his young adult life is obscure. There had been the high fever in 1798, and while at medical school, he had experienced one or two minor indispositions, a severe bump on the head in late 1803, as well as the seven or eight scalpel wounds that had worried his father.[18] He later said that by 1808 he had begun to suffer daily from "asthma," "hypochondria," and a "thousand nervous mishaps." Sometimes, he was so severely breathless that he could not tolerate the weight of his clothing and would have to strip to the waist in order to keep working at his desk.[19] In his late twenties, he claimed to have experienced the pains of angina pectoris; by age thirty-one he had written his will;[20] and before he was forty, he had suffered at least two attacks of gout and excruciating headaches with vertigo. The first attack of gout occurred in 1813 in the carriage en route to Couvrelles; the second in 1817. His uncle demanded to know how someone as active as his nephew could contract this "cruel disease of the lazy."[21] He was thin, he coughed, he often had palpitations and fever; his chronic feelings of weakness prevented him from rising early in the morning. But until much later in his life, this paragon of physical diagnosis firmly resisted all attempts to find tuberculosis in himself; and he may well have been right. His intensely personal experience with the restorative power of vacations offered existential evidence of the psychosomatic nature of his illness and its healing; he refused to believe that he had phthisis.

As Laennec completed his studies, he heard from his mother's cousin, Anne-Marie Audoyn de Cosquer de Pompéry (1762–1820). Cultivated, clever, devoutly Catholic, and expert in the eighteenth-century arts of conversation and letter-writing, Madame de Pompéry had been a popular hostess and owner of one of the two pianos in Quimper during the Revolution. Her letters from Finistère were published by an adoring grandson, who cast her as a latter-day Mme de Sévigné.[22] In 1804, her husband inherited a chateau at Couvrelles, in the region of Soissons, northeast of Paris; the family moved there with their three children in early summer 1805 (fig. 4.1). She professed a fear of loneliness, but contended that there would be better opportunities for her two sons closer to the capital. Placing herself at the center of a small enclave of displaced Bretons, she found support in two women: her friend, Mme de Laubrière, who owned a large manor at the nearby hamlet of Bruys; and her paid companion, the twenty-five-year-old widow of Pierre Argou (also spelled Argoult), Jacquemine Guichard (1779–1847). Many years later, Mme Argou would become the wife of doctor Laennec.

In September 1805, Laennec left his ailing brother to his own devices and went to visit his mother's newly transplanted relative. At Couvrelles, the concerts, parties, and charades continued as they had done in Quimper, but now they were interspersed with strolls in the orangerie, or walks by the reflecting lake, and hunting in the surrounding park. Mme de Pompéry was forty-three years old, but even at that age, historians say, "she had kept intact her wit and charm."[23] Laennec was smitten at first sight with his cousin and her world: "At the edge of a village . . . I saw a beautiful house ending in two pavilions, a vast courtyard surrounded by very tidy stables, sheds, and barns. The gothic bell tower of an old church rose above these buildings. Behind the chateau could be seen woods surrounded by walls." And of his hostess, he wrote to his father: "I will not tell you Madame de Pompéry is charming: you know her even better than I do. She has the head of a man and the heart of a woman. Her affinity for religion, her talents, her spirit, made me discover a sweetness in her company that I have not known since my exile in Paris where I have lived for the friendship of scholars and the commerce of books. We played music, toyed with proverbs, wrote verse . . . and sang motets in the parish church of Couvrelles. Charles [her oldest son] and I killed rabbits, partridges, hares, and quails."[24]

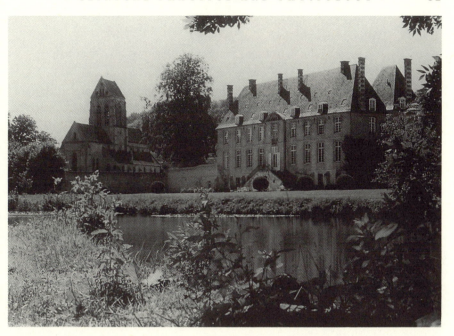

Figure 4.1. The chateau at Couvrelles near Soissons, formerly home of the de Pompéry family, where Laennec spent at least four long September holidays walking, hunting, playing music, and writing poetry. He associated these vacations with improved health. View from the park. Source and photograph: With permission of the present owner, the Centre International de Rencontres, DOSNAN.

The carefree warbling, writing, rhyming, and eating well were precisely to the father's taste, and Laennec treated him to minute descriptions of the plays and poems of Couvrelles. The three weeks in Soissonais had been his first holiday in four years and had replaced the remembered conversations in the political cafés of Nantes as the "happiest days of [his] life." He would vacation there again in the late summers of 1806, 1808, and 1813, and after each visit, returned to Paris "big and fat," and filled with a sort of romantic exaltation. He asked repeatedly for portraits of his parents to hang in his new apartment and for a lock of his mother's hair.[25] Since March 1805, he had been trying to "relearn" the Breton language; now it was a passion, encouraged by Madame de Pompéry and nourished by his father, who was charged with sending Breton grammars, dictionaries, songs, and bibles.[26] In early 1807, the medical flautist-poet was elected member of the Société de Belles Lettres of Soissons in recognition of his enthusiastic contributions to local culture. His passionate (but mediocre) "Canticle to False Philosophy" may have been written for a soirée with Madame de Pompéry: in medical metaphor, he expressed his disapproval of the political and religious sentiments in the postrevolutionary world:

Like the fatal wind that poisons the atmosphere
With the germ of destroying plagues,
The voice of the corruptor [Napoleon] has flown over the earth
And taken hold in every heart.[27]

Above all, Laennec's health had improved. With vigorous walking at Couvrelles, his asthma and gout disappeared, and his appetite improved, provoking a dramatic change in his physical well-being. He vowed to take a holiday every year, and would insist that his young cousins avoid the mistake that he had made of studying without interruption. "Less fortune, more health; now there's a precept that you will find just as philosophical as I find medical," he told his father.[28] He came to think that he needed six or seven hours of walking a day in order to avoid the nervous ailments that had become his bête noire. His fondness for hunting did not stem from a love of killing things, he explained, but from the fact that it was the "only activity sufficiently engaging to carry one far enough."[29] Some years later, when he could not leave the city, he would try to substitute hospital gardening for hunting, but decided that exercise of the arms was not as beneficial as that of the legs.[30] Long after Madame de Pompéry had left her beautiful chateau, Laennec would hunt in the rolling countryside of Soissonais in pursuit of a psychic cure for his bodily ills.[31]

Healing by intellectual stimulus, physical exertion, and inner contentment confirmed all that Laennec and Bayle would maintain about disease and the limitations of pathological anatomy for its explanation. The belief in psychosomatic causes and cures, through the mediation of an active life force, did not originate with them, nor was it merely a sophist solution to the inadequacies of their technology. W. R. Albury has shown that this ancient idea had been rejected by their teacher, Corvisart, who thought that the life force could be only palliative at best.[32] But for Bayle and Laennec, it was a physiological tenet for which they collected a mass of evidence from their own lives and those of others. Bayle would teach Laennec how to read his experience at Couvrelles (see below).

PATIENTS IN THE CITY

The lack of steady income from the *Journal* and the unwillingness or inability of his father to make regular contributions in support of his nonlucrative research forced Laennec to take his first paying patients in the summer of 1805. His clients came from a well-circumscribed circle that related to his origins and to his political and religious leanings. Christophe told his mother how he felt miserably outclassed in this milieu: "My dear cousin, . . . whom you know has a little grain of vanity, has launched himself uniquely in nobility. He introduces me as a musician and I have been politely received. But you must imagine the sad figure I make in the midst of German barons covered in cordons and crosses, Italian Monsignors, bishops, etc."[33]

The practice began slowly, but Christophe reported that an asthmatic man reliably paid four livres at each visit and another settled a bill for thirty-six livres.[34] By 1806, Laennec claimed that he was owed four hundred francs from his practice, and soon discovered that well-off patients could be the least reliable in meeting their medical debts.[35] In 1807, he broke his vow about annual holidays for fear of losing fiscal momentum: having already earned twelve hundred francs that year, he expected an equal amount more if he stayed in Paris. He expressed his regret to Christophe: "Unless someone else perpetrated more hostilities on them than I have done, the partridges of Soissons and the hares of Reims were left in tranquillity to roam the places where Julius Caesar, *Frédègonde*, and *Brunehaut* made so much noise and dust in bygone days, just like you and I."[36] He earned twenty-four hundred francs in 1807, close to thirty-six hundred in 1808, and by 1809 was able to engage his own cook and servant, because his stomach could no longer tolerate the food of the restaurateur and his patients found it "very disagreeable" to be received by the doorman. His cook, "*la bonne* Angélique," stayed for many years and the doctor called her his friend, but her reception of patients may have been no warmer than the doorman's. One visitor described her as "a sort of female Cerberus," who watched the doctor's door, which she would open "only at fixed hours," and who was indifferent to the plight of clients kept waiting in an austere oratory furnished with only a low chair and a crucifix.[37]

Christophe had to admit that his cousin was temperamentally unsuited for the intrigue required to launch the coveted academic career; he belonged in practice, and his patients loved him.[38] By late 1808, Laennec was consulting by letter for more than twenty different physicians in various towns of France; his Paris clientele included several well-known personalities, aristocrats, and clergymen, some directed his way through his connections in the church.[39]

PHYSICIAN TO THE CLERGY

Shortly after his religious conversion, Laennec befriended the young abbé and future archbishop of Paris, Quélen. The priest had been a student at the Saint Sulpice seminary, one of the spiritual homes of the Congrégation, but in 1806 he was sent to the Breton town of St. Brieuc. Recalling "many agreeable evenings together at the home of a lady of their common acquaintance," Laennec sent greetings to Quélen through his father, who was once again in St. Brieuc pursuing his wife's lost inheritance.[40] Given the entrée, the father did not hesitate to cultivate the abbé and seek his advice on his legal matters.[41] By 1807, Quélen was attached to the household of Napoleon's uncle, Cardinal Joseph Fesch (b. 1763) at the *Grand Aumonerie* in Paris.[42] Through Quélen's recommendation, Fesch appointed Laennec his "*premier médecin*," in the spring of 1809. Rouxeau claimed somewhat unconvincingly that Laennec had to overcome his "natural repugnance" to such situations in order to accept, but clearly he had no repugnance for the annual retainer of 3000 francs.[43] This salary compares favorably with the estimated annual income for rural practitioners of nine hundred francs.[44] There were some expenses: five hundred francs in outstanding fees for his education and seven hundred francs for essentials such as the *costume de cour, chapeau à claque*, and sword—official attire for the Cardinal's retinue. But the young doctor felt that his new title would enhance public confidence; judging by his subsequent rise in fortune, he seems to have been correct (see Appendix B).[45]

Fesch is said to have been difficult: he was preoccupied by the vagaries of his political fortune and insisted on daily medical visits, but he liked his doctor, gave him gifts—a bust of himself and a crucifix—and when he had to travel, allowed him the freedom to remain in Paris to look after sicker but less illustrious patients. Laennec was equally respectful: during his bid for the chair of Hippocratic medicine, he said, the Cardinal "is the best man in the world and the least exigent. Not even a place in the medical school would console me of the loss of such a patron, if circumstances force him to leave Paris definitively."[46] Laennec served Fesch for an initial three years until March 1812, when the Cardinal fell into disgrace with his Emperor-nephew for opposing (with Quélen) Napoleon's plan to place himself at the head of a national church. Laennec returned to Fesch's entourage for a few months in 1814 before the cardinal left Paris for Rome in 1815.

The early connection with high-placed clergy made Laennec a doctor of choice for ailing men of the cloth. A file entitled, "Consultations of the Cardinals," contains the case histories and autopsy reports of Cardinal Eriskin (d. 1809) and of Cardinal Vincenti (d. 1811). Eriskin, who had been in good health except for "two or three attacks of urinary retention" died at 70 with sudden hemiplegia, but his autopsy concentrated on the changes in his bladder. Vincenti died at 75 of pneumonia, which Laennec had treated with bleeding.[47] Another seventeen-page report, in Latin and dated "The Ides of March," 1810, describes the sickness and treatment of sixty-six-year-old Cardinal "X", possibly Monsignor Fabrizzio Ruffo, who fell ill of angina while visiting France.[48] Rouxeau contended that the Latin consultation was written for the cardinal's doctors back in Italy; but its learned discussion of the various theories of angina pectoris probably formed part of Laennec's Latin essay, read at the Société de l'Ecole de Médecine in 1810 (see chaps. 3 and 8).[49]

For at least ten years, Laennec served a strict religious community of women in Paris as consultant physician, and his observations on the effect of stress on the development of phthisis would form part of his treatise on auscultation.[50] During or before 1814, Laennec also attended a fellow Breton from Saint-Malo, Félicité de Lamennais. This liberal philosopher-priest attempted to reconcile church and throne, and when the project failed, he tried to cultivate a bond between the church and the people, independent of the state. He may have chosen Laennec as his physician because of his openly avowed religious and royalist leanings, but later it appears that he preferred Fizeau. Laennec, he said, was "overly stern and expensive" and smitten with "certain systematic ideas," in spite of being an "excellent clinician," with "strong principles, and remarkable spirit."[51] What exactly Lamennais meant by "systematic ideas" is not clear. It may have been Laennec's use of the stethoscope, which some contemporaries found excessive to the exclusion of other modalities of diagnosis. Alternatively, it may have been his practice of using high-dose antimony emetics, or his obvious royalism at a time when Lamennais was disillusioned with the crown.

Certainly patients chose their doctors, but it seems evident, in this case, that the doctor chose or, at least, maintained an interest in his patient. When Lamennais published the second volume of his *Essai sur l'indifférence en matières de la religion* (1820), Laennec wrote him a congratulatory letter concerning the section on the rise in insanity with the decline in religion. Laennec explained the futility of physical methods in treating moral diseases, and he expounded on the relationship between emotional ills and political unrest. The comments could be summarized as, a healthy mind results from a healthy, strong society. Lamennais printed the unidentified letter "by one of the most capable doctors in Paris" in subsequent editions.[52] The doctor had become a participant in the life work of the patient, but the reverse is also true. For his own Collège de France lectures on mental illness, Laennec made remarks that bear a Mennaisian stamp: he called for more order and authority, and he thought that political and moral chaos were both product and cause of insanity.[53]

After the Restoration, Laennec remained a devout Catholic, but his popularity as physician to Parisian clergy appears to have waned when his connection with Fesch had dissolved and his bond with aristocracy strengthened. The change may reflect his allegiance in the growing rift between church and throne. His friendship with the Bishops of Quimper, however, was unshaken and would continue to be useful till the end of his days.

PHYSICIAN IN SOCIETY

From 1808 to 1815, Laennec served as an adjunct physician in the fourth dispensary of the Société philanthropique, an eighteenth-century benevolent society that had been resurrected in 1803 to offer food and medical treatment to the indigent poor of Paris. House calls were made as necessary, and outpatient care was provided on Mondays and Thursdays from noon to two o'clock. The ordinary physicians were paid out of a fund established by the patrons of the society, but adjunct doctors, like Laennec, received nothing. He referred to this service as "unpaid and onerous" work, which he could not refuse in 1808 because he had volunteered for it in 1802.[54] The Congrégation doctors Buisson, Fizeau, and Bayle had preceded him into the society and, as Dora Weiner has observed, many members saw the work as an

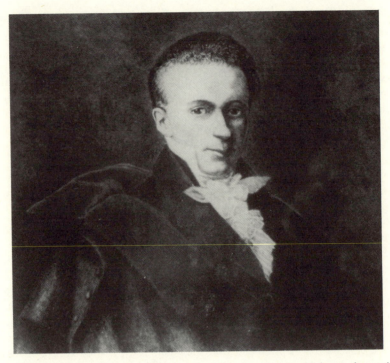

Figure 4.2. Laennec, engraving based on the Dubois portrait which now hangs in the entrance to Kerlouarnec, Ploaré. Source: With the kind permission of the owner, M. A. Halna du Frétay. Photograph: Joshua Lipton-Duffin, 1995.

extrapolation of Christian charity; patrons included royalists and aristo-crats.[55] Laennec's annual patient load for the Société philanthropique ranged from a low of five in 1816 to the maximum of forty-three, and was usually more than fifteen. In 1809, he reported that he had been making house calls on forty-three dispensary patients, most of whom had chronic diseases: twenty-two had been cured, ten were sent to hospital, nine were still being treated, and two had died of phthisis.[56]

Among Laennec's paying patients figured artists, actresses, musicians, and students of law and medicine. Remuneration was sometimes creative: in 1812, Alexandre Dubois (later known as Dubois-Drahonnet), a popular but struggling artist, painted a full-sized life portrait of the doctor in return for medical services rendered (fig. 4.2). The result so pleased the subject that the portrait was shipped to Brittany, preventing the dismayed artist from enter-ing it in the Paris salon until the following year. Laennec told his cousin to warn any young woman who might fall in love with the man in the picture that the artist had flattered his subject. [57]

Delicate problems were sometimes discussed in correspondence with other physicians. In the case of an eighteen-year-old "nymphomaniac," Laennec wrote, "the causes were almost always entirely moral," and he added, "the disturbance of the mind and the heart usually precedes that of the body."[58] At the death of a thirteen-year-old girl of "a very limited mind without idiocy," an autopsy was performed with special attention to the brain.[59] This case and those of the cardinals show that postmortem investigation was not reserved for people dying in hospitals.

The patients whom Laennec encountered in his practice did not have to die in order to become subjects for communication to the academic world. Three women, two "ladies" and a "domestic," provided the case histories for his essay on fever complicating convalescence; all recovered after following Laennec's advice, which for one woman had constituted a trip to the country—yet another example of psychic healing.[60] But in spite of his best efforts, many patients died. In the spring of 1812, Laennec lost an unidentified woman patient of "rank and fortune" of whom, he said, he had grown "very fond, because she had great confidence in me." Like Madame de Pompéry, she had a "strength of soul and a solidity of character that were rare even in men"; she died "after long sufferings" that required almost constant medical care. He had spent nearly forty consecutive nights in her house and was aroused two or three times each night.[61]

Better-known patients were the Breton writer, statesman, and politician, René de Chateaubriand (fig. 4.3), and his spouse, Céleste Buisson de la Vigne (1774–1847) (fig. 4.4). Chateaubriand had hidden during the Revolution, but rose to prominence under Napoleon, who granted him state appointments and sent him as ambassador to Rome in 1804. Together with Cardinal Fesch, Chateaubriand had been assigned the difficult task of encouraging the Pope to appear for the imperial coronation. He eventually broke with the "tyrant" Bonaparte and supported the return of the royal family and the old aristocracy, of which, conveniently, he was a member, though he was never financially secure. Chateaubriand married for money and ignored his wife for the next decade, but she and a network of mistresses and patrons supported and encouraged him in his opinions and his art. Narcissistic and given to fits of anger or depression, he indulged in ill health for many years. At the end of his life, he was virtually immobilized by gout. Possibly through the "Brittany connection" or perhaps through devotees of the Congrégation, Chateaubriand first encountered Laennec sometime before 1812. In that year, he was afflicted with palpitations and, because some physicians suspected an aneurysm, he feared the worst. His wife wrote this account, testimony of their love-hate relationship:

> The palpitations of Monsieur increased to the point that he was convinced he suffered from a fatal disease. As he did not lose any weight and his color was good, I was fairly certain that he had a nervous condition. This didn't prevent me from being anxious all the same and I implored him to see Laennec, the only doctor in whom I had any confidence. . . . I let him leave, but my anxiety was so great, that he had gone no more than a quarter of a league, when I left myself and arrived only moments after he did. I hid until the end of the

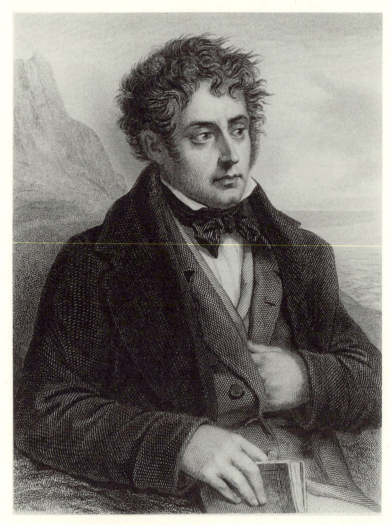

Figure 4.3 René de Chateaubriand, author, statesman, royalist, and Laennec's patient. Source: From *Chateaubriand* n.d., *1*: frontispiece. Photograph: Queen's Medical Photography Services.

consultation. Laennec arrived: after a long narrative, in which he [Chateaubriand] did not minimize his woes, the doctor told him that he had nothing wrong; Monsieur de Chateaubriand gave him a complete list of his ailments; Laennec was firm and would prescribe nothing, except, perhaps, that he take his hat and go for a stroll. "But what if I placed a few leeches?" said my husband. "If that would make you happy, you can go ahead," said Laennec "but I advise you to do nothing." I can't describe how I suffered until he left. I watched for the doctor in the passage way and asked him what was the matter with my husband: "Nothing at all," he replied and bidding me goodnight, he disap-

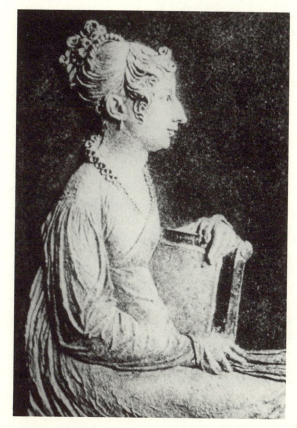

Figure 4.4. Céleste Buisson de la Vigne, Madame de Chateaubriand, 1812. Like her husband, she was also a patient of Laennec. Source: *Céleste Chateaubriand* 1929, frontispiece. Photograph: Queen's Medical Photography Services.

peared. Five minutes later, I heard the patient, charmed and cured, come down the stairs singing and laughing that certain persons had wanted to bury him alive; and when he came home around eleven o'clock, he was delighted to find me there so he could tell me that Laennec had found his state so alarming that he didn't even want to use leeches: he had only a small rheumatic pain . . . his imagination, working on a pain to which he wouldn't have paid the least attention at another time, had created for him a real disease.[62]

As the writer indicated, the formulation of disease through the working of a nervous mind—especially an intelligent, sensitive mind—would always be a medical reality for Laennec.

Madame de Chateaubriand and her physician continued to see each other often. She suffered from a bronchitic condition, possibly bronchiectasis, and her capricious health forced her "from time to time to heave great sighs in the direction of the little doctor." Laennec was her "*petit secco*" (little dry stick), but when he left Paris in 1819, she vowed she would have no medicine other than common sense and asses' milk. Twelve years after Laennec's death, she was still praising his skills and mourning her loss.[63]

Once again, the interest seems to have been mutual. The name of Madame de Chateaubriand figures in Laennec's lecture notes and in his personal letters. The nature of her illness fascinated him. In 1818, she would contract all the signs of pulmonary consumption, and one colleague was convinced she would die. Laennec reminded himself of this illness on several occasions, as an example of the unreliability of clinical signs and as a reason for hope in phthisis.[64]

As Roy Porter has observed, little is known of patient loyalties in medical history.[65] The late ambivalence of Lamennais and the fidelity of Madame de Chateaubriand show that some "doctor shopping" took place in postrevolutionary Paris and that the choice was influenced by a physician's politics, religion, and position, as much as by his personality, comportment, and medical accomplishments. Politics and philosophy seem also to have combined with practice in the frequently recognized link among Lamennais, Chateaubriand, and Bonald, who had been the psychologist-inspiration of Buisson. Bringing Laennec into the same political picture was Chateaubriand's enthusiastic review of Laennec's treatise on auscultation, the work of a "knowledgeable Breton compatriot"; it was immediately followed by a combined review of new works by Bonald and Lamennais.[66] Order in living, order in government, order in the mind, and order in the soul—a recipe on which these men could agree for the bodily health of individuals and collectivities.

FAMILY DIFFICULTIES: DEATH BY CHAGRIN

In November 1807, Michaud Laennec decided to give up his job in Beauvais and return to Brittany, stopping on his way to visit his brother in Paris. The alarming bouts of hemoptysis had persisted, and despite his efforts to ignore them, they brought ominous premonitions. He intended to devote some time to sorting out his father's myriad debts and legal processes.[67] After several weeks of wading through a labyrinthine collection of lawsuits, certificates, deeds, notes, and accounts, Michaud realized that his father had squandered all his own money and was indebted to his children for most of the twenty-five thousand-franc estate they were supposed to have inherited through their mother. In April 1808, Michaud asked his brother to do without the allowance, which he had been receiving since 1801, and devised a plan by which the father would forfeit all his belongings in property and liquid assets to his children who would then forgo their inheritance in order to pay his debts. Michaud confided in his aunt about his disgust for his parents' behavior: the step-mother's endless court battles and her gambling at dinner parties; the father's indulgence for "bad" women. In this matter of family honor, Michaud's concern was the future security of his siblings, both of whom he feared were "dupes," unequal to the task of managing their own money.[68]

At the same time, the father lost the position he had held for two years as counselor in the prefecture of Quimper, and in late spring 1808, he went to Paris where he taxed the patience of his doctor-son by writing poems for distribution to the high bureaucracy in the hope of finding new employment. "Fortunately," Laennec told Christophe, "he did not stay too long."[69] Laennec *père* was reinstated only to be dismissed again in January 1814; he would remember his son's reception during the 1808 trip to Paris with bitterness.[70] A permanent chill set into their previously warm and mutually indulgent relationship. Initially, the father was anxious for Michaud to come to his rescue, but he soon realized that the planned solution would alter his lifestyle and decided to oppose it. The family was shocked to learn that on 28 August 1809 the Quimper court witnessed the spectacle of an impecunious old lawyer making "ridiculous arguments" against his younger son who was wracked by the late stages of consumption. Michaud told his aunt of his exasperation when the roundly defeated father had immediately turned his misfortune into paternal pride: on leaving the court, he proclaimed, "My son argued like a angel!"[71] The agreement was signed on 14 October 1809. Laennec offered to give his father a voluntary pension of six hundred francs a year, but refused to formalize the commitment to do so.[72]

Having finished this difficult and financially disadvantageous task, Michaud's little remaining strength unraveled completely; he died on 9 or 10 January 1810 in Quimper. Laennec, who had long been expecting the outcome and had fretted over his brother's cavalier attitude to religion, was consoled by the report that Michaud had died shriven and with Christian feelings: "he had a thousand good qualities that would easily pardon a few character flaws."[73] Christophe comforted their aunt de Miniac, telling her that Michaud had "always thought of her as his best friend"; the chagrin of the legal proceedings, combined with worry for his brother and sister, had been the cause of his death.[74]

Little perturbed by his son's demise, the father complained about Michaud, now transformed in paternal estimation from "angel" to "monster." He accused his dead son of having stolen his papers in order to exaggerate his debts; he failed to understand how the sale of his children's house and furniture constituted anything less than personal robbery.[75] Three years would pass before he would agree to relinquish his claim on the small estate of Michaud, allowing the 1809 settlement to proceed.[76] The recriminations and reduced circumstances led to a temporary separation between the father and the stepmother, whose selfishness and stupidity was, in Guillaume's opinion, the reason for their ruin.[77] At times, Laennec *père* was inclined to agree: "O unthinking marriage!" he moaned, professing fatigue over the endless squabbles with his "crazy companion"; however, once he was reunited with his "sovereign Julie," he lauded her patience and charity.[78]

The father spent the next fifteen years claiming that Laennec's voluntary offer of a pension had been a promise of a greater amount, and he whined to his son, notary, nephews, sister, and brother, when it was not paid. To Guillaume, he invoked the ultimate insult, "My son is pursuing me just as Dupuytren chased his father, mother, and brother out of Paris."[79] Laennec defended his brother's memory and reassured his father about his continued affection, describing the obligations that prevented him from giving more: "Rest assured, *cher papa*, that I will always share with you so that your condition is no worse than mine."[80] But sometimes he would be obliged to explain the circumstances to a dunning relative, temporarily convinced by Laennec *père* that the son had neglected a "*dette sacrée*."[81] The father's unjustified assaults on his children, both living and dead, became so tedious that many years later Guillaume decided to establish yet another pension in his brother's favor, not because it was deserved, he said, but in order to have some peace.[82]

Michaud's death and the financial restructuring meant that Laennec *père* could abandon any semblance of providing for his daughter, Marie-Anne. Laennec's sister was the most enigmatic person in his sphere: all who have written about her imply that she was somehow dull or sick and incapable of looking after herself; and no one was inclined to care for her. Sent at the age of eighteen months to a maternal aunt, she had been restored, at the age of eleven years, to her father and stepmother in Quimper with Michaud and her young aunt. The father resented her pallor, her habits, and her inability to learn, and placed her for short periods in the Ursuline convent and with several different "ladies." He had also tried to send her to his physician brother in Nantes, but Guillaume protested that he already was raising two nephews with four sons of his own and could not cope with the addition of the third of his brother's children.[83]

In the fall of 1803, Marie-Anne contracted smallpox; her father complained of the expense, while Théophile, student of Hallé, demanded to know how the family could have overlooked her vaccination and offered to send vaccine lymph to Quimper: "It is the most beautiful present anyone can give a country."[84] She survived with scars, which may have contributed to her annoying habits of lying late in bed, spending several hours daily on her toilette, and compulsive buying of unneeded items. Only two letters written by Marie-Anne have survived;[85] otherwise, our knowledge of her is filtered through the assessment of her family. Their words suggest mental disturbance: "bizarre," "*gauche*," "*folle*," "manic," "timid," "distracted," "indifferent," with unceasing "tics." Christophe and his father believed that her strange behavior was the result of abusive treatment by her parents, "those tigers" in Quimper.[86]

Christophe was the only person who seems to have harbored some affection for Marie-Anne. He alone could spend a few hours with her without becoming frustrated. She had a good heart, he said, but the Nantes family was disappointed to discover that she would not tolerate any opposition and always preferred solitude to their company. Descriptions of Marie-Anne's behavior defy explanation: in 1820, she was so excited to have a surprise visit from Christophe that she purchased everything for an elegant dinner, including the food, dishes, cutlery, and other tableware, in the space of two hours.[87]

When Laennec was far away from this "most original of sisters," as Christophe called her, he tried to reach out. Fresh from the defense of his thesis, he was "charmed," by reports that she was beginning to care about her appearance; he joked that "Hippocrates, in his chapter on hats, observes that they are a good sign in girls." Because he did not have a fiancée or a mistress, he would send a copy of his thesis to his sister, and he was pleased to hear that she enjoyed reading his poetry. He told his father he would spend some time with her to determine if her "disease" was "physical or moral."[88] Proximity, on the other hand, taxed his patience.

In May 1810, after the legal arrangement with the father and the death of Michaud, the house in Quimper was put up for sale, and Marie-Anne was sent to live with Laennec in Paris. Ostensibly she was to manage her brother's household, but she was inept with a budget, helpless in the kitchen, and miserable. She caused more expenditures than she could prevent. She wanted only to live in a convent, to which her skeptical brother said he might consent, if she could prove herself capable of managing her affairs for at least six months.[89]

Eventually Laennec realized that his sister needed some form of protection, and he arranged a legal settlement similar to the one that Michaud had constructed for their father. He would buy all Marie-Anne's properties, manage the income (with the help of an advisor), and give her a lifelong pension sufficient to sustain a modest existence. The Nantes family approved, his sister agreed, and the papers were signed on 1 December 1812. To his great relief, she left Paris at the end of the month for her own small house in Quimper. Now it was possible to receive the cousins, Ambroise and Mériadec.[90] The combination of his sister's obligatory pension of twelve hundred francs and the voluntary donation to his father of six hundred francs (or more) limited Laennec's savings for many years.

Christophe announced his forthcoming marriage to Claire Marion de Procé in 1813. In congratulating him, Laennec confided that "fear" had made him reject a lucrative offer to wed a pretty seventeen-year-old with an annual income of twelve thousand francs. He was happy as a single man about Paris, and none of the women of his acquaintance suited his character or met his requirement that a future wife must be willing to move to Brittany. He realized that his resistance to the women whom he knew already might make him seem "a bit difficult to those whom he did not know yet." But if Christophe would only give him some nephews and nieces, then he would ensure that the "species of old bachelors did not go extinct like the *paleothères* and other antediluvian animals found by Monsieur Cuvier in the quarries of Montmartre."[91]

SOLDIERS: PSYCHIC CURE (AGAIN)

By the end of 1813, Napoleon's domination of Europe was threatened by a string of failures: the disastrous campaign in Russia in the winter of 1812–13; a defeat at Leipzig in October 1813; loss of control over the long guerrilla war in Spain; and finally the collaboration of his former victims into a strong allied opposition. Even in France, support was soft, and the Emperor resorted to restrictions on the press and the conscription of children. From all sides, his tattered armies retreated back across the natural borders of France with the allied enemies in pursuit.

Laennec would recall 1814 as the worst year of his life. Paris was in chaos; private citizens fled from town and countryside for fear of the *cosaques*. Even the intrepid Madame de Pompéry abandoned her chateau to the care of a solitary and terrified Madame Argou. Laennec's family begged him to return to safety in Brittany; instead, he sent Christophe his will and two trunks full of his most precious belongings, including his medals and the prize amputation set, and he settled down to wait for the allies in the capital.[92] Paris fell on 31 March 1814, and Napoleon would leave for Elba in mid-April, making way for the king's return a few weeks later.

By February 1814, the military hospitals overflowed with injured soldiers, and public hospitals were needed. Typhus was rampant. According to J. P. Kernéis, eighteen thousand men crowded into the twenty-two hundred beds of the Salpêtrière hospital, and a third of the seven hundred doctors and nurses working in Paris that year, succumbed, including Laennec's associates, Savary des Brulons and J. J. C. Legallois.[93] Christophe's brother-in-law, the young doctor Pierre-Martin Marion de Procé (1788–1854), developed a high fever; Laennec tended him daily, writing regular reports to the family in Nantes until his recovery.[94] In 1814, at both hospitals where Laennec would hold permanent appointments, the Necker and the Charité, the patient mortality exceeded twenty percent and was the highest in more than fifty years.[95]

During that difficult winter, Laennec volunteered at the Salpêtrière hospital where his charges included many Breton soldiers, whom he made his private concern. Some could not understand French, and they pined for home in the stench and confusion of the enormous city hospital. The men seemed to improve emotionally and physically when they were grouped together, and their Breton doctor conducted a small research project on what might anachronistically be called the "psychosomatic" aspects of care. He sought and obtained permission to create a special ward for these men, recruited three Breton doctors and a visiting Breton cleric, and spoke to the patients only in their native tongue.

The Bishop of Quimper, Pierre-Vincent Dombideau de Crouseilhes (1751–1823), heard of the initiative and wrote to thank Laennec for his concern (fig. 4.5). In his reply, Laennec outlined the program he had implemented and its positive results:

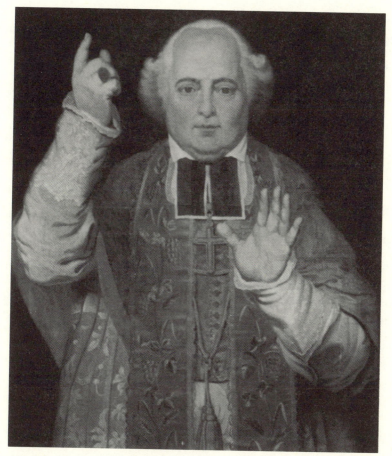

Figure 4.5. Pierre-Vincent Dombideau de Crouseilhes, Bishop of Quimper, Laennec's correspondent and friend. Source: AEQ. Photograph: Joshua Lipton-Duffin, 1995.

What I have done is very little. . . . In this calamitous community, the Bretons had more to complain about than the others. Isolated . . . almost all overcome with homesickness, they fell into profound discouragement and many refused any sort of help. All my colleagues found them even more difficult to understand than the Germans and the Russians because they made no use of sign language. Those that I could assemble in my ward were a little less unfortunate. I had the consolation of losing only one sixth, a terrifying mortality in normal times, but low in this moment. I lost approximately one third of my French patients, which was the average mortality in most of the military hospitals of Paris.

I had also hoped to provide my patients with the spiritual succor that they needed, but it was absolutely impossible. In Paris there was only one cleric who could follow Breton. Monsieur le Floc'h, a deacon of your diocese, visited my patients and Bretons in the other hospitals and several times I saw the benefits of his presence in the courage and health of my patients. On the very the day of his ordination, he administered the last rites for the first time to a Breton soldier who was in a very serious state following the evacuation of almost the entire hospital. Those of my other patients whom I lost were almost all tended by another priest who had the zeal to take on a good work: he read them an exhortation that I had translated into Breton at his request, and he managed quite easily to recite it in a very intelligible manner.

I would fear that I am abusing your patience by going into such great detail if I did not know of your charity and the interest you bear your flock.[96]

Not only could this cultural project heal the body, it might also heal the soul: if the clergy would use Breton, Laennec was certain that religion would return to Finistère.[97]

With the return of peace, this experience and the Bishop's praise, together with the departure of Madame de Pompéry, may have prompted Laennec's journey to Brittany late in the summer of 1814. It was his first trip home in thirteen years, and he used the opportunity to survey the domains that the arrangement with his father had handed over to him. He now owned several small farms near Pont l'Abbé and the dilapidated manor of Kerlouarnec, birthplace of his father and his uncle. He began to plan for repairs to the buildings and for extension of his holdings by the purchase of adjoining properties and the draining of a marsh.

Bayle's Nostalgia versus Phthisis: The Vital Lesion

Of all the cases Laennec witnessed in his early years as a practitioner, the repeated illnesses of Bayle had the most powerful impact. Bayle both suffered from and studied tuberculosis, but he thought of his diagnosis as "nostalgia." The blend of psychic and physical elements in the stories of his health and that of his friend were entirely consistent with their theories of disease and exemplified their lifelong convictions about clinical pathophysiology.

By 1808, Bayle had been appointed one of the four *médecins du quartier* in the Imperial medical service, probably through the continued influence of Corvisart and despite his hatred of Bonaparte. According to one biographer, he left for Spain soon after.[98] Laennec covered his friend's practice during his many absences and illnesses; Bayle did the same for him. In the summer of 1812, Bayle was sick for three months, and the following year, Laennec wrote, "I miss Bayle above all. I could never attempt to travel more than a few hours distance, when he is not here."[99]

Like Laennec, Bayle had published a steady stream of scholarly papers, mostly in the field of pathological anatomy. In the eight years following his thesis, he gathered clinical and autopsy material for his 1810 book on pulmonary phthisis (tuberculosis) and for another book on cancer, which did not appear until after his death.[100] His work on tuberculosis is often cited as an important step along a continuum toward linking the pathological lesion with clinical appearances and as part of the trend to provide increasingly materialistic explanations of health and disease.[101] Yet, Bayle had more to say about phthisis than appears in the traditional accounts. In the midst of the process to which he contributed, he turned in the opposite direction, emphasizing the limitations of pathological anatomy and developing what could be called a vitalistic theory of disease causation and its treatment, a theory that Laennec embraced.[102]

Bayle's diagnostic priorities had not changed since his thesis. For a diagnosis of pulmonary phthisis, he insisted on three equally important criteria: the characteristic symptoms, the presence of a disorganizing pulmonary lesion, and unremitting progression to death. On the basis of nine hundred autopsies, he reduced the multiple anatomical forms of phthisis to six, describing the changes that could occur in "life" of each type of lesion. All patients must suffer from the characteristic symptoms of fever, wasting, dyspnea, cough, with or without hemoptysis, and regional changes in the percussion sound; inevitably, they died.[103]

Death was an integral part of the diagnostic signature of Bayle's phthisis, just as important as the organic change. A favorable prognosis implied the absence of organic lesions and necessitated a different diagnosis. Since the detection of organic changes in the chest of the living patient was fraught with difficulty, considerable room was left for hope; however, the patient was obliged to hope for a mistaken diagnosis instead of a cure, because a cure for phthisis was impossible. The diagnostic ambiguity allowed Bayle's idea of absolute mortality to persist unchallenged until Laennec would later identify it as an "error."

Symptoms without lesions were not phthisis for Bayle, but they did represent disease. Having studied hundreds of cadavers, he thought that there were some diseases, easily recognized by the pattern of florid symptoms, which left no visible trace on the organs of the body. These included benign disturbances, such as emotional upsets and mild physical ailments, but they also included the more serious and potentially fatal conditions of epilepsy, asthma, tetanus, rabies, fevers, and sudden death, like that of *cadet Rousseau*. These diseases were not associated with any typical organic change, and, Bayle said, pathological anatomy would never provide a complete explanation for them.[104] The opposite situation—organic changes without symptoms—was almost completely unrecognizable, if not inconceivable to Bayle. Here, at least, he agreed with the nosologists: to be physically sick, a person had to feel sick.

When it came to the causes of tuberculosis, most medical contemporaries adopted theories that incorporated various combinations of heredity, constitution, environment, contagion, and emotion.[105] But by 1812, Bayle had constructed a classification of diseases that would compensate for the apparent inadequacies of organic-based medicine to explain the cause of lesions. As Laennec had done in 1803, Bayle used the concept of a psychic or "vital" lesion, an alteration in the functioning of the "life force," potentially as lethal as any organic change.[106] He believed that this vital lesion, if ignored and untreated, could engender a physical lesion, even tubercles.

Bayle extrapolated on his concept of "vital" lesion to devise a new classification of therapy. It included the centuries-old Galenic modes of treatment—cure, preservation, and palliation—and introduced the concept of preventative or "vital" therapy for "vital" lesions.[107] In his opinion, the "vital" disease had to be arrested before the abnormal functional process produced incurable physical change. Bayle's mind-body concept of the cause and treatment of phthisis was an old idea supported by evidence from the new science of pathological anatomy, and from his own case history.

Two versions of Bayle's illness were published. They represent either two different episodes of sickness, or two versions of the same illness, because there are discrepancies over names, dates, and courses of action; however, his identity is certain, and each account provides a vivid description of the patient and exemplifies his concept of disease. The first appeared as one of five cases in the 1806 thesis on "nostalgia," by C. Castelnau. A well-recognized disease in eighteenth-century nosology, nostalgia was taught by Corvisart to have both moral and physical manifestations.[108] It seems to have been actively demedicalized in the 1870s for its lack of an organic basis, although a tradition causally linking nostalgia and consumption persisted in nineteenth-century thought.[109] The following is a summary of what Castelnau wrote:

> A young, thirty-four-year-old doctor of nervous temperament and subject to mucous conditions, was born in a village situated in one of the most dismal parts of the Alps. He left home at the age of thirteen and since then never returned for more than a few months at a time.
>
> In Paris, he had been successful beyond all his dreams, but he was afflicted with a sense of uneasiness and depression. He had done all that was necessary to help him forget his village, but he would wake in the middle of the night thinking about his homeland; he suffered violent heart palpitations; and, quite unbidden, copious tears would flow from his eyes. By the summer of 1804, he began to lose weight and could not sleep at all. His legs were swollen and would contract spontaneously . . . even though he knew his village was not worth so much misery. In July, he suffered violent cramps, and spasms of the legs, his pulse slowed, he was emaciated and he had to stop working.
>
> He returned to his village. . . . As soon as he saw the mountains of his home, he felt better. Suddenly no longer weak, he ran here and there throwing his arms around the trees, weeping tears of joy. By early October, he experienced no more palpitations nor swelling of his legs, and his appetite was restored. Two weeks later, he was cured.

He returned to Paris at the end of October and since then (eighteen months), he has had no recurrence of his disease. But he must avoid anything that can remind him of his home. A half-hour conversation about the Alps suffices to bring on tears and palpitations.[110]

This narrative was known to Laennec as the "nostalgia of Bayle." He referred to it with Bayle's name in his teaching;[111] and it was the subject of a romantic poem that occupied eight closely printed pages in Bayle's posthumous *Treatise on Cancer*.[112]

A second, somewhat different version of Bayle's illness was published by Bayle himself in his 1810 book on phthisis. Case 53 of the fifty-four case histories was included as an example of a condition that had imitated pulmonary phthisis, but could not be phthisis because it resolved. The following is a summary:

> Doctor G.L.B**, a twenty-eight-year-old man with pale skin, light chestnut hair, and a nervous temperament . . . developed a dry cough in early July of 1802. In late July and August, the cough became productive, occasionally with hemoptysis. By September, he began to lose weight, there was a malar flush, he was pale and his palms and soles burned. He had severe night sweats, a rapid pulse, and six loose stools a day. One night he changed his chemise twenty-two times! He and his doctors were convinced that he was suffering from phthisis. He took no medication and put his affairs in order with no anxiety or regret, to end his course at such an early age. In late September, he developed a very high fever and an exacerbation of all the symptoms that lasted for a week. Then his appetite returned, the fever disappeared, and by October he was back to normal. In the eight years since this illness he has had various complaints [perhaps a reference to the 1804 nostalgia], but nothing suggestive of a cold or other lung disorder and he is presently in good health.[113]

In the discussion, Bayle claimed that it was futile to treat a phthisic whose symptoms were as advanced as in this case. If the correct diagnosis had been made and the patient really did have phthisis, nothing would save him; if not, improvement could occur, as happened here, but only if the diagnosis were wrong. A "vital" rather than physical intervention, such as travel, might help a suspected consumptive at this pre-phthisis stage of the disease, when the lesion itself was "vital" and not yet incurably organic—not yet phthisis.

Bayle made at least two other trips to Provence in 1813 and 1814 for pulmonary complaints.[114] With each voyage, his condition improved, and in late 1814 he appeared to recover completely. This improvement coincided with the restoration of the monarchy; however, at the return of the "usurper" Napoleon in March 1815, Bayle was "plunged into a painful despair which took on all the character of a very serious disease." During this last illness Bayle was extremely weak and unable to leave his room for several months; in the final weeks, he was confined to bed. One biographer wrote that the battle of Waterloo had come "too late" to save Bayle. It seems that incurable organic lesions had been detected in his lungs, probably by percussion. There was no longer any question of another journey home, which then, by his own definition, would have been futile. Attended by his wife and two sons, he lingered a year, but in May 1816, he rendered his soul to Providence with "an equanimity and confidence equal to his humility."[115] It is not known if there was an autopsy.

Bayle's experience was compatible with his definition of the disease and his understanding of its cause. He had always maintained that strong passions and deep sadness contributed to a weakening of the constitution and to the origin of phthisis.[116] In 1802, 1804, and perhaps also in 1813 and 1814, his symptoms had been suggestive of phthisis, but on each occasion he recovered with a trip home, and a retrospective revision of the diagnosis to "nostalgia" or something else was necessary. For Bayle (and his biographer), the early episodes had to have been vital or nonorganic because they improved; they were attributable to the pain of homesickness and his reaction to the tyranny of Napoleon. When lung lesions had been demonstrated, he did not attempt a journey home in the months that remained. The lack of action was tantamount to refusing therapy, an admission of futility in the presence of incurable, organic change.

And so Bayle died like Michaud, a victim of torment. Laennec drafted an obituary of his friend, and he rose in a meeting of the Société de l'Ecole to announce the "painful loss." Strangely hinting at further projects on the part of Bayle, he "promised to provide some information about the investigations, which his disease could inspire, if he could obtain it from those who propose to do the research."[117] The familiar domino effect was already taking place. To Christophe, he wrote, "[Bayle's] death and that of another hospital physician have resulted in a movement in the hospitals."[118] But Laennec said that he would not apply for the vacancies, since he had decided that such work was well beyond his strength. Nevertheless, the Restoration had come, "too late" perhaps for Bayle, but in good time for Laennec.

By 1815, Laennec was widely known in academic circles as an excellent pathologist, while in the royalist-Catholic and Breton enclaves of Paris, he had become the consultant of choice. His life was full: a large private practice with obligations to absent colleagues; public clinics and voluntary house calls on the indigent poor; research, reading, and writing every evening to sustain his contributions to the weekly meetings of his academic and religious societies. His infrequent vacations offered the only opportunity for the vigorous exercise and the cultural pursuits of music and literature which he loved so much. He had no time nor use for marriage. And even as he conducted his investigations into pathological anatomy, he was continually reminded of its differences from the experience of disease as suffered by individuals. These perceived inadequacies of the "new science" may have made his manuscript treatise seem less interesting and can be added to the other reasons for why it was never finished.

Laennec's own sicknesses, together with those of patients, family, and friends, taught him about the relationship between psychic pain and physical ills. Bayle's concept of a vital lesion gave him a quasi-scientific vehicle to convey these ideas. The illness experiences drove home a message that had hovered in the background of his medical life since its inception: pathological anatomy had serious limitations. It dealt only with "morbid appearances," death and the end stages of disease; it did not address cause of disease, nor did it examine its living evolution from disturbances in function to alterations in structure. A clinical physiology conjoined with a clinical anatomy was essential for a full comprehension of disease. These physiological precepts were anchored in the study of the sick, not the cadaver. They had little to do with the actual discovery of mediate auscultation, but they strongly influenced the direction in which he took his stethoscopic research. And they would pose major problems for his contemporaries and for his biographers.

The Restoration: Politics, Hospitals, and Patients

Frenchmen, let us abjure these monstrous doctrines, no longer . . . ought we to slit each other's throats over words.

—Laennec, 1815b, 34

I know better than the Wolf of La Fontaine that I am only a butcher, and as a result, since the little excursion into politics that you saw not long ago, I will stick to my butchery . . . I have had quite enough [of politics], for I have it up to my neck *usque ad nauseam*. I would not go back into politics, which in reality suits me better than theology, unless circumstances arise that can all too easily be imagined, in which one would have no other option but to calmly let them happen or make reason with gun in hand.

—Laennec to his father, 21 April 1818

LAENNEC was thrilled by the return of the king and the promise of peace and prosperity. During 1814 and 1815, he sent a string of breathless letters to his cousin Christophe reporting in rhapsodic terms on the final "short reign of him who has reigned too long," and on the approach of Wellington, the military actions of medical students, Napoleon's One Hundred Days, and the return of the king "who alone can bring peace and good order."[1] The stubborn opposition of another cousin failed to sway his views and he became a contributor to royalist propaganda. The Restoration had a direct impact on the fortunes of his family: it almost destroyed the uncle Guillaume, but it brought Laennec his first official appointment in a Paris hospital, where the work quickly consumed all his energies. Soon, as is indicated in the second epigraph above, he grew tired of intrigue, though he continued to "prefer politics to theology" and to accept the use of force to preserve order.

POLITICAL DEBATE: DOMESTIC AND OCCULT

With the advent of peace, Guillaume Laennec's second son, Ambroise, came to Paris to complete his studies in medicine in the fall of 1814. Following in his older cousin's footsteps, Ambroise had begun his studies at the Hôtel Dieu hospital in Nantes, but in December 1808, he had been conscripted into Napoleon's army as an eighteen-year-old surgeon third class. Guillaume was tortured with worry by his son's four years in occupied Spain, where he survived wounds and two serious fevers. Only through Laennec's influence with the prominent surgeons Larrey and Desgenettes, was his cousin Ambroise transferred to the imperial guard and sent to Prussia as a medical aide, accepting a demotion for the opportunity. He seems to have been captured in late 1813 and was held in the military hospital at Dresden.[2] Five months after the peace, Ambroise finally returned to France with money borrowed from Laennec; he decided to round out his six years experience in military medicine with a thesis at the Paris school.

Laennec and Ambroise did not get along: they disagreed on political matters, and the young soldier seemed lazy and uninterested in clinical medicine. After six years of army service, Ambroise shared the opinions of his fellow veterans and was strongly Bonapartist. The domestic arguments were described as painful and amusing, and they mirrored the divisions of the entire city. The younger man would sometimes vanish without explanation in the company of people whom Laennec thought of as thugs and hooligans. In turn, Ambroise made fun of his cousin's piety, his royalism, and his sympathy for the English allies; Guillaume sympathized with him on those points.[3] During Napoleon's return in the One Hundred Days of spring 1815, the cousins barely spoke to one another. Ambroise reenlisted with other medical students and joked about the skirmish that had caused his relative and colleague, Marion de Procé, to be grazed on the head by a bullet. On 22 June 1815, the day of Napoleon's final abdication, Ambroise disappeared again, reappearing three weeks later, in the company of a "sad specimen" of a man with "such a bad air that the porters and domestics were astonished to see them together."[4] Because of their apparent eagerness to oppose the Restoration, students in law and medicine fell under police surveillance.

Unlike Ambroise, Laennec seemed little disturbed by the English and Polish allies who occupied the city. During the One Hundred Days, he refused to leave the city, and after Waterloo, his ebullience stood in stark contrast to his misery of the winter before: "We Parisians are good, peace-loving people who do not get upset over little things and who cannot imagine any event that could prevent us from going to the café for a demi-tasse, or having a small game of dominoes, topped off with a stroll round the Luxembourg or through the Tuileries. On 30 March last year all that was going on to the sound of cannon."[5] He assumed Christophe shared his views and was hungry for news: in order to save time he sometimes dictated his letters while shaving.[6] If Laennec had any reservations about the direction of events, he did not express them, and we do not know if he had mixed feelings about the honorable burial that royalists insisted on giving to the recovered remains of Cadoudal, the Chouan leader against whom he had once been enlisted to fight in the Vendée. After his execution in 1804, Cadoudal's body had been dissected by medical students; at the Restoration, his skeleton was supposedly found hanging in the closet of Napoleon's surgeon, Larrey.[7]

And Laennec, who had once been scandalized by his father's pamphleteering in favor of Bonaparte, resorted to the same tactic himself on behalf of the emperor's opponents. In May 1815, an anonymous, forty-five-page pamphlet was published by the Royal Printer in Ghent where the Bourbons had fled: "*On Feudalism; or Essay on the Question: Is the Reestablishment of Feudalism More to Be Feared under the Government of the King than under the Empire of Buonaparte?*" Rouxeau claimed that the essay had been merely an evening's pastime, not intended for distribution; he contended that Laennec's friends in the royalist party must have had it published to the great embarrassment of its author. It is clear, however, that the generous biographer was far more embarrassed than his subject. Laennec proudly sent copies "from the author" to royalist friends and to family, including the de Miniacs and Christophe, in whom he confided that the pamphlet had been published at his own expense for distribution in Burgundy. Ambroise was disgusted and took it as a sign that his cousin was beginning to despair of winning the hoped-for royalist favors.[8]

Political tracts had long been an important vehicle for influencing public opinion in France. A few weeks earlier, Chateaubriand had published a pamphlet that, according to Louis XVIII, had done more for his Restoration than an army one hundred thousand strong.[9] Laennec's pamphlet attacked and analyzed the threat of royalist feudalism that pervaded Napoleon's speech read at the Gulf of Juan where he landed from Elba on 1 March 1815. Avoiding the taint of "feudalism" was a justification for ridding the country of monarchs, Bonaparte maintained. The idea was much talked about in the press; it also echoed in medical circles, reeling from a reactionary proposal by the restored royalists to separate medicine and surgery once again—a plan that was intended to tighten up perceived laxity in professional training.[10] Laennec wrote that his reflections were those of "a citizen who was equally opposed to license and tyranny" and had no "personal interest" in the outcome of the debate; "I can be wrong, but I hate lies."[11] Returning to the ironic style of his medical journalism, the author began with an analysis of the Latin derivation of the terms. Then, he patiently traced the social and legal history of feudalism from Ur of the Chaldees and compared its abuses under a constitutional monarch with those of the Empire. Confident in his political positivism, Laennec claimed that the old-fashioned brand of feudalism was a problem only for states in their infancy.[12] He concluded that greater deprivations of freedom and a more elaborate and oppressive hierarchy had emerged

nder Napoleon. The "usurper's" threat of a return to feudalism was a severe
ase of the pot calling the kettle black, and it was reflected in the uniden-
ified, untranslated epigraph chosen to adorn the title page: "*Quis tulerit
Gracchos de seditione quaerentes* [Who could stand the Gracchi making accu-
ations of rebellion]."[13] Although he had not used it in his medical articles of
he previous fifteen years, Laennec returned to Old Regime orthography, for
xample, "*étoit*" for "*était*," etc. His Bonaldian rhetoric surely contains
races of the arguments that he had marshaled against his Bonapartist cousin
uring their strained life together.

Obliged to his uncle's wayward son and still without an academic position,
Laennec used his contacts in the Société de l'Ecole to arrange for Desgen-
ttes to preside over Ambroise's thesis on epidemics; he hoped that the old
oldier would look benignly on a young one's mediocre efforts to master a
opic that was far too broad.[14] Laennec did not attend the defense on 10
April 1816—possibly because of Bayle's illness—but the following day, he
eported to Christophe, that the newly graduated physician had said, "I
on't give a '*f...*' [sic]. I pulled through with honor, because I ought to have
een hung and was only whipped and scarred."[15] Laennec observed to his
ncle, "Here he is '*docteur*,' but so little '*docte*' [learned]. . . . I will be sure
o take him to see some patients and give him a few lessons in clinical prac-
ice."[16] Grudgingly, Ambroise stayed on.

WHITE TERROR, NANTES: A LAENNEC LOSES HIS HOSPITAL

The history of the Restoration has been steeped in an ambivalence that
vaxed and waned with French political changes over the last century and a
alf: some historians seem to participate on the side of one faction or an-
ther; others treat it like a period of shame following the "glory" of the
Revolution and Empire. Rouxeau's influential biography bears signs of his
iscomfort; as a result, the extent to which the advent of the royalists
rought the Laennec family *both* profit and strife has not been appreciated.
Despite Laennec's personal satisfaction at the return of Louis XVIII, his rela-
ives suffered from the political change before they derived any benefit.

Guillaume Laennec, once confined by Carrier on suspicion of being an
nemy of the Revolution, now became a victim of the "White Terror" that
ollowed the Restoration. In early March 1816, he was denounced to the
ninistry of the interior as an antiroyalist and a "dangerous person" by his
urgical colleague, Pierre-François Blin, and a handful medical associates.
Blin has been called a "true weathervane," for his wide swings in political
llegiance, from "fiery revolutionary," through "ardent imperialist," to "ex-
lted royalist."[17] His personal allegiances seem to have been equally loose: he
wed his career to Guillaume's lawsuit against the University thirty years
arlier; however, he now reasoned that professional security lay in a conspic-

uous demonstration of royalism; he decided to jettison his old friend in order to preserve himself. Guillaume was swiftly removed from his position as founding director and professor of the medical faculty at Nantes. With him went another of Laennec's former teachers, chief surgeon J.-B.-A. Darbefeuille (1756–1831).

Laennec was warned by a "royalist friend" of his uncle's denunciation in March 1816, long before the rest of the family had heard. He immediately went to the ministry of the interior, taking along another "royalist friend" and armed with a petition, which protested the possible dismissal and demanded to see the charges. Anticipating the type of antiroyalist, anticlerical charges that might have been trumped up against his sixty-eight-year-old uncle, he told the authorities that the aged and ailing doctor may have an "easy elocution," but it sprang from his "honest spirit of opposition to arbitrary acts of government," which had been just as obvious in the days of the "usurper" as it was now. His uncle was above all else "a zealous defender of good order," with a respectable record of loyalty and service. Laennec reminded the minister of his uncle's Revolution: prisoner of Carrier, provider for a priest-brother, patron of religious schools where he educated his sons. During the Empire, Guillaume had never taken advantage of the émigrés or of the English, and had always spoken of the King with respect.[18]

But when Laennec heard the evidence, which amounted to reports by students and patients of sarcastic puns and clinical jokes—remarks that hovered just on the edge of political decency—he began to despair. Of one patient, Guillaume had supposedly said, "His pulse is like the government; it rises and it falls;" and to another, "You are lucky, you'll soon have legs like L[ouis?]." A nervous woman was said to have the "disease of the D[uchesse] d'A[ngoulême]."[19] Flippant remarks like these were precisely the kind of thing that his uncle was wont to say and Laennec knew that the "evidence" would be impossible to disprove and difficult to forgive in the climate of growing intolerance. He recommended that Guillaume accept the forced retirement and apply instead for recognition as an emeritus professor with the associated pension. Then he might be able to encourage other family members to replace him in the faculty: Christophe's brother-in-law, Marion de Procé, or perhaps his own son, Ambroise; the latter idea might have seemed more than a bit premature to Laennec who continued to express grave doubts about his cousin's political orientation and his commitment to clinical practice.[20]

Added to the rather thin evidence against Guillaume was the professional lobbying and jealousy of younger colleagues, especially the doctor Julien Fouré (1769–1855), who leapt to fill the academic vacancy. Not surprisingly, the authorities passed over Marion de Procé and young Ambroise, who had only just defended his undistinguished thesis. Soon after, the local council of the prefecture in Nantes took further action and stripped Guillaume of his remaining privileges and position as chief physician at Hôtel

Dieu hospital.[21] Unlike the academic insult, which originated in Paris, this local maneuver did seem to be worth a fight, and Guillaume's nephew joined in the fray.

In the summer of 1816, Laennec dined several times with his friend François-Louis Becquey (1769–1849), newly appointed undersecretary in the ministry of the interior in charge of the Assistance Publique. During the Revolution, Becquey had supported the constitutional monarchy and opposed legislation against clergy who, like Laennec's uncle, were non-juring. During the Directory, he was a "crypto-royalist" working for the Restoration of Louis XVIII, but he seems to have softened his stance during the Empire and was appointed councillor of the University. By 1815, he was the elected deputy for his native department of Haute-Marne and would serve in that capacity and as commissioner of roads and bridges for fifteen years.[22]

When and how Laennec met Becquey is unknown. The connection may have been religious or academic, or it may have been through Madame de Pompéry, as Becquey hailed from near Soissons. In approaching his bureaucratic friend, Laennec hoped to help his uncle by arranging a pension and advancing the cause of Marion de Procé and Ambroise; however, he warned, it had become difficult to reach Becquey now that he was installed in "*les grandes affaires*," and it was awkward to ask for favors. Becquey complained to Laennec that his powers were limited; he could not secure a nomination for his relatives if the local committees did not place them at the top of their own list of candidates.[23]

Embittered and lonely, Guillaume fumed over his misfortune; his facility with words, sarcasm, and tendency to self-pity pervade his cynical letters to the family in Paris. Here it is easy to find a resemblance to his flighty brother, Théophile-Marie. His wife had died after a long illness in the summer of 1813, and his formerly crowded home now seemed empty with only his mother-in-law and his youngest son to share it. He raged at the stupidity of the authorities who based their decisions about the hospital on the religious and political credentials of practitioners: "In the minds of the administrators . . . the medical care given by graduated doctors who have not been to confession in the previous eight days cannot possibly expect to have the blessing of Heaven."[24] He prevailed upon his nephew and sons in Paris to visit potential allies who were perceived to have influence, and to report back on how sympathetic they had been. The young men delivered letters and requests to a host of eminent doctors, politicians, bureaucrats, and journalists; they asked the leftist mayor of Nantes, Louis-Marie Rousseau de St. Aignan (1767–1832), to act as an intermediary.[25] St. Aignan was concerned with Guillaume's lack of discretion. His sons also feared that their father's "lively imagination" and "immoderate transports of joy" might lead him to confide his fears, hopes, and projects to the first person who came along.[26] Four years would elapse before the problem could be solved to Guillaume's entire satisfaction.

WHITE TERROR, PARIS: LAENNEC AT THE NECKER HOSPITAL

It was on 5 June 1816 at a dinner with Becquey over the problems of Guillaume that Laennec first learned of his own possibilities in a Paris hospital. He had asked for the meeting to discuss his uncle's prospects, but Becquey raised the issue of the hospital vacancies created by the recent deaths of Bayle and two other doctors. Indeed, the choice of Laennec was part of what Jacques Léonard has described as the "elitism and selection" of the royalist attempt to "combat materialism" and to resist "the expansion of ideas and new social forces."[27] Later, Laennec claimed that he had asked for two days to ponder the offer of a salaried position as a hospital doctor while twenty eager candidates were kept waiting. He feared that his health would not permit him to take on the strain of additional clinical activities, and he did not want to set aside his vague plans to move back to Brittany. Administrative confusion and delays meant that he did not take over the service at the Necker hospital until early September 1816. By that time, his misgivings seem have to evaporated and the one-time medalist and longtime whirlwind of research and journalism plunged enthusiastically into his first academic appointment, twelve years after finishing his degree.[28]

The Necker hospital, or officially the *Hospice de [la] charité des paroisses de St. Sulpice et du Gros Caillou,* was named for its benefactress, Suzanne Curchod Necker (1739–1794), wife of the minister of finance and mother of the famous author, Germaine Necker Mme de Staël (1766–1817). It was her popular husband's dismissal in 1789 that unleashed the furor that led to the storming of the Bastille. In 1778, Mme Necker had secured funding from the king to establish her institution in a building vacated by the Benedictines of Notre-Dame de Liesse. She ran the one-hundred-bed hospital for male and female patients as a model of efficiency and hygiene, excluding people with the "unclean" diagnoses of madness, pregnancy, and venereal disease. Cabanis and Jacques Tenon (1724–1816) cited its size and management as ideals worthy of emulation.[29]

At the Necker, there was no shortage of clinical material for research in pathological anatomy. During the years of Laennec's affiliation, the hospital was full: one thousand patients were admitted annually, of whom approximately 20% would die (see tables 5.1, 5.2). In her detailed study of the archives of the Assistance Publique, Lydie Boulle found that the mortality in the Necker hospital ranged from 140 to 190 per thousand admissions in the years from 1816 to 1823.[30] This mortality was greater than that of the general population but about average for Parisian hospitals; however, statistics from hospitals in rural areas and other countries compare favorably with those of Paris.[31]

Hospital patients were used as subjects for teaching and research; if they died, their bodies were autopsied. This "clinical contract," as Toby Gelfand has called it, survived the Restoration, despite its revolutionary origin.[32]

TABLE 5.1

Hospital Movement at Necker Hospital during Laennec's
Presence, 1816–1819

	1816*	1817	1818 †	1819 ‡	Totals
In hospital 1 Jan	?	?	122	?	
Total admissions	932	955	1099	1217	4203
Laennec present	302	955	912	990	3159
Total deaths	201	208	240	233	882
Laennec present	68	211	151	176	618

Sources: Registes des Entrées de l'Hôpital Necker, 1816–1819, Archives de l'Assistance Publique, Paris, 34 1Q2.19–22; Registres des Décès de l'Hôpital Necker, 1816–1819, Archives de l'Assistance Publique, Paris, 34 3Q2.3–5. (Registre des Décès for November–December 1818 is missing.)

* Laennec began 4 Sep (admissions and deaths before that date not included).

† Laennec absent 7 Aug to 12 Nov 1818 (admissions and deaths for that period are not included).

‡ Laennec retired to Brittany 8 Oct 1819 (admissions and deaths after that date are not included).

TABLE 5.2

Hospital Movement at Necker Hospital during
Laennec's Presence, 1821–1822

	1821*	1822	1823 †	Total
In hospital 1 Jan	100	107	113	
Total admissions	915	1183	1340	3438
Laennec present	127	1183	229	1539
Total deaths	174	210	218	602
Laennec present	6	182	47	235

Sources: Registes des Entrées de l'Hôpital Necker, 1821–1823, Archives de l'Assistance Publique, Paris, 34 1Q2.24–26; Registres des Décès de l'Hôpital Necker, 1821–1823, Archives de l'Assistance Publique, Paris, 34 3Q2.6–8.

* Laennec returned to Necker hospital 15 Nov 1821 (admissions and deaths before that date are not included).

† Laennec transferred to Charité hospital 17 Mar 1823 (admissions and deaths after that date are not included).

While Laennec conducted his earliest research on auscultation, some four thousand people were admitted and nearly nine hundred died. He was present for the majority of these admissions, and some of their case histories have been preserved in manuscript. The extant records are rarely in Laennec's own hand, although he dictated and occasionally annotated them. The writing was assigned to students, who were required to provide a detailed history and, if the patient died, an autopsy report. As many as three or four different accounts of the same case can be found, presumably because Laennec assigned interesting patients to several different students.[33] Some documents, written in Latin, are daily entries, while longer accounts, in French, are case summaries. A detailed history of medical, psychological, and social circumstances surrounding the illness was provided, and reference was often made to the patient's temperament.[34] The clinical and autopsy diagnoses were written on the top of the first page of every case as a title (see also Appendix A).

Laennec quickly became very busy. He soon allowed his medical activities to consume the energy that he had once spent on politics, and he declined an offer to serve Quimper in the Chambre des députés because of his hospital teaching.[35] In a letter to an old friend he described the pattern of his daily life six months after his appointment:

> I get up at seven or even eight o'clock, because I need a lot of sleep. Most often, I dress while giving consultations. I make rounds at Necker hospital followed by a little clinical instruction for the students who come with me. This brings me to ten-thirty and already I am pressed for time to reach home for lunch. Then I begin a round which lasts until five o'clock, and after dinner, that is to say around eight o'clock, I begin another until ten o'clock. I have only the hour before I go to bed and occasional moments before meals to bring my correspondence up to date, to correct and organize the observations collected by the students in my hospital, and to deal with small matters, etc.
>
> This picture gives you only a vague idea of what the bustle of life in Paris does to all types of relationships for a man who is a bit busy, however careful he may be to keep things simple.[36]

The reluctant Ambroise stayed in Paris another year and was cajoled into the Necker work. The experience seems to have had softened his resistance to medicine and to his cousin. Just as he was about to go back to Brittany, he wrote to his older brother, Christophe, "If Heaven had granted a hospital position to my cousin the first year of my stay, I would be leaving Paris as a learned doctor."[37]

Guillaume's third son, twenty-year-old Mériadec, had arrived to study medicine by the spring of 1817, a few months before Ambroise left. Thirty-six-year-old Laennec was now established at the Necker hospital, and Mériadec applied himself with great energy to clinical studies, regretting the time that his father had caused him to waste in Nantes. Seven years younger and more deferential than Ambroise, Mériadec tried to engage in the political arguments, but he usually lost. He also joined in hospital gardening, which was his cousin's surrogate exercise for the more time-consuming hunting. Mériadec "works like the devil," reported an astonished Ambroise, and he predicted that some day his young brother would replace their cousin.[38] Mériadec became Laennec's most devoted student, accompanied him on private consultations, researched a successful thesis on auscultation, and worked as his *chef de clinique* in two Paris hospitals. If Christophe was the best friend, Mériadec became his "son," through blood and common profession, strengthened by the intensity of a shared adventure in a new realm of diagnostic technology.[39] The correspondence with Mériadec is the most important source of information about the later years, and it was to him that Laennec would bequeath his scientific papers.

LAENNEC'S HOSPITAL PATIENTS

Laennec's records demonstrate that the postrevolutionary hospital was much like its eighteenth-century predecessor. The presence of teaching and research notwithstanding, it catered to the working-class sick, seldom the destitute, never the rich. Hospital patients tried to carry on with their occupations, even when they were severely ill, and some had recourse to self-help and nonexpert treatments before turning to an institution. For example, in his comparison of late eighteenth-century hospitals in Copenhagen and Berlin, Arthur Imhof proposed that an increase in the intermediary (noninstitutional) levels of care might explain why people admitted to hospital appear to have been much sicker than those in either contemporary cities or later hospitals.[40] As a result, Laennec's hospital may have held only a minority of the urban sick.

The hospital records raise possibilities for the demographic and disease history of Paris. Indeed the ambient diseases, the "pathocenosis," of early nineteenth-century Paris had a role to play in the discovery of auscultation.[41] But making generalizations can be risky because several features of Laennec's record collection may have skewed the selection: patients most likely came from the neighborhood of the hospital; wards were for women or men only; the records of patients who had died were probably preserved more often than those of the people who were discharged; Laennec's growing reputation as a lung specialist may have meant that people with other diseases went elsewhere. Nevertheless, some comparisons can be made between the group of people defined by Laennec's case records and the demographic analyses of contemporary Paris.

For 662 of the 770 patients described in his case records an occupation was given. There were 189 different occupations, some so precise that they defy the usual classification, but the pattern corresponds to other demographic studies of early nineteenth-century France (see table 5.3).[42] Almost one-quarter of the male patient population worked in the construction industry, the most common occupations being mason and stonecutter (involving 41 individuals). The most frequent employment among women was dressmaker (34), followed closely by maid (30), and lingerie maker (27). The sewing of clothing concerned a total of 75 of the 662 patients. The flavor of early nineteenth-century Paris is vividly evoked with special mention of activities such as pin maker, ribbon maker, flounce maker, shepherd, spaghetti maker, junkman, bottle seller, mule keeper, fan painter, chimney sweep, midwife, lamplighter, writer, male nurse, and ropedancer, each represented by one patient. There were six water carriers, two teachers, two female gardeners, and three each of lemonade salesmen, butchers, lapidaries, and weavers. Laennec's hospital patients also included jewelers, coachmen, milliners, printers, bakers, pastry chefs, students in law and medicine, theater workers, and dancers, but there were no musicians, aristocrats, politicians, lawyers, or doctors.

Of the 662 patients with occupations, 234 were women, only 10 of whom were described as "housewife." Those with no occupation given were not always women, but for these individuals, many other details are often lacking, including the name and sex. One important group of workers was the day laborer, as often female as male. At least half of the domestics were male, and some of the heavier jobs, such as porter, were occupied by females. Perhaps because they could work at home, married women tended to do laundry leaving the outside domestic jobs to single women. Some of the workers were quite young: a twelve-year-old girl, who died, was identified only as a "mattress maker"; a sixteen-year-old carver recovered from his disease, but a seventeen-year-old milliner and two eighteen-year-old masons were not so fortunate.[43] Other workers were quite old: an eighty-year-old woman, who died of pneumonia after five weeks in the hospital, was found at autopsy to have been suffering from widespread cancer; on admission, she had been described as a laborer.[44]

From 1816 to 1826, there was a trend to more faithful recording of employment, which may reflect an increasing consciousness of occupational disease. Sometimes the mine or the factory was specified, as in the cases of four workers from the white lead factory at Clichy, north of Paris.[45] Three of these men were diagnosed as having lead poisoning; one died. Other workers (masons, copper smelters, and lapidaries) were also thought to have "*colique métallique*," although their symptoms were mild.[46] Laennec became interested in the relationship between dusty work environments and the physiological mechanisms that protected against lung disease. He later commented on the ability of workers to adapt to their environments and speculated on a relationship between stone dust and the formation pulmonary concretions in lapidaries and marble workers.[47]

This trend to more reliable reporting of occupation suggests that the doctors of postrevolutionary Paris, who had been instructed in hygiene by Hallé, were so attuned to the possibility of labor-related illness that when confronted with any patient at risk, they could diagnose little else. It also contrasts with the apparent lack of sensitivity to work-related illness observed at the end of the eighteenth century and suggests that the Revolution may have sensitized the medical gaze with respect to the laborer. In her detailed study of French hygienists, Ann La Berge has situated the French awakening to

TABLE 5.3
Occupations of Six Hundred Forty-Six Patients in Laennec's Hospital Records
(Necker and Charité Hospitals, 1816–1826)

Occupant	Number	Occupant	Number
Agriculture		Commerce, Arts, Public Servants	
Gardener	10	Merchant	34
Farmer	5	Office	19
TOTAL	15	Military	12
Building and Quarries		Postman	5
Mason	34	Student	4
Joiner	22	Artist	3
Painter/plaster	14	Teacher	2
Carpenter	10	TOTAL	79
Stone cutter	7	Equipment and maintenance	
Digger	5	Metal worker	37
Welder	4	Carriageworks, etc.	26
Roofer	3	Fine craftsman	18
TOTAL	99	Porcelain & cutlery	7
Alimentation		Saddler	7
Chef	20	Jeweler	5
Baker & pastry	19	Cooper	3
Water, juice seller	10	Sweep	1
Butcher	5	TOTAL	104
Wine/beer	5	Unskilled labor	
Kitchen maid	3	Laborer female	34
Refiner	1	male	30
TOTAL	63	Domestics female	37
Textiles and fashion		male	16
Dresses/lingerie	75	Housewife	10
Shoes	30	Concièrge, huissier	4
Tailor	13	Colporteur	3
Laundry	10	TOTAL	134
Hats	11		
Weaving/spinning	6		
Bedding	3		
Hair Dresser	2		
Dyer	2		
TOTAL	152		

Source: Patient records in ML, MS, Cl. I, Cl. II, and Cl. III.
Note: Categories after Henry 1980. For 662 patients, an occupation was given, but in sixteen cases the employment did not correspond to Henry's classification.

work-related illness in the 1820s and 1830s, and described it as a reaction to the effects of industrialization in Britain. Analysis of these diagnostic preoccupations through a comparative study of patient records from eighteenth- and nineteenth-century hospitals has yet to be made, but might shed some light on the impetus for medicalization of work.[48]

SAMPLE CASES

Laennec's private clients have attracted the attention of historians, but his research owed more to the hospital patients. Many examples can be found of antemortem diagnosis confirmed by autopsy, but there are others, in which the autopsy results came as a surprise or in which the patient left the hospital alive. Four case histories are summarized here to set the stage for the conditions under which the earliest investigations into auscultation were conducted.

The first sample history was that of a woman admitted to the hospital 12 October 1816 at about the time Laennec claimed to have discovered auscultation:

Wife Dumont, a sixty-one-year-old woman of good constitution and sanguine temperament, . . . suffered confluent smallpox at the age of seven, which left only a few permanent scars on her face. Her menstrual periods appeared at age nineteen, she married at twenty and bore eleven children, six of whom are still alive. She reached menopause without complication at the age of fifty. Sent at an early age to work at a painful [*pénible*] occupation, she often sought oblivion in wine. Her character was irascible; her food quite healthy. Ten years ago, she noticed that carrying a heavy load or becoming very angry made her heart beat harder than usual. Eight years ago, she was treated with violet and honey tea for catarrh, but she did not stop working. She notices that her cough improves in summer and worsens in winter. Lately, her palpitations have been more frequent accompanied by a choking sensation and violaceous changes to her nose and lips especially when in the cold. Exposed to all the atmospheric vicissitudes of this season, her respiration became labored, her cough much worse, and, abandoning her usual occupation, she presented herself to the Necker hospital on 12 October 1816.

On physical examination, she was a well-nourished woman with yellowish skin and smallpox scars. The nose was very large and dark purple in color especially at the tip. There was a scar on her right leg from an old injury and there were several varicosities. Respiration was short and noisy [a judgment made at the bedside apparently without the stethoscope] and was sometimes interrupted by choking and coughing spells productive of frothy sputum. Percussion of the thorax was mediocre over the back and in the region of the heart. The pulsations of the heart were tumultuous and easily felt over the base of the sternum. The pulse was rapid by intervals, but equal in both arms. The jugular veins were distended and in the one on the right, there was a marked trembling. The tongue was moist but the patient complained of severe thirst and bitterness in her mouth. The abdomen was distended and tender to deep palpation. There was constipation, the urine was scant and dark, but intellectual functions were intact. The breathing worsened and delirium caused the patient to try to leave her bed several times. She died at 5:30 in the evening.[49]

Even without auscultation, the clinical presentation was entirely consistent with the postmortem findings of enlarged heart and tricuspid valve abnormalities, which could have been anticipated by Corvisart and may or may not have been predicted by her attendants—the record does not indicate. The lungs and liver were engorged with blood. There were signs of previous pleurisy, and the uterine cervix was obliterated by a polyp.

The second patient was examined with the stethoscope, but his doctors were mistaken about the nature of his problem until a subsequent admission. The case history was entitled "Boulimia":

Herbé, a twenty-two-year-old soldier . . . in the colonial regiment, with pale skin and red hair, was admitted to the hospital in December 1818 for aching pains in his legs and emaciation, despite a voracious appetite which he had trouble satisfying. His illness went back two years and appeared to begin with a venereal condition, which he had contracted in Martinique and for which he had been given a lengthy treatment this winter, consisting of, so he said, sixty-four bottles of Van Swieten liquid and many frictions [of mercury]. Since this therapy, he had no symptoms of syphilis, he did not masturbate, and he did not have any commerce with women. His principal symptoms on admission were an extreme thinness so that his arms and legs resembled those of a six-year-old child and an insatiable appetite. . . . *[H]e did not cough at all* [emphasis in the original].

Toward the end of December he noticed an increase in his urinary volume, out of proportion to the amount of liquid he drank. We verified this phenomenon and thought he had diabetes, but it disappeared in a few days without treatment.

On 24 and 25 December he had two nervous attacks, or convulsions. . . . [but he improved and] . . . still with his great appetite, left hospital at the beginning of January.

One month later he was readmitted with a cough, and doctors used the stethoscope to make a diagnosis of tuberculosis, which was confirmed at an autopsy.[50]

The third case, labeled "Nostalgia," demonstrates that the physiological view of phthisis, as expressed by Bayle and Laennec, was a clinical reality in the wards of the Necker hospital in 1819.

A young girl, eighteen years of age, with fair complexion and chestnut hair, was admitted to hospital . . . with no particular localizing symptoms. She was weak and unhappy with facial pallor and dark circles around her eyes. . . . She was so depressed that it was thought she was suffering from nostalgia. In fact, she had been in Paris for only a short time and longed to return to her native village near Amiens. The pulse was regular, but weak and rapid. The chest resounded a little less than normal on the left, but respiration was clear on both sides. . . . She continued in the same condition for a few days; then, the depression and sadness deepened. Then, diarrhea and fever appeared, which became continuous and increasing; the abdomen was slightly tender; she developed the Hippocratic facies ["*grippé . . . tiré*"]. . . . Her mental faculties were altered and she drifted into stupor. . . . leeches were applied. . . . her condition worsened and she died [almost three weeks after admission].

On autopsy, tubercles were found in the right lung and the peritoneum. The cerebral convolutions were flattened, and there was increased serosity in the pia mater and ventricles.[51]

The fourth case, labeled "Quartan fever?," was the history of a man admitted to the Charité hospital where Laennec transferred in 1823; however, the patient appears to have been malingering.

Joseph Fleuret, a forty-seven-year-old locksmith, was admitted with a five-week history of quartan fever on 8 May 1824. Each attack began at three A.M. The patient had had the disease before. The skin was yellowish, the spleen perhaps a little enlarged. All other functions . . . [were] . . . in good condition and [he had] a very big appetite.

Today, 10 May the day an attack should have occurred. The patient maintained that he had a brief chill at three A.M. and more abundant sweating than usual. At six A.M., there was no evidence of fever and the skin was only slightly moist as is normal after sleep. We have doubts about this fever.

The 11th. Displeased about the doubts raised concerning the existence of his fever and finding that he is not being given enough to eat, the patient insists on leaving the hospital. Agreed.[52]

A general study of patient records and record keeping has yet to be made. This sample is too small to be fully representative of Laennec's practice, and it is not known if these records are similar to those that were kept in other Paris hospitals at the same time, much less those in other countries. But the cases do offer a glimpse of the vast range of hospital experiences and they demonstrate the record-keeping formula of Laennec's staff: an interest in the old-fashioned constitution and temperament; a focus on emotional and personal events; an emphasis on details of physical examination; and an attempt to establish a relationship between clinical appearances and autopsy. They also give the life histories of people who were not usually able to leave their own record, as told by members of a different social group preoccupied with the search for specific signs. Often, the "story" of the patient's life was intimately connected to the account of her illness. Laennec's work contributed to a shift in how patients' stories would be retold by their doctors in a way that could map the individual's illness onto a new theory of disease.[53]

With the Restoration, Laennec finally managed to obtain a long-awaited place in the Paris medical establishment, while in Nantes, his uncle was stripped of his academic and hospital positions. Laennec's consummate skill as a pathologist is often cited as the major reason for the successful development of auscultation; the skill was essential, but the hospital position was equally important, if not the sine qua non. Only in a ward full of chest patients could he gather the clinical and pathological experience necessary to establish the meaning of the lung and heart sounds with speed and accuracy. A master of pathology, an astute clinician with an interest in the physiological relationship between emotions and physical ailments, Laennec was now provided with large numbers of patients and ready facilities for postmortem examination. These were the intellectual, social, and practical underpinnings for his research in auscultation.

PART TWO

Auscultation

To be able to explore is, in my opinion, a large part
of the art.

—*Hippocrates*, Epidemics III, *cited by Laennec,*
Traité *1819 and 1826, epigraph*

The Discovery

[Buisson] distinguishes two sorts of hearing, the passive or
audition, the active or *auscultation*, a division based on
equally exact observations, and on which is based the
difference between the words, *to hear* and *to listen*.

—*Laennec 1802f, 176*

Words will often fail me to describe them [on rales].

—*Laennec,* Traité *1819, 2:1*

Observation is less independent of the dominant systems in
each epoch than we like to think; we easily see what we
want to find, and we often neglect, as inconsequential, that
which has no rapport with our favorite theories.

—*A. L. J. Bayle, 1856, 42*

RARELY does a discovery occur in an instantaneous flash, although accounts
by inventors often make it seem that way. A discovery is a complex process.
It can follow a long prehistory and emerges—sometimes quite slowly—
within a receptive milieu that holds at least an inkling of what might constitute a useful application. It cannot be a product of chance alone, although it
may profit from accidental circumstance. Most moments of discovery pass
undocumented, and the stories are constructed retrospectively by the discov-
erers or their associates. Despite the best of intentions, post hoc accounts are
never innocent; they are written with full knowledge of the ultimate significance of the event. Laboratory notebooks are essential for the historical reconstruction of a scientific discovery, and, as Mirko Grmek and F. L. Holmes
have observed, many case studies are needed to elaborate and test the general
theories of discovery as they apply to life science.[1]

Laennec's discovery of mediate auscultation—or the practice of listening via an instrument ("mediator") to explore the state of the organic structures concealed within the chest—offers no exception to these generalities. For him, as for other clinical researchers, the "laboratory" was the hospital; the "notebooks" were the patient records published in his treatise or kept with his papers.[2] References to the new technique in the personal correspondence are disappointingly scarce: either he wrote many fewer letters during the period of his intense labors, or the letters that he did write in those critical years cannot be traced (see Appendix A). This chapter is a case study in discovery: the recognition of signs of anatomical change that could be derived from listening to the human chest with an instrument. When words failed him to express his findings, as they often did, he invented new ones.

Laennec's fullest account of his first attempt at mediate auscultation in the clinical setting appeared in both editions of his treatise, and was scarcely changed from a version he read at the Académie des Sciences in February 1818. He said that he had "for a long time been in the habit of sometimes placing an ear directly on the patient's chest, when it was practicable in a difficult case." The word "sometimes," included in 1818, was deleted from the later published versions. But direct auscultation was problematic: "distaste alone made the incommodious technique impractical for hospital patients; and it was scarcely to be suggested for most women patients, in some of whom the size of the breasts also posed a physical obstacle." He had not seen the technique recommended by medical authors, but the idea was so simple that it must be very old, possibly Hippocratic in origin. His justly famous account is notoriously vague about the conditions of who, what, when, where, and how:

> I was consulted, in 1816, for a young person [*jeune personne*] who presented with generalized symptoms of heart disease, and in whom palpation and percussion gave few results because of plumpness [*embonpoint*]. The age and sex of the patient [*la malade*] prevented me from conducting the type of examination I have just described; I recalled a well-known acoustic phenomenon: if the ear is placed at one end of a log, the tap of a pin can be heard very distinctly at the other end. I imagined that this property of bodies could be applied to the case at hand. I took a paper notebook, made it into a tight roll, one end of which I applied to the precordial region, and, putting my ear on the other end, I was just as surprised as I was satisfied to hear the beating of the heart in a manner that was clearer and more distinct than I had ever heard it by the direct application of the ear.[3]

Later in the treatise, Laennec gave references to Hippocratic passages on auscultation; he had read them many times, he said, but it was the "memory of a few physics experiments," which may well have taken place in his youth, that had prompted him to try mediate auscultation.[4] K. Keele has shown that

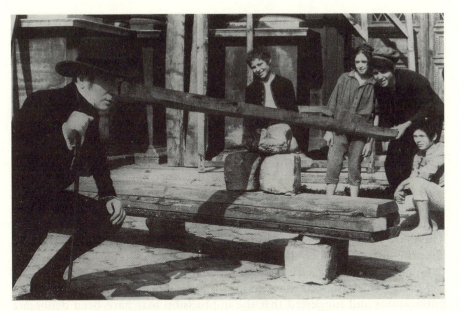

Figure 6.1. Laennec, played by actor Pierre Blanchar, listens to the transmitted sound of a boy tapping on the far end of a beam lying in the courtyard of the Louvre. The scene is based on the unsubstantiated recollection of Kergaradec. Source: From the 1949 film by Maurice Cloche, in Bernard-Luc 1949. Photograph: Queen's Medical Photography Services.

these experiments were also known to Pliny in antiquity; Laennec cited Pliny on other topics, but he did not refer to that passage.[5]

Former students and associates embellished the tale. The neurotic, A. B. Granville, possibly taken in by his mediocre French and an impressive demonstration on ward rounds, claimed to have witnessed the actual moment of discovery, which he situated in the Necker hospital on 13 September 1816.[6] In 1868, the former associate Jacques-Alexandre Le Jumeau de Kergaradec (1788–1877) recounted an anecdote, omitted from his 1826 obituary of Laennec, that he said he had heard from the inventor himself: on the way to visiting the *jeune personne* with heart trouble, the doctor had watched children playing the acoustic game with logs in the courtyard of the Louvre—an entirely plausible event since the recent Restoration meant the palace was under repair.[7] So frequently has this vignette been attached to Laennec's own account that it has merged with the original to form a captivating legend with a resiliency all its own. In Maurice Cloche's 1949 film, Laennec is invited by urchins to participate in their game with a log; he kneels, listens, and in a voice heavy with meaning, solemnly pronounces the immortal words, "J'entends!" (I hear) (fig. 6.1). With its alternative meaning, "I understand," the phrase sets up an elegant double entendre.

WHEN DID THE DISCOVERY TAKE PLACE?

Most histories of auscultation accept the basics of Laennec's account, and place the moment of discovery in 1816; some specify the month of October. In February 1818, he located the moment in 1816, "toward the end of the year," but the specification was deleted in the subsequent publications.[8] He had taken up his duties at the Necker hospital in early September 1816, and former students testified to his stethoscopic research there in early 1817. Granville was confident of the date 13 September 1816, "for [he] took note of it," but he admitted to being baffled by Laennec's apparent disagreement with him.[9] The Breton, Adolphe Toulmouche (1798–1876), said that he had found Laennec engaged in stethoscopic research when in he arrived in Paris with his fellow student, Mériadec Laennec, in "the fall" of 1816.[10] There are serious problems with these sources: they were written decades after the discovery, when the legend was already well established; and errors in Granville's account, especially, imply that it was partly fabrication.[11]

Mirko Grmek noticed the deletions that Laennec had made for his later publications and suggested that the imprecision may have been deliberate obfuscation to shore up his claim to priority.[12] When it came to publications, François Double (1776–1842) had recommended direct (or immediate) auscultation first. In the second volume of his treatise on clinical signs published in early 1817, he wrote that "the ear should be brought against the thoracic wall" in order to appreciate the intensity and the location of the noises inside.[13] Double also referred to sounds made in other parts of the body: voice, speech, and stomach, but he did not provide parameters for normal and abnormal sounds of the chest or other parts, and his discussion of circulation focused almost exclusively on the pulse and he did not refer to auscultation of the heart.[14] Nevertheless, Laennec may have found inspiration in his remark; certainly existing records cannot disprove this hypothesis.

Laennec made a few changes in his account of the discovery for the second edition of his treatise in 1826, possibly because Double or his associates had complained: he repeated the story of the *jeune personne*, but in the later version he gave the credit for direct auscultation to his dead friend Bayle as well as Hippocrates. Laennec's own notes, taken as a student, confirm that Corvisart, too, sometimes "heard" the heart beat; however, in 1826, Laennec stated categorically that his recently deceased professor may have held his ear "very close" to the patient's chest, but he had "never" practiced direct auscultation.[15] In Buissonian terms, then, Corvisart listened only passively; while he, Bayle, and Hippocrates listened actively. Rolling back claims of priority to dead predecessors has been recognized in other disputes.[16] But of Buisson—who was credited by one author for having "introduced the word auscultation into physiology" and whose 1802 thesis had led Laennec to contemplate the meaning of auscultation and the exploration of the human voice—of Buisson, he wrote not a word.[17]

The idea of using a mediator to transmit sound may have come, as Laennec said, from his physics experiments in school—or, as Kergaradec suggested, from the urchins at the Louvre—or, as others have wondered, from his knowledge of Pliny. But a closer, and somewhat more tangible inspiration can be found in the 1810 muscle experiments of William Hyde Wollaston (1766–1828) of London, who had used a long "stick" to transmit sounds from his foot to his ear, which he had covered with a "cushion." In his first edition, Laennec did not cite Wollaston, claiming later that he had not known of the work. In 1826, however, he commented on only one experiment—"ingenious" though "devoid of significance"—but he did not mention Wollaston's stethoscopic stick.[18]

The identity and outcome of the first patient to have been auscultated by Laennec is not known. Only one undated manuscript seems to represent an attempt at mediate auscultation during 1816 or early 1817: the private consultation for "D. Argou, age 37"; it contains the words: "*pulsationes cordis [+ in praecordiis] mediocres, sonum absque impulsio[nibus? or ne] dantes sub clavicula sinistra non perceptibiles*" (moderate pulsations of the heart [+ in the precordium], giving a sound without impulsion[s?], not perceptible beneath the left clavicle).[19] These words, and the fact that the record was kept in a file concerning angina pectoris, led Rouxeau to wonder if the prototypical *jeune personne* had been Laennec's future wife, Jacquemine Guichard, widow of Pierre Argou, who would have turned thirty-seven in the fall of 1816. Laennec had known her as a friend and distant relation since their first meeting at Couvrelles in 1805, and he had treated her for illness on other occasions.[20] Privacy and friendship may have made him comfortable enough to attempt a new and bizarre form of examination. The personal relationship could also represent an additional reason for concealing her identity.

Always careful to substantiate his statements, Rouxeau did not publish his reasonable and intriguing speculation, perhaps because he thought a thirty-seven-year-old woman was too elderly to meet the description of a *jeune personne*. In any case, the notes of a student who followed Laennec's lectures in 1823 suggest that the young person was "almost pubescent," a condition that would disqualify the middle-aged future wife from having been the first to be auscultated with a paper stethoscope, without diminishing the significance of the early date on her record. The student notes specify that the "young girl" lived in a "boarding house" to which Laennec had been summoned, and that he had used a "paper roll" that happened to be lying on her bedside table; the "next day" he examined "all" his patients in the "Necker hospital" with a similar paper roll.[21] No date was given.

The case records point to early 1817 as the onset of stethoscopic research. The earliest reference to auscultation in the published observations is the case of the forty-year-old chambermaid, Marie-Mélanie Basset, first examined with the stethoscope on 8 March 1817 and autopsied on 2 June 1817.[22] Auscultation was not mentioned in either of two other patients seen in 1816 whose histories were published in the treatise for their important findings at autopsy.[23] Laennec claimed that the relevant information concerning an additional two patients, examined with the stethoscope in May 1817, had been lost because his assistants were unaccustomed to keeping such records.[24] Of the thirty-seven patients who had been examined with the stethoscope and whose complete case histories appeared in the first edition of the treatise on auscultation, two were examined in 1817, twenty in 1818, and fourteen in the first half of 1819; one case was undated. Sixteen of the twenty cases from 1818 had been attended before the end of August (see Appendix C).

Evidence from late eighteenth-century Britain and early nineteenth-century America suggests that experimental and student procedures were withheld from affluent patients until they had been tried on the poor. For example, when William Withering (1741–1799) began to use digitalis, he tested it on charity patients.[25] In contrast, Laennec claimed to have made his first rudimentary stethoscope in a private setting and did not hesitate to experiment with it on paying patients. Modestly performed through the clothing, auscultation was painless, harmless, and singularly noninvasive. Within a year of his discovery, he boldly used his stethoscope to examine a famous private patient: the dying Mme de Staël, daughter of the Neckers who had founded the hospital where he worked.

The consultation for Mme de Staël in mid-1817 brought Laennec's activities to the attention of the medical and popular press for the first time. Her fame, as daughter of the Neckers and author, was enhanced by Napoleon's displeasure over her account of the Revolution (which she had welcomed) and the birth of his Empire (which she had not). Exiled to Switzerland, she had maintained a liberal, artistic forum. The notoriety that she had enjoyed during the now defunct Empire piqued interest in her death among supporters of the newly restored throne. For several months, she suffered from breathlessness, jaundice, and swollen legs. Having previously suffered from scarlet fever, her dropsy and breathlessness may have been due to what would now be called rheumatic heart disease.[26] In his defensive and indiscreet account of this last illness, her lifelong physician, Antoine Portal, suggested that his menopausal patient fell victim to her own therapeutic adventures, her stubborn resistance to following his mild recommendations, and her lack of faith in him alone. His extended role at her bedside was cast as a continuous mopping-up exercise to rectify the damage done by other consultants and the patient herself. He described a consultation with Laennec, which took place in June 1817: "She complained of a squeezing pain in the upper part of the chest over which a newly graduated doctor placed a large blister. Another well known doctor [Laennec], using a horn of paper, which he placed with one end on a part of the thorax and the other in his ear, believed he diagnosed a hydrothorax and could even hear a sort of undulation. One can well understand that I considered this method of investigating the interior of the chest to be very strange, and I did not share his opinion, in spite of the regard I might have for him."[27] Portal scoffed at Laennec's recommendation that the patient be treated with two magnetized plates on her chest.[28] Her son-in-law, the Duc de Broglie, who also thought that the advice had been "of little use," observed that Laennec was a man of "a lofty mind with a weak appearance" who "stood himself in great need of medical care."[29] Mme de Staël died on 14 July 1817, and a postmortem examination failed to demonstrate fluid in the chest; however, Laennec gladly accepted the attention and publicity given his new method by Portal's widely circulated account, which he cited in his presentation to the Académie des Sciences.[30]

Manuscript records for the five earliest stethoscopic cases published by Laennec cannot be located; the Necker hospital manuscripts do not mention auscultation until November 1817. The family correspondence is even less helpful about the date of the discovery. The first reference to the "new method to diagnose chest diseases" appeared in a letter from the cousin, Mériadec, to his older brother, Christophe, on 30 December 1817.[31]

On 23 February 1818, Laennec gave a detailed presentation on auscultation to the Académie des Sciences (fig. 6.2). He had made no secret of his research, he said, but was prompted to speak "sooner than he would have preferred" because others, whose independent verification he claimed to welcome, were now beginning to publicize, comment, and draw conclusions that might benefit from his own observations. He referred to an earlier demonstration by his "friend" and fellow Congréganist, Joseph-Claude-Anthelme Récamier (1774–1852) of Hotel Dieu hospital, who "had agreed to verify [the essential features of the technique] in front of a large gathering of medical students."[32] Portal, who had so publicly expressed his doubts eight months earlier, was assigned by the Académie to study auscultation with P. F. Percy and Philippe Pelletan (1747–1829). At their examination, Laennec presented a few patients with phthisis and allowed the evaluators to make independent confirmation of the transmission of respiratory and cardiac sound. On 29 June 1818, the committee delivered a favorable opinion, which Laennec later printed in his treatise.[33] Portal's original skepticism had melted away.

The Académie lecture was followed by four others delivered at the Société de l'Ecole de Médecine between 1 May and 9 July 1818.[34] On 4 August 1818, Laennec told his uncle that the formal presentations had been "very favorably received" and that his book on the "cylinder" was nearly complete.[35]

To summarize the apparent sequence of events: the first case was auscultated with the stethoscope no later than the winter of 1816–1817; Laennec was aware of possibilities in the phenomenon for at least a few months before mid-1817 when he began his intense investigations that peaked in early 1818. The structure of his book was defined by mid-1818, although, as will be shown below, some details were still being explored.

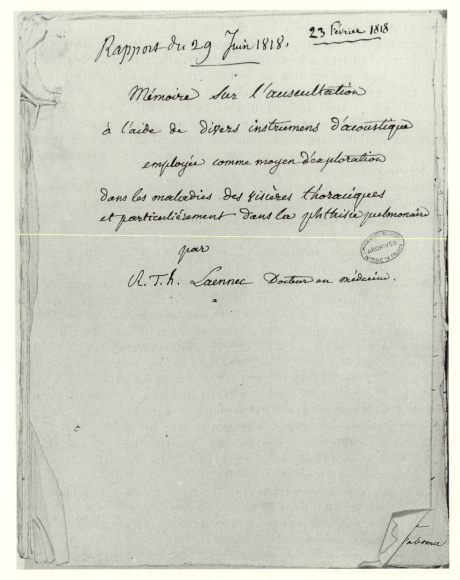

Figure 6.2. Title page of the essay read by Laennec on 23 February 1818 at the Académie des Sciences. "*Memoire sur l'auscultation à l'aide de divers instrumens d'acoustique employée comme moyen d'exploration dans les maladies des viscères thoraciques et particulièrement dans la phthisie pulmonaire.*" Source: AAS. Photograph: Jean-Loup Charmet, Paris.

THE STETHOSCOPE

The first stethoscopes were cylinders, one foot long, one and a quarter inches thick, and made of three tightly rolled notebooks wrapped in gummed green paper. The ends were filed. Initially, Laennec tried unsuccessfully to obliterate the central canal, but he soon came to realize that the unwanted hole enhanced "exploration" of the voice; a solid cylinder was better for listening to the heart. Respiration and rattles were heard to advantage if the patient-end of the cylinder was hollowed in a funnel shape. He set up a lathe in his apartment and experimented with different shapes and densities of wood and other substances. Metal and glass were too heavy and too cold for the patient's comfort. Very dense and very light wood did not transmit sound well. He preferred paper or a wood of medium density, such as rattan.[36] Laennec continued these experiments in his home for the remainder of his life: at the sale of his estate, two lathes, woodworking tools, ivory, and a large amount of dried wood suitable for turning were disposed of by auction; Récamier bought a lathe for 305 francs, the second-highest price paid for any of his possessions.[37] The Académie Nationale de Médecine in Paris and the Musée Laennec of Nantes both possess stethoscopes turned by Laennec.

According to his former student Toulmouche, Laennec was still using paper instruments in late September 1817, but at least by February 1818 and possibly earlier he was using a stethoscope similar to the illustration in his treatise of the following year. It was a wooden cylinder about one foot long with a quarter-inch central canal, a break in the middle joined by a screw, and a funnel-shaped hollow in the end. The only modification that took place before the 1819 publication was the addition of an obturator, which allowed the instrument to be converted from one with a hollow end (for respiration and rattles) to one with a straight cylindrical canal (for voice and heart) (see fig. 6.3). Laennec's stethoscope was to be used through light clothing.

The instrument does not appear to have received the name of "stethoscope" until mid-1818, when it appeared in a student's thesis, defended on 27 June.[38] Laennec preferred to call it "*le cylindre*"; he said that he "had not imagined it would be necessary to give a name to such a simple device, but others thought differently." He had heard his invention referred to as a *sonomètre, pectoriloque, pectoriloquie, thoraciloque*, and *cornet médicale*; his uncle once called it a "*thoraciscope.*" Laennec said that these terms were all "improper," and some "barbarous," especially those featuring an infelicitous conjunction of Latin and Greek. "If one wants to give it a name," he said, "the most suitable would be 'stethoscope.'"[39] The word was derived from two Greek words: στῆθος (chest) and σκοπεῖν (to examine, to explore). The choice is telling: Laennec was proposing to use his ears to investigate or "see" inside the chest, to practice an autopsy before his patient became a cadaver. It was a technological extrapolation of Corvisart's "gaze" through the ears instead of the eyes. Already familiar with telescope (for seeing far) and micro-

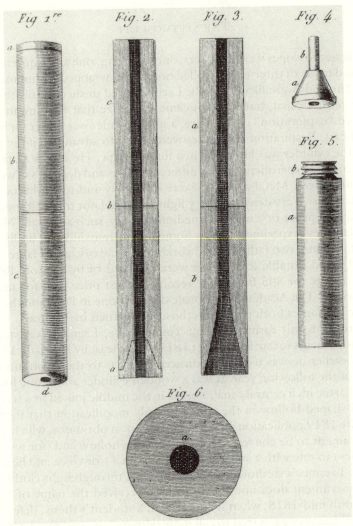

Figure 6.3. Laennec's stethoscope from *Traité* 1819, 1: plate I. Photograph: Queen's Medical Photography Services.

scope (for seeing small), doctors quickly associated the new instrument with these visual tools and its name with visual connotations.[40] The stethoscope would serve the "better eye." But to emphasize "seeing" over "exploring" was etymologically incorrect, as Laennec's cousin Mériadec reminded readers of his thesis defended 16 June 1821.[41] Nevertheless, the inventor's concession to the penchant of his colleagues did little to stop their creativity, and the barbarisms persisted: "stetoscope" and "sthenoscope" could soon be added to the list of offending words.[42]

WHAT DID LAENNEC NOTICE FIRST?

The investigation leading up to the first edition of the treatise on auscultation proceeded in several stages that reflect Laennec's concerns and his
realizations: heart sounds, rattles (or bubbles), pectoriloquy, succussion,
metallic tinkling, emphysema, and egophony. The first two stages resulted
in interesting information, but scarcely altered existing diagnostic practices. Beginning with pectoriloquy, however, each of the last five stages represented a mini-discovery or breakthrough, with immediate conceptual
and practical implications. They provided escalating impetus to Laennec's
investigation.

Cardiac Auscultation

In keeping with the conditions ascribed to the discovery itself, early case
records suggest that the former student of Corvisart was initially preoccupied
with the application of his new technique to the study of the heart. For example, the 1816 apparently pre-stethoscopic case of "Wife Dumont" (cited in
chap. 5) reflects a preoccupation with the heart.[43] Similarly, on 6 April 1817,
Laennec had his freshly graduated cousin, Ambroise, record the history of
eighteen-year-old Amand Guérin, who had been admitted to Necker Hospital on 2 February 1817. The stethoscope and auscultation were not mentioned specifically, but the history refers repeatedly to the "pronounced,"
"tumultuous," and "strong" heartbeat and a precordial thrill (*"battements"*
and *"frémissement"*) that could have been detected either with the stethoscope or by application of the hand, it is not clear which. Ambroise's two-
and-one-half-page report on Guérin's autopsy devoted one-and-a-half pages
to description of the heart, but the lungs were not mentioned at all.[44] Shortly
after Guérin's death, Ambroise recorded the case of Jean Millet, who also
does not appear to have been auscultated, although his aortic aneurysm was
presented to the Société de l'Ecole de Médecine and featured in Laennec's
treatise.[45] Perhaps the new technique had been used in these cases, but verbal
conventions to relay that fact did not yet exist.

The initial cardiac focus is also evident in the case history of chambermaid
Basset of early 1817, in which the author referred to the beating of the heart,
although no interpretations were applied to the sounds. But that of Marie
Potel, examined six months later, described the heart sounds with an interpretation. Potel's case centered on the antemortem detection of cardiac
changes with autopsy findings of "globulous vegetations," hypertrophy (increased muscle thickness), and dilatation (increased volume) of the right
ventricle of the heart. After examining Potel on 18 November 1817, Laennec wrote confidently about the "ventricular and auricular sounds," designations that he must have established prior to that date and to which he

would always adhere (see chap. 8).[46] In the preamble to his presentation at the Académie des Sciences, and in both editions of his treatise, he said, "It is especially in diseases of the heart that a desire is felt for a sign that is more certain and more constant than that provided by percussion."[47]

Respiration and Rattles

The heart sounds were sometimes drowned out by noisy breathing. Early in the research, Laennec defined the sounds of healthy respiration, inspiration (breathing in), expiration (breathing out), yawning, snoring, and coughing, but his cases do not allow this work to be dated. He recorded variations in the quality of healthy breath sounds heard in different parts of the chest: the "bronchial" sounds heard over the main airways and the "vesicular" sounds heard over the distant lung tissue. He also compared the sounds heard in children with those heard in adults and defined "puerile" respiration as a louder, more efficient type of breathing, which he would later view as an acquired sound in illness (see chap. 7). A greater obstacle to cardiac auscultation would have been the loud bubbling that emerged from the chests of the hospital patients, many of whom were dying of pneumonia, pulmonary phthisis, or heart failure. These distractions eventually became Laennec's focus. After making his preliminary interpretations of the heart sounds, he appears to have turned his attention to "exploration" of these rattles, or as they are called in French, "*râles.*"

Laennec quickly distinguished several types of rattles: crepitant, mucous or gurgling, sibilant, sonorous, and cavernous. Because these words were comprehensible to patients and possibly frightening, he described them in Latin at the bedside: "*râle*" became "*rhonchus*" modified by various adjectives, including "*crepitans, sibilans, sonorus.*"[48] The hospital records confirm that the statement reflects his practice, but the duplicate names resulted in confusion over the nomenclature of the respiratory sounds, especially in English.[49] Laennec tried to associate each type of bubbling sound with a specific pathological condition, and this preoccupation spilled over into the theses of his students. For example, his student, Baume, claimed that an experienced physician could recognize "the different types of rales that characterized other lung diseases"; in one case, he said that he had been "greatly surprised to a hear a rale the nature of which was still unknown."[50] For diseases of the airways, Laennec followed the nosological divisions of Pinel, a classification that took into consideration the quantity and texture of the secretions. The result was cumbersome: if Laennec's complicated rales promised only to bring bedside diagnosis back to the symptom-based framework of Pinel, it was difficult to perceive any advantage in the new technique. The sections of the treatise devoted to catarrh contain no clinical examples, and his earliest critics complained of the abundant nuances and excessively thick prose.

This early stage in Laennec's research led him to expand on the ancient diagnosis of pneumonia (Laennec used the classical term *péripneumonie*) and to refine the definition of a new pathophysiological entity, pulmonary edema. Pneumonia or inflammation of the lung tissue was common, and Laennec claimed that his experience in auscultation had been enhanced by an outbreak of pneumonia in the winter of 1816–17. The claim cannot be confirmed, because no clinical case observations were provided in this part of the treatise, although several patients whose cases were used elsewhere in the treatise had died of pneumonia at other times. Instead, he wrote of the pathophysiological stages of pneumonia defined by "anatomopathologists," who were largely unnamed with the exception of Bayle: (1) engorgement ("*engouement*"); (2) "hepatization," consolidation, or inflammation of the lung tissue; and (3) resolution.[51] Laennec said that Bayle had designated the first stage of pneumonia as "*engouement*"; however, according Laennec's own student notes, their teacher, Corvisart, had also used the words *engouement* and *hepatisation* in the same context.[52]

The diagnosis of pneumonia was already relatively easy with the existing methods of examination, but auscultation made it possible to follow the progress of the disease through the stages that previously had been detectable only at autopsy. In the first stage, percussion was equivocal, but breath sounds and crepitous rattles could be heard; in the second stage, percussion was noticeably dull and breath sounds were absent, but occasional rattles might be heard; in the third stage, percussion would be equivocal, but breath sounds would return with a bronchial quality and the "*râle de retour.*" Laennec emphasized the importance of combining both techniques and gave detailed instructions on how to perform percussion.[53] But in this early research, when he was concentrating on distortion of breath sounds, he did not notice the now well-recognized possibility of an increase in the sound of the transmitted voice overlying lung tissue in the second stage of pneumonic consolidation or hepatization (see below). Nevertheless, pneumonia was no longer a symptomatic diagnosis and a static autopsy finding; it had both a structural and a physiological progression that could now be defined in the living patient.

Pulmonary edema, or swelling of the lung tissue, was first described by Laennec in the autopsy of Marie-Mélanie Basset, the chambermaid whose case history is the earliest definite record of mediate auscultation. She had suffered from shortness of breath, swollen legs, and anasarca; her breath sounds were diminished. Autopsy revealed serous infiltration of the lower lobes of the lungs, or pulmonary edema, but there is no evidence that the findings had been anticipated before her death.[54]

The unexpected postmortem finding in Basset may have prompted Laennec to seek the stethoscopic signs by which the same changes could be identified before the patient's death. In this endeavor, he was only partially successful. Rattles were not mentioned in Basset's case, but "slight" or "crepitant" rattles, "less loud" than those heard in early pneumonia, were heard in the two other published cases of pulmonary edema. Even in these patients, who came along later in his research, the rattles were not essential to establishing a diagnosis. For the first patient, seen in April 1818, the diagnosis sheet had been lost and Laennec relied on his memory; in the second case, from May 1819, the patient was "sad and difficult," and auscultation could scarcely be practiced on her because of her "deafness and morosity." The key findings in all three patients with pulmonary edema came from the autopsy, not from auscultation.[55] Laennec credited Bichat with having been the first to draw medical attention to pulmonary edema.[56] Inexplicably, he failed to cite either of the two essays by Rostan on cardiac asthma, one of which he could not deny having read because he had been asked to comment on it at the Société de l'Ecole de Médecine in early May 1817.[57]

In pneumonia and pulmonary edema, a fairly reliable anatomical diagnosis could already be suspected on the basis of the patient's symptoms and the doctor's examination by observation, palpation, and percussion. The stethoscopic findings from these early physiological and clinical experiences were interesting, sometimes even confirmatory, but they were not essential to making a diagnosis. As will be shown in chapter 7, Laennec probably knew that he was dealing with pneumonia in most of these early cases before he began to listen.

THE BREAKTHROUGHS AND CLINICAL NEOLOGISMS

Breakthrough 1: Pectoriloquy (summer 1817)

Grmek has shown that it was only after Laennec recognized the powerful significance of what he called "pectoriloquy" that he began to appreciate the full potential of his discovery and started to work fervently at his research on auscultation.[58] Pectoriloquy (or "pectoriloquism," as John Forbes translated it)—meaning "the chest speaks" as ventriloquy means "the stomach speaks"—was the word Laennec gave to the exaggerated intensity of the patient's voice heard by the listener through the chest wall (fig. 6.4). The observer could judge the isolated increase (or decrease) in transmitted voice sounds by listening and comparing at many places over both lungs while the patient was speaking. Pectoriloquy was usually confined to a single well-defined site, and Laennec quickly associated it with a cavity in the underlying lung. It was the first of several neologisms that Laennec created to convey his new medical semiotics, predating even the new word, "stethoscope," and capturing the imagination of early commentators on auscultation, several of whom referred to the instrument as a "pectoriloque."[59] The recognition of this new sign took place not long before early September 1817 and corresponds well with the dates of the cases published in his treatise.

The first patient in whom Laennec claimed to have observed the phenomenon of pectoriloquy was a twenty-eight-year-old woman with fever and cough. Perhaps she was speaking instead of breathing quietly when the doctor was listening to her chest; he did not explain what had prompted the "examination of the voice." She displayed exaggerated intensity of voice over

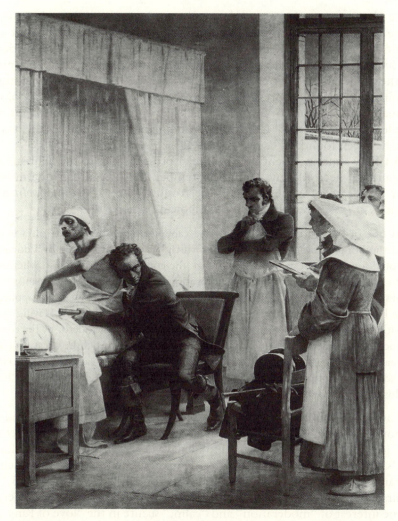

Figure 6.4. Laennec practicing direct auscultation on a patient at the Necker hospital. Mural by Théobald Chartran (1849–1907), Sorbonne. Normally Laennec preferred to use the stethoscope for a more comfortable posture. He also appreciated the polite distance that the instrument established between the physician and patients of differing sex and class, especially those with sweaty, smelly, and sometimes lice-ridden bodies that he described as "disgusting." Source: by permission of Sorbonne, University of Paris.

one square inch of chest wall just below the middle of the right clavicle. At that spot her "voice seemed to come directly from the chest and pass completely through the central canal of the cylinder." Buoyed by the discovery, Laennec proceeded to examine "most of the other patients in the [one-hundred-bed] hospital and found that twenty others displayed the same phenomenon. Most were in an advanced state of phthisis, but two or three had absolutely no other symptoms. "From that moment on," he said without specifying a date, he suspected that the sound was due to cavities in the lungs produced by the softening and evacuation of tubercles. Since many of the hospital patients eventually died, he was able to gather autopsy confirmation of this impression on numerous occasions.[60] The story of this woman was central to Laennec's February 1818 presentation at the Académie des Sciences.[61] Unfortunately no manuscript record of the pivotal case has been found.

An early announcement in the popular press testifies to the heuristic importance of pectoriloquy. On 26 September 1817, less than two months after the death of Mme de Staël, the royalist journal, *Annales politiques, morales, et littéraires*, published the following report:

> At one of the scholarly societies in the capital a report was made on a new method of physiological investigation, which has been introduced by a doctor noted for esteemed works. To recognize the conditions of the chest, whether there are alterations and what is their location, he makes use of the transmission of sound by the intermediary of a conducting body, one end of which is applied to his ear, the other to the parts of the thorax of the sick person. Having the patient speak, the sounds of the voice are transmitted to the doctor by the conductor when there are cavities and alterations in the organs of the chest. In the healthy state, it is only through the mouth that the sounds can be transmitted, and they cannot be heard through the thorax. The most useful conductor for this ingenious test is a simple roll of several leaves of paper.[62]

Laennec was probably aware of and may even have drafted or edited the announcement himself, although the turn of phrase belies that conjecture. The journal's editor, Mathieu G. F. Villenave (1762–1846), had been Laennec's teacher in Nantes, and had already invited him to contribute when he began publication in support of the Restoration on 16 December 1815.[63] In its first issue, Villenave stated the aims of his periodical: to use "wise energy" in the interest of "moderation" and "calm," secure in the "love of King and country."[64] I have been unable to determine which "scholarly society" heard the report on auscultation and who gave it, unless it was Récamier's aforementioned public demonstration "to a large gathering." But Laennec's remarks at the Académie des Sciences, five months later, suggest that the "scholarly society" may have heard from someone who, in Laennec's opinion, had an imperfect understanding of his research: "Several of my colleagues have taken the opportunity to offer verbal communications on the subject at diverse societies without me . . . newspapers and medical journals and even political papers have gathered incomplete ideas."[65] The report in the *Annales politiques, morales, et littéraires* may have been an attempt by Villenave, or by Laennec, to set the record straight.

For Laennec, pulmonary excavations were always associated with pectoriloquy, and he began to use the words interchangeably. The English visitor,

Charles Scudamore (1779–1849), told how an autopsy failed to confirm Laennec's diagnosis of a tuberculous cavity in one of the upper lobes. Laennec insisted on "making a closer inspection" of the pulmonary tissue himself and "discovered that a small part of the upper lobe had been left inside the chest; and upon its removal, the ulceration was found exactly as he had predicted."[66] Laennec recounted a similar story, possibly about the same case, citing Récamier as a witness.[67]

Gradually Laennec was forced to realize that all cavities may be associated with pectoriloquy, but not all pectoriloquy implied a cavity. By December 1817, he began to suspect that the new disease bronchiectasis, or dilatation of the large airways, might also result in pectoriloquy. To illustrate the possibility, he offered the brief example of an anonymous fifty-year-old woman who died in the Necker hospital in December 1817; possibly, she was the first and only patient he had encountered with the newly recognized pathological entity of bronchiectasis since he had begun his research into auscultation.[68] Two longer case reports, both provided by Jean-Bruno Cayol (1787–1856), came from patients examined long before the stethoscope had been invented: a three-and-a-half-year-old boy who died on 15 February 1808 at the *Hôpital des Enfans Malades* (Laennec had been invited to examine the child's lungs), and a seventy-two-year-old piano teacher who had died at the Charité on an unspecified date, which was prior to mid-1816 because Bayle had attended her autopsy.[69] At the Collège de France and in his second edition, Laennec was more explicit about the priority of Cayol for the anatomical description of bronchiectasis; in the interval he had, with Laennec's support, become a professor.[70]

Laennec seems to have resisted the possibility of pectoriloquy in bronchiectasis or in other conditions. His student René-Marie Rault (1794–1866) defended his thesis on 27 June 1819, shortly after closure had been invoked on the manuscript of Laennec's first edition. Rault claimed that, in dilatation of the bronchial airways, the voice was louder and more resonant, but true pectoriloquy was absent; however, he wrote, the subtle distinction could confuse the unpracticed ear.[71] A greater challenge came from Victor Collin (b. 1796) who claimed in his medical thesis, defended in December 1823, that he had heard pectoriloquy over the consolidated or hepatised portions of lung in the second stage of pneumonia.[72] This lesion bore no structural similarity to a cavity at all; in fact, quite the opposite was true. To cope with these manifestations of pectoriloquy in settings that were not cavity, Laennec later invented a completely new term, "bronchophony," which did not appear in the first edition of the treatise, but was described in the second with clinical case examples (see chap. 7).[73]

Back in his early research, however, Laennec did not foresee these later complications and subtleties; he was greatly excited by his discovery of pectoriloquy and thought that, being specific to cavities of the lung, it was also specific to phthisis. In February 1818, he devoted more than half his address at the Académie des Sciences to pectoriloquy. He described the physiological and pathological conditions in which it would be "evident," "imperfect" or "doubtful," and the physical properties of instruments that could enhance or diminish its appreciation. He ended with a powerful statement: "Art XXVI: From all that precedes, I must conclude that Pectoriloquy is a true pathognomonic sign of pulmonary phthisis and that it detects the disease with certainty long before any other [sign] can raise suspicions. I ought to add that it is the only sign that can be regarded as certain."[74]

The following year, Laennec reproduced this passage word for word in his treatise.[75] Rarely had any doctor dared to make such a confident assertion about an internal organic condition, especially in the absence of symptoms. The implications for tuberculosis and for all of medical practice were tremendous.

Breakthrough 2: Hippocratic Succussion (25 January 1818)

The second significant breakthrough occurred at the end of January 1818 with the recognition of succussion splash, or the sound of free fluid and air in the chest. The thirty-year-old army veteran, J. M. Potu, was auscultated on the day of his admission, 3 November 1817 and died on 26 February 1818, three days after Laennec had read his report to the Académie des Sciences. Potu's history, recorded by Laennec's Breton intern, René-Marie Rault, is the earliest published case for which a manuscript can be found. It is presented here both to explore the succussion breakthrough and to exemplify the method that Laennec applied to his research on auscultation.[76]

Potu was of "good constitution with a lymphatico-sangine temperament" and had been born of parents who were still alive and well. While a prisoner in the Russian campaign, he had suffered fever and earache, but he recovered and, at the peace of 1814, returned to Paris to work as a porter. He stopped working in May 1817 because of a cold, which steadily worsened over a month until he developed shortness of breath, a severe cough, and weakness. By August, he spent three weeks in the Charité hospital, but was discharged unimproved. Two weeks later he entered the Hôtel Dieu, which he left after two months, sicker than before.

On 3 November 1817, Potu was admitted to Necker hospital. On examination that day he was found to be "pale, very thin, with shining eyes, hot skin, rapid pulse, short respiration, and a heavy cough productive of thick yellow sputum." The percussion note of the chest was "less resonant on the right, especially the upper anterior portions," but was normal elsewhere. With the aid of the cylinder, respirations were heard throughout the chest, but a little less distinctly under the right clavicles. Pectoriloquy was present in a "slightly doubtful manner below the right clavicle and in the axilla." The contraction of the ventricles gave a "long, dull sound, and a certain impulse"; the contraction of the auricles was "brief and loud." Potu's appetite and thirst were moderate, his stomach soft and not tender, and he passed two or three liquid stools each day. "In consequence of these signs, he was given the following diagnosis: Pulmonary phthisis; heart in the natural state."

Over the next few days the patient's condition was unchanged, and the stethoscopic findings of louder respiration on the left and pectoriloquy on the right became more distinct, leading the physicians to suspect tuberculous excavations in the upper right lobe of his lung. By 18 November, when the patient spoke, coughed, or took a breath, a new ringing sound of uncertain significance was heard and called "metallic tinkling."

The report describes the evolution and treatment of the Potu's illness over several weeks, until a significant event. On 25 January 1818, "the patient said to M. Rault that for a few days he seemed to hear a knock (*choc*) of liquid in his chest when he rolled over. Informed of this circumstance, I [Laennec] had the patient sit, and, taking him by the shoulder, I shook the trunk. A fluctuation was heard like that produced by the shaking of a half-filled bottle. With the naked ear, it was difficult to establish from which side the sound was coming; but when the cylinder applied to the right side, the fluctuation was clearly heard when the shaking was stopped, while on the left no such sound was heard."

The patient's condition remained unchanged until 14 February

> when he was seized with a severe coughing spell that produced six ounces of sputum in fifteen minutes. . . . The patient began to insist that the doctors remove the liquid in his chest by an operation. After consulting several colleagues, including Messieurs Leroux, dean of the Faculty, and Récamier, I believed I ought to comply with his desires. . . . The operation was performed on 14 February by M. Baffos, chief surgeon of the hospital. Before the procedure, the chest was explored again by percussion and auscultation. . . . [T]he skin was stretched so that there would be no parallelism between its opening and that of the muscles. In twenty minutes, two pounds of a purulent, opaque liquid flowed from the chest mixed with bubbles of air. . . . Immediately after the surgery, the metallic tinking was louder. . . . [T]he respiration seemed no better, although the patient was relieved.

Five days later, the patient complained of the puncture site, although it appeared healed, and he became very weak, his skin was hot, and his abdomen distended. Loud rales were heard between the fourth and fifth interspace on the right and the jugular veins were full. His condition steadily worsened until his death on 26 February. In addition to Récamier and Leroux, a great number of doctors including Cayol, Fizeau, Gallot, Landré-Beauvais, and Ribes had seen the patient and verified the findings with the help of the cylinder.

The autopsy on 28 February was attended by M. Landré-Beauvais, Lucas, and Mac-Mahon. Before proceeding, Laennec repeated the commotion with the same results as before. Percussion of the thorax gave a clear note on the left and anterior portions of the right chest, but was dull over the right side and back. The right chest was larger than the left. Five pages were devoted to the postmortem findings, which included two pints of yellow green liquid in the right chest, exudate over the right parietal pleura, a collapsed, adherent right lung, and tubercles in the lung and peritoneum.

Potu seems to have been captivated by the research taking place around him: he volunteered his own impressions about the noises in his chest; he seemed to understand their significance, learned of possible therapies, and participated in decisions about his management. Had the physicians ignored his observations, they could not have made the discovery. On 5 February 1818, ten days after he first observed succussion, Laennec announced to the Société de l'Ecole de Médecine that he had a patient in the Necker hospital who when "shaken lightly" presents "the sign indicated by Hippocrates of fluid in the chest."[77] Laennec gave at least three Hippocratic references to succussion, but it appears in several other passages in the Hippocratic writings.[78]

Laennec collected records of the succussion sound from predecessors, including Ambroise Paré (1509–1590), Thomas Willis (1621–1675), G. B. Morgagni, and noticed that it had always been the patients who had noticed the sound first.[79] But he did not cite Corvisart's reference to the neglected practice, possibly because his former teacher had implied that Hippocratic succussion was so cumbersome that it deserved its oblivion.[80] Few physicians had troubled to verify it for themselves; most discounted it completely. Laennec admitted that the sound would be absent in effusion or empyema unless there was also a pneumothorax, which meant that free air would combine with free fluid in the chest. A year later, he accurately predicted the possibility of Hippocratic succussion in at least three cases before the patients were shaken.[81]

Potu's case, more than any other, made Laennec appreciate his participation in a great tradition of medical observation that had begun with Hippocrates. And by demonstrating that Hippocrates had been right, Potu allowed the Father of Medicine to partially redeem himself for what Laennec seemed to view as an incomprehensible error in a reference to direct auscultation: Hippocrates had said that water could be distinguished from pus if a sound like boiling vinegar could be heard when the ear is applied to the chest.[82] Laennec engaged in a philological discussion about the merits of various translations, in which he recognized the importance of manuscripts. He could not refrain from drawing the rather concrete conclusion that Hippocrates had made a mistake. The redemption, through having recognized succussion, was only partial because Hippocrates did not state that an additional effusion of air, added to fluid, would be needed to produce a sound.[83]

One year later, Laennec let Rault perform a similar thoracentesis operation on the twenty-two-year-old Savoyard shoemaker, Pierre Moineau, who died four hours later. The patient was in extremis before the procedure began, and pus did not flow from the wound, although the autopsy demonstrated that the incision had been made in the right place. In the published version of the case, Laennec concealed the identity of the young surgeon, not because he had actually done anything wrong, but because, "in the eyes of the public, a surgeon is always wrong when he fails to attain the immediate goal of his operation," and he quoted a similar sentiment from Hippocrates.[84] Despite the elegant defense, Laennec also made it clear that the unnamed Rault had misunderstood his orders, but the patient would have died had the intern followed his instructions perfectly. Little perturbed by his harrowing experience, Rault closed the thesis that he had been preparing by asking if thoracentesis was dangerous and concluding that it was not.[85] In the 1820s, the role of the stethoscope in planning and positioning of thoracenteses operations became Laennec's preferred means of combating critics.

Potu's case exemplifies the method used during the period of intense investigation. Patients were auscultated frequently if not daily, and the hospital record in Latin was kept for future use in preparation of the final report.[86] The evolution of physical signs throughout the hospital admission now became a standard component of the records. Any unusual findings were confirmed by Laennec together with his students and demonstrated to as many other physicians as possible. Witnesses were invited to attend the post-mortem examination. Techniques that did not depend on the cooperation of the patient, such as percussion and succussion, were repeated on the cadaver before the autopsy, which followed a regular sequence: general description of the cadaver, then the detailed findings in the head, thorax, and abdomen, in that order. The final report was written in French by one of Laennec's students or assistants (on the right-hand side of the page only, leaving room for annotations). The title on the first page could be the diagnosis, an important anatomical lesion, or a stethoscopic sign. For a time, Laennec seems to have conceived of the anatomical and stethoscopic findings as equivalent: in the place where the diagnosis would normally be written, he would sometimes supply the name of the stethoscopic sign instead of the name for a disease or an organic lesion. A table of lesser findings usually from the autopsy or the history would follow on the left side of the first page. Some of these reports are corrected and annotated by Laennec himself. Physiological events in the life history of the patient, in the physical examination, and in the progression of the disease were emphasized in the written descriptions.

Breakthrough 3: Metallic Tinkling and the Antemortem Detection of Cavity (3 February 1818)

Metallic tinkling was a particular ringing quality to auscultated respiration, voice, or cough that sounded like "a little bell that had just finished ringing or a fly buzzing in a porcelain vase."[87] Laennec said it resulted from a sort of echo in the chest and was a pathognomonic sign either for pneumothorax with a small quantity of fluid, or for a vast cavity in the lung. Metallic tinkling could be heard with respiration, he said, but it was more obviously associated with the voice or cough. Evidently he did not recognize this sign until after the discovery of pectoriloquy, when his attention had turned to the voice. By the time he published the first edition of his treatise, Laennec claimed to have heard metallic tinkling and accurately predicted the autopsy findings on only four occasions.[88] Two of these four observations were published, and will be summarized below. The first is the earliest case in which he could prove the significance of the sound; the overlap with his exploration of succussion is interesting. The second is the final case to be collected before he went to press.

On 29 January 1818, four days after Potu had invited his doctors to appreciate the succussion splash, the Necker hospital admitted Mme N***, a forty-year-old woman who had suffered from a cough for five months. She was discovered to have pectoriloquy in the middle and upper left chest, and by 3 February Laennec also heard "metallic tinkling" in the same place, a sound he had been following in Potu since late November. Eager to test the new observation being investigated in Potu, the doctors also shook Mme N***, but no succussion sound was heard. Laennec concluded that she had a "vast excavation in the middle of the left lobe" with only a "small quantity of liquid tuberculous matter." She died on 8 February, two and a half weeks before Potu would die and three days after Laennec had made his announcement to the Société de l'Ecole about succussion. Her autopsy the following day confirmed his predictions.[89]

The second case is that of the fifty-year-old laundress, Marie Levas, whose physical condition made her appear twenty years older. Laennec heard pectoriloquy and metallic tinkling when she coughed, and predicted a vast excavation in the right upper lobe of the lung. He narrowly missed collecting autopsy confirmation in this, the last observation gathered for the treatise, because he was obliged to expel Levas from the hospital for "having seriously disrupted the good order of the ward." Six weeks later, she was readmitted with her "physical condition unchanged." One cannot help but wonder if her mental state, at least, had shifted to contrition, or if negotiations had taken place between the nurses, who were obliged to care for an uncooperative patient, and the doctors, who wanted to complete one final research observation. She died on 6 June 1819, and once again autopsy confirmed Laennec's predictions.[90]

Like pectoriloquy and succussion splash, Laennec believed that the sign of metallic tinkling had a diagnostic power that could not be matched by any other modality in the clinical setting. To emphasize his point he referred to Bayle's treatise on phthisis that had included five cases of pneumothorax, none of which had been recognized before the autopsy. He eulogized his dead friend's superior clinical skills, his religious faith, and his rigorous attention to duty, but said that "a man cannot see everything and is not equally apt for observations every day." He continued, "using only percussion, it is morally impossible to recognize pneumothorax."[91]

Breakthrough 4: Antemortem Detection of Emphysema (July 1818)

Emphysema of the lung was a pathological alteration that involved expansion of air cells and loss of tissue. Laennec cited a few anatomical descriptions, including a case seen by Magendie and a long description by Matthew Baillie (1761–1823), but he claimed to be the first to write about emphysema as a separate entity. He said that he had noticed it long before he discovered auscultation, although he had thought it to be quite rare. Use of the stethoscope allowed him to recognize its presence in still-living individuals and had caused him to change his mind about its frequency.[92]

In a person with emphysema, the chest might be inflated and cylindrical, the percussion note would be resonant, but the breath sounds would be diminished. Not only did Laennec have to convince his readers of the potential for its detection before a patient's death, he had to convince them of the very existence of this organic change as a distinct entity. In contrast to the absence of cases for the ancient and well-understood conditions of pneumonia and catarrh, five case observations and a plate of illustrations were provided in the discussion of new disease of pulmonary emphysema. Even though he had taken the anatomical pieces to the engraver, along with his drawings and those of Toulmouche, he was dissatisfied with the illustrations of emphysema (fig. 6.5).[93]

The first observation used in the treatise was that of Marie C***, a woman who had died at the Charité hospital in 1802 during Laennec's studies with Corvisart. She was likely the first patient Laennec had ever seen with pulmonary emphysema. The second case was J. B. Cocard, a thirty-seven-year-old farmer admitted to Necker hospital on the first of three occasions on 25 May 1818 in the midst of Laennec's most intense research. The man's swollen feet and genitals, shortness of breath, and bluish skin led the doctors to think of heart disease. But by the first week of July, the resonance of his chest and the absence of breath sounds made Laennec predict the finding of emphysema, which was confirmed by autopsy when the farmer died of smallpox in October 1818. The cardiac condition was considered secondary to the chronic changes in the lung.[94]

Cocard was probably the first patient in whom Laennec had accurately predicted the postmortem finding of emphysema. The three other emphysema cases in the treatise were collected shortly after and quickly, within a three-week period ending 11 January 1819. The frequency with which Laennec was beginning to recognize what he had thought was a rare condition made him wonder if he was beginning to hear simply what he expected to hear. In the final patient, fifty-two-year-old chambermaid Jeanne Jolivet, he had been confident of the presence of an excavation in the right upper lobe; however, he hesitated to record an additional diagnosis of emphysema, despite the suggestive findings. He "suspended his judgment," he said, because he was "somewhat astonished at the number of patients in whom [he] was

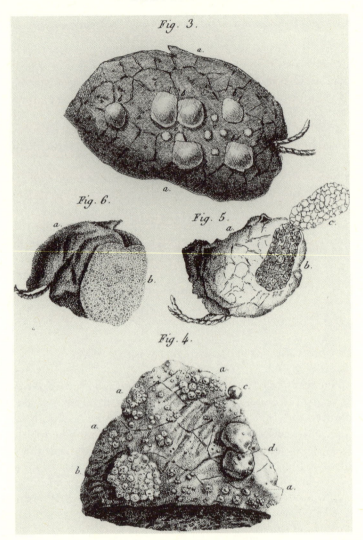

Figure 6.5. Views of pulmonary emphysema. Laennec had difficulty rendering the thin dilated air cells. Dissatisfied with his own drawings and those of his students, he took the anatomical specimens to an engraver whose pictures, he thought, were no more successful. Source: *Traité* (1819, 1: Plate III). Photograph: Queen's Medical Photography Services.

finding signs of this disease since [he] had begun to pay special attention to it."[95] But the autopsy showed that his clinical impression had been correct. On 3 June 1819, he drew attention to this new discovery in pathological anatomy, by presenting the Société de l'Ecole de Médecine with "portions of the lungs of an individual who had been subject to a sort of emphysema about which he propose[d] to speak in a book he is now having printed."[96]

*Breakthrough 5: Egophony and the Antemortem Detection
of Pleural Effusion (Early 1819)*

Laennec did not fully appreciate the distinctive sound he eventually called
"egophony" until early 1819. "Egophony," another neologism—referring
to the bleating voice of a goat—referred to the distinctive nasal quality of the
voice heard through the chest wall overlying the upper level of a collection
fluid in the thoracic space. The word was not mentioned in his February
1818 report to the Académie des Sciences, in which he described a "type of
pectoriloquy" that he might later have called egophony: "choked-sounding
like a ventriloquist with a sort of vibrating as if blowing across a cracked
reed."[97] Nor did the word "egophony" appear in any published account until
Rault's thesis, defended July 1819, in which it was used interchangeably with
"salpingophony, as if someone were speaking through a trumpet."[98] Eventually, egophony became equivalent to a diagnosis of acute pleural effusion,
just as pectoriloquy had come to signify cavities of the lung.

The prototypical case of egophony may have been sixty-year-old Marie-
Magdeleine Grigy, daughter, wife, and mother of soldiers, who was admitted
to the Necker hospital seeking shelter rather than treatment, on three separate occasions between 3 February 1818 and February 1819 (fig. 6.6). The
doctors' special interest in her case may have made them tolerant of her presence. In mid-February 1818, they detected "pectoriloquy" under the spi-
nous process of her right scapula, and a peculiar quality to her voice—"*vox
agrota*" and "*beaucoup plus aigue.*" During Grigy's admissions, the unusual
sound was labeled simply "pectoriloquy"; however, her hospital record was
later labeled and "diagnosed" by Laennec as "egophony perhaps together
with pectoriloquy."[99] She survived her experiences and autopsy confirmation
of the significance of egophony had to be found in others. Similarly, a post
hoc diagnosis of "egophony" was also added by Laennec to the case report
of the sixty-year-old shawl maker Jacques Dumesnil, who had been admitted
12 February 1819 and whose autopsy showed small pleural effusions.[100]

In his published discussion of egophony, Laennec admitted that he had
initially conceived of it as a variation of pectoriloquy and had long "confused" the two sounds. By late March 1819, he reconsidered the diagnosis
given to the still-living, forty-seven-year-old Jean Edmé, when he found
"pronounced egophony" with a "bleating" quality to the voice under the left
scapula—a sound that had not been "heard" at admission two weeks earlier,
although all other signs pointed to an effusion.[101] Three weeks later, Laennec
was so sure of his distinctive, new sign that he was able to claim that
"egophony was extremely evident" at the tip of the left scapula of forty-two-
year-old veteran Simon Villeron at his admission on 23 April 1819.[102]

The diagnostic pattern in the preceding four cases clearly shows that Laennec invented the concept of egophony between 12 February and late March
1819. He ascribed its recognition to the fortuitous outbreak of pleurisy in
the spring of 1819, during which he claimed to have found the new sign

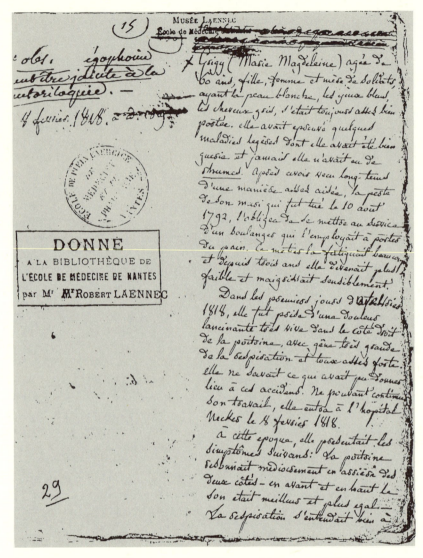

Figure 6.6. Title page of the six-page case history of sixty-year-old Marie-Magdeleine Grigy, February 1818, annotated at the upper left in the hand of Laennec: "*obs.*[ervation] *égophonie peut être jointe à la pectoriloquie*" (observation of egophony possibly combined with pectoriloquy). Source: Musée Laennec, MS Cl. I (b), f. 29r–31v. Photograph: Queen's Medical Photography Services from photocopy.

several times. He did not recall hearing it in any of the numerous cases of pneumonia that had been admitted to hospital in the winter of 1816–1817. Failing to ascribe the same limitation to his own powers of observation that he had found in those of Bayle, he confidently said, "a phenomenon as striking as egophony would not have escaped my attention."[103] He concluded that the sound had simply not been there to be heard; he, unlike his dead friend, could not possibly have missed an obvious physical sign.

Laennec was convinced that egophony had not been present in 1816–1817. Indeed pleural effusion was (and still is) essential for its observation, but another equally important epistemological ingredient may have been lacking. Would Laennec's mind have been prepared to take advantage of chance observations in a surfeit of pleuro-pneumonics before he had isolated and named pectoriloquy and begun exploring the voice? He displayed a vague awareness of the psychological precondition of a "prepared mind," supposedly enunciated much later by Louis Pasteur.[104] For example, Laennec said that he would have found egophony in two patients whom he had examined in late 1817 and July 1818, if only he had "looked for" it.[105] He made a similar references to the psychological importance of prior definition and description on at least three other occasions: when he accounted for the failures of his interns to keep track of certain details in the earliest observations of emphysema; when he worried about having overdiagnosed emphysema in the case of Jolivet; and when he made a retrospective revision of pectoriloquy to egophony.[106]

The notion of "prepared mind" raises important questions about the impossibility of liberating scientific observations and their interpretation from prior assumptions; these interrelationships extend to the metaphorical baggage of scientific language.[107] Laennec had to invent language to express the sounds and their anatomical significance, and once he possessed the words, the ideas became objects to be sought. Each stethoscopic sign was a tiny theory that came to influence his subsequent observations, in the manner described in the epigraph of Bayle's nephew at the beginning of this chapter.

THE PUBLICATION AND THE RETREAT

As Laennec's research moved through its increasingly hectic stages, his fatigue grew and his wish to retire to Brittany became a resolution. Even before he had discovered pectoriloquy, his days were exhaustingly full, and opportunities to escape to the country had vanished. In April 1817, during the admission of Marie-Mélanie Basset, he apologized to a friend for his delay in writing and confided his desire to leave Paris: "I have often been surprised that you and other colleagues retired to very small towns. Today I strongly approve and congratulate you and (just between us) I myself am longing to arrange my affairs so that in a few years I can retire to Lower Brittany. If I had what I am owed here, it could be today."[108]

TABLE 6.1
Theses of Laennec's Students and Other Associates, 1818–1823

Author	Subject	Date of Defense
Beaugendre	apoplexy	27 June 1818
Baume	pneumonia	5 June 1819
Rault	diagnostic signs in the lung	27 June 1819
Mazet	phthisis	3 July 1819
Dalbant	arteritis	29 July 1819
Noverre	aortic aneurysm	15 Jan 1820
Toulmouche	diagnostic signs in the heart	10 Feb 1820
M. Laennec	auscultation	16 June 1821
Vyau de Lagarde	antimony (tartar emetic)	1822
Bouillaud	aneurysms	23 Aug 1823
Collin	auscultation	20 Dec 1823

By the end of April 1819, Laennec told his cousin that he had sold a projected thirty-five thousand copies of the first two editions of the *Traité de l'auscultation* for a total of seven thousand francs and that the work was being printed for release in July. "I was astonished by the price I obtained, compared with that of first editions of other successful medical books. . . . Bichat sold the four volumes and the rights to his *Anatomie général* for only 3000F, and me, I will keep the rights."[109] To his father, however, he understated by five hundred francs the amount that he would receive from the sale of the first edition.[110]

Ambroise and Mériadec were joined by other young doctors who participated in the clinical work, several of whom would write theses on the stethoscope and chest disease.[111] If students did not concentrate on auscultation, they would at least mention the technique, refer to it in cases, and announce the forthcoming book.[112] Before the release of Laennec's treatise, the faculty had approved five theses in which auscultation had been given a prominent place—one in the summer of 1818 and four in June and July of 1819 (see table 6.1). There may have been some professorial objections to this flurry of activity over the new technique: Toulmouche recalled that Laennec had had his old rival Dupuytren removed from his examining board, for his hostile refusal to approve the topic.[113] Praise for one's instructor was de rigueur and Laennec's students conformed to this rule: they were "honored" and "glorified" to be pupils of the "celebrated practitioner"; one student found a generous measure of Corvisart's "*tact particulier*" in Laennec; another said that he had surpassed the goals of Hippocrates.[114] After Laennec's *Treatise* had appeared, auscultation would creep into the dissertations of other students, one of whom, J. B. Bouillaud (1796–1881), said that the technique was more effective in diagnosing aneurysms than Laennec himself realized.[115]

As the research slowed and printing began, Laennec planned the details of his escape. He would repair Kerlouarnec and derive an income from the Pont l'Abbé farms, which would be enlarged by draining the marsh. He could keep his hand in medicine by consulting and working on subsequent editions of his treatise of auscultation. Perhaps he could finally publish the long-neglected treatise on pathological anatomy. He knew that what he was doing might seem odd: "After nineteen years of very tedious work, I am leaving Paris without a fortune and without even being assured of the necessities, at the very moment my dreams are to be realized. If my nerves had allowed me to stay another four or five years, I would have left with twenty or twenty-five thousand francs of savings. My book would have given me the first vacant chair in medicine." But his health simply would not permit him to be a professor who spends his life "getting out of an armchair only to climb into a cabriolet." He had been planning on an early retirement for at least a decade; now it was time. His greatest regret was to leave Mériadec alone in Paris with his studies incomplete.[116]

The family was horrified. Preoccupied by his own misfortune, the uncle Guillaume blamed Laennec for spoiling his plans. He predicted that the homesick nephew would eventually be bored in the country; life in the provinces was a "veritable hell"—no one would chose to live there if he had any means of escape; he must keep a small place in Paris. Laennec's father felt waves of anticipatory grief for the money the son would not earn. The brothers corresponded with each other, with Théophile, and with his cousins over the madness.[117]

Laennec consoled them all: "I have never been bored in my life," he told his uncle, "except perhaps once at school when Mr. Tardivel kept me after class." And he agreed that it was "a pity that auscultation was not the discovery of someone who would know how to make a lot of money from it." To his father, he tried to explain his financial situation and the importance of the wretched attacks of "asthma" that could keep him in bed for five days at a stretch unless he took regular and strenuous exercise.[118] Two brief hunting trips in the summer of 1819 strengthened the convictions about his needs, but the benefits of each journey had evaporated after only a few days back in Paris.[119] Only Mériadec understood the emotional and physical reasons for the departure.[120]

In mid-July 1819, Laennec delivered a printed copy of his *Traité de l'auscultation médiate* to the faculty of medicine, with a letter requesting permission to include an accompanying Latin dedication to its professors. He did not expect his discovery to have the same utility as that of the "illustrious" Jenner nor the same impact as that of Auenbrugger and the "eminent" Corvisart; but he dared to hope that in simplifying the matter of anatomical diagnosis, doctors would be able to concentrate on cures.[121] Desgenettes, Royer-Collard, and Duméril were assigned to study the matter, and on 5 August, they reported that the offer of respect and recognition should be accepted.[122] By 19 August the final copy with its dedication had been delivered to the faculty and was available from the publisher, nine hundred pages divided in two volumes, which sold for thirteen and sixteen francs each. A stethoscope would cost the buyer two or three francs more.[123]

The following month Laennec donated his anatomical specimens to the medical school, sold all his possessions with the exception of a hundred books, and gave up the apartment in the rue du Jardinet, where he had lived for nearly fifteen years.[124] On 4 October 1819, he set out for Brittany, for at least a year, he said, "possibly forever."[125]

CHAPTER SEVEN

The Treatise on Mediate Auscultation: The Lungs

Pathological anatomy is without doubt the most certain
light to guide the physician . . . but . . . it is not easy
to appreciate that which is healthy and that which is
sick, that which is cause of the disease and that
which is merely its effect.

—*Laennec,* Traité *1819,* 1*:xxi–xxii*

No pathological case presents with more obvious characteristics of an ailment due to a simple disturbance in
nervous influence than does shortness of breath with
puerile respiration.

—*Laennec,* Traité *1826, 2:75*

As HE HAD INTENDED, Laennec's book on auscultation was understood as a
contribution to pathological anatomy as soon as it was published. Less evident however, both then and now, was the author's additional intention that
auscultation should also be accepted as a contribution to physiology. In this
chapter and the next, we will leave the thread of Laennec's life to analyze the
ideas in his most important publication. I will review the status of his treatise
as a contribution to pathology and the attendant shift in disease concepts,
especially as they pertain to the chest. Without refuting the general view that
the *Treatise on Mediate Auscultation* can be read as a text in pathological
anatomy, I will show that Laennec also conceived of auscultation as a physiological process with physiological applications, and that he believed it could
reach beyond and compensate for the limitations of pathological anatomy.
This vision of auscultation as a multidisciplinary tool and its interplay with
older disease concepts influenced the theory of disease that he would elaborate at the end of his life.

The two editions of the *Treatise on Mediate Auscultation* were separated
by seven years and contain a number of differences; however, most of the
changes for the 1826 edition were not retractions, but rather expansions and

modifications to clarify the opinions he had held in 1819 or to shore up his authority as a master of the new technique. For this reason, both editions will be used in the following analysis. To illustrate the blend of pathology and physiology in Laennec's concept of disease, special attention will be given to the sections of his treatise devoted to tuberculosis, pneumonia, bronchial dilatation (bronchiectasis), asthma, and heart disease; the stethoscopic signs discovered after 1819, such as bronchophony, pathological "puerile respiration," and pericardial friction rub, are also included. This chapter deals with the lungs; the next chapter, with the heart. At the end of chapter 8, I summarize the clinical reasoning used in Laennec's construction of stethoscopic signs. The reviews and his reactions to them will be more fully addressed in chapter 9 where we once again pick up the thread of his life.

AUSCULTATION AND THE PATHOLOGY AND PHYSIOLOGY OF DISEASE

Auscultation, combined with percussion, brought pathological anatomy from the morgue to the ward, and it did so in a manner that bridged the transition from philosophical sensualism to scientific positivism. The mysterious changes inside the "bony cage" of the patient's chest (στῆθος) could now be brought to view—explored or examined (σκοπεῖν)—through the doctor's hearing. The stethoscope eliminated speculation about the range of possible diagnoses through "signs" that indicated organic "facts," independent of the physiological circumstances that had been their cause.

The *Treatise on Mediate Auscultation* introduced a diagnostic method that endorsed and consolidated the new way of thinking about disease, a method that had been on the agenda of medical research in Paris and elsewhere since the end of the eighteenth century (fig. 7.1). The stethoscope made it possible to reveal physical changes before the patient died. Disease no longer had to be defined by subjective symptoms felt and described by the patient; it could now be defined and classified as a physical change detected objectively by the doctor, sometimes even without the patient's knowledge. As a result, concepts of disease could be reformulated to incorporate anatomical observations. The stethoscope had finally ruptured the epistemological barrier that had prevented the seemingly useful pathological anatomy from finding applications in the clinical setting. The conceptual shift from symptoms to organs was reflected in new names for diseases: shortness of breath, cough, coughing of blood, chest pain, and fever would become characteristics of the narrower and more structurally committed entities of pleural effusion, pulmonary edema, emphysema, bronchiectasis, and tuberculosis. With his meticulous, even classic descriptions of the newly recognized organic diseases of the lung, Laennec was an active participant in this trend.

Laennec also saw his invention as a boon to physiology. Ever since Buisson's 1802 thesis on the classification of physiological processes, he had been

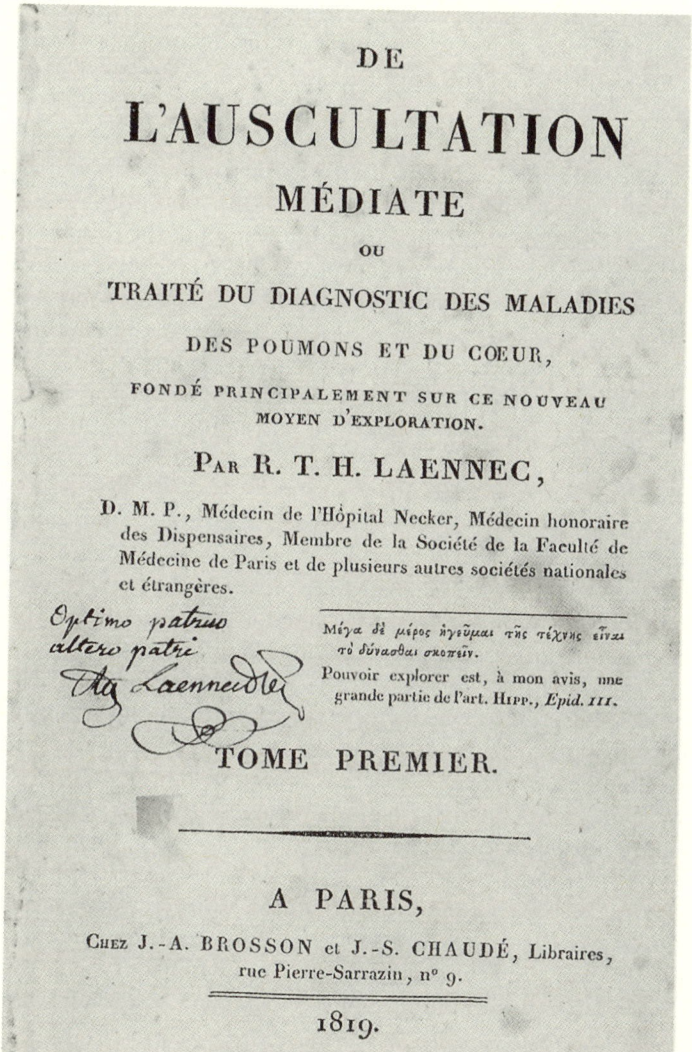

DE

L'AUSCULTATION

MÉDIATE

OU

TRAITÉ DU DIAGNOSTIC DES MALADIES

DES POUMONS ET DU COEUR,

FONDÉ PRINCIPALEMENT SUR CE NOUVEAU
MOYEN D'EXPLORATION.

PAR R. T. H. LAENNEC,

D. M. P., Médecin de l'Hôpital Necker, Médecin honoraire
des Dispensaires, Membre de la Société de la Faculté de
Médecine de Paris et de plusieurs autres sociétés nationales
et étrangères.

*Optimo patruo
altero patri*
Laennec

Μέγα δὲ μέρος ἡγοῦμαι τῆς τέχνης εἶναι
τὸ δύνασθαι σκοπεῖν.

Pouvoir explorer est, à mon avis, une
grande partie de l'art. Hipp., *Epid. III.*

TOME PREMIER.

A PARIS,

CHEZ J.-A. BROSSON et J.-S. CHAUDÉ, Libraires,
rue Pierre-Sarrazin, n° 9.

1819.

Figure 7.1. Title page of the first edition of Laennec's treatise on mediate auscultation, August 1819. This copy was dedicated and signed by the author for his
uncle "*optimo patruo, altero patri*" (to the best godfather; to my second father).
Photograph: Medical Historical Library, Yale University School of Medicine, New
Haven, Conn.

aware of the difference between hearing and listening. The word "auscultation" implied an active physiological process that required both human intelligence and sensory perception.[1] Not only did stethoscopy make use of the
examiner's physiology, but it also required a living patient, often one who
would cooperate. Breathing, speaking, coughing, sighing, snoring, yawning,

and the beating of the heart, were not to be found in the dead. In fact, with auscultation, Laennec could not emulate his professors' percussion practice of eliciting signs before an autopsy: in a cadaver, life functions had ceased and there was nothing to hear.

Laennec's vision of physiological applications for his technique was evident before he published his book. In the earliest press releases it was touted as "a new method of physiological investigation," and at the Académie des Sciences, he announced that his study of the voice and the heart was strongly linked to "physics and physiology."[2] Above all else, the structure of the first edition of the *Treatise on Mediate Auscultation* proclaimed its physiological purpose. It was organized in sections, not by disease, nor by anatomical alterations, but by the "exploration" of four physiological processes: voice, respiration, rales, and circulation. Again it was in the thesis of the uncited Buisson where Laennec had first encountered the physiological possibilities in "examination of the voice," which, with its attendant sign of pectoriloquy, opened the door for auscultation.

In the structure of Laennec's first edition, diseases were subservient to the physiological processes that allowed their diagnosis. For example, pectoriloquy, the altered sound of the transmitted voice, was the pathognomonic sign of phthisis; therefore, phthisis was discussed as a disease of the voice. Similarly, pneumonia was associated with rales—bubbling or silent respiration; it became a disease of rales. This conceptual classification helps to explain how Laennec could have overlooked what now seems to be the obvious presence of pectoriloquy/bronchophony in the hepatization stage of pneumonia. The disease declared itself by its symptoms; being a disease of rales or absent breathing, it need not be investigated through the voice. Support for this explanation comes from the chronology of his discovery: Laennec said that his work on pneumonia had been conducted during an outbreak in the winter of 1816–1817; his recognition of pectoriloquy and his interest in the voice did not take place until the following summer or fall (see chap. 6).

Clinical practice had instructed Laennec in the limits of the new science of pathological anatomy. Pathological physiology could take over where pathological anatomy left off, and the stethoscope would contribute to both. His concept of altered physiology was constructed on the model of anatomical change, and it had its origin in "Bayle's nostalgia" and their shared notion of a vital lesion. His teacher, Corvisart, also held strongly psychosomatic views, but, as W. R. Albury has shown, Corvisart rejected the ancient notion of *vis medicatrix naturae* (healing power of nature). For him, life brought about its own end and the psyche could only damage the soma.[3] For Corvisart's more conservative students, however, the life force could both harm and heal. Laennec held these views before 1819, but he articulated them more strongly in the second edition, possibly because he thought that they had been misunderstood in the first.

Of the fifty complete case histories in Laennec's treatise, at least fifteen displayed psychological preconditions with their physical ailments. Among the many other shorter histories, ten patients—five in the first edition, nine in the second, four in both—had also experienced psychic distress (see Appendix C). The Revolution had stripped three people of secure employment in opulent houses; many others had suffered privation and fatigue in the subsequent wars. Seven patients, including a female, had been attached to Napoleon's armies, and two had been taken prisoner. One woman's ailment followed the fright she experienced in the battle of Brienne; another fell ill after the death of her husband. Psychological preconditions could also act in a positive sense: two patients, one who survived and another who lived longer than expected, were said to have a special "equanimity." And Laennec said that he "knew a man," whose health had broken at age twenty-two after prolonged studies and who was cured by vacations in the country or vigorous walking; in 1812, the pressure of the man's work in Paris forced him to abandon exercise and brought back his symptoms.[4] I think that this un-named man was Laennec himself. This case illustrated the nonorganic nature of angina pectoris. Its deletion from the second edition, published in the year of Laennec's death, tends to suggest that by 1826 he realized that his chronic "nervous" illness had finally become organic.

LAENNEC'S TUBERCULOSIS: PATHOLOGY AND PHYSIOLOGY AT WORK

The word "tuberculosis," said to have been coined by Johann Lukas Schön-lein (1793–1864) in 1830, was derived from the name of the anatomical lesion that typifies the disease. It arose as part of the reformulation of disease naming—from symptom-based to lesion-based terminology—that had been unleashed by Laennec's discovery. Nevertheless, artistic, literary, and paleo-pathological studies confirm that tuberculosis is a condition of great antiquity. Until the early nineteenth century, it was identified exclusively by the symptoms of fever, sweating, and wasting—the pattern graphically named, "consumption" or "phthisis." With the advent of anatomoclinical medicine, the disease was linked to the presence of certain changes in the internal organs of the body, and the diagnostic concept shifted to embrace the presence of organic lesions. It was not until after the work of Jean-Antoine Villemin (1827–1892) and of Robert Koch (1843–1910) that long-suspected ideas about its communicability were proven. As a result, the concept would change once again to conform to the pattern of an infectious disease as defined by the newly elaborated germ theory.[5]

Tuberculosis is thought to have been the single most important cause of death in early nineteenth-century Paris. Laennec claimed that one-third of the people in the city's hospitals suffered from phthisis.[6] Nevertheless, retrospective determination of the mortality owing to this disease is difficult. Contemporary estimates of the annual death rate from pulmonary tuberculosis in Paris range between 400 to 500 deaths per 100,000 population; in Britain it may have been higher, on the order of 500 to 600 per 100,000 population. Because extrathoracic manifestations of tuberculosis were not usually recognized as variations on the same pathological process, the "real" death rate from what might now be called tuberculosis would likely have been much greater than those published in contemporary sources. Similarly, there seems to have been considerable imprecision in diagnostic terminology. For example, tuberculosis is generally thought to have been endemic to rural France, but its effects are necessarily obscured in the contemporary categories of "periodic fever," so-called *paludisme* (malaria), and *affections des voies respiratoires* (disease of the airways).[7]

Pathology: Unification

In contributing to the anatomical shift in disease concepts, Laennec is frequently said to have "unified" tuberculosis.[8] "Unification" well describes the pathological anatomy in his views about phthisis, but it ignores his physiology. Before the stethoscope, physicians made distinctions between elements that are now considered two aspects of the same thing: on the one hand, there was the febrile wasting disease, called phthisis or consumption; on the other, there was the anatomical presence of tubercles. The existence of one did not necessarily imply the existence of the other. For centuries, the diagnosis of phthisis had been based on the distinctive symptom pattern of wasting leading to death, but there were many variations within the category. Some patients who wasted had fever; others did not, but they might have other symptoms such as polyuria, diarrhea, or tumor. In the late seventeenth century, Franciscus de la Boe, called "Sylvius" (1614–1672), had attempted to restrict the diagnosis of consumption to only those patients who wasted with fever and symptoms of chest dysfunction, preferably with tubercles in the lung.[9] Since it was impossible to determine the organic state of the lung before the death of the patient, other conditions, which might now be classified as chronic infections and cancer, met Sylvius's criteria for phthisis.

While attempts were being made to restrict the symptomatic diagnosis of phthisis to fevers accompanied by chest problems, physicians who were interested in anatomy also began to narrow the postmortem diagnosis of consumption. Acknowledging the diversity of the anatomical changes that could accompany consumption, Richard Morton (1637–1698) had described seventeen different clinical and pathological types in the lung, in addition to the consumptions of other body parts.[10] More than a century later, Portal, early investigator of Laennec's auscultation, had identified fourteen anatomical types of pulmonary consumption.[11] The new preoccupation with organic change in disease was reflected in three clinical consultations given for a single patient in 1772: references to a presumed "tuberculous state" of the left lung figured prominently in the doctors' statements, but their conclusions were derived from the patient's symptoms of pain, fever, breathlessness, and hemoptysis, not from an examination of the chest.[12] The three consultants each displayed a remarkable degree of optimism concerning the powers of medical art, but it seems that their optimism was not shared by their patients, whose gloom typified popular attitudes about consumption.[13] Portal lamented that without knowing the nature of the changes inside the lungs, doctors almost always made the diagnosis after the disease had progressed to an advanced state. He cited a phrase from Giorgio Baglivi (1668–1707): "*O quantum difficile est diagnoscere morbos pulmonum!*" (Oh how difficult it is to diagnose diseases of the lung). Laennec would also cite Baglivi's lament in his Latin preface, hoping, he said, to put it to rest; but it became a popular epigraph among his students and other medical writers in the early nineteenth century.[14]

Laennec's friend, Bayle, had moved into this realm of overlapping terminology with his 1810 treatise on pulmonary phthisis.[15] On the basis of organic appearances, Bayle reduced the anatomical types of phthisis to six: granular, miliary, ulcerous, calculous, cancerous, and melanotic. But by 1819, Laennec rejected the latter two categories because they represented types of malignancy, of which, he believed, he had written the original descriptions. As for the remaining four types, his complaint was reminiscent of Bayle's attack on Pinel: the difference between them was no greater than that between "ripe fruit" and "green fruit."[16] In chiding his meticulous colleague for not having paid enough attention to morbid changes, Laennec became the first of many to describe Bayle's "failure" or "error," which some historians explain as having resulted from a lack of imagination and/or a penchant for observation over definition.[17] These criticisms lack epistemological sensitivity: given Bayle's priorities and his clinical technology, his diagnosis of phthisis—like that of Sylvius—could not be more precise. Bayle had been striving for an organ-based method of diagnosis that could be applied at the bedside, yet it was impossible for him to perceive the nature of the internal lesions before the patient died. All six categories reasonably belonged to Bayle's phthisis because they were associated with the uniform clinical picture of wasting, chest symptoms, often with fever and hemoptysis, percussion signs of thoracic alteration, and, as shown in chapter 4, they always led to death.

Laennec was provided with many opportunities to examine cadavers containing tubercles. The chance discovery of pectoriloquy that led him to envisage the power of auscultation as a tool for the diagnosis of organic change had been made in a patient with phthisis. His detailed descriptions of tubercles, cavities, and other organic alterations were considered by his critical contemporaries to be prolix, but careful observation combined with auscultation allowed him to appreciate the tubercle as a unit lesion with a life history.

From the earliest days of his career, Laennec had insisted that there was only one type of phthisis, that accompanied by tubercles. Over the years, the number of different forms that he ascribed to tubercles would decrease. In his 1803 course on pathological anatomy, he had said that tubercles appeared in six forms: "enkysted;" "non-enkysted;" "in organs;" "in mucous membranes;" "infiltrating;" and "scrofulous."[18] In 1819, he said there was only one type of tubercle with three patterns of evolution: one typical ("isolated") and two atypical ("enkysted" and "infiltrative"). He illustrated the point with plates showing a lung with the lesions at various stages of development (fig. 7.2). Tubercles found in lymph nodes and other organs were identical to those found in the lung. These statements were repeated later in his lectures at the Collège de France, where he ascribed several nonpulmonary conditions to tubercles in other parts of the body, including idiotism, epilepsy, carreau, abscess, lumbar caries, scrofula of lymph glands, slow apoplexy, and a fatal disease simulating hydrocephalus.[19]

In 1826, for the second edition of his treatise, one final and stronger reduction was implemented: now there was one tubercle with only two patterns of development ("isolated" and "infiltration"), each having two stages (before and after softening). "Whatever the form in which the tuberculous matter develops, it begins as a grey, semitransparent matter that little by little becomes yellow, opaque, and dense. Then it softens, and slowly acquires a liquidity like pus, and, when it is expelled through the airways, it leaves cavities, commonly called ulcers of the lung, that we will designate as tuberculous excavations."[20] In short the evolution of the tubercle was constant, "whatever the form" or site of the tubercle.

The decreasing number of forms and stages of evolution of the lesion represents Laennec's "unification." One historian, who was enthusiastic over this insight, was "unable to imagine" how Laennec had "hit on the facts" and suggested that he was "either a superlative guesser or gifted in superlative degree with the power of generalization."[21] But Laennec's unification of tuberculosis was an insight provided by auscultation. With stethoscopy and percussion, he was able to delineate the location and texture of tubercles in the lungs and follow their precise evolution, their life cycle, as they progressed through caseation, evacuation, cavity, calcification, or miliary spread. He made his clinical observations over months and years and was able to relate the perceived organic changes to the state of the patient.

Pathology: Absence of Inflammation

Beyond unification, Laennec's pathological anatomy of tuberculosis contained two other important features: first, absence of inflammation either as a physiological process or as a concomitant finding; and second, emphasis on "perfectly lined" cavities in the case of a cure. Since at least 1803, Laennec had grouped the tubercle with the "nonanalogous accidental productions," the class of lesions that he had disputed with Dupuytren. For him, inflammation and tubercle were independent pathological entities; the one had nothing to do with the other. As a result, pleurisy, which Laennec defined as the disease resulting from pleuritis or "inflammation of the pleura," had only a peripheral role in his clinical picture of phthisis. But pleural effusions and chest pain

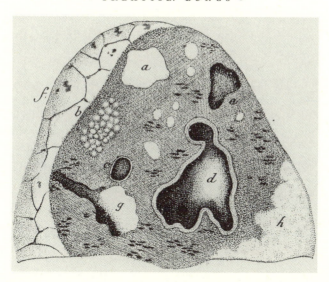

Figure 7.2 Several stages in the life history of the tubercle shown in a single lung. *a*, early, yellow tubercles; *b*, groups of incipient tubercles; *c*, cartilaginous cyst containing tuberculous matter; *d*, tuberculous cavity lined by two membranes; *e*, a small tuberculous cavity, which is empty but not lined by a membrane; *f*, surface of the lung; *g*, softened and evacuated tubercle. Source: *Traité* (1819, 1: Plate II, fig. 1). Photograph: Queen's Medical Photography Services.

occur frequently in people who suffer from tuberculosis. How did he reconcile the coincidence of pleurisy with tubercle that he must have seen on many occasions? In three ways: first, he said that tubercle in the pleura led to "hydropsy," a form of effusion without inflammation; second, tubercles could be situated within a zone of inflammation, itself secondary to the presence of tubercles or other causes; and third, all debilitated patients, including consumptives, were "subject to" pleurisy.[22] Elsewhere, Laennec enumerated the predisposing causes of pleurisy and effusion, but tubercle is notably absent.[23]

Several factors may have contributed to Laennec's reluctance to group the two lesions, inflammation and tubercle, into a single disease. At the outset, his early work on peritonitis may have led him to seek isolated diagnoses for inflammatory conditions of other membranous structures like the peritoneum and the pleura. When pleural effusion accompanies tuberculosis, tubercles are not necessarily found in the pleural membrane; therefore, in a phthisic patient, pleural effusion could be seen as an inflammatory process, independent of the tubercles contained in the lung.

Next, after the discovery of auscultation, Laennec tended to ascribe a single disease to each auscultatory sign, as is shown at the end of chapter 8. For example, the sign of egophony became equivalent to inflammation of the pleura; the sign of pectoriloquy meant phthisis. Two signs; two diseases. This specificity of auscultatory signs was an important aspect of Laennec's clinical reasoning. Just as it could operate forward in the construction of signs, it could also work backward in the fine-tuning of the diseases that the signs were supposed to represent.

Finally, Laennec was struck by the observation that tubercles are almost always surrounded by healthy tissue. On the rare occasions when inflammation *was* present, Laennec thought it may have been induced by the prior existence of tubercles and not vice versa.[24] This opinion was welcomed with enthusiasm by his translator, but it was in direct opposition to that of Broussais, who cited irritation and inflammation as the physiological cause of almost all lesions.[25] The animosity between the two physicians may have caused Laennec to lean further away from pathophysiological explanations based on inflammation (see chap. 9).

Pathology and Physiology: Cure and Perfectly Lined Cavities

Laennec's interest in perfectly lined cavities and well-organized scars stemmed from his unorthodox opinion about the possibility of healing in tuberculosis. His first edition was criticized for not addressing treatment for phthisis, a problem he tried to remedy in the second. The oversight arose from his idea that only nature could cure this disease. The belief was diametrically opposed to the opinion of many others, including Bayle, who had maintained that phthisis could be defined by its inevitable fatality. The insight about structure and cure, like that concerning the life cycle of the unit tubercle, came from auscultation.

Laennec reminded his readers that "the destruction of a portion of lung tissue was not necessarily a fatal situation, because even wounds of this organ could heal."[26] The words chosen to describe healed lesions suggest that he was intrigued by the relationship of the morbid appearances to cure. For example, at autopsies of people with "healed phthisis" (i.e., when the patient had died of another disease), he found "cavities, lined by a membrane, . . . that do not contain tuberculous matter," "a smooth, thin, even membrane," "a very smooth membrane as if it were polished," "a well-organized cellular tissue," "a full and solid scar."[27] On the other hand, in patients who died with symptoms of phthisis, he sometimes observed "incomplete" or "uneven" lining of old cavities. For example, in the postmortem examination of Nicolas Herbé, who died of phthisis in March 1819, Laennec observed excavations with a thin, irregular lining, which "cried out when scraped with the scalpel."[28]

Healing may have anatomical properties, but it was a physiological product of nature, not of the art: "to remedy the destruction caused by tuberculous matter, nature . . . seems to produce this healing substance with seemingly exuberant abundance." And with respect to associated pleural effusion, "a cartilaginous cuff . . . seems to be the method used by nature to prevent effusion of tuberculous matter into the pleura."[29] These "completely scarred" excavations took on powerful significance in their promise of cure.

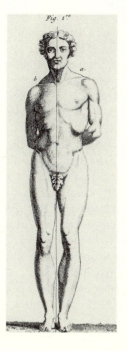

Figure 7.3. Man cured of chronic pleurisy with retraction of the chest; parts *a* and *b* draw attention to the different shoulder heights. Laennec was intrigued that significant lesions in the lung and elsewhere could persist without the slightest functional damage. He described this condition in M***, a distinguished Paris surgeon, who was in "very good health" and could lecture for two hours daily "without tiring." Source: *Traité* (1819, 1: Plate II, fig. 1; see also *Traité* 1819, 1: 369–377). Photograph: Queen's Medical Photography Services.

Physiology: Latency and Etiology

Identification of the presence of tubercles through the diagnostic signs of rales, bronchial breath sounds, and pectoriloquy was essential to the diagnosis of phthisis. Laennec also recognized the symptoms of wasting, periodic fever, hemoptysis, malar flush, chest pain, and breathlessness. Some patients who had been sick with tubercles could recover, but he also began to realize that patients who demonstrated signs of fresh tubercles were not always sick. The subjective experience of the patient was becoming an epiphenomenon of the disease.

With his stethoscope, Laennec, was the first clinician not only to imagine but also to diagnose serious organic alteration in the absence of symptoms (fig. 7.3). For both physicians and their patients, he implemented the medicalization concept that had originated with Corvisart.[30] Laennec had "unified" tuberculosis from the standpoint of pathological anatomy, but he continued to envisage two stages in its physiological evolution, reflecting two stages in development of its organic lesion. The first stage was latent and incurable; the second was associated with symptoms and could be cured, but only if the natural organic process moved to softening, complete evacuation, and a "completely cicatrized" cavity.

The meaning of "latency" wandered in the early nineteenth-century terminology. In 1825, P. C. A. Louis (1787–1872) would describe what he called "latent phthisis" in six patients who had not suffered the usual symptoms of the disease before their deaths and in whom autopsy revealed tubercles. This "latent" phthisis had insidiously claimed their lives without making them sick.[31] Louis's latent phthisis was not the same as that of Laennec, who would have searched for another explanation for the death of these patients, especially if he thought that the damage caused by the tubercles was "insufficient" to provoke death.[32] The phthisis was indeed latent, but, as such, it could not be the cause of death. Laennec's latent phthisis may not have been curable, but it did not kill.

The stethoscope indicated the presence of tubercles and/or scars in the lungs of patients who had no symptoms or whose illness had resolved, signs inaccessible to Bayle. When a patient with symptoms of phthisis recovered, Bayle and the prestethoscopic Laennec revised the diagnosis retrospectively to something else, such as nostalgia or chronic catarrh. But the older Laennec believed that some patients were cured. He collected histories in which symptoms of phthisis had disappeared with the persistence of signs; when the patients died later of some other problem, he performed autopsies hoping to demonstrate "scars" and "completely lined cavities" produced by nature from previously active tuberculosis. One of these cases had been published by Bayle as an example requiring a retrospective revision to nonphthisis. With the stethoscope, the same patient was found to have had a form of pulmonary consumption that had healed spontaneously with a perfectly lined cavity.[33] Without naming the patient, Laennec also referred to Bayle's account of himself (case 53) as another example of healed phthisis.[34] But his friend had labeled that illness "nostalgia," not phthisis, and in 1819, with Bayle already dead three years, the "healing" could well have been disputed.

When it came to causes of disease, Laennec, like his teachers, was reluctant to commit himself. In 1819, he said only the following: "the existence of tubercles is the cause and the anatomical characteristic of pulmonary phthisis." Because he defined phthisis as the presence of tubercles, this statement about its origin could be reduced to tautology: the cause of tubercles is tubercles.[35] Laennec did not reveal his understanding of the cause of tubercles until 1826, but he had held the ideas for a long time.

In his second edition, Laennec reviewed the etiological theories of contagion, heredity, climate, and environment and found fault with all. As for inoculability, he mentioned his own experience with an accidental slip of the saw that cut his finger in 1806; a tubercle appeared at the site of injury, but it slowly disappeared after he cauterized it, and, he confidently added, "I have never felt the slightest sequelae from this accident."[36] Here was evidence that tubercles could be inoculated, and that inoculation did not always lead to consumption. Laennec, whose brother and priest-uncle were thought to have died of phthisis, also considered the heredity theory. It was refuted, he said, by the observations that in some families with healthy parents, all the children were consumptive, and by the corollary that in others with consumptive parents and grandparents, the children were healthy.[37]

After the preamble, Laennec revealed a pathophysiological mechanism for phthisis: "among all the occasional causes [of phthisis], I know of none more certain than sad passions, especially when they are profound and prolonged."[38] He illustrated the statement with his decade-long experience in a strict, religious community of women. The unnamed order had not received official sanction and was barely tolerated by the Church because of the austerity of its dietary practices and its fixation on the "most terrible truths of religion." When a novice developed signs of phthisis, Laennec would advise her to leave: "almost all those who heeded the counsel were cured." The population of the community "turned over two or three times" with the successive loss of its members either to phthisis or to its preventative treatment. Those who were spared included the mother superior, the cook, the concierge, the gardeners, and the nurses—the only members who were allowed to go out.[39] Similarly, the observed differences in urban and rural statistics on phthisis were explained by the "fact" that city living was more depressing and stressful than country life. Laennec had twenty years of evidence from his own illness experiences and those of patients to support his theory.[40]

The cause of phthisis for Laennec was mediated by the same pathophysiological mechanism as Bayle's nostalgia: the concept of a vital lesion. In short, psychological pain acting physiologically could induce organic lesions, which could progress quickly to death or remain static for years (see fig. 9.7). When organic illness developed, there was the possibility of a cure, if and only if the physiological efforts of nature, supported by careful diet and rest, brought about complete evacuation and scarring of the tubercles. As shown in chapter 9, the earliest reviewers of the treatise in Paris thought that this causal mechanism was reactionary, and the idea of cure, almost quaint.

Bronchophony versus Pectoriloquy in Bronchiectasis and Pneumonia

What was bronchophony and when did Laennec first notice it? Bronchophony—voice of the airways—was an "imperfect" form of pectoriloquy that depended on the quality of the sound and its location. Like pectoriloquy, it indicated the louder-than-usual sound of the patient's voice heard by the examiner through the chest wall. Instead of the whole "chest speaking," however, it was only the airways, or "bronchi," that "spoke." Laennec insisted that the difference between the two sounds was more than one of intensity: in pectoriloquy, the patient's voice would leap directly through the cylinder; in bronchophony, the transmitted voice was not quite as loud, and it did not make that subtle leap. An observer with only "mediocre experience" would readily distinguish bronchophony from pectoriloquy.[41]

Bronchophony had not been part of Laennec's first edition in 1819, but he had coined the word for his teaching by early 1824. It would become a sign of both bronchial dilatation (or bronchiectasis) and of hepatization of the lung in the second stage of pneumonia.[42] But his understanding of this new sign evolved through several stages, stimulated by the discoveries of three young physicians, Rault, Andral, and Collin. Laennec certainly invented the word "bronchophony," but his claim to having discovered the phenomenon in bronchiectasis and pneumonia is considerably weakened by the testimony of his papers and his revisions to them. Exploration of the manuscript evidence pertaining to bronchophony reveals some personal foibles, and it sheds more light on the psychology of his discovery. First, we examine his use of bronchophony as a sign of bronchial dilatation, discovered by Rault and Andral; then, we turn to its use as a sign of second-stage pneumonia, discovered by Collin.

During Laennec's retirement to Brittany, young enthusiasts for his method soon discovered that pectoriloquy could occur in some conditions that were not phthisis. The first observer to refer to the possibility of pectoriloquy in a condition other than phthisis was the student, Rault, who defended a thesis in June 1819, just before the release of Laennec's first edition. Setting the stage for the elaboration of a separate, new sign, Rault indicated that inexperienced observers might be fooled by the louder and more resonant voice in bronchial dilatation, a sound that was like pectoriloquy, but not "true" pectoriloquy.[43]

Laennec was amenable to a relationship between pectoriloquy and bronchial dilatation, probably because of the architectural similarity of hollows in both dilated airways and the cavities of phthisis. For the second edition of the *Treatise on Auscultation*, he wrote that in bronchiectasis, the examiner did not hear pectoriloquy, but bronchophony. He referred to two cases of bronchial dilatation, published by Gabriel Andral in 1824; he would also collect two new cases of his own.[44]

Rivalry for priority with Andral seems to have had a role to play in his development of the new sign. During Laennec's two-year absence, Andral had completed his medical training and plunged immediately into a promising career. With the much older N.T. Lerminier (1770–1836), he practiced auscultation and dissection in preparation for their 1824 volume on chest diseases. After Laennec's return to Paris, Andral continued his stethoscopic research, collecting numerous observations, many of which Laennec would cite. For example, in the two cases of bronchial dilatation borrowed by Laennec, he had purported to have heard a new sound, which he had called "*respiration bronchique*," differing from Laennec's use of the same term.[45] Andral did not bother to attend the inventor's clinics and lectures, and Laennec seems to have been vexed by the younger man's incursion into his domain. In a sulky passage of his 1826 preface, he complained about Andral's "bizarre" decision to ignore his teaching, and he inaccurately and unjustifiably postdated by two or three years Andral's "efforts" to understand the signs that Laennec had invented, including "the resonance that I [Laennec] call *bronchophony*."[46]

The two new cases that Laennec added to the section on bronchiectasis from his own collection do little to shore up his claim to priority, nor do they contribute to the distinctive identity of the new sign. The first was that of an unidentified man of unspecified age who died "in the winter of 1821–1822."[47] The date placed his observation earlier than Andral's cases; the vague description is reminiscent of the imprecision surrounding the mysterious, prototypical *jeune personne*. I have been unable to find a corresponding manuscript. The second was the history of René-Marc Chopinet, a forty-one-year-old coach-driver, who died 24 April 1825.[48] Two manuscript versions of Chopinet's case have been preserved, one heavily annotated by Laennec. The words "pectoriloquy" and "imperfect pectoriloquy" appear in several places, but "bronchophony" was written once, only to be deleted in the final versions.[49] In other words, as late as 1825, Laennec himself was not always capable of making distinctions between pectoriloquy and bronchophony in the clinical setting.

Laennec may not often have employed the word "bronchophony" on the wards, but he did use it in at least two of three lectures, delivered in March 1824 at the Collège de France.[50] Bronchophony is clearly written in his notes for the lectures on bronchial dilatation and on pneumonia; however, in the notes for the first of the three lectures (on auscultation), the word appears twice and only in marginal notations (one of which is crossed out), suggesting that it was added as part of a later revision for the second cycle given two years later. A student who heard the auscultation lecture the first time it was read in 1824 did not record "bronchophony," although he did record it as a sign of bronchiectasis and pneumonia in the second and third lectures, given a few days later.[51] In other words, the sign became a general tenet of auscultation, as a product of observations in specific diseases: its occurrence in pneumonia was crucial, because no cavities or hollows were involved; rather, it indicated increased lung density.

Why might Laennec have been preoccupied with this new sound in early 1824? I believe that he had been provoked by Victor Collin, another young doctor who had defended his thesis on 30 December 1823. Collin claimed to have heard "pectoriloquy" in six Necker hospital patients who suffered from pneumonia in the second stage; Cruveilhier had confirmed his findings.[52] By March 1824, the aforementioned student's notes show that Laennec had either misread or disagreed with Collin, whom he did not cite. The new sign of "bronchophony" was an "imperfect pectoriloquy," emphatically "not pectoriloquy," which occurred in dilatation of the airways, but also at the end of the *first* stage of pneumonia.[53] Laennec's own notes on the pneumonia lecture were revised, possibly two years later: bronchophony moved from being a sign of the first stage of pneumonia to a sign of the *second* stage or hepatized lung.[54] This alteration indicates that Laennec had quietly come to accept Collin's observation, with only one difference: pectoriloquy had been replaced by its "imperfect" new variety, bronchophony. In his second edition, Laennec adhered to the view of bronchophony as a sign of second-stage pneumonia;

it continues to serve in that capacity to this day. But he did not admit to his earlier oversight and/or error, and still he did not cite Collin.[55]

"Bronchophony" allowed stethoscopists to avoid using the special sign "pectoriloquy" in situations that were not phthisis. It seems to have been, however, little more than a face-saving device, a convoluted and unnecessary splitting of verbal hairs, a mere variation of degree, similar to the distinctions that Bayle had disputed with Pinel two decades before. In the creation of this sign, Laennec had been taking his cues from others. Bronchophony was coined only after Collin had published his observations on pneumonia and after Andral purported to have heard a new sound in dilatation of the airways. Even with all his "experience," the inventor himself sometimes had trouble distinguishing between the two sounds.

Laennec's unjustified attack on Andral and his apparent lack of charity in failing to credit Collin with priority for his astute observation in pneumonia (and also in pericarditis; see chap. 8) seem to have been motivated by jealousy or pride. Auscultation was such a success that by the time he returned to Paris, many people were conducting research and claiming expertise; some young upstarts did not bow to his authority. The neologism "bronchophony" declared his superior clinical acumen and the subtlety of his greater and longer experience. Its invention could simply have been a way of subconsciously holding on to what had been his and his alone until he had retired to Kerlouarnec.

There are at least two other psychological explanations for Laennec's need to invent another neologism; both emerge from the conceptual priorities to which he had committed early in his investigations. First, Laennec would always be inclined to find a different sound/sign for each organic lesion/disease (see chap. 8). Second, to notice something, an observer must be prepared to look for it. To hear pectoriloquy (or bronchophony) in a patient with pneumonia, it is necessary to listen for it by asking the patient to speak. In his new physiology-based classification of chest diseases, Laennec thought of pneumonia as a disease of breathing, not a disease of voice. His initial failure to notice this rather obvious sign indicates that, in most pneumonia cases, he had probably already made the diagnosis before he picked up his stethoscope. In pneumonia—until Collin reminded him to do otherwise—he listened only to breathing.

ASTHMA AND THE MEANING OF "PUERILE RESPIRATION"

Laennec's auscultation was not confined to the investigation of clinical illness and organic pathology; he believed that it could also be successfully applied to the study of normal human physiology. This preoccupation is most evident in his exploration of the sound he labeled "puerile respiration."

Medical students in postrevolutionary Paris had been taught by the chemist Fourcroy that respiration involved the uptake of oxygen or "vital air" and

he release of heat (caloric). These ideas built upon the work of Antoine-
Laurent Lavoisier and Lazzaro Spallanzani (1729–1799) on the relation-
hips among respiration, combustion, and the new element, oxygen. Re-
earch focused on the site and control of gaseous exchange, and the prospect
of oxygen therapy was fascinating.[56] Laennec was aware of these studies and
ad incorporated them into his concept of physiological control: the connec-
ion between psyche and soma in sickness and health. The sign "puerile res-
iration" became a justification for his ideas.

Medical historians have been fond of pointing out that Laennec had man-
ged to describe most of the auscultatory terms pertaining to respiration in
ess than three years. Not all his signs were destined for posterity; ausculta-
ory vocabulary actually decreased after his death. "Puerile respiration" is
ne expression that fell into relative disuse: medical dictionaries continue to
efine it; however, in the last half century, manuals of physical diagnosis
iscarded "puerile respiration" both as a physical sign and as a description of
ncreased intensity in breath sounds.[57]

For Laennec, "puerile respiration" had three distinct meanings. First, it
epresented the louder type of respiratory sound heard in most healthy chil-
ren; hence, the name. He reasoned that because children are growing and
ave relatively large alimentary needs, the enhanced respiratory sound was
roportional to their greater "need" for oxygen and reflected the physiolog-
cally more "efficient" nature of each infant breath. Second, he thought that
uerile respiration also occurred in some healthy adults as their usual type of
reath sound. Third, he believed it could be acquired as an accessory change
n certain pathological states and could serve as a diagnostic sign. The long
escription of puerile respiration was identical in both editions of his treatise;
owever, the second edition contained more information on its use as a sign
of disease.[58]

Laennec said that adults who retained puerile respiration into old age were
of nervous temperament and their characters retained aspects of the "irasci-
ility" of childhood. Displaying a vague notion of gaseochemical homeosta-
is, he postulated that the blood of normal children or of sick adults with
uerile respiration was chemically different from and probably contained
nore oxygen than that of normal adults. He denied that the sound was due
o variations in thickness of the chest wall, because it could be heard in mus-
ular males and through the female breast.

For Laennec, "puerile respiration" indicated a type of breathing that ex-
racted more than the usual amount of oxygen from the atmosphere. It was
he sign of a "perfect" or "complete" breath in response to an increased
need" originating elsewhere in the organism. When it was heard in appar-
ntly healthy adults, it translated a variation in ambient nervous tone (my
xpression). During illness, it represented the extra work being done to sup-
ly the organism's increased demand for oxygen, a demand resulting from
he presence of an organic change in another lung or from an increase in the
ntire body's physiological need for oxygen.

Laennec's younger disciples emphasized the difficulty in recognizing puerile respiration. None reduced it to a simple increase in intensity; there was an additional nuance in quality, the detection of which required vast stethoscopic experience. Cayol showed Laennec a patient in whom they were both convinced that puerile respiration could be heard through an effusion of air.[59] A student wrote that puerile respiration was "never caused by a lesion of the lung or part thereof"; it was heard in the "healthy lung where the action is momentarily increased to supply the unhealthy parts"; it had been "observed in portions of lung which were found to be invaded by pneumonia on the following day."[60]

Laennec said that the best evidence for the effect of nervous influence on the soma came from those states associated with puerile respiration. No anatomical lesion could be found, yet the patient was sick. "If respiration is puerile, dyspnea can be attributed only to a particular state of the 'nervous fluid,' or 'vital principle,' or, if you will, to an exaggerated need for increased oxygenation of the blood over what occurs in health."[61]

The realization that puerile respiration could be a pathognomonic sign for a *lesionless* state may have struck Laennec just as forcefully as his accidental discovery of pectoriloquy, a sign that had become his sine qua non of phthisis. An illness associated with puerile respiration was for him the "most easily" detected of all pathological states, as indicated by the statement used as an epigraph for this chapter. Puerile respiration was objective, audible to any educated observer, but it was special: it indicated functional, not structural, change. It was to be the first indisputable sign of purely physiological alteration, a nonanatomical but nonetheless perceptible change in the "life force" or "vital principle."

Laennec associated his sign of puerile respiration with one disease in particular: asthma. At the beginning of the nineteenth century, the ancient term, asthma, had come to mean simply shortness of breath with no emphasis on its cause. Many different disease states—cardiac, pulmonary, metabolic, and febrile—can produce rapid and labored respiration. For example, the broad description of asthma by William Heberden (1710–1801) contained a case of mitral stenosis and another of emphysema, both of which Laennec would have detected by 1819.[62] Similarly, in 1818, Rostan had challenged the traditional idea that asthma of the elderly was a nervous affliction and suggested that it was caused by edema in the lungs.[63] With the increasing emphasis on dissection and the advent of percussion, the category of asthma was shrinking as an appropriate diagnosis for breathlessness; it was being reserved for "lesionless" dyspnea only. Nevertheless clinical "reality" forced a continued acknowledgment that some breathless conditions could not be associated with physical signs or postmortem findings sufficient to account for the distress or death of the patient. Therefore, some doctors found it useful to define asthma as a disease of the lungs without organic change, or as a nervous condition.[64]

Asthma was conceptually problematic for anatomoclinical medicine. Like the "essential fevers" or "mental alienation," it was clinically recognizable, but anatomically obscure.[65] However, the controversy that surrounded fevers and insanity as apparently nonorganic diseases does not appear to have extended to "lesionless" asthma, possibly because the shrinking dimensions within which it was confined meant that it was rarely fatal. Reflecting asthma's popular reputation as a benign diagnosis, four of Laennec's patients with organic changes diagnosed their own ailments as asthma, although their physicians did not.[66] Asthma was perceived as merely an ancient term fast on its way to obsolescence with the "progress" of pathological anatomy.[67] Attempts to isolate organic correlatives for a vague, rarely fatal, and possibly nonexistent disease may have been seen as a waste of time.

Laennec recognized the problems with asthma: "there are few terms which are more abused in medicine and by which as many different diseases are designated."[68] His description of asthma was intimately linked to puerile respiration as a diagnostic sign. In the first edition of the *Treatise on Auscultation*, he described it as a nonorganic manifestation of "chronic catarrh," which was diagnosed far more often than it occurred.[69] By 1826, however, he waxed eloquent for almost thirty additional pages on "asthma." He described two different types based on two physiological mechanisms: the first, called "puerile" asthma, was due to an augmentation in the baseline "need" or "want" for air; the second, called "spasmodic" asthma, could be attributed to bronchiolar muscle spasm.[70] Both were nervous conditions indicated by puerile respiration.

Laennec's puerile asthma consisted of an increased need for oxygen and could be further subdivided into primary or secondary forms, corresponding roughly to the sequence of symptoms, or types that might now be called "acute idiopathic" and "superimposed on chronic." The physiological circumstances in this type of asthma were likened to the increased oxygen demand and altered nervous tone that Laennec postulated in individuals who displayed puerile respiration as their healthy breath sound. No specific cases were provided, but once again evidence came from his own health: his cousin Mériadec claimed to have heard puerile respiration on listening to Laennec's chest in 1819.[71]

The second form, "spasmodic" asthma, was a complication of chronic illness and included the periodic forms of breathlessness that might now be labeled "extrinsic" or allergic asthma. Spasmodic asthma was to be recognized by a temporary decrease in the breath sounds in the setting of an inflated chest. If, however, these patients were induced to "increase their need for respiration" momentarily by prolonged coughing, Valsalva maneuver, or rapid, loud recitation of prayers without taking a breath, the first inspiration following the exercise would be "puerile." The spasm seemed to be under both voluntary and involuntary nervous control, "because even healthy men can make soundless inspirations."[72]

Laennec used anatomical and physiological explanations to explain spasmodic asthma. He speculated that the underlying mechanism was spastic contraction of the bronchiolar musculature, described in 1803 by Franz David Reisseissen (1773–1828).[73] He believed that both the bronchioles and the air sacs were covered with muscles and that owing to these muscles the lung had its own action ("*action propre*"), independent of the costal and diaphragmatic respiratory movements. If both bronchial and alveolar muscles were to contract, the lung would not be able to absorb oxygen in spite of great exertion from the skeletal musculature. This theory seemed to explain the situation in asthmatics, who were exhausted by their efforts to breathe; yet, they appeared to have no organic lesion in their lungs. Laennec did not address the seemingly obvious question emerging from his hypothesis: what filled the extra space between the contracted air cells and the inflated chest wall?

Two new cases were included to illustrate the role of the mental state in the production of spasmodic asthma: a horse-rider, who developed breathlessness every time he left his home town; and a certain octogenarian, "M. le comte H ***" (identified in lecture notes as the eighty-two-year-old Count d'Hanache) whose thirty-year history of asthma depended on the inadvertent absence of his night lamp or on a closed window.[74] Laennec observed that light, fresh air, and closing the eyes produced a beneficial effect and that emotional stress or the exposure to certain "smells," especially tuberose and heliotrope, could provoke an attack. In a sensualist fashion, he equated anxiety with odors, because both were mediated by the "nervous" or sensory systems, the one "internal," the other "external." Here was further evidence for the nervous or "vital" nature of the disease. Open to a physicochemical explanation of these immaterial effects, he cited "atmospheric electricity" as a potential mediator.[75]

Laennec considered several therapeutic modalities, including the use of pure oxygen, but his conception of the altered physiology led him to recommend the newly isolated narcotics for asthma in order to "decrease the need for respiration."[76] He was aware of the experiments of his fellow Breton, the physiologist J. J. C. Legallois, who had demonstrated that a lesion in the medulla oblongata could arrest respiration, but the neurological effects of morphine as a respiratory depressant were still poorly understood.[77]

The section on asthma was almost devoid of clinical observations. The two "nervous" men were both alive when Laennec went to press, and there were no autopsies on asthmatics from his own practice, although he referred to autopsy cases published by others.[78] To explore Laennec's clinical experience with increased respiration, I searched the manuscript records for observations pertaining to asthma or puerile respiration (see table 7.1). I have found seven cases, but do not pretend that the search was exhaustive. Of the seven, only one patient had a suspected diagnosis of asthma, but his physical examination was not recorded. The rarity of asthma among these patients tends to suggest that it was not considered severe enough to warrant hospitalization.

or that being a strictly symptomatic diagnosis within the trend to anatomic diagnosis, asthma was being demedicalized. In six other patients, puerile respiration was detected over one lung in conjunction with evidence of organic alteration in the other. It seems that the changes on the diseased side were so great that breath sounds overlying it would have been diminished or virtually absent, making the sounds on the healthy side seem exaggerated in contrast. This survey also suggests that puerile respiration appeared as a clinical sign more frequently after May 1824.

The context in which Laennec formulated his explanation of puerile respiration as a response to a need can now be reconstructed.[79] It is possible that the sounds were absolutely increased in intensity because of the increased depth and rate of inspiration. Laennec may have been aware of this easily demonstrated effect. In most cases, however, it is not necessary to postulate an absolute increase in intensity of sound to explain his findings. He "heard" increased breath sounds in the healthy lung, because the opposite and ailing lung offered no breath sounds at all. The result of comparing auscultation of the two sides of the chest would be a relative augmentation in respiratory sounds on the healthy side. Laennec would have disputed this simple analysis. For him, the increase in respiratory sound was absolute, not apparent, and it was combined with an alteration in quality, which reflected increased physiologic work performed by each breath. The healthy lung could be seen as maintaining the basic needs of the whole body by performing "twice the work" of its normal state through "more perfect" breathing.[80]

But Laennec also "heard" puerile respiration in people who were not sick. The nervous but healthy persons in whom he found puerile respiration may have hyperventilated, especially if their attention had been directed to their breathing by the conspicuous use of a new diagnostic instrument. Hyperventilation may not augment the intensity of the breath sound, but it could cause an attuned physician to think of puerile respiration. When confronted with a breathless patient whose lungs and heart were apparently normal, Laennec may have found puerile respiration because he anticipated it. For healthy individuals, no records have survived, and it is not possible to investigate the experience that led Laennec to his claim.

Laennec believed his auscultatory research on asthma had provided another important breakthrough, one that seems to have ripened between the two editions of his treatise. With puerile respiration, he thought he had discovered a diagnostic sign for asthma, a nervous and "lesionless" condition. Here was clinical indicator that was inextricably linked to the living patient's physiological state, a state about which the autopsy could provide no information at all. The existence of such a sign was support for his conviction that some diseases did not leave organic lesions, but they were still real diseases that made people sick. This "physio-clinical" (rather than "anatomoclinical") arrow pointed to an alteration in the vital principle; as such, it seemed to confirm the existence of the life force and its alteration.

TABLE 7.1

Clinical Records Pertaining to Puerile Respiration and Asthma

Date	Occupation	Sex	Age	Symptoms	Stethoscopic Signs	Autopsy	Diagnosis
Nov 1821	cooper	m	67	cough, swelling	puerile left anterior	yes	lungs engorged posteriorly; cancer stomach
May 1824	saddler	m	26	fever, dyspnea	puerile left	yes	pneumothorax right
June 1824	tailor	m	18	fever, dyspnea	puerile right	yes	pneumonia left
June 1824	mason	m	31	fever, dyspnea	puerile right	yes	pneumonia left
Oct 1824	boot maker	m	28	chest pain right	puerile anterior; heart murmur	yes	lungs engorged posteriorly; mitral valve disease
Dec 1824	laborer	m	71	fever, dyspnea	puerile right	no	pneumonia left
Apr 1825	draftsman	m	59	dyspnea	no record of exam	no	chronic catarrh, asthma?
July 1825	laborer	m	27	dyspnea	almost puerile right	yes	pneumothorax left

Sources: ML, MS Cl. I, lot c, f. 5–7; Cl. II, f. 272–275, 360–361, 370; Cl. III, f. 57, 212–216, 319, 388–392.

That a serious disease could exist without an organic lesion was not new or surprising to Laennec, long-time custodian of the case of *cadet Rousseau*. Who could argue the existence of the life force, if an objective sign of its alteration had been found? In 1826, he addressed the following to those for whom lesionless disease was becoming intolerable: "But now, even as doctors are very attentive to this point and while many educated men doubt the possibility of any life-threatening disorder depending solely on a disturbance in nervous influence without serious, primary, organic lesions, I have seen many cases in which, in spite of the most meticulous searching, it was impossible for me to find an organic lesion to which asthma could be attributed."[81]

Laennec's continued enthusiasm for the potential value of auscultation in physiology is apparent in a pamphlet published only a few weeks before the second edition of his book as part of his bid for the Montyon Prize. He announced that simple experiments with auscultation had proven certain "new facts:" among them, that the "need to breathe . . . is variable, according to age . . . and according to individuals; [and that] the purely physiological augmentation of the need to breathe was sufficient to cause asthma."[82]

Puerile respiration was an important discovery with powerful implications. It made the lesionless, but nevertheless pathological, state recognizable in the living, even when it could not be identified in the dead. It vindicated Laennec's stance that a disease did not need to be caused by, or even associated with, a solid, organic lesion; this, he knew, was an ancient idea, but he gave it a new slant. Being perceptible to the senses and to the "better eye," puerile respiration was neither immaterial, nor theological, nor metaphysical; it was positive. It was an indicator of the psychoneurotic tonus of the individual and the state of the vital principle where, he thought, lay the origin of all disease. It was to become the first step in a new type of clinical physiology, free of the limitations imposed by pathological anatomy and whose equivalent in modern medical practice can only be described as a strange combination of blood gas analysis, basal metabolic rate, and the psychocybernetics of brain waves.

The Treatise on Mediate Auscultation: The Heart and Clinical Reasoning

On 13 March 1824, I was consulted by a lady in whom I found a few signs of pulmonary phthisis . . . I lent my ear attentively . . . as a result, I noticed the tune that follows.

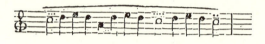

—*Laennec,* Traité *1826, 2:424–425*

I would have gladly attended the arterial concert.

—*Cruveilhier to Laennec, 13 April 1824*

THE HEART

The Big Mistake

Laennec's medical successors and historians have criticized his research on the heart in different ways, all mostly inadequate and ranging from open ridicule to bemused indulgence. Words, like "wrong," "inferior," or "less excellent," have been applied to his cardiac semiology and he has been accused of leaving the study of heart disease in a hopeless "snarl."[1] Sometimes, the fact that he ever listened to the heart at all has been treated as pardon for his "mistakes," but usually his cardiac research is neglected in favor of his more "successful" work on diseases of the lungs. What was the error? His interpretation of the sounds of the beating heart did not correspond to our own. Few historians have explored the reasons for Laennec's interpretation of the heart sounds; nor have they tested the predictive value of his misinterpreted signs.

In its early stages, Laennec (fig. 8.1) considered his work on auscultation of the heart to be just as important as that of the lungs. It was for the express purpose of a cardiac examination that he created the original, paper stethoscope.[2] His early research in mediate auscultation was focused on the heart, and in one of his introductory speeches, he said that it was "above all in

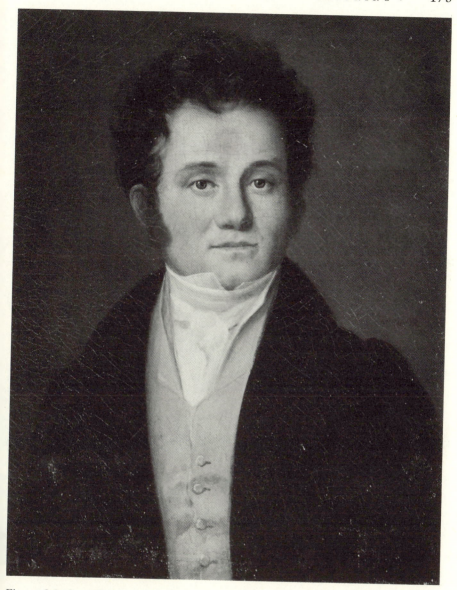

Figure 8.1. So-called portrait of Laennec, labeled and signed by J. J. Ansiaux. This fine portrait differs considerably from other more familiar but rather ectomorphic images of the inventor. There may be doubt about the identity of the subject, but a number of elements bring the artist into Laennec's sphere. In 1820s Paris, Ansiaux was a popular painter of royalist, Catholic, and medical subjects, whom he was said to have customarily "fattened" for a healthy glow. Ansiaux's brother was a medical graduate of Paris, known to Laennec, who cited him at the Académie de Médecine. The extant correspondence does not mention this portrait, but Ansiaux's portrait of the Laennec in-law, Marion de Procé, has been in the family since it was painted. Photograph: François Puget (owner), Quimper.

diseases of the heart that signs which are more reliable than those provided by percussion are needed."[3] Laennec heard and described most of the sounds generated by the heart in health and disease. Some sounds became signs of hidden organic changes; others he rejected. But the specific lesions that interested him had little to do with those that became important to physicians after his death.

Here I show that, at the time of Laennec's investigations, the most important and most obvious organic changes of the heart were those of size and muscle bulk; changes on the valves and in the coronary arteries were not yet a major preoccupation, although they would soon come to dominate cardiac pathology. I also examine Laennec's interpretation of the heart sounds in health and disease. My study shows that his interpretation may not have been revolutionary, but it was plausible. It also corresponded to the philosophical, physiological, and anatomical concerns of his contemporaries. Moreover, his physical signs could sometimes actually predict the organic changes that he sought.

Examination of Laennec's cardiology allows us to rectify a historiographic imbalance by completing the litany of successes with understanding of the "failures," which, in the case of great scientists, as Alexandre Koyré said, "are not only instructive; they reveal the difficulties that had to be conquered, the obstacles that had to be overcome."[4] Laennec's work on the heart reveals the psychological and epistemological priorities governing an early nineteenth-century physician's use of evidence. As in his formulation of pulmonary signs, the decision-making criteria he imposed on this ensemble of inductive evidence expressed an inkling of statistical probability, typifying one whose existence straddled the sensualist philosophy of the late eighteenth century and the dawn of positivist thought. That Laennec's interpretations were "inaccurate" by late twentieth-century standards should not deter us from an assessment of his priorities. In fact, the gaps between his interpretations and those of the present—his so-called errors—permit a certain enhanced clarity in appreciating his method, a clarity that is difficult to achieve for his work on the lungs, which appears to conform to present standards and tempts us to assume that it had the same significance. His heart signs and their evolution, however, defy reduction; they are not simple, but the effort to understand them competes against unwarranted assumption. At the end of this chapter, I analyze Laennec's clinical reasoning in establishing auscultatory signs for both heart and lung.

ORGANIC DISEASE OF THE HEART IN THE EARLY NINETEENTH CENTURY: STRUCTURAL CHANGE, FUNCTIONAL CAUSE

Cardiology did not emerge as a specific discipline until much later in the nineteenth century with other specialties.[5] The concept of a disease of the heart was plausible by 1800, but symptoms and signs that could indicate cardiac lesions were few. For centuries, the phenomena usually associated with disease of the heart were palpitation, chest pain, and sudden death. Other symptoms that are now more frequently related to cardiac dysfunction, such as fainting, shortness of breath, and swelling of the legs, were not so obviously linked to the heart; they appeared to be problems situated in the brain, lung, or kidney. Saul Jarcho commented that records must be unearthed from "unexpectedly diverse hiding places" in order to make a longitudinal study of a modern cardiac concept.[6] It is not my purpose here to make a longitudinal study, but rather to describe the status of knowledge concerning the anatomical pathology of the heart and the methods used to detect it at the moment Laennec began his work.

As Victor McKusick observed, there is a "dearth of recorded interest" in the physical diagnosis of the heart before Laennec.[7] The reason is clear: eighteenth-century physicians were not looking for signs of heart disease any more than they were looking for signs of any other organ-based disease, perhaps even less, because of an ancient tradition against the notion of a sick heart.[8] Practitioners who were familiar with pathological anatomy might suspect structural alteration in the hearts of some patients, but suspicion did not constitute method; being able to identify and treat a heart lesion in a living patient was almost inconceivable. Corvisart's work on percussion and Laennec's on auscultation provided methods for identification.

Anatomical lesions of the heart had been recognized in most compendia from Bonet to Baillie.[9] Raymond Vieussens (1641–1715) wrote an anatomical-physiological treatise devoted solely to cardiac structure and movement. He mentioned, but did not emphasize structural alteration as part of disease and suggested that these lesions could result from alterations in the quality of the blood.[10] Some thirty-five years later, Jean-Baptiste Sénac (1693–1770) associated diseases of the heart with changes in cardiac muscle and the pericardium, the membrane tissue around the heart; he also described lesions of the valves, coronary arteries, and great vessels.[11] Sénac considered sadness to be a cause of heart disease, but thought that alterations of the heart were rare, and he lamented the impossibility of trying to link variable symptoms to organic changes before the patient died.[12] In 1804, Portal addressed the same problem, suggesting that clinicians were not good pathologists and pathologists were not good clinicians.[13]

As Laennec began his career, British physicians had developed a special interest in angina pectoris, and some tried to link that condition with a specific cardiac change. William Heberden left a classic description of the symptoms, but he was unable to connect angina to a specific lesion: of more than one hundred patients who had consulted him for this problem, only one had been autopsied.[14] Soon, however, angina was linked to "ossification" (bone formation) in the coronary arteries by John Fothergill (1712–1780), John Hunter (1728–1793), Caleb H. Parry (1755–1822), and Edward Jenner.[15] In angina, the subjective symptom of a specific pain became a sign of a specific organic change; acceptance of the notion was neither immediate, nor universal, however. Baillie stated cautiously that the pain of angina "would seem to be intimately connected to ossification" of the coronary arteries, but he readily admitted that for other organic changes, such as those on the heart valves, "no observations have yet been made by which practitioners may be led to conjecture what set of valves is diseased."[16]

In the early nineteenth century, several works appeared that sought to combine clinical presentation with structural changes in the heart. In France, the best known was Corvisart's *Essay on the Organic Diseases and Lesions of the Heart and Great Vessels* (1806) followed two years later by his translation of Auenbrugger's *Inventum Novum*, in which he expanded on the value of cardiac percussion. Both books were being researched during Laennec's studies, and the former pupil reviewed Corvisart on percussion for the *Journal de médecine*.[17] Corvisart's *Essay* on the heart was divided into six parts: five more or less concerned the different sites of organic alteration, while the sixth dealt with etiology, diagnosis, prognosis, and treatment. Case histories illustrated the commentary on pathological lesions. Corvisart associated failure of the mitral valve to open completely (stenosis) with a palpable "thrill," a vibration ("*frémissement cataire*" or catlike purring) felt by the doctor's fingertips on the patient's chest.[18] He described clinical conditions that led to angina pectoris, but was unaware of, or unwilling to credit, the coronary theory expounded across the Channel. Given his position in Napoleon's household, there may have other reasons for this opinion; Laennec once hinted that the "motives" behind his former teacher's rejection of classical languages and authors may have been political.[19]

Notwithstanding the ingenious observation of palpable mitral thrill, Corvisart's main concern and that of his contemporaries was the accurate prediction of cardiac enlargement, which he called "aneurysm" and subdivided into "active" (thickened muscle) or "passive" (thin muscle). To detect aneurysm he laid his palm on the patient's chest to feel the heart beat, or he percussed the anterior thorax to determine the extent of cardiac dullness.[20] An enlarged heart would be associated with an increased area of dullness; a thickened cardiac muscle would give a stronger impulse than usual.

Corvisart acknowledged that the changes in the heart could not always be distinguished from those of the lung.[21] Like Sénac, he thought that heart diseases came from "the passions," such as "a fit of anger" or the distress owing to the "horrible times" of the French Revolution. Unlike Sénac, he thought that they were common, perhaps even increasing in frequency because of recent hard times.[22] Both physical and emotional causes acted in a mechanistic fashion to produce organic changes: narrowing of the outflow through the aorta meant greater work for the heart muscle to pump against increased resistance; emotions also increased heart work. "This organ is the point in which the effects of all the moral affections, gay or melancholy, seem to be concentrated. No moral affection can be experienced without acceleration, diminution, or other derangement of the motion of the heart. . . . The unexpected news of pardon strikes a criminal dead who was going to be executed. A lover dies at the very moment the flame of his passion was to be satisfied; the one is destroyed by terror; the other apparently thunderstruck with a paroxysm of passion."[23] Removal of the emotional cause might stabilize the problem, but as Albury as shown, Corvisart did not believe that it could effect a cure.[24]

Later observers contended that Corvisart held a sentimental and antiquated view of the heart as the seat of the emotions; the frequency of heart diseases had not increased, they said, but Corvisart's sensitivity to the psychological stress in his unstable, political environment caused him to look at the heart more closely, seeking (and finding) anticipated, organic change.[25] His words lend some credence to the claim: "The bloody scenes of the revolution, ruin of fortunes, emotions, and chagrin which followed, do, at this period, furnish numerous proofs of the influence of the moral affections concerning the evolution of the organic diseases in general, and those of heart in particular."[26]

In his 1809 treatise, the Glaswegian surgeon and anatomist, Allan Burns (1781–1813), displayed many of the same preoccupations, including an interest in active and passive enlargements and the coronary artery theory of angina, but he seems to have been unaware of Corvisart's book and did not practice percussion.[27] Burns rejected the concept of "acrimonious humors" and accused his contemporaries, including "the venerable Portal," of offering only vague conjectures about etiology.[28] He developed a mechanistic theory of back pressure to explain dilatation and cardiac edema, but he, too, was unable to commit to purely mechanical causes for the dilatation of the heart. He also rejected the observation of the Bath physician, C. H. Parry, that dilatations tend to occur in those parts immediately proximal to an obstruction. "Suffice it to say," Burns said, "that, in general, the dilatation is not caused by any mechanical agent. We know that individuals are predisposed to certain diseases, and that these different affections are produced by similar exciting causes."[29]

Laennec was not familiar with Burns's work until after 1819, but he cited Antonio Giuseppe Testa (1756–1814) and Friedrich Ludwig Kreysig (1770–1839). Testa accepted the coronary artery theory of angina and, like Corvisart, envisaged vitalistic causes of organic heart disease.[30] Kreysig's prolix, four-volume work was a compendium of anatomical abnormalities found in the heart. He, too, adopted the coronary theory of angina, the valvular significance of palpable thrill, and once mentioned having "heard" a swishing sound, but he did not use percussion. He devised a nosological classification of diseases of the heart with two broad categories: physiological (*"Dynamische"*) and anatomical (*"Organische"*). Above all, he, too, was preoccupied with the obvious changes of hypertrophy and dilatation.[31]

Early nineteenth-century interest in the organic changes of the heart can be summarized in four points: first, illness could be attributed to organic changes in the heart; second, most authors conceived of physiological and psychic causes for organic changes; third, the study of these organic lesions emphasized enlargement of the heart and its muscle; and finally, clinical signs indicative of the pathological change were scarce. Only a few signs, like the palpable thrill and changes in percussion note, did not depend on the patient's perception and description. Many, like the pain of angina pectoris, were intimately related to the patient's subjective experience of illness. Most, like dependent edema, dyspnea, and cyanosis, were not specific for heart ailments. Virtually all practitioners acknowledged that the detection of organic heart disease in the antemortem setting was problematic. Corvisart's "gaze" and "tact" were the senses that a seasoned practitioner must use to select the correct organic diagnosis among many possibilities suggested by a complex and imprecise ensemble of observations.[32]

LAENNEC'S ORGANIC PATHOLOGY OF THE HEART

From his student days, Laennec joined in the contemporary enthusiasm for anatomical study of the heart and devoted his earliest publications to that topic.[33] He retained Corvisart's classification of heart lesions, substituting only the words "hypertrophy" and "dilatation" for his teacher's "active" and "passive" aneurysms (see table 8.1). He pointed out that hypertrophy of the myocardium could exist in the absence of dilatation. Use of the word "hypertrophy" led to yet another small priority dispute, this time, with his old "friend," R. J. H. Bertin (1757–1828), who said that he had coined it first in his communication to the Institute on 8 August 1811, commented on by Corvisart.[34] In response, Laennec said that he had used "hypertrophy" for some time, but admitted that he had not invented it. He would not accuse Bertin of plagiarism, he said, and he suspected that they had made a mutual discovery: "it is quite natural that in a matter of pure and simple observation, two men carefully examine the same object and see the same." Once again, he resolved the debate by ascribing priority to distant predecessors; the idea was recognized earlier but not yet named by others: Morgagni, Covisart, Burns, Kreysig, and Burserius.[35] Bertin's claim to having coined the term "hypertrophy" seems to have been justified. Laennec was still using Corvisart's word "aneurysm" in his 1803 course, but by 1812 he had switched to the etymologically more satisfying "hypertrophy," meaning exaggerated growth and corresponding well to his idea of "increased nutrition."[36] The relationship between Laennec and Bertin seems to have been long-standing; many years earlier, Laennec refused to comment on the quality of a translation by the much older Bertin, because his praise would be construed as a sign of their friendship.[37]

Laennec classified both hypertrophy and dilatation with diseases of "nutrition": more heart was present than in the normal state and no other prior organic change was implicated as a cause. His emphasis on the independence of structural changes in each of the chambers was coupled with a characteristic silence on the physiological circumstances that produced them. Like Cor-

Myocardium (heart muscle)
    Nutrition: Hypertrophy: left, right, both
                    Dilatation: left, right, both
                    Dilatation with hypertrophy
                    Partial dilatation
    Texture: Hardening
                    Softening: violet, yellow, white
                    Atrophy
                    Gangrene
    Displacement
    Prolapse
    Congenital abnormalities
    Carditis
    Communication between right and left heart
    Rupture
    Fatty degeneration
    Ossification of the myocardium (Laennec had never seen a case)
    Accidental productions: Tubercles
                                 Cancers
                                 Cysts: serous, acephalocysts
    Inflammation of the internal membrance
Valves
    Induration and ossification
    Detached eustachian valve
    Mitral aneurysm
    Polyps
Pericardium
    Pericarditis: acute, chronic
    Hydropericardium
    Pneumopericardium
    Accidental productions
    Ossifications
Lesions of the vessels
    Aorta: narrowing, incrustations, inflammation
    Pulmonary
    Coronary
Neuralgias
    Heart
    Vessels

Source: Traité 1826; Collège de France, lessons 44–53, 1823–1824, as recorded by James Kitchen, "Leçons de Laennec," MS HMCP.

visart, Laennec observed that atrial dilatation usually occurred in conjunction with diseased atrioventricular valves; however, in keeping with the etiological reticence of his school, he did not speculate on a causal relationship between the two conditions. He treated them as separate entities.[38]

Laennec shared the fascination of his eighteenth-century predecessors for volume changes of the myocardium. He took care to notice the size of the heart relative to the size of the individual: a natural heart should be slightly larger than a person's clenched fist. Without knowing of Burns, he also imagined that a heart too small for a body made an individual susceptible to disease of that organ.[39] He noted the relative volume of the four heart chambers and the texture, color, and thickness of the cardiac muscles and septum: normal thickness was between three and four "lines" (a "line" was one-twelfth inch, the width of a line drawn by a quill).

In autopsy reports, Laennec occasionally commented on the state of the atrioventricular valves and the great vessels. He wrote a possibly original description of a type of valvular change called "globular vegetations or excrescences," the cause of which still remains obscure.[40] He recognized two forms of congenital heart disease: patent ductus and septal defects. In the majority of clinical cases that he would diagnose as heart disease, however, he used the words "hypertrophy," and/or "dilatation."

In keeping with the ideas of his contemporaries in Britain and in France, Laennec's views on the causes of heart lesions were a blend of psychosomatism and mechanical physiology. Like Corvisart, he said, "The energetic and frequently repeated action of all muscles causes them to increase in volume . . . as the arm of a soldier or the hands of laborers. . . . As a result, one realizes that palpitations, even if they are only of nervous or emotional origin, could lead to a true augmentation in the substance ("nutrition") of the heart, if they occur too often."[41] The link between emotion and cardiac muscle in the pathophysiology of heart disease remained entrenched in later medical thought. By the mid-twentieth century, physicians were less inclined to ascribe organic changes to emotional states, although recently such causal links have been revived.[42]

Modern physicians are surprised that Laennec excluded valvular changes as a cause of enlarged hearts. The role of heart valves in volume changes was still not understood, and valvular disease was a new concept. Corvisart's palpable thrill had made it possible to detect stenosis of a valve. On the other hand, the possibility of a valve's failure to close completely (insufficiency) was not recognized until 1831.[43] The "mechanical" obstruction posed by persistent elevation of systemic blood pressure had not been imagined as a pathological entity: it was undetectable at the bedside, invisible in the cadaver, and as yet had no place in medical pathophysiology.

Laennec disputed some ideas of his predecessors. Corvisart had suggested that all valvular lesions were due to syphilis, but Laennec thought that other processes were involved.[44] He criticized Corvisart's emphasis on coarctation (narrowing) of the aorta as a source of heart disease, because it was too rare.[45]

Above all, he rejected inflammation as a cause of heart lesions or valvular change. But inflammation was soon to be endorsed as a cause of heart trouble by Bertin, whose young assistant, J. B. Bouillaud, would become an expert in "endocarditis," or inflammation of the heart.[46] For Laennec, valvular alterations were due to long-standing chronic illness and could themselves cause other organic changes, such as dropsy in the legs, edema in the lungs, and hemorrhages, but they did not arise from inflammation.[47] Similarly, Laennec said that redness in blood vessels did not imply inflammation.[48]

Although Bertin devoted the largest section of his treatise to hypertrophy of the heart, he did not think inflammation should be neglected. He accused the "celebrated observer," Laennec, of "exaggerating" his claims against inflammation, which Bertin said would be justified "if it were necessary to demonstrate pus in order to diagnose [it]."[49] Laennec may have been provoked by a wayward student, Eloi Dalbant, whose thesis had contained many examples of circulatory redness that had been construed as arteritis; moreover, Dalbant had annoyingly dedicated his work to Dupuytren.[50] In 1826, Laennec described an experiment to "prove" that arterial redness was the result of blood left standing after death and that it had nothing to do with inflammation.[51] He also added sometimes critical, sometimes complimentary references to Bertin's two-year-old treatise; however, his hostility was clearly directed against the editor, Bouillaud, and his ideas on inflammation, which, according to Laennec, even Bertin seems to have disavowed.[52] This vendetta against inflammation in the heart, which was similar to his campaign against inflammation in tuberculosis, led Laennec to ignore endocarditis, the condition first described by Bouillaud, surely coincidental to his relationship with Broussais.[53]

AUSCULTATION OF THE HEALTHY HEART: PHYSIOLOGY

When Laennec first listened to the heart, he was seeking signs of the most important organic lesions cited above: hypertrophy and dilatation. First he had to interpret the meaning of the sounds he heard in health; then he tried to relate variations in those sounds to hypertrophy and dilatation. His investigations into the heart took him on a little-known journey into physiological experimentation. Inconclusive and ultimately unfruitful though it may have been, this journey merits our consideration for two reasons: first, it exemplifies Laennec's physiological interests; second, it furthers our understanding of his conceptual priorities.

But before embarking on Laennec's cardiac auscultation, a caveat is necessary: present-day cardiac concepts cannot be avoided in a discussion of his auscultatory signs of the normal and diseased heart. This vocabulary may be criticized as "presentist," but it is the only vehicle for the exploration of his observations—not only to discover whether or not he made good observations and thereby practiced "qualitatively better or worse science"[54] —but more specifically, to determine what aspects of heart disease were important to him and how he came to make his decisions. There were no other words for these concepts prior to Laennec, and it was only after his death that consensus was reached and conventions were established to facilitate communication between scholars—literally—through conferences devoted to that cause. I will abide by those conventions.[55]

The normal heart beat consists of two narrowly separated sounds, imitated on the wards as "lub dub": the first sound is synchronous with closure of the valves between the atria and the ventricles (i.e., mitral and tricuspid valves); the second, with the closure of the valves between the ventricles and the main arteries (i.e., aortic and pulmonic valves, which Laennec called "sigmoid"). The double beat is followed by a pause, then the next beat begins. The exact physical cause of the sounds can be debated, but synchrony with valve closure is well established. For Laennec, however, the sounds made by the heart had nothing to do with movement of the valves; they were the sounds made by the contractions of the muscular chambers of the heart: the first of the ventricles, the second of the atria.

Laennec's interpretation of the heart sounds has astounded some observers, who have called it his greatest "blunder." How is it possible, they marvel, that the inventor of the stethoscope could have been unfamiliar with the work of the man who discovered circulation? Long before the stethoscope, both William Harvey (1578–1657) and Albrecht von Haller (1708–1777) had known that the atria beat "first" and the ventricles, "second"; and Laennec had cited their work.[56] In seeking to explain the "incredible" errors, Rullière suggested that Laennec simply had no flair for physiology and that he over-emphasized pathological anatomy.[57]

Laennec's interpretation of the heart sounds was accomplished by October 1817 (see chap. 6). The reasoning proceeded as follows: he heard the first sound at the same time as he felt the rise in pulse of the carotid artery in the neck and the beat of the apex of the heart just below the left nipple; he noticed that the point of maximal loudness was over the apex. According to Harvey, Laennec knew, the apex beat represented ventricular contraction; he was skeptical of the so-called Cartesian view that cardiac dilatation was active.[58] From his accurate observation and his knowledge of Harvey, he concluded that the first sound must be due to the muscular contraction of the ventricles, and called it the "*bruit ventriculaire.*" He *assumed*, then, that the second sound was due to the contraction of the atria, and called it the "*bruit auriculaire.*" The assumption was supported by the accurate observation that the second sound was loudest high on the sternum and by an extrapolation of the erroneous first conclusion: if ventricular contraction was audible, then all muscular contractions should be audible. He said that von Haller had overlooked the long rest period after the contraction of the atria.

Laennec analyzed the work of the heart, attempting to time the duration of the sounds: although the heart seemed to be in perpetual motion, he concluded that in every twenty-four hours, the ventricles were actually at rest for twelve hours and the atria for eighteen.[59] The entire period of what we now think of as diastole was what Laennec meant by "the rest period after auricular contraction" overlooked by Haller. This nomenclature explains how he could reconcile his so-called "reversal" of the order of atrial and ventricular contractions. These observations, made with only a stethoscope and a watch, are surprisingly accurate; they could neither be confirmed nor disproved without the as-yet-undeveloped technologies of direct vision and kymographic recording.

Using this interpretation of the heart sounds, with his knowledge of anatomy and repeated physical examinations, Laennec then delineated the boundaries of the normal audible heart beat and determined the best site on the chest to hear the "contraction" of each chamber. He established a list of sites to which augmented sounds would progress and from which diminishing sounds would recede: left side of chest to axilla and the stomach; right side of chest to axilla; left back; right back.[60]

After 1819, Laennec continued to refine his understanding of cardiac physiology by studying muscle action. A few revisions were made for his lessons at the Collège de France and the second edition. While in Brittany, he experimented on the sounds of muscle contraction in the hand, arm, jaw, chest and back.[61] He accepted the still controversial notion that contractions of skeletal muscle could be heard with the stethoscope, an observation that tended to bolster his conviction that cardiac contraction was audible. Taking advantage of gruesome clinical opportunities, he listened to the muscles of "several" patients with the lockjaw of tetanus and of a young woman with "*catalépsie*"; their rigid, involuntary contractions seemed to be relatively silent when compared to voluntary contractions. He tried to distinguish between small muscle contractions, which resulted in both movement and sound, and isotonic contractions, which did neither. Only Barthez, he said, "among all physiologists," had written about isotonic contraction, which he called "force of the fixed situation."[62] Unfortunately, in the one surviving manuscript record bearing a diagnosis of "tetanus," the stethoscope was not used to study the patient's trismus (lockjaw).[63] Laennec read a paper on his muscle experiments at the Académie Royale de Médecine on 19 April 1825, but the manuscript cannot been found.[64] This line of physiological investigation fell dormant for decades, because the sound heard over contracting muscles was attributed to secondary circulatory changes or friction between tissue planes; however, in the 1990s acoustic myography is thriving once again, in the hands of researchers who ascribe priority to W. H. Wollaston.[65]

In 1826 and at the Collège de France, Laennec cited the work of Erman (also "Hermann") of Berlin and W. H. Wollaston of London;[66] however, I found no evidence that he was aware of the studies on turbulence and sound made by his contemporaries and compatriots, Félix Savart (1791–1841) or Jean-Louis-Marie Poiseuille (1799–1869).[67] Erman spoke of two simple experiments of listening at the wrist of a man who is making a fist, or of placing the ear and jaw against a pillow while biting repeatedly on a knotted handkerchief; the two muscle experiments result in the same sound. Erman's work later attracted the attention of C. J. B. Williams (1805–1889) and R. B. Todd. Laennec, however, had not known of the experiments until Erman wrote to thank him for donating a copy of the *Treatise on Mediate Ausculta-tion* to the Academy of Prussia, of which he was secretary for the section on physics. Erman and Laennec exchanged letters about the possibility of tim-ing the alternating or "rotating" contractions of muscle fibers in order to develop an auscultatory assessment of the strength of muscle action.[68] In 1810, Wollaston had described similar experiments with an elbow resting on a board and the thumb of the same arm over the ear; and he had rigged up a system for counting discrete noises, which Laennec judged "ingenious" but invalid. This project was frustrated, Laennec said, because it was impossi-ble to count more than seven or eight discrete noises per second, although he could hear that there were many more. Wollaston had also used a long stick to transmit sounds to his ear, much like Laennec's cylinder; however, the inventor ignored that precedent.[69]

During the same period between the two editions of his book, Laennec was an enthusiastic witness of the ambitious experiments on the cardiovascu-lar physiology of animals performed by his British friend, David Barry (1780–1835).[70] Born in Ireland with a medical degree from Aberdeen, Barry was already a distinguished military surgeon and Extra-Licentiate of the Royal Society in London (Physiology) when he came to Paris. The experi-ments that he conducted between 1822 and 1825 for a thesis were directly related to Laennec's studies, which Barry lauded as the "admirable" and "brilliant" accomplishments of a "great physician."[71] Laennec in turn de-scribed Barry's achievement as "the most remarkable" discoveries since those of Harvey, his "illustrious compatriot."[72] Barry was interested in the effects of changes in atmospheric pressure and in respiration on blood flow. Harvey and his successors had studied the heart's motion through direct vision, but they had opened the thorax and sometimes also the pericardium. Their interventions had necessarily altered the physical environment of the heart, resulting in conditions that did not reflect the situation in life. Barry pro-posed to study heart action without altering the pericardial void (*"vide"*) in which it worked.

Barry's 1827 thesis described seven experiments that he had conducted in 1825 on living and dead animals—mostly horses—obtained from the veteri-nary school at Maisons Alfort or the insalubrious abattoir of Montfaucon.[73] Barry's first experiment involved tracheal intubation of a living horse: he inserted his arm through an incision into the horse's abdomen, then through the left diaphragm to the left and behind the beating heart, which he held in his palm for twenty minutes without opening the pericardium. He studied the effects of alternately compressing the aorta and the venae cavae with his fingers and noticed the variations in flow within the great vessels with respira-tion. The second experiment repeated the first, but on the right. In the third experiment, Barry used the heart and great vessels of a recently killed ewe to study the pressures required to move fluid through the heart. The fourth, fifth, and sixth experiments were designed to measure pressure changes relative to the atmosphere within the pericardial sacs of recently killed horses. The last experiment was done on another living horse and involved canulation of the left ventricle via the xiphoid, and of the brachial artery via the leg. By closing and opening the two canulae, Barry noticed that expelled blood would not flow back into the ventricle; he concluded that dilatation of the ventricle was a passive event, since blood should have been drawn back if it were an active phenomenon.

Two of Barry's other conclusions seriously contradicted Laennec: first, Barry decided that the audible sounds made by the heart were not due to contraction, but to dilatation and passive filling of the chambers; second, he claimed that the first sound was made by expansion of the atrium and the second, by expansion of the ventricle. Neither man went out of his way to emphasize their differences. Laennec accepted most of Barry's observations about increased atrial filling during inspiration. He may have reconciled the differences by imagining that the atria dilated while the ventricles contracted, and that the ventricles dilated while the atria contracted; hence, the physical cause of the sound might have been under dispute, but the timing of the events was not. Barry continued to praise the physiological importance of auscultation, and requested a letter of reference from the dying Laennec to carry with him back to Britain where it would "establish his reputation."[74]

Historians who are critical of Laennec's cardiology tend to describe his interpretation of the heart sounds as a "reversal" of the correct sequence of contraction. But the heart sounds are not caused by muscular contractions; Laennec's interpretation is neither corrected nor improved simply by switching his nomenclature to label the first sound "auricular" and the second, "ventricular"—a terminology that corresponds less well to the physiological events observed. Moreover, Laennec's so-called "reversal" of the sequence of contractions may be more apparent than real. If every ventricular beat is preceded by an atrial beat, it must also be said that every ventricular beat is also *followed* by (and therefore precedes) an atrial beat, albeit displaced considerably in time. Laennec did not think that his description of the heart sounds was inconsistent with the work of Harvey, von Haller, or Barry. The sequence of the contractions seems to have been less important to his predecessors than the fact that the contractions alternated. For example, Sénac, who cited Harvey frequently, placed no special emphasis on the sequence of chamber contraction. Similarly, Barry concluded that one of his experiments had proven that Harvey was correct: the "atria contract *alternatively* with the ventricles," but he did not declare which contraction came first, and which, second.[75]

More support for this reconciliation between Harvey and Laennec can be found in the work of William Stokes (1804–1878), who published a short treatise on auscultation in 1825.[76] Stokes adopted Laennec's interpretation of the heart sounds, and was the first to use the terminology, "first sound" and "second sound"; however, his ordinal nomenclature was the direct opposite of present convention. Stokes's "first" heart sound was the one now called "second" and vice versa. Why did Stokes create this curious grouping of the sounds giving a longer pause between the two components of each heartbeat (first sound or atrial contraction, then a long pause, then second sound or ventricular contraction) than between the end of one beat and the start of the next? I believe that he was trying to strike an accord between the plausible observations of Laennec, including the rest period "overlooked by Haller," and the undisputed work of Harvey.

AUSCULTATION OF THE DISEASED HEART: PATHOLOGY

Having established the parameters of the normal heart sounds, Laennec began to study how they would change with disease and contribute to the existing signs of cardiac alteration. In diagnosing organic heart lesions, he already recognized the general symptoms of dyspnea on exertion, orthopnea, dependent edema, anasarca and palpitations. Unlike his British colleagues, he rarely timed the pulse, but he did notice quality and rhythm and startling variations in rate, which he sometimes tried to characterize. For example, in the case of Marie Potel, he described "two or three regular pulsations followed by several others that were very frequent."[77] He claimed to have felt a pulse slower than fifty beats per minute without symptoms, but he set less store by these examinations than had Corvisart.[78] He also resurrected swollen jugular veins as an indicator of enlarged right heart (hypertrophy and dilatation), the sign that had first been described by Giovanni Maria Lancisi (1654–1720) and rejected by Corvisart.[79] The disagreement about the jugular veins may have originated in Laennec's student days: the patient described in his first publication had pronounced beating in the jugular vein together with the pathological finding of dilated right heart.[80] Laennec thought that percussion was less useful in examination of the heart than it was in the lungs, but like his teacher and Burns, he relied heavily on the value of palpation of the chest wall: exaggerated impulse was a sign of enlargement; thrill, a sign of valvular disease. Auscultation merely enhanced the utility of the older methods in the diagnosis of the heart.[81]

With his predecessors and contemporaries, Laennec was interested more in enlargement of the heart and its chambers than he was in the state of the valves or arteries. Hypertrophy and dilatation were the most obvious, and seemingly the most common, anatomical alterations of the heart, and they dominated his clinical research on that organ. The most useful diagnostic signs would be those that could reliably and precisely indicate hypertrophy and dilatation of cardiac muscle. Signs of valvular disease, coronary disease, and pericarditis were less important. From a present-day perspective, hypertrophy and dilatation may be the most obvious findings at autopsy, but they are usually thought to be secondary to some other pathological change, be it anatomical (such as valvular lesions, lung disease, and infarct) or metabolic (such as uremia, toxemia, and hypertension). Laennec described sounds that would now be considered diagnostic of these primary conditions, but his concern was to associate the sounds with the ultimate changes in size and volume of the heart.

Alteration of the Heart Sounds

Laennec assumed that variations in the quality and intensity of the heart sounds must reflect organic changes in the myocardium, rather than in the other components of the heart. This assumption may have been fostered by his musical literacy, which suggested a relationship of loudness to strength; it was supported by his physiological investigations on skeletal muscle. Initially the duration of the heart sounds was considered an indication of enlargement: several case reports from 1819 or earlier mention "short" and "long" heart sounds.[82] Later cases, however, do not mention the duration of the sounds, except in conjunction with murmurs.

The final criteria established by Laennec involve an inverse relationship between acoustic events and muscle bulk: distinct or loud heart sounds implied dilatation of the ventricles (thin-walled, enlarged chambers); silent or absent sounds implied hypertrophy (thick-walled chambers of any size). Laennec also relied on the location of the sounds and their extension to unusual locations. The impulse of the heart on the chest wall felt by the examiner's outstretched hand, precordial lift, was an important consideration; sometimes, the impulse was carried to the side of the examiner's head through the stethoscope as a movement rather than a noise (see table 8.2).[83] Barry and Bertin both confirmed Laennec's finding of louder heart sounds in cardiac dilatation and softer sounds in hypertrophy, although Barry's experiments do not appear to have given him the opportunity to test their validity.[84]

At first, Laennec seems to have been confident of his heart signs. In both editions of his treatise and in the thesis of his student Adolphe Toulmouche, the stethoscopic signs of heart disease are described in enthusiastic terms proclaiming the advantages of auscultation over "equivocal" symptoms: he used phrases like, "the only sure sign," "the only constant and truly pathognomonic sign."[85] When he employed these superlative modifiers for the lucidity of his technique, however, he indulged in some of the muddiest prose in his book; the interpretation summarized in the preceding paragraph is derived only with difficulty. For example, he said that the signs of right ventricular hypertrophy "are exactly the same as those for that of the left except that the ventricular beat is less soft."[86] Then he said that the signs of hypertrophy of both ventricles "consist in a unification of the signs of hypertrophy of each ventricle, but with an almost constant predominance of

TABLE 8.2
Laennec's Criteria for Diagnosis of Cardiac Hypertrophy and Dilatation

Lesion	Impulse	Percussion	First Sound	Second Sound	Other Signs
LV hypertrophy	great	dullness	soft, short	soft, increased	pulse
RV hypertrophy	great, lower sternum	—	soft, but less than in LVH	soft	jugular distent
LV dilatation	decreased	—	clear, loud	loud	pulse soft, wea
RV dilatation	—	unreliable	loud over lower sternum	loud	jugular distent
L & RV hypertrophy	Combination of the signs described for LV hypertrophy and RV hypertrophy				

Source: *Traité* 1819; *Traité* 1826.
Note: R, right; L, left; V, ventricular.

those of the right."[87] But the only explanation of "those [signs] of the right" in the second citation was the unrevealing statement in the first citation—a meaningless circle of words! Such confusion made excellent fodder for his detractors who would complain, not inappropriately, of "the overabundance of detail, and excessive nuances of perception."[88]

Murmurs and Rubs: Disease or Not Disease

Another of Laennec's great cardiac "errors" was his failure to appreciate the significance of heart murmurs, which are extra sounds that are relatively easy to hear even by a novice stethoscopist. They are now thought to occur in any situation that entails turbulence in blood flow, either because of structural changes, such as holes in the heart wall or diseased valves, or because of functional states of high cardiac output, including pregnancy, fever, anemia, and thyroid dysfunction. Diseased heart valves can usually be recognized without difficulty at autopsy. Consequently, it might now seem probable that an anatomically oriented clinician should have been able to make the correlations between murmurs and altered valves quickly and easily. But the physiological alterations in heart function caused by pregnancy, fever, anemia, and thyroid dysfunction leave no trace in the cadaver heart, although they can result in murmurs during life. The fact that murmurs can occur both with and without organic change is important.

Laennec heard and described murmurs, relating them to the familiar objects of bellows, wood files, grates, and saws; he did not know their significance, however. In 1819, he said that murmurs represented diseased valves, but he thought ossifications and excrescences on the valves were rare.[89] When the mitral valve was ossified, he said, "the auricular sound becomes much longer and more muffled and is slightly choked and brusque, reminiscent of a file on wood [*bruit de lime*]; sometimes this sound is similar to that of a bellows closed abruptly [*bruit de soufflet*]."[90] He did not associate a murmur with ossification of the aortic valve.

Laennec tried to distinguish between different organic changes on the heart valves by the different tonal qualities of the murmurs. For example, he associated the "file sound" with valvular ossification.[91] A "muffled noise" synchronous with the second sound was correlated with atrial enlargement, because it seemed to represent a prolongation of the atrial contraction (the second sound).[92] The muffled noise may have been due to stenosis of the mitral valve, which is often associated with left atrial hypertrophy as a secondary change.

Laennec soon began to reconsider his initial interpretations of murmurs, or as one historian put it: his thinking on the subject "deteriorated" into "curious aberration" in the "wrong direction."[93] In 1823, at the Collège de France, he retracted the original interpretation. Citing Erman's experiments, he said "[there are] many varieties [of murmurs]: file, grate, bellows, saw . . . [they] indicate spasm only. I used to believe they indicated a obstacle [to blood flow], but [it is] obvious from exper[ience or experiment?] that [this is] not so."[94] Confusing the issue in the same lecture, he continued to say that Corvisart's old sign of precordial thrill was a reliable sign of ossification of the valves that "never" appeared without a murmur.

In 1824, Victor Collin, Laennec's junior colleague at the Necker Hospital, published his thesis of late the previous year, including the observations about pneumonia and some of the experiments that had caused Laennec to retract his opinion in part. Collin claimed that the bellows sound or murmur could occur "in nervous individuals, hysterics, hypochondriacs, in the presence of hemorrhage often without any change in the structure or function of the heart," and "at autopsy no consistent organic changes are found." He reported that Laennec now thought of the murmur "as the sign of a simple spasm in the circulatory system," and he described four observations to support this new opinion:

1. its analogy with forced muscular contraction, as one places the elbow on a table, the hand on the ear and repeatedly contracts the jaw (inspired by Erman's experiments);
2. the ease with which it appears upon compression of the arteries of healthy people;
3. its existence over arteries delivering blood to a hemorrhage;
4. its existence in the palpitations produced by anemias.[95]

Collin did not reject all murmurs as signs of physical change. He reaffirmed the grating or file murmur as a sign of valvular narrowing, and emphasized Laennec's concern for distinguishing between different valvular changes on the basis of the quality of sound: "Mr. Laennec regards this murmur as a reliable sign of valvular narrowing by ossification, vegetation, or any other cause. The site and timing of the contractions in which [the murmur] is heard indicate which orifice is affected."[96] While the "file" sound indicated a change on the valve, it was due to muscular spasm upstream of the lesion.

In his second edition of 1826, Laennec did not cite Collin, but now he added a long discussion concerning abnormal sounds: a modification, if not a retraction, of his original opinion.[97] All murmurs indicated spasm, or prolonged contraction of a cardiac chamber, and he included Erman's example of the contracting jaw muscles. His reassessment was directly related to the work on noisy and silent muscular contractions. The same blend of physics and observation resulted in perhaps the most disarming passage in his entire opus: music, complete with staff, notes, slurs and clef, to describe the sounds he heard in the carotid artery of a woman with phthisis who had consulted him on 13 March 1824. He said, "The melody rolled on three notes separated by an interval of a major third; top note was wrong and a little too low," he said, "but not low enough to require a flat."[98] The exhilaration of his musical finding made such an impact that he promptly described it to Cruveilhier whose reply is cited with the memorable passage in the epigraph above.[99]

Laennec now questioned the value of the murmur associated with Corvisart's precordial thrill as a sign of organic change; he even doubted the significance of the thrill itself. Murmurs are "remarkable," he said; "they are the only auscultatory sounds that are not related to any organic lesion in which one can find their cause." He said that the bellows sound resulted from spasm; neither it nor the associated thrill implied any organic lesion in the heart or its arteries. It was "extremely likely" that they were "due to a specific modification of innervation," because they occur in "young hypochondriacs," people "with fever," and "above all in those with palpitations of purely nervous origin."[100] Having originally considered murmurs as signs of valvular disease, Laennec had now abandoned all murmurs as signs of structural change; they were the result of the altered physiology of muscle spasm.

Two cases, one from May 1820 and another from November 1823, illustrate the change in Laennec's interpretation of murmurs and its awkward implications. The first, a thirty-five-year-old woman, with a palpable thrill and a murmur "softer than a file sound," led her examiners to predict the mitral valve ossification, which was confirmed by autopsy.[101] The second was a twenty-five-year-old cabinet-maker, named Jean Juelle, with a left precordial lift and a file-sound murmur synchronous with the first heart sound, in whom the initial observer predicted ventricular hypertrophy and ossification of the aortic valves. But when Laennec examined Juelle the following week, he heard the same murmur and a crepitant *râle* and made the additional diagnosis of "pulmonary edema—spasm of the arteries." Autopsy proved beyond question the presence of left ventricular hypertrophy, but the student-writer seems to have tried to minimize the valvular findings that he had predicted successfully but his teacher had not. He wrote: "one of the sigmoid valves of the aorta was entirely ossified at its base and open [*"béante"*]; nevertheless it reduced the caliber of the artery only a little at this point" and the rest of the aorta and other arteries were "perfectly healthy."[102] The valvular change was confirmed, but spasm, being a phenomenon of life, could be neither demonstrated nor disproved by autopsy.

Laennec's revised opinion about murmurs was not unjustified. Given the incidence of tuberculosis with its complications of fever and anemia, it is probable that he often heard murmurs in the seemingly "lesionless" physiological states of fever and anemia. Arterial bruits can also occur with hemorrhage or in anomalies of physical architecture that have no pathological significance, as Collin's experiments had demonstrated. Laennec's familiarity with the findings of his friend, Kergaradec, concerning the murmur overlying the normal human placenta probably further clouded the apparent significance of all murmurs.[103] Heart murmurs seemed to be like puerile respiration, a sign of physiological change that may or may not be associated with physical change.

Friction rubs, like heart murmurs, are distinctive, additional sounds, similar to the noise made by creaking leather. Easily heard, they are now associated with inflamed or roughened tissues sliding over each other with the natural movements of circulation and respiration, especially in pericarditis, pleuritis, and following infarctions of the lung, heart, or spleen. But they can be confused with the noise made by clothing brushing against the skin. Laennec does not appear to have heard the friction sound before the first edition of his treatise. In 1820, one student said that his teacher had seen pericarditis "many times with no clinical signs to which he would dare to accord the slightest degree of certitude."[104] In 1823, however, the aforementioned Collin, wrote the first clinical description of the rub in pericarditis.[105] Collin's description was confined to two patients: the first he had personally examined, but without autopsy; the second had been attended and autopsied by an intern at the St. Antoine hospital who had also examined the first patient. But in 1826, Laennec did not name Collin and mentioned the sound only to reject it: "I thought for a while that this sound could be a sign of pericarditis, but since then, I have been convinced that it is not."[106] The failure to cite the younger man on friction rub was later criticized by Bouillaud as a lack of charity.[107] His rejection of the sound appears to be yet another of Laennec's "mistakes" that seems to invite justification.

In 1823–1824, Laennec was receptive to the idea of the rub as a sign and said, "I believed I heard a noise like that of leather in a convalescent case, but I cannot confirm it."[108] A problem lay in the differing frequencies of the lesion and the sound. Pericarditis was "quite common" in Laennec's experience, and it appeared often in his autopsy reports. The friction rub was heard far less frequently at the bedside than pericarditis appeared in the morgue. Now it is accepted that the rub appears only in some varieties of pericarditis and rarely in those associated with large effusions or tuberculosis.[109]

By 1826, Collin's evidence for rub as a sign of pericarditis may have seemed too tenuous for inclusion in the treatise; it was based on only one case with postmortem confirmation. Shaky evidence in other situations had not deterred Laennec from including new observations by his associates; perhaps he meant to slight his former *chef de clinique*, because he and Collin did not always agree on how to teach or popularize auscultation. Collin had been the first to suggest that pectoriloquy occurred in pneumonia, something Laennec did not accept until he had devised the new sign bronchophony (see chap. 7). Collin also appeared to endorse the criticisms of some reviewers about the inventor's lengthy descriptions. He advised that a stethoscopist should "avoid tedious detail and infinite subdivisions, convinced that the many nuances belonging to the major stethoscopic sounds can be appreciated only by attentive and repeated observation and that even a very long description gives only an incomplete idea of their nature."[110]

Angina Pectoris and the Absence of Sounds: A Lesion of Physiology?

By the time Laennec published the first edition of the *Treatise on Auscultation*, the coronary theory of angina had been accepted by medical writers in Britain, Italy, and Germany, but those in France were skeptical. In October 1809, the Société médicale de Paris had held a competition for the best essay on the controversial topic. The judges were dissatisfied with the first entries and prolonged the deadline until February 1813. None of the essays submitted were deemed worthy of the prize, but three received special mention: two in Latin and one in French, which was later published.[111] The three competitors had been aware of the coronary theory, but only one granted it any place in his classification. In the meantime, Eugène-Henri Desportes (1782–1875) published his theory of the nervous origin of angina, which he supported by invoking the unmistakable relationship between anginal pain and emotions.[112] In France, angina was a nervous disease.

Laennec did not mention the coronary arteries in his 1803 course in pathological anatomy, but by late 1810, he was aware of the coronary artery theory and its critics. His Latin lecture on angina pectoris read at the Société de l'Ecole de Médecine in December 1810, may have been one of the unsuccessful entries for the competition of the rival society; unfortunately only part of the manuscript is preserved (fig. 8.2).[113] In it, he wrote that the arguments "of Jenner and other observers" were refuted by autopsies: ossified coronary arteries could be found in persons who died without ever having experienced the symptoms of angina; conversely, normal coronaries were found in others dead of what he considered to be unmistakable angina.[114] As a result, the causal relationship of coronary ossification to angina pectoris could not be proven, and he continued to think that angina was of nervous origin. The loyal biographer, Rouxeau, intimated that some rivalry existed between Laennec and Desportes over priority for the neuralgia theory; he hinted that Desportes may have been inspired by Laennec without giving him his due. Even without Laennec's obscure essay, the nervous theory already had many adherents.[115]

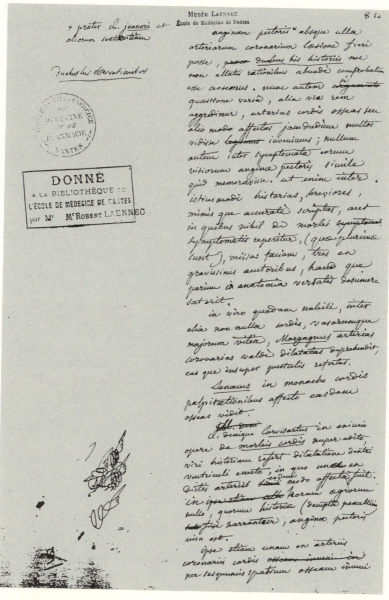

Figure 8.2. A page from Laennec's incomplete Latin essay on angina pectoris read in December 1810 at the Société de l'Ecole de Médecine. The coronary theory is mentioned at the upper right, with a reference to Jenner in the upper left and to Morgagni, Sénac, and Corvisart lower on the page. Source: ML, MS Cl. 7, lot e-2, f. 9r.

With Laennec's essay on angina are several clinical records, including a manuscript case-history entitled "angina pectoris?" The patient, fifty-year-old Nicolas Millot, was thought to have suffered angina pains ten to twelve times a day for six years, but he died of erysipelas of the right chest in November 1810. At autopsy, Millot was found to have a slightly enlarged heart, but the valves and great arteries were "natural," and the coronary arteries had "not the slightest trace of ossification." This case served Laennec as evidence against the coronary ossification theory. It may have been a poor choice, however, because some features of Millot's chest pain did not correspond to the descriptions of angina that had already been accepted for some time.[116]

As for his observations on puerile respiration, some clinical evidence about angina came from Laennec's own health. Along with asthma, hypochondria, and gout, he diagnosed angina pectoris in himself on various occasions from 1806 to 1819. He referred to his own angina in his Latin manuscript and in the case history, which I believe to be his own, printed in the first edition of the *Treatise on Mediate Auscultation*. It describes intermittent left-sided heaviness in the chest and emphasizes the beneficial effect of strenuous exercise.[117] A person suffering from an organic lesion of the heart could neither tolerate nor improve with vigorous effort, he thought.

Laennec's reservations about the coronary theory predated auscultation by at least seven years, and his opinion would not change after the stethoscope.[118] The absence of definite auscultatory abnormalities in angina tended to consolidate his opinion. For him, persistence of normal sounds implied the absence of organic change. Therefore he continued to describe angina as a nervous "lesionless" disease, or "*névrose*," localized to the heart—a disease that bore no constant relationship to the state of the coronary arteries or to the myocardium. Reports of autopsies performed after the invention of the stethoscope rarely mention the coronary arteries, as if he had given up testing the theory. This disease, like asthma, was a lesionless condition; no objective sign, however, could be found for detecting angina.

CARDIAC SIGNS IN PRACTICE: CLINICAL CASES

Belying the superlative adjectives to the contrary, Laennec seems to have been discouraged by his attempts to sort out cardiac auscultation. The evidence marshaled in support of his stethoscopic signs of the heart is unconvincing, and he cautioned his readers not to place too much confidence in the stethoscope in diagnosis of the heart. Uncharacteristically, he dwelt on the value of other modalities in diagnosing heart disease and he thought the stethoscope could do little to detect aneurysms.[119] The first edition closed with a discussion of aortic aneurysms, in which the unreliability of auscultation was emphasized—an opinion shared by one of his students.[120] A few cases were added to this section for the second edition, with little change in the conclusions, and he ignored the 1823 thesis of Bouillaud, who had said that auscultation was better in detecting aneurysms than the inventor had thought.[121] Some claimed that Laennec tended to emphasize the stethoscopic signs of the heart in public more than he did in his own practice, a habit that earned him the nickname of "cylindromanic."[122]

To explore Laennec's practical use of the stethoscope in heart disease, I have examined thirty-six published and unpublished clinical records on cardiac cases (see table 8.3). Only a few case observations were published in the chapters on the heart; they changed little between the two editions. Sometimes they failed to support Laennec's claims. In the 1819 edition, only six of a total of fifty complete case observations concern the heart and great vessels: Ponsard, Potel, Villeneuve, Lefebvre, an unidentified thirty-five-year-old laborer, and Millet.[123] Four had been examined with the stethoscope, five had been examined by autopsy. Lefebvre, who had died in 1803, was a prestethoscopic case selected because of the spectacular postmortem findings on the valves. Potel, a thirty-nine-year-old woman who died in early December 1817, was found to have loud heart sounds, which were correlated with the autopsy findings of cardiac dilatation, pulmonary tuberculosis, and an enlarged liver. Villeneuve died in 1819, but auscultation of his loud heart sounds had failed to predict the pericarditis found at autopsy. The case of the thirty-five-year-old laborer, who had died in April 1819 with a murmur, was used to illustrate the diagnosis of ventricular hypertrophy by variation in the intensity of the heart sounds. Ponsard's loud murmurs were attributed to diseased valves, but he was still alive in 1819. No mention was made of auscultation in the case of Millet who had died in May 1817 of a dissecting aortic aneurysm with left ventricular hypertrophy.

In 1826, a few brief clinical examples were added in the chapters on heart disease, but no new complete case histories appeared, although Laennec had revised some interpretations. Again there were six complete cases out of a total of fifty-one: Ponsard, Potel, Lefebvre, the unidentified thirty-five-year-old laborer, Millet, and Dirichard.[124] The seemingly new case of Dirichard had already been published in the 1819 edition in the section on lung diseases.[125] The unsuccessful predictions concerning the case of Villeneuve were removed, as were cross references made in 1819 to another five cases, in which the heart sounds had been unreliable in florid disease of the lung.[126] There was an update on the still-living Ponsard, who had returned to visit Laennec in 1822: still without autopsy and still with his loud heart murmurs, his case and that of the thirty-five year-old laborer were both left as examples of mitral valve disease, although in Laennec's revised semiology, "murmur" now meant spasm, not obstruction.

In addition to the seven cardiac cases published in the two editions of the treastise, twenty-seven manuscript records and two cases published elsewhere in the treatise have titles that indicate heart disease (table 8.3). Sometimes, Laennec's diagnostic signs could predict hypertrophy or dilatation with success. Once, for example, Laennec's cousin Mériadec was embarrassed to discover a greatly hypertrophied heart, after he had ignored

TABLE 8.3
Diagnosis of Heart Disease in the *Traité de l'auscultation* and the Manuscripts

Date	Reference	Name	Ausc	Perc	Palp	PM	Accur
n.d.	MS I b 195	Anon.				pm	
20 July 03	2:675	Lefebvre			pal	pm	
2 Feb 17	MS I b 17	Guérin		perc		pm	
22 Apr 17	2:696	Millet				pm	X
30 Oct 17	2:636	Potel	a		pal	pm	√
6 Dec 17	MS I b 21	Chaudron	a			pm	X
14 Apr 18	2:302 (1819)*	male 62 yr	a		pal	pm	par
12 June 18	MS I b 78	Rocha	a		pal		
30 Jan 19	2:382 (1819)	Villeneuve	a		pal	pm	X
8 Feb 19	2:642	Dirichard	a		pal	pm	par
11 Feb 19	2:582	Ponsard	a		pal		
10 Apr 19	2:623	male 35 yr	a		pal	pm	par
5 May 19	MS I b 178	Mercier				pm	
23 Oct 19	MS I d 1	male 65 yr	a		pal	pm	X
20 Apr 20	MS I d 6	female 35 yr	a		pal	pm	√
15 Nov 21	MS I c 5	Moissenat	a			pm	par
18 Jan 22	MS I c 16	Brasard	a		pal	pm	√
29 Jan 22	MS I c 31	Piron		perc	pal	pm	par
21 Mar 22	MS I d 13	Schmidt	a		pal	pm	X
8 Nov 23	MS II 80	Juelle	a		pal	pm	√
13 Mar 24	MS II 168	Duvinage	a		pal	pm	X
20 Mar 24	MS II 509	Troncin	a		pal		
16 Apr 24	MS II 201	Lepaul	a		pal		
30 Apr 24	MS II 188	Boulaud	a		pal	pm	par
n.d. ca. July 24	MS II 385	Guillio	a			pm†	
4 Sep 24	MS II 466	Taguel	a		pal	pm†	par
18 Oct 24	MS II 488	Bouquet	a	perc	pal		
11 Dec 24	MS III 61	Magdelain	a		pal	pm	X
24 Jan 25	MS II 454	Claudel	a		pal	pm	X
1 May 25	1:518*	Richard	a		pal	pm	par
18 May 25	MS III 271	Charon	a		pal	pm	X
1 June 25	MS III 261	Laurent	a		pal	pm	X
3 July 25	MS III 372	Desabau			pal	pm	X
6 Aug 25	MS III 412	Anon.			pal		
7 Dec 25	MS III 448	Millet	a		pal	pm	par
Feb 26	MS III 490	Prevost	a		pal	pm†	par

Note: MS, Musée Laennec code for document, Classeur, lot, page; a, use of auscultation; pal, palpa of the precordium; perc, percussion of the precordium; pm, autopsy examination; part, partially cor prediction; X, incorrect prediction; √, correct prediction.

* Published case for which a manuscript record is also available, e.g. *1*:518.

† Indicates an incomplete autopsy.

Laennec's teaching and predicted a "weak" heart on the basis of soft sounds.[127] In another patient, he seems to have had better results in using auscultation and the presence of a thrill to predict hypertrophy and mitral valve disease, but Laennec's annotation, "it is useless to use it," implies that Mériadec had hoped that his successful diagnosis would be published, but Laennec had refused.[128]

Four of the thirty-six cases in the survey had findings at autopsy that had been correctly predicted before death, but in two of these, the prediction of change in the mitral valve relied more on the presence of a palpable thrill than it did on auscultation. Ten other diagnoses had been predicted with partial success, but the stethoscope had not made the diagnosis: in two, cardiac enlargement had been recognized by palpation and percussion alone; in one (Piron) the stethoscope had not been used; and two (Taguel, Prevost) had presented with murmurs, but the heart valves were not mentioned in the autopsy report. Sometimes it seems that words used in the final write-up were carefully selected to match the predictions. The pathology report on Moissenet, a sixty-seven-year-old male, justified the clear heart sounds suggestive of dilatation: "heart not very large . . . [but] cavities were perhaps a little larger than the walls were thick."[129] Similarly, an anonymous sixty-year-old man had a heart, that was "a little bigger" than his fist, the right ventricle "quite large," and the left "a little more vast than it ought to have been."[130]

Eleven cases of the thirty-six in the survey resulted in postmortem findings that were precisely the opposite of what Laennec's cardiac signs should have predicted; in none did the author openly declare the signs to have been inaccurate. As had been done for the reports on Moissenet and on Juelle, failures in diagnosis were occasionally softened by manipulating the phrases used to describe the autopsy. For example, in the case of Charon, hypertrophy had been implied, but dilatation was found: the student wrote, "the right and left ventricles were of a capacity perhaps more than double what they should have been; the walls were not thinned, those of the left ventricle were perhaps even thick." Similarly for Laurent, hypertrophy also seems to have been expected, but the report stated, "the walls of the ventricle did not seem thick but, because of the large capacity of the cavities, they truly were thickened because they were in proportion to the increase in capacity." And for Magdelain, "cavities of the heart were vast, the walls of a mediocre thickness compared to the size of the cavities, but nevertheless thicker than in the natural state."[131]

The remaining eleven cases, which were labeled heart disease, afford no opportunities for anatomoclinical correlation: either they lacked a record of auscultation or they lacked an autopsy or an adequate autopsy; and one patient was diagnosed with heart disease without autopsy or auscultation. Four were given a postmortem diagnosis of heart disease, which had not been suspected before death. In six others, heart disease was diagnosed on the basis of history or physical examination, and all were still alive at the time of the report; in none of the six had the stethoscope provided the reason for the clinical diagnosis: three had irregular heart beats, two had precordial impulsion, one, a thrill. In one case, that of Françoise Guillio, the patient was auscultated and her cadaver autopsied, but the reporter failed to record the pathological findings in the heart.

Comparison of the manuscripts with the published versions of case histories is instructive. For example, the manuscript of the report on the twenty-two-year-old weaver, François Richard, contains no antemortem diagnoses; however, the published version provided several diagnoses at different stages throughout his clinical course. Moreover, the auscultatory signs in Richard's published case seem slightly different from that on his hospital admission record.[132] Although this case was entitled "heart disease," it was published as an example of resolving pneumonia.

This survey suggests that Laennec's confidence in cardiac auscultation was on the wane. The cases after 1824 that contain a clinical diagnosis had been attended in Laennec's absence by his colleague, Cayol, and the antemortem cardiac diagnosis, if it appeared at all, was not based on auscultation.[133] Laennec's efforts to establish auscultatory signs for the heart seem to have been largely abandoned by the mid 1820s, and many of the brief cases added to the heart section of the second edition of the *Treatise on Mediate Auscultation* had been published elsewhere by others.

CARDIAC AUSCULTATION AFTER LAENNEC

Attacks on Laennec's cardiology by his physician-colleagues began with the first edition and continued, with unceasing vigor, during the debate over the interpretation of heart sounds after his death. Even the translator, John Forbes (1787–1861), referred readers to Burns and other works on heart disease, saying that the "paramount importance of auscultatory diagnostics in [Laennec's] mind has rendered this epitome too brief . . . [it is excellent] as far as it goes."[134] These early assaults may explain mysterious lacunae in his papers. Few of the complete histories published in the section on heart disease in Laennec's treatise now exist in manuscript, although many lung cases do. The cardiac sections of his 1803 course on pathological anatomy are missing.[135] The aforementioned Latin lecture on angina pectoris is also incomplete. Similarly, all but one of the ten lessons on diseases of the heart given at the Collège de France have been lost or destroyed—an exceptional omission in an otherwise complete collection.[136]

The first interpretation of the heart sounds as products of valve closure appeared in the 1832 thesis of J. Rouanet (1797–1865), but the hypothesis could not be proven until the advent of experimental cardiac catheterization (F. Magendie and C. Bernard 1844) and a technique for measuring intracardiac pressures (J. B. A. Chauveau and J. Marey 1861), work conducted in horses and dogs.[137] In the meantime, the valvular hypothesis was rejected by some of the luminaries of physiology, including Magendie, Dominic Corrigan (1802–1880), and Joseph Beau (1806–1865).[138] In Britain the second sound was "proven" to be synchronous with aortic and pulmonic valve closure by the experimental work of C. J. B. Williams and James Hope on donkeys poisoned with curare and stunned by a mallet.[139] Williams had studied with Laennec at the Necker hospital in 1825, and the following year Hope worked with A. Chomel (1788–1858), Laennec's successor at the Charité. Williams and Hope became rivals for priority for the new, but equally erroneous, interpretation that the first sound was muscular because of ventricular contraction and the second was valvular. Nevertheless, the debate continued on both sides of the Channel, each side in apparent ignorance of what was happening on the other.[140]

Heart murmurs were linked with changes of the valves within Laennec's lifetime, despite his reservations and long before the interpretation of the heart sounds had been resolved. Bouillaud became thoroughly convinced of the reliability of thrill and murmurs in predicting valve lesions and was not in the least troubled by the numerous cases in which murmurs could be heard without organic lesions. Friction rub was adopted equally quickly as a sign of pericarditis, and the fact that the sign had been described by an associate of Laennec has somehow insulated the inventor from criticisms on this point from most writers, except Bouillaud.[141] As for angina pectoris, the debate over the coronary artery theory would continue well into the twentieth century, and some of Laennec's favorite ideas, including spasm, were eventually resurrected, although his theorizing about them had long been forgotten.[142]

Historians who are preoccupied with bolstering claims to priority miss the epistemological diversity within a protracted controversy. When the debates over the heart sounds finally ended, Laennec had been on the losing sides of all. Nevertheless, his observations were accurate, his reservations justified, and his opinions irrefutable with the evidence and technology at his disposal. The precision of some of his observations was not confirmed until the 1970s, probably because the lesions that were important to him had not been important to his successors. For example, the inverse relationship between the amplitude of heart sounds and the thickness of the heart muscle (quiet sounds in hypertrophy) has been established once again.[143] This analysis confirms the observations of Reidar K. Lie that medical theories are adopted (and rejected) in the face of good evidence and tenable theories to the contrary.[144]

CLINICAL REASONING IN THE TREATISE ON AUSCULTATION

In this and the two preceding chapters, we see how Laennec constructed diagnostic entities out of the sounds he heard through the stethoscope. But it is clear that the perceptual activities involved in both the construction of these signs and their application went well beyond listening. These entities were more than sounds; they incorporated visualization, imagination, calculation, and theory. Laennec did more than simply listen through his stethoscope.[145] The remainder of this chapter is devoted to Laennec's reasoning as he established his new elements of diagnosis. Except for the rather straightforward example of percussion, there were few precursors and no rules for the handling of objective, clinical evidence. What were acceptable limits of accuracy for the link between a noise perceived by the doctor and the physical change inside the patient's body? Was there a tolerable margin of error? Were there thresholds?

Laennec moved through this uncharted domain, apparently oblivious to the new methods in acoustics, mathematical probability, and statistics that might have provided preliminary guidelines for his decisions concerning the utility of a sign.[146] He also seemed to ignore, perhaps deliberately, any consideration of the degree of pathophysiological disruption required to generate (or obliterate) the abnormal sound and he seems to have been unaware of at least two French physicians' work in fluid dynamics and sound. C. J. B. Williams determined that his former teacher had a poor understanding of acoustics.[147] Nevertheless, Laennec set rigid standards for his stethoscopic signs. Using the patient records and the changes made for the second edition of the treatise, it is possible to reconstruct the epistemological priorities in his decision-making process.

At first, Laennec considered the organic lesion a necessary cause for each abnormal sound: whenever he heard the sound, the lesion had to be present. He was inclined to ascribe one and only one lesion to each stethoscopic sign; initially, he grouped diseases under the physiological process that allowed for their diagnosis (voice: phthisis; respiration with bubbles: pneumonia, etc.). Gradually, he came to accept the possibility that, for some sounds, one or several lesions could be sufficient cause of the abnormal sound: whenever he heard the sound, a limited range of pathological lesions was implied. If a sound could be associated with more than one type of lesion, he usually rejected it as a sign of anatomical change, but he would consider whether it indicated a physiological alteration. His concept of diagnosing pathological physiology was modeled on that of pathological anatomy and was centered on detection of lesions (see table 8.4).

Laennec's priorities can be restated in terms of the "specificity" and "sensitivity" of twentieth-century decision-making vocabulary. The self-conscious application of these terms to medical decision-making and their ultimate incorporation into medical vocabulary appeared in the first third of the twentieth century as a vehicle for speaking about potential inaccuracies in laboratory testing for venereal disease and tuberculosis.[148] As for my discussion of the heart and lung sounds, I use this twentieth-century vocabulary to elucidate—not evaluate—a methodological process that entered medicine ahead of the words that are now used to describe it. These words are conceptual tools of analysis that can be applied to the past as well as to the present. The purpose of the exercise is not to demonstrate that Laennec thought as we do, but to explore the evolution of his clinical reasoning. What exactly made him accept or reject a stethoscopic sign? A hypothesis?

TABLE 8.4

Correlation of Auscultatory Evidence with Pathology and Physiology: Clinical Examples

thoscopic m?	Anatomical Pathology: Organic Lesion (patient sick or well)	Pathophysiology: No Organic Lesion (patient sick)	Physiology: No Organic Lesion (patient well)
	phthisis = pectoriloquy	asthma = puerile	nervous = puerile
	effusion = egophony	spasm = murmur	pregnancy = murmur
	ossified coronary arteries	fever	health
	aortic aneurysm	angina pectoris	

Laennec insisted that, in order to be reliable, a sign must be specific. Specificity means that a sign is peculiar to one condition only and that, whenever the sound occurs, the lesion is present. If a sign is not specific, then it can occur in conditions other than the one for which it is intended to be an indicator; the result is a false positive. Specificity was not Laennec's word for this priority; he used the words "*pathognomonique*" and "*constans.*" Nevertheless, the concept of specificity held absolute control over his formulation of auscultatory semiology. He abhorred the false positive.

Laennec also insisted on a certain level of sensitivity. If a sign is sensitive, then it will appear in every example of a condition, even if the change is minimal. If a sign is not sensitive, there may be cases that escape detection: false negatives. Sensitivity is independent of specificity. For example, a sign may be sensitive to a certain condition, but not specific; it will result in many false positives but no false negatives. Laennec assigned less importance to sensitivity than to specificity.

Each of Laennec's new signs was a tiny theory about the anatomical or physiological status of his patient. He rejected a sign if it could be "falsified," usually by having predicted a false positive occurrence of the lesion; sometimes he rejected it if it produced an abundance of false negatives—a practice that tends to adhere to Karl Popper's theory of falsifiability–falsification in scientific change and demarcation.[149] If an idea or a hypothesis is formulated in a postulate that is falsifiable, it is scientific; if it can be proven wrong—falsified—it is rejected. Laennec seems to have supported this principle, whereas a generation earlier, Lavoisier did not.[150] These priorities will be illustrated by a few examples from the material already presented.

The heart murmur provides a good example of a sign that was sensitive but not specific. For Laennec, heart murmurs were sensitive to valve changes, but they were not specific and resulted in many false positives. Valvular alteration was a sufficient cause for a murmur, but not a necessary cause. Murmurs could also be heard when there was no valvular pathology, in anemia and tachycardia, and in the heart of a healthy, pregnant woman or overlying her placenta. Murmurs could also be produced experimentally by compression of healthy vessels, or accidentally by injury and hemorrhage. Laennec rejected the reliability of murmur for the recognition of organic changes on the valves, because false positives occurred too frequently to fulfill his standards of specificity. He did not reject murmurs as signs, however.

In situations of false positive murmurs (when no valvular change had been present), patients had usually been sick or otherwise altered from their usual healthy or nonpregnant state. He proposed that murmurs were signs of spasm (trembling of a heart muscle) that may or may not have been associated with a concomitant change in a valve. If murmurs indicated spasm, then confirmation could not be found in the cadaver. They pointed to a physiological change, which sometimes, but not necessarily, was associated with lesions on the valves.

The sound of friction rub offers the example of too many false negatives, or a lack of sensitivity. Pericarditis had been found at autopsy far more often than the rub was heard at the bedside. Laennec seems to have been more tolerant of false negatives than of false positives, or at least willing to suspend judgment until he had convinced himself one way or the other. For example, after he recognized egophony in some but not all effusion, he waited and wondered until he was confident of its meaning. But the rarity of instances in which the friction rub had been heard contrasted markedly with the large numbers of patients in whom autopsy revealed pericarditis. In other words, the friction rub may have been specific, but it was not sensitive.

Examples of these criteria for the acceptability of stethoscopic signs are not confined to auscultation of the heart. Like the murmur, puerile respiration was a sign of physiological alteration in which Laennec had confidence. He believed that it was specific for a certain type of respiration that could occur in health or disease, but distinguishing between the two states required the further input of the patient's subjective feelings of sickness or well-being.

Laennec's distrust of the false positive is especially apparent in his consideration of the causes of pectoriloquy. For him, pectoriloquy was an absolute indicator of tuberculous excavation; it was equated with a diagnosis of phthisis. This conviction was demonstrated in the clinical vignette in which he insisted on reexamining a cadaver lung to prove that the sign had accurately predicted a cavity that had been missed by careless dissection.[151] Laennec tried to establish degrees of pectoriloquy to correspond to different lesions. When he found that this single sign seemed to appear in a second condition, bronchiectasis, he justified his findings at length with emphasis on the anatomical similarities of the two conditions. When the newly graduated Collin pointed out that it could also exist in a third condition, consolidation of the lung in pneumonia (hepatization)—a condition that bore no anatomical relationship to the other two—he made no comment. Finally, he had to create a "different," new sign, "bronchophony," a form of "imperfect" pectoriloquy that was supposed to occur in enlargement of the airways or in consolidation of the lung.[152] The specificity of pectoriloquy could then be unchallenged.

Laennec's description of pulmonary catarrh or bronchitis also illustrates the one sign–one lesion principle. He named many different types of rales, each corresponding to clinical variations of bronchitis, based on sputum color, quantity, and texture—variations that may reflect what might now be considered differing bacterial or viral pathogens.[153] These subdivisions might have had some explanatory power, but they were subtle and cumbersome. Because they did not correspond to any reliable clinical or therapeutic distinction, they garnered early criticism and fell into disuse.

Similarly, egophony always represented pleural effusion for Laennec. He knew that some effusions were not associated with the sound, and accepted occasional false negatives of less than perfect sensitivity. Andral was unable to convince him, however, that egophony could exist under false positive circumstances, when there was no effusion at all.[154] In Laennec's auscultatory work, there were no exceptions to the priority of specificity.

The same priorities governed Laennec's reasoning in domains other than auscultation, including the conceptual realm of etiology. For example, he had rejected the coronary artery theory of angina by 1810, because he believed he had seen good evidence against it in the single case of Nicolas Millot: the man felt the pain, but his cadaver did not have the lesion.[155] In other words, Millot's case was an example of a false positive in a diagnostic system that tried to link the pain of angina with a change in the arteries. For Laennec, one case was sufficient to prove that anginal pain was not a specific sign of coronary ossification. Therefore, coronary disease could not be the cause of, or associated with angina, even if they sometimes occurred in conjunction with each other. In angina, he also had evidence of the false negative and claimed to have seen ossified coronary arteries in people who had never suffered anginal pain. A single example to the contrary was sufficient to erode the whole structure of a theory, and he virtually gave up examining coronary arteries possibly because the lesion could not be associated with a definitive clinical syndrome. Here again, Laennec's practice conforms to the "logic" described by Popper.

When it came to the cause of phthisis, Laennec thought that the heredity theory was refuted by the observations that the children were healthy in some families with consumptive parents and grandparents (false positive), and all the children were consumptive in other families with healthy parents (false negative). Therefore, a parent with phthisis did not reliably predict the disease in offspring.[156] Likewise with inflammation: unless a lesion could be shown to have the classic findings of *rubor, dolor, calor, tumor*, and *laesio functionis*, it was reductionist to impute any organic change to inflammation simply because it existed. Again with "latency": Louis may have seen tubercles in the lungs of his dead patients, but tubercles were ubiquitous and their presence did not imply that they had caused the death or even the illness experienced by the patient.

Finally, Laennec rejected the presence of illness as a necessary sign of physical change. He thought that lesions could be absent, and the patient could be seriously ill. He was among the first to appreciate that anatomical changes could occur in health (false positive); but he did not forget that they could be absent in sickness and the patient still might die (false negative). Anatomical changes were not causes of disease; like the symptoms of illness, they were the result of some prior insult, which was the cause of the disease. Laennec believed that younger practitioners of pathological anatomy did not pay sufficient attention to the evidence provided by clinical situations. They were beginning to see organic lesions as causes of all disease, but he disagreed. Even if a lesion could be linked to illness, it was not necessarily a cause. Auscultation went beyond the barriers raised by anatomical etiology. Yes, it could reliably predict the presence of organic changes in the chest, but Laennec also saw it as an indicator of the physiological state in health and disease.

In both editions of his treatise, Laennec defended the utility of pathological anatomy, but he also warned about its limitations in pathophysiology.[157] A good clinician should not ignore the realities of false positives and false negatives. Only a fool could forget that the lesion itself must have had a prior cause.

Laennec's colleagues embraced his invention and the method it proclaimed, and they busily began identifying lesions for many clinical syndromes in a movement that sought to link all diseases to internal organic changes. But Laennec remained firm in his commitment to the principles of specificity and sensitivity, and he would combat medical theories that pretended to ignore the physiological reality of the sick patient in the absence of anatomical signs. He enunciated the same ideas with increasing stridency in his later years as he reacted to the reception of his treatise.

PART THREE

Disease

I have tried to place the internal organic lesions on the same plane as
the surgical diseases with respect to diagnosis.

—*Laennec,* Traité *1826,* 1*:xxv*

I am far from denying the utility of studying anatomical species of
disease. I have scarcely worked on anything else, and this book itself
is entirely devoted to the subject. It is the only basis of positive
knowledge in medicine, I believe, and one should never lose sight
of it in etiological research for fear of chasing chimeras or creating
phantoms to combat. . . . But I also believe that it is dangerous
to study local conditions exclusively and to the extent that their
difference from the causes on which they depend is lost from
view. . . . The necessary shortcomings of a limited outlook is often
to take the effect for the cause, or to fall into the even greater error
of considering them as identical. . . .
This mistaken view, which appears to have been adopted by several
practitioners of our time, seems inconceivable to me. Perhaps it is a
result of mediocre and superficial application of pathological
anatomy. But I think that it would be impossible for any man to
persist in this misconception for very long, if he is endowed with
a good mind and practices this science carefully and repeatedly.

—*Laennec,* Traité *1819,* 1*: 413–414; 1826 2:233–234*

Reception and Impact of Auscultation: Reviews, Diagnoses, and Broussais

> In spite of all his faults, the name of Laennec will remain in science and be honorable for his homeland. What he has done will be used to advantage, and his mistakes, which people will grow tired of criticizing, will fall into oblivion.
>
> —*Broussais,* Examen *1834, 4:334–335*

LAENNEC'S TREATISE received immediate attention at home and abroad. Auscultation and the conceptual changes it subtended had a prompt impact on diagnosis and on the conceptualization of disease—an impact that was soon felt in the medical literature and at all levels of hospital practice, including record keeping. Most observers recognized the work as a contribution to pathological anatomy and to the detection of organic lesions. Laennec's ideas about physiology and etiology, however, had little resonance for his contemporaries, and they were largely ignored, except by his rival Broussais, who accused him of plagiarism. From his retreat in Brittany, Laennec watched the reception of his book, pleased with the praise and annoyed by the criticisms, until the taunts of Broussais drove him back to Paris in late 1821.

THE EARLY REVIEWS

A myth revolves around medical circles that Laennec's work received no praise when it first appeared. This distortion is a product of the late nineteenth-century romanticization of Laennec as an unsung hero. Nothing could be further from the truth. The stethoscope was one of the first medical inventions to attain an international profile in an impressively short time. Reviews of the *Treatise on Mediate Auscultation* were published quickly, and most were favorable. A few doctors joked about the instrument and the strange physical posture demanded of its adepts, but evidence for their slights is largely indirect: Laennec's allusion to the tendency of his contemporaries to laugh at innovations in his Latin preface, his associates' defensive comments, and their defiant recollections.[1] It is easy to confuse mockery of the stethoscope with that of its inventor, especially for his politics, character, and mannerisms; and for that kind of mockery, the evidence is more concrete.[2] In any case, ridicule of auscultation melted away within a year.

The first review appeared one month after the treatise. The young L. L. Rostan admitted that he had yet to develop the knack of listening to the chest, and he ignored the diagnostic implications of auscultation; nevertheless, he said, his review would substitute as a manual of mediate auscultation, saving doctors the trouble of having to read what he thought was an overly prolix book. The future high priest of organicism was the first in a long line of physicians to maintain that Laennec's pathological anatomy was his "most considerable" contribution. Rostan disputed many of Laennec's claims: the possibility of natural cures in phthisis; its definition as the presence of tubercles; the existence of emphysema as a disease; the retention of the old-fashioned notion of catarrh. He objected to Laennec's failure to cite his own work on asthma, accurately describing their differences on its etiology as structural (Rostan) versus functional (Laennec). He said that Laennec had "allowed himself to make conjectures that a less lively imagination would have seen fit to repress or at least to present with more skepticism." But, he concluded, "in spite of its defects" the work was that of "an attentive, laborious, and patient observer." He promised to pass judgment on the diagnostic value of auscultation when he had had time to test the signs; but the promise was not kept.[3]

A few early reviewers lauded the physiological applications of auscultation together with the pathological anatomy, among them the medical journalist J. B. Nacquart. In 1818, Nacquart had made snide remarks about the stethoscope (as well as its inventor): he likened the stethoscope to a "kaleidoscope," at the same time confessing "to his shame" that he had yet to try it; and he had also proclaimed his animosity toward "pious," "gaunt" physicians, presumably like Laennec, who reaped "favors" and "distinctions" with the Restoration.[4] In his review of 1819, Nacquart joined Rostan and others to criticize the overabundance of detail in the clinical descriptions and the lack of attention to therapy. But Nacquart complimented Laennec's skills as an observer and his ingenuity in linking external signs with internal organic changes, and he readily admitted the implications of auscultation for pathological anatomy, clinical practice, and physiology. He said "this book proves how useful it will be for science to have physiology . . . march side by side" with the clinic and with the study of anatomical change.[5]

The *Revue médicale* opened its January issue of 1820 with the first half of its 140-page appreciation of Laennec's book. The reviewer justified the "infinity of details" in the *Traité* as being "indispensable" to the new method of investigation, which could not be reduced to a handful of general principles. Other writers expressed some doubt about auscultation, but their judgments cannot be described as hostile.[6] Isidore Bricheteau concluded that "the discovery of pectoriloquy and of auscultation would hasten progress of the art" and place the author in "a distinguished rank."[7]

The most detailed review of the *Treatise on Auscultation* was the work of the Breton, Jean-Alexandre Le Jumeau de Kergaradec (1788–1877). His assessment appeared in a series of five articles over the course of a year and filled more than one hundred pages. In preparation for his review, Kergaradec conducted an independent verification of the new technique with Adrien-Jacques De Lens (1786–1846) at the Hôtel Dieu hospital.[8] He later claimed that his admiration for the potential of the stethoscope led him to seek the friendship of his fellow Breton.[9] It is difficult, however, to believe that the Breton Kergaradec did not already count himself a friend of the inventor: they shared strikingly similar life histories, joined in collaborative work on the *Dictionnaire des sciences médicales*, and had been fellow members in the Congrégation for more than a decade.[10] Initially, Kergaradec had planned to test and counter the criticisms of detractors; however, in the year that elapsed between the first and final articles, such a defense—like Rostan's promised evaluation of diagnostics—had become "superfluous"; most serious practitioners were using the stethoscope already. Kergaradec concluded that Laennec's treatise was "one of the most remarkable works to have been published on positive medicine."[11]

Kergaradec soon extended stethoscopy to the pregnant belly. Despite at least one letter warning not to invade the sanctity of mother and child (not to mention the domain of the *accoucheur!*), he soon described the fetal heart beat and the placental souffle, which is the murmur of blood pulsing in the vessels of the placenta.[12] His associate, De Lens, went on to contribute a favorable entry, correctly entitled "*Stethoscope*," for the *Dictionnaire des sciences médicales*, which compensated for the less enthusiastic, erroneous but longer account, entitled "*Pectoriloque*," that had appeared two years before (fig. 9.1).[13]

Within a year of its publication, Laennec's auscultation was being cited in the work of researchers who had known nothing of his investigations, while the theses of his students attracted the attention of journals.[14] The faculty of medicine awarded a degree to Laennec's intern who proclaimed that, "in inventing the stethoscope," the teacher who had yet to be a professor "was luckier than all his predecessors and had attained and even surpassed the goals of the Old Man of Cos."[15] Auscultation was firmly established in France and was beginning to spread over the western world.

In November 1819, Matthew Baillie wrote to thank Laennec for his gift of the treatise, of which he had read a "considerable part with the highest satisfaction"; he had already presented the work to the Prince Regent whose "gracious answer" was enclosed in his letter.[16] Laennec had also sent his treatise to academies in Vienna and Berlin. In January 1820, a British journal published a "highly favorable" analysis and by the following year, John Forbes had completed his English translation, which also received reviews before the year was out.[17]

Forbes abridged Laennec's nine-hundred-page, two-volume work to less than five hundred pages, boasting that he had excised half the prose with no

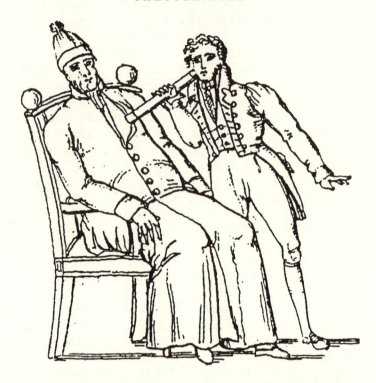

Figure 9.1. An early image of mediate auscultation, published with a diagram of the stethoscope as part of the dictionary article on the "pectoriloque" by Mérat. Original is only one and a quarter inches high. Source: Mérat 1819, plate between pages 34 and 35. Photograph: Queen's Medical Photography Services.

loss of substance. More importantly, he dramatically restructured the book to reflect his opinion that its contributions to pathological anatomy outweighed the significance of the diagnostic gimmick of auscultation. The English title, *A Treatise on Diseases of the Chest*, had been Laennec's subtitle, and the contents were reorganized into two unequal parts: "Pathology" (280 pages) and "Diagnosis" (100 pages). The physiology, which had been Laennec's leitmotiv, had all but disappeared.[18]

　　Forbes engaged with the text. He agreed that emphysema was a new disease (discovered by the English), but he did not think that bronchiectasis should constitute a separate entity: rather it was a variation of "bronchitis." He also added notes about the merits of Laennec's contributions and English-language bibliography. It was, he said, "extremely discreditable" for Laennec to have claimed priority for the recognition of encephaloid (medullary tumor) when British authors had already described it; similar remarks were made about the failure to cite English works on the heart.[19] In abbreviating the text, Forbes excised details about the patients' occupations, personal lives, feelings, and autopsies, especially the psychological antecedents of illness. He made one exception for the case of the Englishman, "G***." According to Laennec, the man had been released from captivity in 1814 and subsequently traveled widely in pursuit of orgies and other debauchery; Forbes left out the man's pastimes and referred to G*** as an English "gentleman" who had been "detained in Paris as a prisoner of war."[20]

Forbes never refrained from nationalistic editorializing, but he came to regret the radical changes. Two years later, he apologized to Laennec for the "great liberties," admitting that the "only substantial excuse" he could offer was his "conviction" that a lengthy translation would not have been read. To make amends, he would translate a second edition more faithfully, and he published his own small treatise on stethoscopy in 1824, in which he supplied "original English cases" because of yet another "conviction" that they were "absolutely necessary to produce the proper impression in favor of the stethoscope."[21] But the label of pathological anatomy had been applied to Laennec's opus; subsequent anglophones have been obliged to grasp his ideas through a veil first erected by the translator.

A letter from Forbes indicates that Laennec did not read English.[22] He may not have been aware of the extent to which Forbes had altered his book, although he kept a French translation of a British review that had compared the original work to Morgagni and criticized Forbes for abridging it.[23] The first English edition attracted the attention of editors in Britain and abroad. Within two years, all five hundred copies had sold, an "unprecedented" success, Forbes proudly told the author, that already exceeded the sales of Corvisart in translation.[24]

In January 1821, Laennec had been told that "all medical Germany has its ear to the stethoscope;" six months later he was gratified to learn that independent observers in Madrid had confirmed his findings, and the following year similar news came from Edinburgh, Bonn, Berlin, Barcelona, and Boston.[25] A Viennese doctor wrote that he had hoped to translate the book, until he discovered that he was too late.[26] A German edition of the *Treatise on Auscultation* was published in 1822; a Latin dissertation on the stethoscope was defended in Utrecht in 1823 by a Dutchman who had studied with Laennec.[27] The first American edition appeared in 1823; the first Belgian edition in 1828; and a four-volume Italian edition in 1833–1836.[28] Scholars have shown that this attention to auscultation in the literature was translated into practice at the bedside.[29]

IMPACT ON PRACTICE AT THE NECKER AND CHARITÉ HOSPITALS

Much has been made of a relative indifference to auscultation in France compared to Britain and other countries, but it is difficult to find evidence for such a claim. Jean-Pierre Kernéis and his colleagues have shown that French medical students and their advisors clamored to apply the stethoscope to the study of the chest. By 1825 the stethoscope had been used in all the clinical

TABLE 9.1

Admission Diagnosis of Patients Who Died in Necker Hospital, 1816–1823

	1816*	1817	1818 †	1819 ‡	1822 §	1823
Fevers	32	116	76	40	31	35
Catarrh	12	30	23	80	22	29
Pneumonia	0	2	1	2	5	11
Pleural disease	0	2	3	2	7	9
Phthisis	0	0	0	0	38	46
Emphysema	0	0	0	0	3	0
Pulmonary edema	0	0	0	0	1	1
Organic heart disease	0	0	0	0	7	12
Subtotal	44	150	103	124	114	143
Total deaths in same period	68	211	151	188	210	218

Source: Registres des Entrées de l'Hôpital Necker, 1816–1819, AAP, 1Q2.19–22, 1Q2. 25–26.

* Laennec began early Sep (admissions before that month not included).

† Laennec absent 7 Aug to 12 Nov 1818 (admissions in that period not included).

‡ Laennec retired to Brittany 8 Oct 1819 (admissions after that date not included).

§ 1822 includes patients already residing in hospital on 1 Jan.

cases discussed in the thirty-nine medical theses devoted to pneumonia in Paris from 1820. By 1828 P. A. Piorry (1794–1870) wrote that the stethoscope was "generally considered to be indispensable" to medical practice.[30] Several independent studies with new applications of auscultation were published in Paris before Laennec had completed his second edition. He had yet to see Itard and other educators of deaf-mute people reap the benefits that he had predicted on the basis of his own experiments; however, the new work included Kergaradec on pregnancy, Lisfranc on orthopedics, Piorry on the pleximeter, Louis on phthisis, Bouillaud on the diagnosis of aneurysms, Collin on auscultation, and Andral on diseases of the chest. Laennec approved of, advised, and cited the first three, barely mentioned Louis, ignored Bouillaud and Collin, and criticized Andral.[31]

Further evidence for a prompt impact on diagnostic practice can be found in the admission records of the Necker hospital where Laennec had conducted most of his research. With the stethoscope, an anatomical diagnosis could now be made on the basis of a physical examination at the time of the patient's admission to hospital; autopsy merely provided confirmation. The trend is exemplified by the relatively quick replacement of admission diagnoses based on symptoms with those based on anatomical change in the hospital records (table 9.1). Phthisis had been rare as an admission diagnosis in 1816. Most patients were admitted with various forms of symptomatic "fever" or "catarrh" (especially "*catarrh pulmonaire*" and "*chronique*"). During 1816, only two patients, both of whom were eventually discharged, had been given an admission diagnosis of "consumption"; no patients were

TABLE 9.2

Comparison of Admission and Postmortem Diagnoses for Patients Who Died in
the Necker Hospital, 1822 and 1823

Diagnosis	1822		1823*	
	Admission	Postmortem	Admission	Postmortem
Fevers	31	9	1	6
Catarrh	22	1	5	2
Pneumonia	5	14	6	7
Pleural disease	7	9	3	2
Phthisis	38 (21%)	70 (33%)	9 (19%)	20 (38%)
Emphysema	3	3	0	0
Pulmonary edema	1	2	0	0
Organic heart disease	7	11	3	5
Subtotal	114	119	27	42
Total deaths in period†	182	210	47	53

Source: Registres des Entrées de l'Hôpital Necker, 1822–1823, AAP, 1Q2.25–26; Registres des Décès de l'Hôpital Necker, 1822–1823, AAP, Paris, 3Q2.7–8.

* Laennec transferred to Charité hospital 17 Mar 1823; deaths after that date are not included.

† Totals from Death Register for a given time period differ from those derived from Admission Register. Admission Register contains those who died from a cohort admitted after 1 Jan. Totals from the Death Register included those who died within the year, including those who were already in the hospital before 1 Jan.

recorded as having had "phthisis" or "pleurisy" on admission.[32] Shortly after the publication of the *Treatise on Mediate Auscultation*, however, phthisis became the most frequent admission diagnosis in the Necker hospital, although "fever" and "catarrh" continued to appear often. The transition seems to have taken place during the two years that Laennec resided in Brittany. "Phthisis" had appeared as an admission diagnosis by April 1821; in the early summer, it was frequent.[33]

The patient's course in the hospital and the autopsy further emphasized anatomical diagnosis. For example, in 1822 the symptomatic diagnosis of fever was more frequent as an admission diagnosis than it was as a postmortem diagnosis. Unfortunately the same comparisons cannot be made for the years 1816–21 because the Necker registers did not indicate the cause of death in those years, possibly yet another indication of the rise in the importance of autopsy after 1821. Anatomical diagnoses on admission increased steadily. For example, in 1819, none of the patients who eventually died in the Necker hospital had been diagnosed with phthisis on admission. In 1822 and 1823, however, approximately twenty percent of patients who eventually died had been given an admission diagnosis of phthisis, while the postmortem diagnosis of phthisis was even more frequent (table 9.2).

The dramatic change in the apparent incidence of phthisis in the Necker hospital from 1816 to 1822 was not due to an outbreak of the disease but

TABLE 9.3

Diagnosis of Heart Disease at Admission among Patients Who Died
in the Necker Hospital during Laennec's Presence, 1816–1823

Diagnosis	1816	1817	1818	1819	1822	1823
Organic disease of heart	0	0	0	2	6	2
Aneurysm	0	0	0	0	0	0
Hypertrophy	0	0	0	0	1	10
Dilatation	0	0	0	0	0	0
Total	0	0	0	2	7	12

Source: Registre des Entrées de l'Hôpital Necker, 1816–1823, AAP, 34 1Q2.19–26.
Note: Laennec absent from 1819 to late 1821.

rather to the infectious nature of a new form of discourse. Doctors now felt competent to label the structural nature of patients' symptoms at the time of presentation; fever and catarrh were being sorted into various anatomical categories.

Other diagnoses in the Admission Register also tell of the efforts to link illness to anatomical change during the period of Laennec's intense investigations. For example, "organic fever" was the admission diagnosis of an eighteen-year-old woman who entered the Necker hospital on 16 July and died on 30 September 1818.[34] In 1819, several patients were admitted with "organic fever," "chronic organic disease," and "organic disease" of the lung, heart, or uterus.[35] Of these vague but anatomically committed designations, only "organic disease of the heart" remained in both the Admission Register and the Register of Deaths for 1822.

The "new diseases" of emphysema, pulmonary edema, and hypertrophy of the heart first appeared in the Admission Registers soon after Laennec's return from Brittany.[36] In 1822, "hypertrophy of the heart" was diagnosed at the time of entry in one of the seven patients who had been given admission diagnoses of heart disease and who eventually died. The following year, ten of the twelve patients who died with admission diagnoses referring to the heart were diagnosed with "hypertrophy" at admission (see table 9.3). The same trend with a lag of two or three years can be observed in the Death Registers of the Charité Hospital, site of the *clinique interne*, where Laennec went to work in 1823 (see table 9.4). The figures seem to suggest a rise in heart disease, especially cardiac hypertrophy, but once again, they are the result of an epidemic of new vocabulary following the movements of the inventor and the application of his technique.

For old diseases there was an increase in semantic precision without neologism: I will use the example of pleurisy, shown by Russell Maulitz to serve as an effective marker for the codification of new disease concepts.[37] In the Necker hospital before 1819, effusions of fluid in the chest were variously diagnosed as "hydrops," "hydrothorax," or "fluxion." In March 1819,

TABLE 9.4

Final Diagnosis of Heart Disease in Patients Who Died in the
Charité Hospital during Laennec's Presence, 1823–1826

	1823 †	1824	1825	1826 †
Organic disease of heart	2	15	9	17
Aneurysm	6	7	22	1
Hypertrophy	0	6	11	10
Dilatation	0	3	4	0
Total in period studied	8	31	46	28
Corrected annual total*	19	31	46	67
Total deaths in year	561	560	714‡	743
Organic heart disease as a percentage of total deaths	3.4%	5.5%	6.4%	9%

Source: Registre des Décès de l'Hôpital de la Charité, 1823–1826, AAP, 3Q2.19–22; Boulle 1986.

* For 1823 and 1826, estimate of the twelve-month incidence of heart disease as a final diagnosis based on the five months studied in each year.

† 1823 begins 1 Aug when Laennec arrived to take up the service; 1826 ends 30 May when Laennec resigned.

‡ 1825 death register after 20 Aug is missing; total estimated on 454 deaths to that date.

Laennec's preferred term of "pleurisy" was first used as an admission diagnosis.[38] By 1823, it was the only diagnostic word used for pleural disease. Similarly, attending physicians revealed their use of stethoscopy when they diagnosed "left-sided pneumonia with effusion" in a patient residing in hospital on 1 January 1822.[39]

Clearly, Laennec's work had made an impact on the diagnostic practice of the medical staff of the Necker hospital even in his absence and probably in competition with other concerns. For example, an exceptional cluster of five patients with "gastritis" were admitted to the Necker hospital from 4 to 11 July 1822, suggesting that a member of the medical staff may have just completed a rotation with Broussais at the Val de Grâce.[40]

How quickly similar changes in admission diagnoses appeared in other hospitals remains to be investigated. Analysis of the registers of the Charité suggests that the change may have been less abrupt and less complete in that hospital, where it appears that the stethoscope was little used until Laennec's arrival. For example, in the thesis of the Canadian student, Pierre de Beaubien, who was at the Charité in 1819, auscultation appeared only once.[41] It seems reasonable to predict that, in each institution, the changes in disease conceptualization would track the advent of auscultation in diagnosis. With his stethoscope, Laennec had indeed altered the detection and the status of the "internal organic lesions," putting them on a plane with the externally visible surgical diseases and turning them into diseases themselves.[42] Corvisart's long-hoped-for "better eye" had been opened through the ear.

Meanwhile Back in Brittany

From his retreat in Finistère, Laennec watched the reception of his book with great interest. He corresponded with Mériadec over the reviews, and their reactions to the criticisms would become the focus of the cousin's dissertation, "Can Mediate Auscultation Contribute to the Progress of Practical Medicine?" Mériadec had been sent to work with Récamier and De Lens at the Hôtel Dieu hospital; drafts and revisions of his dissertation were sent through the mail.

Mérat's 1819 article entitled "*Pectoriloque*" in the *Dictionnaire des sciences médicales* had made Laennec laugh, "I especially like the disadvantages that [Mérat] finds in a purely mechanical technique, which will tend to turn physicians away from skillful conjectures over the pulse, the facies, and excrement. It is the same as refusing to dash around Paris in a cabriolet for fear of losing the ability to tiptoe over droppings in the street."[43] The same idea, packaged in a different metaphor appeared in Mériadec's 1821 thesis: objections to a mechanical technique are "like advising men to renounce the use of boats in order to improve their skill at swimming." The defense of his thesis, was a success.[44]

Laennec was more annoyed by the criticism that he dealt inadequately with the treatment of chest diseases, and he was frustrated by reviewers who failed to appreciate the utility of precise anatomical diagnosis. Why did medical books always have to justify themselves with references to treatment? Other physicians had immediately appreciated the potential of accurate anatomical diagnosis. One was James Clark (1788–1870) who had toured the Necker hospital with Cayol, as Laennec's replacement; in his report, Clark defended the value of precise diagnosis.[45] If a therapeutic application was needed to prove the utility of his method, Laennec would apply his stethoscope to the surgical cure of one of the anatomical conditions it could detect: empyema (pus in the chest).

Doctors generally agreed that the ancient procedure of thoracentesis operation to drain the pus in a patient's chest could be lifesaving; however, as Larrey and others readily admitted, it was difficult to determine the right time and the right site.[46] Laennec believed that the stethoscope had solved the problem. His correspondence reveals a preoccupation, if not an obsession, with justifying the therapeutic applications of auscultation in surgery and beyond. For example, Laennec said of a thoracentesis case, "The utility of auscultation was perfectly verified for indicating the lifesaving stroke of the bistoury that one would never have dared to use without [the stethoscope]."[47] Similarly, he joked with Christophe that if he would visit, they could pass him off to the doctors as "a '*pectoriloque*' cured by our treatment."[48]

In June 1821 while still in Finistère, Laennec used the stethoscope to diagnose empyema in a patient of his friend, the Paris-trained, Quimper physician Georges Ollivry (b. 1778).[49] Together they performed a thoracentesis operation, and Laennec told Mériadec what happened: "Ollivry's face went pale as a sheet and . . . at the moment he was to plunge the trochar into [the patient's] chest he looked at me with eyes that spoke of his fears. To reassure him I had to say, 'Bring the basin.' Two and a half pints of pus flowed from the patient's chest." The man was recovering quickly with a drainage tube in place: "he eats a lot and would drink more if only we would let him." Laennec now had a survivor to add to the less fortunate thoracentesis cases he had seen with Rault and published in his treatise (see chap. 6). He asked his newly graduated cousin to pass along reports of the man's continued progress to Cayol and Récamier and happily planned to present the case to the medical community as "living proof of the utility of the stethoscope."[50] The inventor may have been convinced, but later in the century the value of surgery in empyema was still a subject of debate, although the stethoscope was used to detect it.[51]

During his retirement, Laennec gave medical advice to the local peasants who paid for his services in cod, turbot, and lobster. He took advantage of clinical situations to observe and modify his opinion about various stethoscopic sounds. After hearing from Erman of Berlin, he investigated the sounds of contracting muscles, relating them to the heart sounds (see chap. 8).[52] At Brest, he gave lessons in auscultation to naval doctors who apparently picked up the technique with alacrity. "Forced often" by the state of his health "to interrupt his work and run after hares and snipe," he spent long days hunting with his two spaniels, Kiss and Moustache, and human companions, too, if they could keep up. He carried a small gun at all times—except in church—and would shoot at any creature that moved, including foxes, crows, magpies, and swallows. But even in the woods, stethoscopic preoccupations were not far from his mind: a hunting partner recalled that while they were resting at the side of a ditch, Laennec suddenly grabbed the tired man's equally tired hound and began auscultating and pounding the animal with vigorous percussive "blows."[53]

Laennec contemplated a permanent life in Brittany. He embarked on the long-needed and expensive repairs to the manor of Kerlouarnec, which had become his property with the settlement arranged by Michaud (fig. 9.2). He kept a detailed notebook about trees, gardens, agriculture, domestic architecture—pearls of wisdom that he had gathered from carpenters, farmers, pharmacists, the villagers in Soissonais, and the gardener of the Necker hospital.[54] This previously unknown, one-hundred-page manuscript in Laennec's hand helps to confirm Rouxeau's suspicions that the doctor was the author of an anonymous Breton pamphlet on agricultural practices (fig. 9.3).[55] Unable to do anything on a small scale, he assigned Mériadec the task of finding paints, oils, and varnishes to his precise specifications and having them shipped from Paris. He grew impatient with delays, was angered by costs, and when a shipment arrived in a damaged basket, he practiced Hippocratic succussion on the stoppered bottle of oil and determined that at least

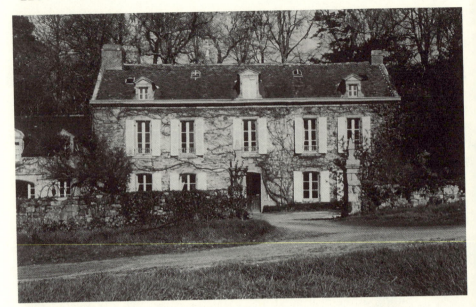

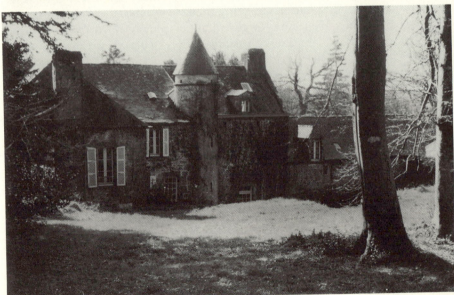

Figure 9.2. The manor of Kerlouarnec at Ploaré: front view (*above*); rear view (*below*). By permission of M. A. Halna du Frétay. Photographs: The author, 1995.

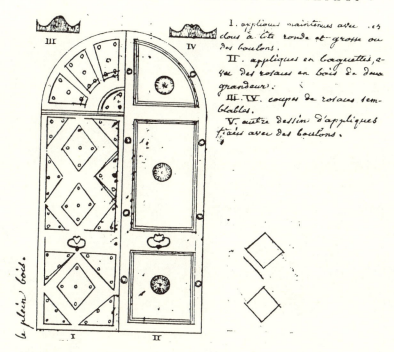

Figure 9.3. Laennec's drawing of a door from his manuscript notebook, "Observations sur les cultures, plantations, et édifices considérés comme objets de décoration et d'utilité," (ca.1820, 77). Source: By permission of Dr. Eric Laennec, Lyons. Photograph: Queen's Medical Photography Services.

half the expensive liquid had run out. Mériadec was sent back to the dealer to demand satisfaction. Laennec designed and built a staircase in a small turreted tower at the back of his house, and he planted hundreds of pine trees. Legend has it that the ground floor of the old manor had been used as a stable, but Laennec left the trapdoor communicating to the upper levels because he thought the fumes of manure were healthful.[56] Because of the repairs, he could not dwell in his house and would board with villagers or at the palace of the bishop of Quimper for weeks at a time.[57] Now he had no domestic help and regretted having to leave Angélique, his "good servant and friend," in Paris, but he was certain that she would never have adapted to Breton life.[58] The Kerlouarnec reconstruction proved to be so complicated that he began to think he should live at Pont l'Abbé.

The small farms northeast of Pont l'Abbé had also been acquired as part of the same settlement. Laennec began studying agricultural methods, joined the local agricultural society, and communicated with his tenants in Breton.[59] He purchased adjoining parcels of land in order to enhance the value and the privacy of his holdings and sold other lots. Four of the small farms surrounded a large marshy inlet off the cove of Poulden near the estuary of the Pont l'Abbé river: two farms (Troliguer and Rosveïgn) on the

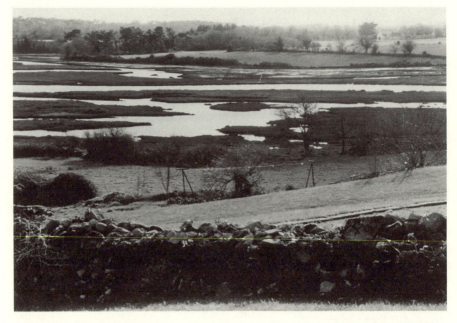

Figure 9.4. The marsh known as Palud de Cosquer, near the town of Pont l'Abbé. Laennec had hoped to increase his income by draining the marsh to reclaim land, expanding the area of the small properties acquired in the 1809 settlement with his father. View from the farm of Troliguer in the north looking southwest across the marsh to the farms of Lande Vallée and le Cosquer. Photograph: The author, 1995.

north shore; two others (Lande Vallée and le Cosquer) on the south; lying between them was the marsh known as the Palud du Cosquer (fig. 9.4). Laennec thought that by investing three thousand francs to drain the marsh, he could double his acreage and derive his entire living from the income of the resulting lands. Work was started in the summer of 1819, but by 1826 the still incomplete project was much over budget, well behind schedule, and the subject of a boundary dispute with a jealous neighbor. Well after Laennec had invested heavily in the project, his neighbor, the sieur de Bohan, challenged his title to the land. The new bishop of Quimper, Poulpiquet, offered to intervene, but Laennec declined, confident that the matter would be settled. A year of legal wrangling resolved the issue in Laennec's favor, but the debate had absorbed so much more time and energy that he demanded that the final decision be publicized in Quimper in the interests of his reputation.[60] In 1919, Rouxeau received a map outlining Laennec's project from a Pont l'Abbé resident, who reverently described Laennec's dike as "a beautiful work with perfect masonry."[61] In 1995, the remains of stone dikes were still visible along the unrelenting tidal marsh.

The family continued to watch the would-be country squire in utter disbelief. The father wanted to know how his "illustrious" son could afford to

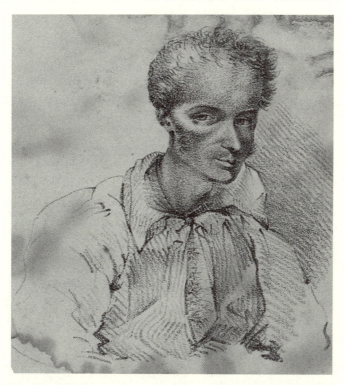

Figure 9.5. Presumed self-portrait of a rather emaciated looking Laennec as the "hermit" of Kerlouarnec, a title he liked to use himself. Lithograph found by Rouxeau in the papers of Laennec, now in the Musée Laennec. Source: Musée Laennec, Nantes. Photograph: M. Certain.

build himself a "castle," while the inadequate pension was making him "die of hunger"; he complained that he was not allowed to visit until the work was done.[62] Laennec scolded Guillaume for lending money to Théophile-Marie: the meddling father would now "go running about the countryside," he angrily wrote, "planting rosebushes that I will have to water."[63] Christophe visited his cousin once and reported to his aunt de Miniac that the "dear doctor," was not so well as he liked to pretend and that he had been too "afraid" of stormy weather to show off his marsh (see fig. 9.5).[64] Guillaume settled down to wait, giving his nephew less than three years before he would tire of "growing his cabbages" and yearn for the glory and excitement of the capital.[65]

Laennec's uncle had mellowed. Four years after his denunciation by the royalists of Nantes, his professional difficulties were finally resolved. In May 1820, he was asked to return to work in the Hôtel Dieu hospital—not because of his many petitions—but because the clinical service had become so heavy that the medical insurgents were overwhelmed.[66] His star had begun its rise: on 17 July, he was named by the king to the *jury médical* of his department; and in September, he was reinstated as chief physician at the hospital above the younger and "sly" Fouré, who had taken his place and with whom he had been obliged to collaborate.[67] The *jurys médicales*, created by the law of Ventôse An XI (1803) to conduct licensing examinations, were normally made up of professors in departments with medical schools; therefore, this bureaucratic assignment was also the first step in his academic vindication.[68] The old doctor was triumphant. He gloated over the errors and misfortunes of his enemies and noted with pleasure how his "civil" practice had grown to enviable proportions despite his age and "dangerous" reputation.[69] With two hundred fever patients in need of his indispensable care, he no longer wanted the more lucrative and less demanding professorship, especially since he could now expect to receive a pension for his previous teaching. In the intervening four years, Ambroise had become a serious practitioner and a good pathologist; he could "slide" into his father's town practice while waiting for a place at the hospital.[70]

The machinations surrounding Guillaume Laennec's dismissal and reappointment seem to have diverted his attention from his nephew's invention, research, and resulting publication. The *Treatise on Mediate Auscultation* had been released in August 1819, but a year later Guillaume was amazed to hear of his nephew's good reputation in Paris; he thought it must be due to the articles he had written as a journalist years before.[71] Several months passed before he finally sat down to examine his copy of the book, which the nephew had inscribed "*optimo patruo altero patri*" (to the best godfather; to my second father [see fig. 7.1]).[72] His uncle's appreciation was not immediate. As a former professor of *materia medica*, he voiced the now familiar complaint that the work needed a third volume for therapeutics.[73] It gradually dawned on him that the discovery was a boon to diagnosis, and he became effusive in his praise: the stethoscope was the greatest achievement in a miraculous "century of inventions" that had witnessed the resurrection of the wisdom of the Greeks and the invention of the "uterine speculum of Récamier." "For at least one hundred years our doctors have written books using only other books; he [Laennec] alone has written *propio sensu* and shown new things, unheard, unknown, useful"; he deserves the "prize of the decade" for his "new creation." Guillaume even attempted auscultation in his own practice in the summer of 1821. To his "very great astonishment" and despite his "deaf ears," he personally verified his nephew's signs in a patient with consumption.[74]

Six months later on 8 February 1822, Guillaume was dead of gastrointestinal bleeding at the age of seventy-three. The reformed Ambroise tended his father through this last illness, informing the family in Paris of the old doctor's painful decline, the Hippocratic facies, and the futile attempts at treatment.[75] Through Laennec's influence with the minister of the interior Jacques-Joseph-Guillaume Corbière (1766–1853), Ambroise replaced his father at the hospital; he would become a professor in 1829. Laennec and his cousins mourned the old man's passing, but he had died with his dignity restored and secure in the knowledge that his wish had come true: his capricious nephew had just announced his decision to go back to Paris. "We have brought about a great victory," Guillaume told Mériadec a few weeks before the end. And he congratulated Laennec for "going to defend [his] honor in person" before the "charlatans, even women and priests" could leap in to profit from his achievement, just as they had from all other inventions. Guillaume knew that the decision had been prompted by the attacks of Broussais. His last orders to his nephew were: "Give a public course, make a noise, a disturbance, a scandal in the Paris School . . . and the house of cards of this charlatan cannot fail to crumble to the advantage of your fortune and renown. Adieu."[76]

THE SYMPATHETIC DUEL

Everything here boils down to a dispute over words

—*Buisson on Laennec, 1804*

One of the few who recognized the physiological aspects of Laennec's work was F. J. V. Broussais (fig. 9.6). As his uncle had indicated, Laennec's strongest criticism came in mid-1821 with the second edition of Broussais's *Examen des doctrines médicale*. Posterity tends to count Laennec the victor of their quarrel, as it elevated his reputation. Until recently, Broussais was relegated to the lowly rank of a mediocre systematist, typified by Ackerknecht's pithy observation that he may have been the "only legitimate offspring" of Bichat, but "medically speaking," he was "an abortion."[77] Perhaps because Broussais was so frequently discredited earlier in this century, historians are now fond of demonstrating that the medical revolution of early nineteenth-century France owed much to his iconoclasm and radical localism. His controversial role, which had been recognized and debated by his contemporaries, was rediscovered and partially rehabilitated in the late twentieth-century beginning with Ackerknecht, Canguilhem, and Foucault. The latter's project to "decenter the actor" was illustrated by a reappreciation of Broussais, as "merely the point of convergence of all these experiences, the form individually modeled out of their collective configuration."[78]

Why did the dispute between Laennec and Broussais take place? Disagreement alone is not an explanation: Laennec conspicuously ignored rather than debated the work of Rostan and others with whom he could not agree, even when they had well-justified claims to recognition. If Laennec saw in Broussais no more than the crude polemicist that later historians tried to make of him, then why did he stoop to wage his own invective? And there can be no doubt that Laennec attacked, too.

I think that there was more than a kernel of plausibility embedded in the thick polemic Broussais hurled at Laennec. His retaliatory jokes and insults

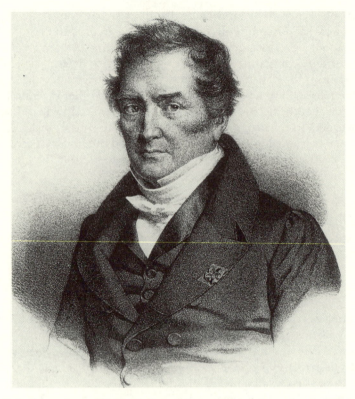

Figure 9.6. Engraving of F. J. V. Broussais, author of the polemical *Examen des doctrines médicales*, in which he criticized pathologists for studying the corpses of their patients instead of the living sick. His 1821 attack on Laennec drove the inventor out of retirement and back to Paris. Source: By permission of M. Valentin. Frontispiece from Valentin 1988; artist unknown.

notwithstanding, Laennec took the criticisms seriously and revised his treatise accordingly. On some points, they even shared a fundamental but tacit agreement of such importance that they argued over who had thought of it first. Indeed, their polemic displays many features of a priority dispute. This intriguing aspect of their competitive behavior can be taken as further evidence for their common ground, but neither man fully understood the agreement.

Broussais and the "Doctrine Physiologique"

Broussais was also Breton from the northeastern town of St. Malo, the home of Chateaubriand, and he, too, trained as a surgical cadet in the revolutionary armies. His parents had been brutally massacred in late 1795 by the royalist Chouans, a tragedy that has been invoked as a psychological explanation for his subsequent behavior. Unlike either Laennec or Chateaubriand, however, Broussais was antiroyalist and anticlerical, and his political senti-ments, though not Bonapartist, were liberal.[79] He was already married and a father when he went to Paris in 1798 to complete his studies with Pinel, Chaussier, and Bichat; the latter, he claimed, was his friend. His 1803 medi-cal thesis had been written in the spirit of nosology on the topic of "hectic fevers" and was cited by Laennec in his own thesis as a reminder—ironic reminder, it now seems—that fevers could occur "without any visceral disor-ganization." Broussais made his career in the army, and in 1812 Laennec considered himself much better off both personally and financially than his military "*condisciple.*"[80]

Broussais founded a doctrine that he called "*la médecine physiologique,*" first described in his *Histoires des phlegmasies* of 1808. This essay contained a collection of case observations gathered during his army experiences and diagnosed as gastroenteritis.[81] All systems of medicine were impractical, he said, because they were abstract and complicated. He deplored their failure to address the two most important aspects of disease: first, the cause; and second, the relationship between cause, organic change, and symptoms. His "physiological medicine" would compensate with a study of causes and their connections to the body, which he labeled "*sympathies.*" He did not com-pletely reject symptom-based nosology or anatomical pathology, but he re-duced them to what he believed were their essential features. Most diseases were the result of chemical, mechanical, or emotional stimuli (such as cold, heat, contagion, or depression), which produced "irritation." This "irrita-tion" most commonly, though not always, led to inflammation, which in turn produced organic changes such as tubercles or cancer. The site of in-flammation was usually the stomach and intestine (Fig. 9.7a). Broussais's medical philosophy has been studied as both materialism and vitalism.[82]

Localization of fever to the gastrointestinal tract was not original with Broussais. Prost had described it in 1804, and its more distant origin was the idea of Roederer and Wagler, cited by Pinel, while some medical observers have equated it with present-day stress ulcers or the side effects of drugs.[83] It may have been endorsed by experiences on the battlefield, where Broussais once told his father, "cadavers were not lacking": every soldier whose fresh wounds allowed internal inspection appeared to have an "inflamed" stom-ach.[84] Broussais recognized the "rapport," described by Cabanis, between the moral and the physical aspects of the organism. Anxiety, fear, and desire often result in altered digestion; therefore, the stomach seemed to be the site for the connection between psyche and soma.

Broussais did not pretend that his concept of irritation could explain all causes of lesions and disease, but he thought it was more realistic than symp-tom-based nosology or pathological anatomy because it did not ignore the existence of a cause that preceded the onset of symptoms and organic change. Causal relationships must become known, he maintained, if medi-cine ever hoped to treat and cure disease effectively. For precisely this reason, the young Auguste Comte (1798–1857) endorsed the notion of irritation as

a) **Broussais's "doctrine physiologique"**

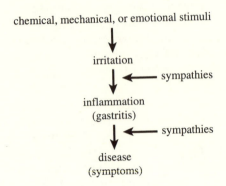

b) **Laennec's "doctrine"**

The body has three components: solid (organs), liquids, and vital principle. Each can be altered to produce disease.

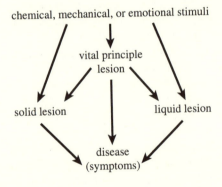

Figure 9.7. Schematic representation of the pathophysiology of Broussais and Laennec. Credit: Valerie Jarus, Desktop Publishing Unit, Queen's University.

a "positive" improvement over "psychology," which was the metaphysical and theological vitalism that had become a "vague and chimerical pursuit" of "the young generation of France."[85]

In contrast to Laennec, Broussais was specially interested in therapy. English and American medical students, who ventured into postrevolutionary Paris, complained that French doctors were more interested in diagnosis than they were in treatment.[86] Broussais was an exception, and his success as a practitioner was related to his enthusiastic embrace of vigorous therapy, dominated by *la saignée* (bleeding by leeches or phlebotomy). His disciple, Bouillaud, would soon promote the drastic "*coup-sur-coup*" form of venesection. Broussais's impact on French medicine has been expressed in terms of a transformation in the French leech trade, from a net export of more than a million leeches per year to a net import of more than twenty million. It has been said that his patients may have enjoyed a better outlook because his therapy protected them from the noxious concoctions of other doctors who used pharmaceuticals, while his confident manner conveyed a powerful, psychosomatic effect.[87] For example, Broussais's former student, Bouillaud, promised that his hardy "*coup-sur coup*" bleeding could save "thousands" of lives in France each year.[88]

An impressive orator, Broussais was gifted with a rare ability to see the truly ridiculous in the medical past and a tongue that knew how to take maximum advantage of his insights. Nothing was sacred, except his own vision of how things ought to be done. He attacked everything and everyone, living or dead, from Hippocrates to Pinel, and he mocked the contributions of his contemporaries by casting aspersions on their integrity. The American student, James Kitchen (1800–1894), kept careful lecture notes on the courses of both Broussais and Laennec. Broussais's lessons were divided into two parts: physiology and pathology; the latter was dominated by discussions of irritation, phlegmasia, and inflammation of various organs.[89] Broussais spoke to a full house, while Laennec's lessons were sparsely attended.

Laennec was not alone in his opposition to Broussais. The reductionist theories were challenged by the faculty of medicine and especially by the medical beneficiaries of the Restoration. Several works against Broussais appeared between 1823 and 1825 and were favorably reviewed in the *Gazette de santé* and in the pro-Laennec, pro-faculty *Revue médicale*; other opponents of his reductionism included Thomas Hodgkin and Elisha Bartlett.[90] To shake Broussais's credibility, a medical society offered a prize for the best essay on the anatomical aspects of the gastrointestinal mucous membrane in health and disease; entries in Latin or French were to be submitted to De Lens.[91] For liberal students, however, Broussais symbolized their anti-Restoration sentiments, and even without an official position, his doctrine commanded the direct attention and the indirect approbation of the faculty. His son, Casimir Broussais (1803–1847), successfully defended a "physiological" thesis on duodenitis and went on to promote his father's system in practice and in print through their journal *Annales de la médecine physiologique* (founded in 1822). Others, including a handful of Laennec's own students, massaged Broussais's philosophy into their dissertations, vicariously drawing academic approval for the "*doctrine physiologique*."[92] After the Revolution of 1830, Broussais was finally admitted to the faculty and the Académie Royale de Médecine. At the end of his career, he turned to the medically chic occupations of psychiatry and phrenology.[93]

Populist factors were important, but they were not the only reasons for Broussais's success. The *Examen* is remarkable both for its bombast and for its insight. Interspersed among the insults, grandiosity, and paranoia are a number of fundamental criticisms that proclaim the author's concern for the suffering patient and the overwhelmed student. As much as he came to be scorned for his diatribes, his intelligent clairvoyance was recognized for bringing some significant if poorly understood contribution to the scientific destiny of medicine. Almost through overstating his case, Broussais had helped to complete the work of organic localization, begun by the pathologists of the eighteenth century. His name commanded respect even from those who eulogized Laennec, including family and friends. Bouillaud would say that Laennec was second to Broussais as "the greatest" medical man of his time.[94] The translator, Forbes, said that "in his total rejection of the doctrines of Broussais, [Laennec] committed a great practical error," which was a manifestation "that he was too much disposed to sacrifice scientific views to empiricism."[95] Laennec's loyal cousin, Mériadec, and his friend, Kergaradec, agreed.[96] More than a generation after the rivals had died, a member of the Académie de Médecine observed that Laennec had been consumed with resisting Broussais "systematically, even in opposition to the evidence."[97]

The Dispute as a Dialogue

Although the fight did not come to a head until 1821, its roots went back many years. Laennec had opposed the reduction of all disease to lesions of the digestive tract long before Broussais wrote his *Examen*. In his 1802 article on peritonitis, he expressed doubts about the relationship of the inflammation to disturbances of intestinal function.[98] Two years later, he criticized Prost's book on gastrointestinal ulcers for incoherence, neglect of earlier authors, and theoretical assumptions. "We must be grateful to M. Prost for drawing our attention to the great frequency of these alterations of mucous membranes in acute disease, especially fevers. But . . . he ought to have limited his observations to noticing the frequent coincidence of the occurrence of these lesions of the intestinal mucosa with the existence of diverse diseases, without insisting on perceiving one as cause and the other as effect: proof of this association requires much longer and more careful observation. . . . One should never hasten to publish a scientific work, especially when one proposes to give it the pompous title of *Medicine, Enlightened by the Opening of Bodies*."[99]

Four years later, Broussais's *Histoires des phlegmasies* supported and extrapolated on Prost precisely where Laennec had criticized. Laennec noticed Broussais's debt to Prost and rejected what he would later call the "imprecise" notion in this "otherwise estimable" treatise, that inflammation was the cause of tubercles.[100]

In their 1812 articles for the *Dictionnaire des sciences médicales*, Laennec and Bayle had presented a classification of organic lesions with a discussion of the methodological problems in identifying diseases solely on an anatomical basis.[101] Their concerns about the limits of pathological anatomy and of nosology were similar to those that had been belabored by Broussais, but they did not cite him, nor did they name inflammation or irritation as a cause of organic change. Laennec saw inflammation as only one variety in a range of lesions.

In 1816, Broussais attacked Bayle, who had only just died, with a section of his *Examen* entitled, "Bayle did not see everything."[102] He criticized the six-fold classification of tubercles in Bayle's 1810 treatise on phthisis and his failure to mention that all six types were caused by irritation and inflammation. Broussais declared himself to be the first to have recognized the failings of the nosological approach and to have introduced the science of localized, organic lesions to medicine. Perhaps he had forgotten, or did not like to remember, that fourteen years earlier while he was still composing his own "Pinelian" thesis, Bayle had challenged Pinel's nosology in public.

Laennec did not object to the localism in the *Examen*, nor did he complain about the emphasis on bleeding, but he was piqued by the slights on Bayle and disapproved of the simplistic pathological anatomy. In his view, Broussais's much-touted localism was a debt owed to Bayle who had seen the local changes first and described them better. Broussais's autopsies were incomplete; his records were too brief, if not falsified; and his conclusions were the product of expectation not observation. Broussais used the terms "inflammation" and "irritation" to express pathophysiological notions. At the same time, Laennec was refining the meaning of these words in the histological sense. "Inflammation" for Laennec was becoming a precise pathological term; Broussais was invoking it for other generalized purposes. Moreover, Broussais's insistence that all fevers depended on irritation and inflammation was "harmful"; because phthisis was not inflammatory, its sufferers should not be bled.[103] Laennec's opinions were supported by his actions.

In 1818, the editor of the *Dictionnaire des sciences médicales* invited Broussais to write entries on "irritation" and "inflammation." In protest, Laennec and fourteen others signed a letter to "disabuse the public" of the notion that a committee of editors presided over the content of the *Dictionnaire*; he then joined a mass exodus of contributors from the collaborative enterprise. From his circle of Congréganist friends only the nephew of Bayle stayed on.[104] A manuscript on "irritation" in his papers may have been written as a substitute entry at the time of this protest, but the articles on "inflammation" and "irritation" were assigned to others, who cited Broussais and his critics.[105] In his treatise of the following year, Laennec alluded to a clinical disagreement with Broussais.[106] He also defended Bayle against the attacks of "a doctor whose opinions appear to me to be poorly grounded only in that they are too general and exclusive." He continued, "No, without doubt, Bayle did not see everything; no one can. But what he did see, he saw very well, and very few books have less to erase than his. One day, when the controversies that are always incited by ideas, which are new or presented in too absolute a fashion, have faded away, this doctor [Broussais] on calmly re-reading what he wrote, under the influence of necessary contradiction, will no doubt realize that he did not always keep himself within acceptable limits; . . . and, together with me, will recognize [in Bayle] a man of modest superiority . . . who died, perhaps without ever having inspired the slightest feeling of hate or aversion in anyone."[107]

The second edition of the *Examen* of mid-1821 devoted one hundred pages to an attack on Laennec and the other "fatalistic" pathological anatomists.[108] The author implied that Laennec and Bayle did not treat their patients in order to augment their supply of autopsy material. Provocatively, he accused Laennec of condescension and of having plagiarized the notion of localization from *Histoires des phlegmasies*. Concerned over possible inadvertent influence, Laennec reexamined the earlier book and was reassured.[109] But some of Broussais's criticisms had hit their mark, and Laennec began to think about revisions to his treatise. The anatomic descriptions *were* exceedingly long. The difficulty of their abundant adjectives and nuances exasperated his translator; Forbes claimed that he had once translated a passage without fully understanding it and speculated that the ambiguities resulted from Laennec's hostility to Broussais.[110] It was true, as Broussais claimed, that Laennec's loyal defense of Bayle was based, not on the latter's science, but on his gentle personality and upright behavior. This strategy was no accident: Laennec, too, had been puzzling over Bayle's "errors," which he thought could not be justified intellectually.[111] It was also true that Laennec had emphasized his stethoscope to the neglect of other modalities and that, as he was so often chided, he had written little about therapy in his first edition. Broussais's criticisms were expressed in immoderate language, but their validity was sufficient to "irritate" Laennec.

In a letter to his uncle, Laennec reflected on the challenge posed by his enemy and discussed his plan for a return to Paris. His dismay mingled with delight because the intended insults could be taken as compliments: "Our new arch-heretic [*hérésiarque*] Broussais . . . does me the honor of calling me the champion of Hippocratic, eclectic, and anatomic doctors. He may be a Breton but I suspect he has committed a '*gasconnade*' in thinking I am more out of action than I am. . . . [W]hen I was a twenty-five-year-old journalist, I would have loved to skewer an author that offered me so much undefended flank and, although the taste for this activity has left me, although writing tires and agitates me, I smiled like a hunter who has just seen the coming hare."[112] In the early fall of 1821, Laennec drafted a sixty-six-page argument against Broussais in the vain hope that it would appear in the *Bibliothèque médicale* early in 1822. He said, "I didn't expect to be obliged to return to the medical 'carrière' for a combat. Nevertheless, it's unavoidable. M. Broussais provokes me without even knowing if I am still living or if his voice can reach a hermit lost in the rocks of Finistère. He defies me, he waits for me . . . he addresses me by private name and collective name and in choosing me somehow [makes me] champion of doctors, who with me profess Hippocratic empiricism, enlightened by the observation of the living and the dead, by the relationship of facts, and by the very reserved use of the inductive method. . . . Only an invalid could refuse to defend such a beautiful cause."[113] Laennec abandoned his Breton retreat to defend his work from the onslaught of Broussais. He took the intended insult of "eclecticism" and conspicuously allowed it to become the name of his own medical doctrine.[114]

In engineering Laennec's return, Broussais had inadvertently brought about the very circumstances that provided his rival with great honors and membership in the elite. From Laennec's perspective, the royalist favors had the satisfying effect of angering Broussais still more.[115] Similarly, the popularity with foreign students, especially the English, became more fuel to Broussais's anti-Jesuit, antiroyalist, anti-Laennec fire. His biographers have vividly portrayed the vicious circle: the more Broussais felt ostracized, the more violently he attacked,[116] and the more Laennec resisted by flaunting and relishing the privileges that so annoyed his enemy.

According to Broussais, Laennec was a "fatalistic ontologist," with a fondness for "old systems" and a "mania" for "poisoning" his patients who eventually became his "victims."[117] Biographers have tried to show that Laennec was a "gentleman" and kept his remarks to polite, defensive statements, within the bounds of professional decorum; they cite his rival's insults to emphasize the outrageous cruelty, as yet another cross to bear for the long-suffering, "good" Laennec.[118] Preoccupied with Broussais's "*brutalité*," Rouxeau collected a large number of the insults for his book and his files.[119] But Laennec indulged in verbal Broussais-baiting, the scope of which may never be known, because only part of it was published. Broussais was like Paracelsus, he said, and amused journalists reported on the "great anger" in reaction from the Val de Grâce: "What language!" came the reply, "It is quite possible that in the eyes of Laennec we all look like drunkards."[120] They bickered over the mortality rates in their practices: Broussais claimed that he lost only one in every thirty patients, but the Val de Grâce hospital statistics revealed the death rate to be one in twelve.[121] Loyal students defended their master who had made an unintentional error; and even after his death, Laennec was criticized for having needlessly belabored the point, especially since the statistics from his own hospital were little better.[122] Some, like Adolphe-Aimé Lecadre and James Kitchen of Philadelphia, dared to follow the lessons of both, and their comparative insights are valuable.[123] The rivals brought out the worst in each other, and, as the dying Guillaume had predicted, their debate was lucrative theater.

The dispute between Laennec and Broussais represents a dialogue between formidable minds: each pronouncement of the one was a response to criticisms of the other. Laennec reworked, rethought, and revised his ideas in answer to Broussais' criticisms, and he too made provocative insults. The best evidence for this idea comes from the revised second edition of the *Treatise on Auscultation*, which can be read as a reply to Broussais's criticisms. Its new preface railed against his enemy with some of the material taken from the unpublished response.[124] But specific remarks in the second edition of the *Examen* about the first edition of the *Treatise on Auscultation* had provoked additions and/or modifications in Laennec's work.

Broussais had said that Laennec overemphasized the stethoscope; Laennec reorganized his treatise from one centered on physiological applications of auscultation to one based on chest diseases. Broussais had observed that Laennec did not address hydrops of the heart; Laennec added a section on hydrops with two new case reports.[125] Broussais had ridiculed Laennec's imprecision about the heart sounds; Laennec removed the passages where he had equivocated and changed passages on heart murmurs.[126] Broussais laughed at the ancient notions of coction and crisis and Laennec's retention of them; Laennec accused Broussais of plagiarizing Hippocrates and set about to prove the utility of the ancient theories of coction and crisis by the new method of statistics (see chap. 10).[127] Broussais had complained that the stethoscope (and its inventor) had done nothing for therapeutics; Laennec added a section on therapeutics to every chapter, expanded the passages on applications of auscultation in surgical empyema and devoted twenty pages to praising the drug, tartar emetic, as a treatment for pneumonia.[128] Did he turn his attention to this controversial remedy because Broussais had accused him of therapeutic nihilism? It seems entirely possible.

After Laennec's death, the 1834 third edition of the *Examen* would swell to four volumes of polemic, with nearly two hundred pages devoted to the arch but now defunct foe. Laennec was "*médico-jésuitique*," a "bad observer," a "bad therapist," "with a brain . . . heated by the all-consuming fever that devoured him, he could be nothing in medicine except a visionary." Laennec had died of his own ignorance, he said, as if "*la médecine physiologique*" could confer immortality on its adherents.[129] Broussais noticed Laennec's revisions, which seemed to have been made in answer to his criticisms, and complained that he had not been thanked for his useful suggestions.[130] He recognized the inventor's rigid tendency to assign one disease to one stethoscopic sign and cited the complexity and futility of the resultant auscultatory method, which sought to differentiate various forms of bronchitis by the color and texture of sputum.[131] He attacked the use of high-dose tartar emetic and questioned the emphasis on the traditional categories of hypertrophy and dilatation, which were the product of altered physiology.[132] He allowed that Laennec had been a good pathologist, but he knew nothing of the clinic, nor of physiology. Above all, he drew in high relief the absurd postures that the "hateful mind" of "the sophist" had adopted in order to refute his doctrine of irritation and inflammation.[133] On inflammation as on many other points, Broussais was right.

In becoming the sworn enemy of Broussais's "irritation," Laennec had also became the enemy of inflammation as a cause. The result was a refusal to admit that inflammation could ever constitute an independent, causal mechanism. Sacrificing lucidity to principle, he constructed verbal labyrinths in an effort to find and highlight alternative organic associations whenever inflammation became a possible candidate for causative process. He baffled some observers by refusing to replace the antiquated word "catarrh" with the newer "bronchitis," favored by Andral, Broussais, and Forbes to indicate inflammation of the airways.[134] As shown in previous chapters, he maintained that inflammation was not part of phthisis except as a secondary or coincidental change, and he excluded the frequently recognized complication of pleural effusion from his concept of phthisis because it was inflammatory. Inflammation of the heart, Laennec said, was "extremely rare" and "impossible" to detect through clinical signs, although a student cited his friend, Récamier, as an expert.[135] Others might overlook these conceptual contortions, but Broussais did not. He said Laennec had cultivated a "vicious habit" of elaborating "specious" hypotheses designed to refute the possible influence of irritation and inflammation in the production of disease.[136]

Laennec and Broussais: Agreement?

According to sociologists of science, "deviant" behaviors such as precipitous publication, plagiarism or, more commonly the accusations of plagiarism, can be described as a response to scientific competition.[137] Priority disputes and closure have been given the most attention in studies of scientific rivalry, probably because they can be taken to signify what the actors themselves consider a "discovery" or the violation and/or reconstruction of scientific norms that identifies a Kuhnian revolution, or paradigm shift.[138]

Working backward, then, can we not ask whether the "deviant" behavior of Laennec and Broussais also signals a priority dispute? Does their polemic mean that they thought they were competing for recognition about a "discovery" that was important to them, although it may be negligible if not imperceptible to us? Is it possible that a priority dispute took place in the absence of what we might now consider to have been a discovery? If so, what might that implied discovery have been? A scientific fight that is neither institutional, nor personal, dwells within the conceptual heart of a matter; each opponent may be making plausible statements that the other is reluctant to admit. Hence, analysis of a seemingly social phenomenon might elucidate a philosophical problem.[139]

Despite their polemic, Laennec and Broussais often agreed; but they admitted agreement only grudgingly, while their colleagues and historians ignored it. Broussais used and praised the stethoscope. Laennec diagnosed gastroenteritis and prescribed leeches far more often than previous biographers cared to admit. They even exchanged compliments: Broussais said, "I am far from disdaining M. Laennec. As a result, I will attack him very vigorously in the best interests of science and humanity"; and Laennec, "I have the highest regard for the talent of M. Broussais in spite of all that I will say concerning his mistakes and his manner of presenting his ideas and attacking his opponents."[140] They shared objections to the observations of Bayle's nephew, Antoine-Laurent-Jesse Bayle (1799–1858), who had linked the neurological condition, now called general paresis, to syphilitic and other inflammation of the meninges: Broussais, because irritation not inflammation was the cause; Laennec, because inflammation could never be a cause (see chap. 12).[141] They both thought that fever was overly divided in nosological classifications and preferred to think of it as a single disease. Neither man wished to preserve Pinel's nosography, but they respected his work as an "*aliéniste*" and embraced the notion of moral treatment with few modifications: Broussais would have added leeches for the well-being of his fellow citizen; Laennec, a straitjacket, in the interests of law and order.[142]

Some have suggested that the dispute centered on a disagreement over therapeutics: the identity of physician as diagnostician versus physician as therapist. Evidence also refutes this claim, however. Laennec may not have written a great deal about therapy, but he drugged, bled, and leeched his patients as often as his contemporaries. He readily complimented Broussais for his service to France in "proving" the benefits of heavy bleeding, and he was a devotee of depletive therapy, which—perversely—he named for Antonio-Maria Valsalva (1666–1723), claiming it had been beneficial in at least five patients.[143]

The most important area of agreement, however, was in the conceptual limitations of pathological anatomy. Laennec's stethoscope helped the movement to localize disease in the organs and, as such, had become an impetus to anatomoclinical medicine. When he refused to conceive of all diseases as a product of organic change, younger physicians—like Andral, Bouillaud, and Rostan—thought the innovator to be peculiarly, even inexplicably, resistant to the logical extrapolation of his own discovery. Broussais approached the issue from a different direction, but ended up in the same position as Laennec. He opposed the pathological anatomists' preoccupation with the dead and material change; their wordy descriptions had little to do with the living patient or with the origin of the organic lesions. His emphasis on gastroenteritis might seem to support a simplified version of their materialism; however, Broussais came to oppose pathological anatomy with his physiology, because it was the abnormal functional process (the sympathies) not the structural lesion, that constituted the disease.[144]

In other words, Broussais and Laennec agreed that the new wave of practitioners were ignoring the causes of disease; diseases were the products of physiological, not anatomical processes. Causes might not be knowable, but it was wrong to pretend that they did not exist. Successful therapies must act through the same mechanisms that had produced the disease, and some fatal illnesses—exemplified by the old case of *cadet Rousseau*—were not associated with organic change. Pathological anatomy could not be expected to explain it all. Broussais's physiological doctrine addressed the unexplained causes of disease, their mysterious link with lesions and symptoms, and the uncertain ways in which to treat. To explode the theories of Broussais, one required a better theory capable of dealing with these unexplained problems. That was precisely what Laennec hoped to do, but with no more success.

Prior to auscultation, Laennec recognized these limitations, but they did not dominate his research; he concentrated on pathological anatomy. After auscultation, the limitations became more apparent with respect to diseases without lesions (angina), disease with physiological lesions (asthma), and causes. As he had stated in his treatise, he was convinced of the value of pathological anatomy, but he also acknowledged the existence of causes and effects even if they could not be known.[145] He and Bayle had long used the ancient notion of "vital force" as the most neutral term to address the "physiological sympathies" defined by Broussais. It offered a great advantage in that it did not necessitate another neologism.

Broussais had couched his concerns in jargon borrowed from pathology and he labeled his approach "physiological medicine." Unable either to accept Broussais's word "physiology" or to use anatomical terminology loosely, Laennec expressed his reservations in traditional, vitalistic words, borrowed from Hippocrates and Montpellier, via Bayle, and rendered scientific with reference to chemistry, physics, and the experimental work of Magendie. Had he chosen his words deliberately to irritate his enemy, the effect could not have been greater. Broussais said that Laennec was "small and nasty in his theory just as he was in his person."[146] Failing to see the ontology in his own concepts of irritation, sympathy, and inflammation, he criticized Laennec's vocabulary for its metaphysics: " 'Vital lesion' is certainly a physiologic term, but it has the air of a catchall used to satisfy a difficult question; a reasoning person does not comprehend what is meant by a lesion of life, which precedes and causes those of the organs . . . all the forces of the Montpellier doctors are little divinities."[147] But in his criticism of Gall's use of the term "*lésion vitale,*" Broussais tellingly acknowledged that it was simply an outdated way of expressing "irritation."[148]

Broussais noticed that Laennec shared his reservations concerning the overemphasis of organic change, but he misunderstood his rival's attempts to speak of physiology, and he flattered himself that these ideas had been stolen from his own doctrine. Inaccurately characterizing Laennec's method as a "complete subjugation of medicine" to a nosology based on pathological anatomy, he portrayed Laennec as possessed of an extreme "medical materialism," which he found impossible to reconcile with his apparent "religious spiritualism."[149] What Broussais mistook for "religious spiritualism," or "poorly defined notions of nervous influence," was Laennec's own version of the physiological doctrine.

Broussais's words "irritation" and "sympathy" dealt with the same notions as the altered "*principe vital*" of Laennec: *pathogenesis* (cf. fig. 9.7). Knowledge of pathogenesis was beyond the reach of early nineteenth-century pathological anatomy, which was restricted to macroscopic observation of the organic lesion without consideration of how that lesion came about. Their immediate successors ignored this theoretical weakness, satisfied with the dictates of radical positivism, which denied contemplation of what could not be known. This positivistic reconstruction of disease created a rift between the clinical and the medical and began to distance the subjective aspects of the patient's illness from the process of diagnosis.[150] Both Broussais and Laennec saw the flaw; few others seem to have agreed. Their shared reservations about the new medicine bordered on this realm of criticism, and it was priority for this "discovery" that they disputed.

Laennec's well-known Catholicism provided a rationale for linking his life force to the soul, thereby placing his vitalism with the retrograde "theological" or "metaphysical" categories in Comte's vision of knowledge— an indictment spared Broussais's physiological doctrine when Comte himself had declared "irritation" to be "positive."[151] Broussais seemed to know what would happen, as his statement in the epigraph to this chapter would suggest, and he predicted Laennec's immortality "in spite of all his faults" and "mistakes."[152]

The many differences between Laennec and Broussais, were fundamentally semantic. Without admitting their common ground, they agreed on a paradigm concerning the problems as well as the advantages of anatomic localization: both emphasized the importance of organic lesions; both also tried to render some recognition and comprehensibility to the aspects of disease that would continue to defy explanation by the anatomoclinical method. The new method had indeed resulted in what Foucault described as a reorganization of medical gaze and discourse, to which Laennec had made a singular contribution with his neologistic stethoscopic signs and the renaming of disease.[153] The nascent clinic was still building its vocabulary, however, and within this unstable environment, there were few acceptable terms in which to frame threatening criticisms.

Thus, in an intellectual form of sociological "anomie,"[154] Laennec and Broussais strove toward a common goal within a conceptual environment that favored reduction and materialism and tolerated neither the preservation of ancient terms nor the creation of neologisms, unless, like stethoscopic signs, the new words stood for material objects—new things, organic changes. Laennec and Broussais both tried to raise criticisms, but the lack of acceptable terms (norms) for the expression of criticism fostered their "deviant" behavior. They chose radically different vehicles to accomplish their task and barely succeeded in defining the problem in the two different vocabularies that reflected their personal, political, and intellectual biases.[155] Neither definition survived, but each man defeated the other's language.[156] When the dust settled, there emerged a less prolix medical discourse, liberated, thanks to Laennec, from the vague terms "irritation" and "sympathy" and wary of the expression "gastroenteritis," but a discourse that had also been purged of the words "vital principle," "crisis," and "coction," thanks to Broussais.

Auscultation was disseminated quickly in France and beyond, and it significantly altered the practice of diagnostics—not only in the technique of physical examination, but also through the conceptualization of disease. The admission records of the Necker hospital show that the names of diseases used in the clinical setting were altered in a short time to reflect the new emphasis on organic localization and medical materialism. The rapid effect of the stethoscope was to displace the subjective accounts of patients from their central role and to make the doctor the central arbiter over the essential distinction between health and disease.

In his treatise, Laennec had warned about the danger of a narrow extrapolation of his technique and overemphasis of pathological anatomy. These reservations were noticed and criticized by Broussais who complained that they had been inspired by his "physiological doctrine" without due credit. Broussais had co-opted the language of "physiology" and joined Laennec's translator in trying to confine his rival into the narrow realm of morbid anatomy. The rivals agreed on one thing: no theory of disease could succeed if it failed to consider the pathogenesis of organic lesions, the suffering of patients, and the stories they told about their ills. Broussais and Laennec may have disagreed about the best way to express this concern, but the preoccupation with building a theory of disease pervaded the remainder of their lives.

Return to Paris: Elite Practice and Professor in the Clinic

To know the nature and extent of a disease is surely
the first step in our progress to the adoption of
rational means of cure.

—*James Clark 1820, 154–155*

People need to have things trumpeted into their ears
several times and from all directions. The first sound
pricks up the ear, the second shakes it, and
with the third, it goes in.

—*Laennec to his cousin Mériadec, 8 June 1821*

BY MID-NOVEMBER 1821, Laennec was back in Paris. He intended to accept
the accolades that he had long believed were his due, and he would rebut his
critics, especially Broussais. The stethoscope was already known throughout
Europe, and its detractors were growing scarce, but he needed to reestablish
his authority over the presumptuous young investigators like Collin and Andral who had challenged the expertise of the inventor. From his room at the
Hôtel du Bon Lafontaine, he returned to the clinical service at the Necker
hospital and served an illustrious private clientele. The death of Corvisart two
months earlier had created professorial vacancies: Laennec busily set about
lobbying on behalf of his friend Récamier and negotiating with the friends of
Magendie over mutual support in upcoming elections at the Institute.[1] He
would play an active role in the royalist coup over the university.

The hospital research that he planned would not be confined to auscultation, nor even to pathological anatomy: he would explore disease and therapeutic interventions with surgery, environmental manipulation, tartar
emetic, and other drugs. Finally, he would do "what no one has ever done"
and test the Hippocratic theory of critical days that had been dismissed by
Corvisart.[2] Students would write theses on these new topics, too. The trea

tise on auscultation would be revised to counter the criticisms of those who had failed to understand the physiological applications of the stethoscope and its potential uses in the treatment of disease. From the perspective of medical posterity these concerns may seem trivial; but for Laennec, they were paramount.

COURT PHYSICIAN AND PROFESSOR AT LAST

Just a few weeks after his return to Paris and through the influence of his former professor, Hallé, Laennec was named physician to the Princess of the Two Sicilies, Marie-Caroline-Ferdinande-Louise, the Duchesse de Berry (1798–1870) (fig. 10.1). She was the widow of the second nephew of King Louis XVIII, the Duc de Berry, who had been assassinated in 1820. Hallé was physician to her father-in-law, the Comte d'Artois, who would be crowned King Charles X in 1824. Seven months after her husband's death, the Duchesse de Berry had given birth to a son, Henri Duc de Bourbon, called the "miracle child." The influence of the Duchesse de Berry at court was considerable; her fatherless child was viewed as a direct heir to throne, and some hoped the unpopular Charles X would abdicate in the child's favor. In 1830, the Duchesse would lead an unsuccessful attempt to replace the next "usurper," King Louis-Philippe, with her son, "Henri V." Among her supporters was Chateaubriand.[3]

Laennec confided in the Bishop of Quimper that Hallé had advanced his cause at court without consulting him first. He felt obliged to accept the new position to avoid embarrassing his mentor, but he worried about the damage that the extra work could do to his health and his independence, until the princess herself assured him "that she did not want his service to her to constrain [his] other occupations."[4] After his presentation on 1 January 1822, he was to attend his royal patient daily in the Pavillon Marsan for a annual salary of four thousand francs, a handsome amount that guaranteed a comfortable existence.[5] As in the days of Cardinal Fesch, he was required to dress in courtly attire complete with a sword. There is a legend that the infant "miracle child" enjoyed riding on Laennec's gold-headed cane. The Duchesse is said to have found her doctor's method of percussion somewhat brutal, but she appears to have liked him: she used her influence on his behalf, gave him an Italian cello, and when he was sick expressed sympathetic wishes for his recovery.[6]

Laennec returned to his former prominence as consultant of choice for Bretons, royalists, and émigrés, more of whom had resurfaced with the departure of Napoleon.[7] The aristocrats were not always rich, and their doctor's dedication stemmed from his respect for their position. His solicitude is revealed in his circumspection about their names: there are records for "Mlle. xxx," the "Duchesse de C. . .," "Monsieur le comte H. . .," and at

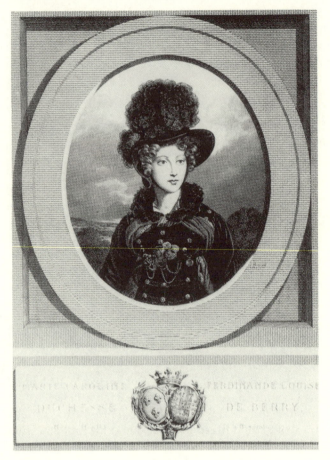

Figure 10.1. Marie-Caroline-Ferdinande-Louise, the Duchesse de Berry. She was the widow of the second nephew of King Louis XVIII, the Duc de Berry, who had been assassinated in 1820. Her father-in-law, the Comte d'Artois, would become King Charles X in 1824. Laennec was appointed her physician in January 1822 and attended her daily at the Pavillon Marsan. Source: Orczy 1936, frontispiece. Provenance unknown. Photograph: Queen's Medical Photography Services.

least three (probably) different people (and surely not Bonapartes) designated simply by the title "N . . . ." From the correspondence, a list of Laennec's noble patients and influential friends can be assembled.[8] Since his Congrégation days, Laennec had known Mathieu Duc de Montmorency, who served as minister of foreign affairs until he was replaced in 1823 by Chateaubriand, Laennec's patient. The doctor also knew the controversial Duc de Doudeauville, Ambroise-Polycarpe de la Rochefoucauld (1765–1841), and he continued to frequent the salon of Mlle Delavau, whose Congréganist brother, Guy Delavau, had become the politically engaged prefect of police. Laennec was pleased with Delavau's appointment, and did not shrink from appealing to him on behalf of various friends. He kept the bishop of Quimper informed of Paris intrigue and the jokes: "upon hearing that the Duc de Doudeauville had been named director general of the post office, a lady from the faubourg St. Germain asked, 'And who has been named the Duc de Doudeauville?' "[9]

While Laennec was in Brittany, the Bourbon administration had been moving increasingly to the right in an attempt to control the influence of subversive forces thought to be lurking in the wake of the assassination of the Duc de Berry and following the failure of the anti-Restoration Carbonari movement. Moderate ministers were replaced with extremists who took measures that have been characterized as expiation of guilt for revolutionary sins. By the time Laennec returned to Paris in late 1821, Joseph Villèle (1773–1854) had been appointed minister of finance and his "boorish" Breton friend, Corbière, became minister of the interior.[10] Laws were enacted to limit freedom of the press, books were suppressed, and the church was given increasing power over education. In 1822, Denis Frayssinous (1765–1841), a former student of the seminary of Saint Sulpice and now Bishop of Hermopolis, became Grand Master of the University; he was chosen to lead a combined ministry of public instruction and ecclesiastical affairs.[11] Laennec's old friend, Quélen, had also donned a miter in Laennec's absence; by 1824, he was archbishop of Paris.[12] The royalists harbored suspicions about members of the medical faculty, many of whom had been sympathetic to the Revolution and had accepted titles in Napoleon's entourage. Partly to counter the influence of the liberal faculty, the Académie Royale de Médecine was resurrected by Louis XVIII in 1820 from its intermediary, the faculty-based Société de l'Ecole de Médecine, and two other medical societies with roots in the Ancien Régime.[13]

Laennec may not have been one of Montmorency's ultra-right Chevaliers de la Foi, whose roots can be traced to the old Congrégation; however, he was a bold participant in what he appears to have viewed as a moral crusade to reestablish order. He had told Christophe that Villèle and Corbière would make him a professor if he wished, and on Christmas Day 1821, an amazed Mériadec reported to his father: "Théophile is in good with the (new) minister of the interior. They met in the street the other day and shook hands like old friends."[14]

Hallé died quite suddenly in February 1822, only a week after Béclard had operated on him for bladder stone and just a month after securing the court appointment for his protégé. His death led to a remarkable series of events that took twelve months to unfold. By April, Laennec had replaced his dead mentor at the Académie Royale de Médecine, through an impressive first-ballot victory over Chomel and Serres, capturing twenty-three of the twenty-seven votes cast.[15] In July, he was named Hallé's successor in the chair of practical medicine at the Collège de France, where he would be expected to give lectures three days a week. He had been nominated by Frayssinous and was appointed by the direct intervention of the King through Corbière and in flagrant opposition to medical voters who were considering Bertin, Magendie, and the areligious anatomist Chaussier; the latter had been elected over Laennec as the candidate of choice by the professors of the Collège de France. Without ministerial interference, the position would likely have gone to Chaussier, who had already defeated Laennec in the another election to replace Hallé at the Institute. Laennec told the Bishop of Quimper that the "liberals" had unsuccessfully tried to promote his "principal opponent, the least of whose defects for teaching medicine was the fact that he had never studied it."[16] Preparation for his new professorial position occupied most of his spare time in late 1822, but by early 1823 he was deeply involved with what can only be described as massive political interference with the faculty of medicine.

The troubles in the faculty exploded with Desgenettes's *éloge* to Hallé delivered on 18 November 1822, the opening day of the medical school. As the published text confirms, the old surgeon was interrupted repeatedly by student hecklers and finally had to abandon his speech at the point when he was describing the tolerant but devout religious sentiments of the deceased professor.[17] Jacques Léonard claimed that the speech had been constructed as a deliberate insult to the increasingly intolerant, royalist regime and that it had inflamed a sympathetic audience.[18] The text itself, however, scarcely seems provocative; it could be that the rebellious students were opposed to venerating the memory of a Catholic servant of the throne. Nevertheless, whether or not Desgenettes had intended the slight, the blame fell on him. The stormy session became a pretext for Frayssinous and Corbière to temporarily close the faculty of medicine in late November, a strategy that had already been imposed on the faculty of law the previous March.[19] Corbière named Laennec with Cuvier and Récamier to the commission charged with restructuring the faculty in concert with conservative goals.[20]

Some biographers, like Kergaradec, were embarrassed by Laennec's part in negotiating the new order; apologetically, they suggest that he allowed himself to get involved only to protect old stalwarts, among them the anatomist, Béclard, and the surgeon, Boyer.[21] Others have distorted the chain of events to suggest that the "underhand maneuvering, treachery and political changes," were directed against Laennec.[22] But his papers make it clear that he was using the system to advance himself and his associates. He and "his friends," both clerical and medical, believed their actions, like the drastic expiatory measures of throne and church, were justified in the interest of a greater public good. For example, Laennec's ecclesiastical friend, Dombideau de Crousheilhes, the Bishop of Quimper, had written to congratulate Frayssinous at the moment of his appointment and to remind him of "all that we expect from him," to heal the "greatest sore" of France, which was its public education.[23] Laennec was a good candidate: his professorial aptitude had been amply proven in two decades of research, teaching, publishing, and practice, during which he had repeatedly been slighted and excluded by liberals and nonbelievers. Here was the final vindication of the brilliant

Congréganists who, like their defunct leaders, Buisson and Bayle, had been shut out of academe.

Those faculty members who were perceived to be too far to the left were expelled. Desgenettes was dismissed along with ten other professors; he wrote to Laennec, beseeching his "courageous and benevolent" help in procuring a pension.[24] It is not known how Laennec responded, if at all. Unlike Béclard, Desgenettes may have seemed to be in a situation every bit hopeless as that of his uncle Guillaume a few years earlier, a situation unworthy of the risk that obvious use of influence might bring. The new medical order had its opponents—for example, the government ordered the police to seize a book of medical biography naming the most notorious royalist collaborators—but Desgenettes was not reinstated until the Revolution of 1830, when Laennec's friends were ousted.[25]

By mid-March 1823, the coup was over. Laennec's devout friends Cayol, Kergaradec, Fizeau, and Récamier became professors. Frayssinous reopened the faculty with a speech about religion and science.[26] With Alibert, Béclard, Roux, and Royer-Collard, Laennec was assigned to work on the curriculum, and he was given the task of preparing a revised set of examination questions in Latin.[27] He resigned from the Necker hospital to take up his duties as professor of clinical medicine and to preside over what had once been Corvisart's domain, the *clinique interne* at the Charité hospital.

HOSPITAL RESEARCH IN AUSCULTATION, THERAPEUTICS, AND HIPPOCRATIC THEORY

The notes of a visitor show that the anatomoclinical research into auscultation continued and allow for a comparison between the Necker and Charité practices shortly before Laennec's transfer. Two British students, William Thomson (1802–1852) and Robert Carswell, visited medical Paris as part of a two-year tour of European hospitals.[28] Between mid-August and mid-October 1822, while the faculty troubles were brewing and Laennec was still waiting to hear about his position at the Collège de France, Carswell attended forty-four autopsies in the Charité and the Necker hospitals. A gifted artist, he was intent on making accurate drawings of anatomical specimens, and his written descriptions of the morbid appearances were to be a guide to his drawings. Often the autopsy was the only information that he recorded about a case, implying, as Stephen Jacyna has suggested, that his interest in the patient was only as a locus of disease.[29] Gradually, however, Carswell began to write a little more about the patients, their symptoms, and their treatment, and these changes occur earlier in his Necker cases than in his Charité cases, inviting speculation about the relative emphasis on patient histories in the two clinics.

At the Necker, Carswell met Laennec in the morgue for at least five cases.[30] The inventor's recent influence can be read in Carswell's references

TABLE 10.1
Hospital Movement at the Charité Hospital (1823–1826)

	1823*	1824	1825 †	1826 ‡
In hospital on 1 Jan	289	301	272	357
Admissions	3552	4010	5185	4933
Total deaths	561	560	714§	743
Deaths while Laennec was present	189	560	464	369

Sources: Registres des Entrées de l'Hôpital de la Charité, 1823–1826, AAP, 1Q2.64–67; Registres des Décès de l'Hôpital de la Charité, 1823–1826, AAP, 3Q2.19–22.

* Laennec was appointed to the *clinique interne* of the hospital in March, but did not take over duties as attending physician until mid-Aug 1823.

† Laennec was absent for three months from Sep to Nov 1825.

‡ Laennec left the Charité hospital in May 1826 because of his final illness.

§ 1825 death register after 20 Aug is missing; total estimated on 454 deaths to that date.

to the new entities of peritonitis, emphysema, encephaloid (cerebriform tumor), and the three stages of pneumonia, as well as in his appreciation of a "healed cavity of tuberculosis."[31] All the lung cases that he recorded during the period were seen at the Necker, where he learned auscultation and its terminology. Carswell also described four cases of liver cirrhosis, a lesion new to him, but did not yet use the newly invented word.[32] At the Charité, Laennec's early discoveries of peritonitis and liver disease were known, but his more recent denominations for heart disease were not yet used, the words "diseased heart" sufficing for a variety of conditions. With Chomel and Lerminier, Carswell saw a number of intestinal and fever cases, but when Laennec came to Charité's *clinique interne*, the direction of research there would change.

Founded in 1798, the *clinique interne* was an elite unit of forty beds, twenty-six for men and fourteen for women, within a huge urban hospice (see table 10.1). Only a few cases selected from the larger hospital were attended in the *clinique interne*, and Clark, who visited the service in 1820, was disappointed to find that the forty patients were all chronic cases being treated with remedies that he considered to be "particularly inert."[33] After Laennec's arrival in March 1823, the pace at the *clinique* and in the much larger Charité seems to have picked up with his continuing investigation of auscultation and his new therapeutic research. The English visitor Scudamore spoke of the enthusiastic students and Laennec's vigorous use of tartar emetic; and the literature contained communications from former students who continued medical inquiry, although they no longer lived in Paris.[34]

During Laennec's tenure, the published *clinique* statistics suggest that the service was not overwhelmed with work: in a four-month period in 1825, 68 patients were admitted, of whom 18 died; for a six-month period in 1826, there were 188 admissions and 37 deaths.[35]

At the Charité hospital, Laennec would continue his Necker practice of gathering clinical evidence to refute his critics, and he would work on the new signs of bronchophony and puerile respiration. As shown in chapter 9, his invention had already brought a marked change in the diagnostic practices of his colleagues during his absence; his restored presence now enhanced their appreciation of the new diseases that he had described. Conspicuously allying himself with British experimental physiologist, David Barry, he refined his interpretation of the stethoscopic sounds in heart and lung for the second edition of his treatise. In response to those who demanded therapeutic applications or had laughed at the idea of cure in phthisis, he conducted clinical experiments on the treatment of tuberculosis and pneumonia. His tests of the Hippocratic theories of coction, crisis, and critical days, were also related to therapeutics, because they explored the healing power of nature.

In its use of statistics, this research modestly paralleled the work of P. C. A. Louis, credited with developing the numerical method with his statistically oriented essays on tuberculosis and bleeding, and it predated the mathematical tools that would be provided by L. A. J. Quételet (1796–1835).[36] Louis was an early user of auscultation, and he worked in the Charité. Some have postulated a bond of friendship between the two men, but Louis's name does not appear in the Laennec papers, and is cited only rarely in the second edition of the treatise on auscultation. Louis later refuted Broussais's charge that he had been the "obsequious pupil" of Laennec, claiming that he had laid eyes on the inventor only twice "for a few minutes each time."[37] The Laennec papers contain an intriguing two-part document, not in his hand, that seems to follow Louis's technique slavishly: it sorts all the symptoms and signs in the cases that had been included in the treatise of Bayle into diagnostic categories and then presents prognostic categories according to Laennec. Its purpose is unknown, but it may have served in Laennec's teaching or in preparation for the treatise on auscultation.[38]

Laennec investigated the action of high doses of tartar emetic, or antimony potassium tartrate, in cases of pneumonia and other diseases. He said he had learned about the technique from doctors who had visited Italy, and he claimed to have put the theories into practice by 1817; however, published and manuscript evidence places the beginning of this research in 1822.[39] The rather exotic drug had a long and complicated history, including bans on its use in Paris and Heidelberg because of its toxic side effects of vomiting, diarrhea, and cardiovascular collapse.[40] Laennec's uncle Guillaume had thought that this emetic "par excellence" was the only useful antimony preparation and that there was "almost no disease" for which it could not provide some benefit.[41]

Laennec cited his own statistical evidence in favor of the observations of Italian practitioners Giovanni Rasori (1766–1837) and Giacomo Tommasini (1768–1846), who had reported that large doses of tartar emetic were effective in pneumonia. The side effects did not always occur, he said, nor were they prerequisite for the drug to be beneficial: in other words, the drug might make some patients vomit or purge, but it seemed to act through an inapparent, physiological mechanism that did not require mechanical expulsion of a toxin. His successes with the emetic in pneumonia prompted him to try it in other inflammatory conditions including, "arachnitis," "acute hydrocephalus," pleurisy, catarrh, chorea, and articular rheumatism; he and his cousin, Ambroise, both used it to "cure" patients with tetanus.[42] Several of his students conducted similar investigations at home and abroad.[43]

In 1826, Laennec said that he had never had an opportunity to study the effects of tartar emetic in peritonitis, the disease he had described as a student. Nevertheless, a case report, which he annotated heavily, shows that he had used the drug in peritonitis, but for some reason this successful outcome was not published in his treatise: "Marie-Louise Usé, a twenty-two-year-old gardener, hysterical ['*hystérique*'] since the age of ten and subject to frequent vomiting, sustained a contusion to her epigastrium on 15 April 1822 and was admitted to the Necker hospital with all the symptoms of intense peritonitis on 9 May. . . . The stomach was tender. . . . [T]here was constipation. . . . She had a smooth red tongue, severe headache, and intense, almost continual vomiting, which aggravated her pains." She received baths, leeches to the groin, and mercury frictions, all to no avail. She developed painful urination. "On 2 July she was treated with orange leaf tea to which had been added tartar emetic. Her vomiting was no worse than before [Marginalia: 'at the end of three days of therapy she felt well and wished to discontinue treatment.'] . . . her fever returned on 22 July, the emetic was started on the 24th, and by the 27th, she was cured. . . . At home she remembered the in-hospital therapy and took a strong dose [of tartar emetic] when needed and was cured the same day."[44]

Antimony therapy earned Laennec sharp criticism from friends and enemies alike, but he forged ahead with his investigations. Jostling with adepts of the physiological doctrine at the bedside of a physician, he gave tartar emetic to Dr. C*** [probably Chauveau] who died after "two new doctors," who "thought they detected gastroenteritis," had prescribed "eighteen leeches to the anus."[45] A Parisian pundit added an ironic twist into the great debate between Laennec and Broussais, by saying that the deaths of both Chauveau and the medical professor A. A. Royer-Collard (1768–1825), brother of the royalist statesman, were iatrogenic—not from the Broussaisist leeching, as the disciples of Laennec maintained—but from gastroenteritis provoked by Laennec's emetic.[46] Broussais and his followers kept up a steady barrage of criticisms for the use of antimony in his journal *Annales de médecine physiologique* and elsewhere.[47] Mériadec Laennec countered the criticism that tartar emetic caused a new disease: "fifty students follow the clinic of

M. Laennec every day . . . none have seen a difference in the state of the intestines of patients who have taken tartar emetic and those who have not."[48] Even friends and eulogists came to denounce the practice, while Bouillaud conducted some retrospective spying on Laennec's service when he had an aide at the Charité hospital, ferret out the less than favorable statistics on Laennec's pneumonia patients, more than a decade after their doctor's death.[49] The drastic side effects of the drug resulted in its decline, and until recently, reasons for Laennec's apparent success with it were unexplored.

In testing tartar emetic, Laennec may have unintentionally skewed his samples, because he compared the treated and poststethoscopic cases with untreated historical cases taken from the period before auscultation. Since the diagnosis of pneumonia is facilitated with the stethoscope, his treated sample may have included cases of mild pneumonia that would have been missed prior to auscultation and that would have healed without treatment. In other words, the historical group was not only untreated, but also sicker than the treated group. These considerations aside, large doses of tartar emetic may actually have had a bactericidal effect on the patients treated.[50]

Extending his interest in therapeutics to other diseases of the lung and heart, Laennec researched new chapters for the second edition of his treatise. He was uncertain of the value of digitalis: "Its effect [as a diuretic] has never been obvious to me." As in the hardy experiments with tartar emetic, he explored the foxglove in large doses, but said it was ineffective "even when the dose was increased to the point of causing vomiting and vertigo." "In short," he said, "I can consider it only as an 'heroic' measure."[51] The high doses went against the warnings of William Withering, who had first brought digitalis into medical orthodoxy.[52] Laennec appeared to accept unpleasant side effects as an inevitable part of any treatment, but the existing case records suggest that the use of digitalis in his own clinical practice was cautious and rare; he used tartar emetic more frequently. For example, Marianne Vicéra, a twenty-four-year-old woman admitted to hospital 22 March 1822 with "cardiac neuralgia," suffered epigastric pains, nausea, and vomiting, which vanished "when one stopped the digitalis and reappeared when it was restarted."[53] He classed digitalis as a poison in his lessons at the Collège de France.[54]

Attempts to explore new therapies did not stop at antimony and digitalis. Laennec had an interest in magnets and animal magnetism, and he experimented with treatments for phthisis in response to statistical observations.[55] Statistics from his clinical experience suggested that the disease was less common and less fatal in rural Brittany than it was in Paris. To investigate the possible role of climactic factors, he conducted a clinical trial in the winter of 1825–1826 with the "creation" of an "artificial marine atmosphere." Cartloads of seaweed were hauled from Normandy beaches and strewn on the floors of a ward accommodating twelve consumptives. Nine of the twelve patients left the hospital, but he admitted that for only one did he entertain any hope of a cure.[56] Laennec's translator, Forbes, viewed this attempt at treatment with scorn: "I cannot pass without remark on the imbecility of this statement. . . . If a 'marine atmosphere' alone sufficed for the cure of phthisis, happy would it be for us and all other islanders, who could so easily enjoy the benefit of its influence in all its natural perfection and without the aid of stinking sea-weed."[57]

Other statistical observations refuted the claims of medicine for curing phthisis and endorsed Laennec's belief in psychic disturbances—Bayle's nostalgia—in the production of the organic disease of phthisis. The etiological concept of a "vital lesion" led him to resurrect Bayle's notion of "vital therapy," with release of stress, rest, and vacations—treatments proven to be effective in his experience. These observations supported Laennec's idea that phthisis resulted from a physiological reaction to psychological stress and privation—a vital lesion—the opinion that had been repeatedly endorsed by his own experiences with the same disease in the Paris nuns, his brother, his friend, and eventually in himself. [58]

Telling remarks made in letters show that Laennec believed that city life was responsible for his own chronic illness: "I risked my life and I knew it when I came back to Paris last year."[59] In the city, he had exposed himself to the risk of tuberculosis, not because of contact with infective patients, not because of the dangerous autopsies he had performed, not because of the unhealthy urban environment, but because of the severe psychological pain of homesickness, unhappiness, lack of vigorous exercise, and overwork—a vital lesion. The same could be said for the many examples of psychological antecedents described in cases of anatomical illnesses in *the Treatise on Auscultation* (see Appendix C).

Laennec's preoccupation with the physiological mechanisms of disease led him to contemplate the physiology of cure and the healing power of nature imputed to Hippocratic texts.[60] He was motivated to disprove the presumptuous claims of Corvisart, Broussais, and the young pathological anatomists, who claimed to know more than the Father of Medicine about how to recognize and predict natural recoveries. In his 1804 thesis, Laennec said that every era had created its own mistaken theories as a result of trying to simplify the effort to understand. He implied that "*les jours critiques*" may actually have been the mistaken theory of Hippocrates.[61] The same idea is found again in the opening lecture at the Collège de France: theories, like Hippocratic coction, could be eliminated from a collection of work to leave meaningful observations.[62] Earlier, Laennec had not bothered to mount a defense for these ancient notions, although the letters show that he respected and utilized them;[63] but at the end of his career, he flaunted their utility. He said, the "only way to put an end to the great debate" over critical days would be to research thoroughly the Hippocratic writings and coordinate the material into a coherent doctrine, something that no one had yet bothered to do.[64] With his professorship, Laennec proposed to do just that, and he would test the doctrine on his patients. As historian Jackie Pigeaud has observed, Laennec "never stopped meditating on Hippocrates."[65]

General diseases, especially the fevers, posed the biggest problem: Broussais had simplified fevers and localized them to the stomach. Laennec also preferred to unify fevers, but he chose not to discard the symptomatic distinctions made by the nosologists or the wisdom of ancient texts. By 1821, he was composing an essay, "On the Fevers According to the Doctrine of Hippocrates and the Findings of Pathological Anatomy."[66] After his return to Paris, he put Mériadec, now his *chef de clinique*, to work investigating Hippocratic tenets. His cousin was smitten with his weighty task: "We work with courage. Théophile teaches with zeal and precision. We have nearly thirty students and they seem pleased with his *modus faciendi*. We have lost none of the ten patients with serious fevers and gastroenteritis in our wards. Almost all had crises, a word that makes partisans of the physiological doctrine shrug; these crises have surprised those of their number who come to see the adversary of their master. We are delighted to be able to prove to them that Hippocrates was not wrong."[67]

Laennec admitted that, according to various Hippocratic texts, many different days could be critical, and he acknowledged the difficulty that clinicians could have deciding where to begin their count. To avoid having medical therapy conflict with salutary crises, he devised a rule to help with the decision: "Keep the count [of days] uncertain until the first critical change; then you will be on the seventh day. Count this day as the seventh and you will see the other multiples of seven and indicators will bring new crises. In summary, according to Hippocrates himself, all days can be critical days, but the seventh and the fourteenth days are most often."[68]

Clinical observations from January to April 1824 show that Laennec was putting his rule into practice; they are annotated with underlined remarks, emphasizing the count of days: "Fever with furious delirium, crisis on day 14?"[69] "Continuous fever, crisis on day 21;"[70] "Continuous fever. Critical diarrhea on day 14;"[71] "Continuous fever with acute gastroenteritis ending on day 44;"[72] "Continuous fever followed by confluent smallpox beginning on day 8."[73] A survey of manuscript case histories diagnosed as "continuous fever" shows that from late 1823, the days of the illness were counted.[74] Mériadec continued to gather observations concerning the ancient ideas after his cousin's death.[75]

PRIVATE PRACTICE IN THE 1820s

Laennec worried about Mériadec's future; three years after his degree, the young cousin was still unable to provide for himself. To extend his experience and his reputation, Laennec arranged for Mériadec to accompany the tedious but amiable Madame de Talaru on a voyage. The letter advising Mériadec on how to prepare for the upcoming adventure tells of his own approach to private patients. He said a "wise man" knows to hold his tongue on matters of politics, "especially when he has no hope of convincing others." Madame de Talaru's "simple and unaffected" husband and their live-in friend would be no problem, but the "greatest inconvenience" will be the patient herself. "It is difficult to speak more boringly, more hyperbolically, more obscurely, and more continually than she does." Because she is "excessively exigent," the young doctor must learn not to allow his life to be governed by her demands for "four, five, or six visits a day." If he could maintain his distance and carry out his duty well, she would be a loyal client and would introduce him to high society.[76]

Laennec was pleased when Mériadec decided to take a chance on his future in the capital and declined an attractive but bourgeois situation in Laon with the added prospect of an advantageous marriage.[77] The family in Nantes urged Laennec to do more for the younger man by giving him one of his own positions, but he would promise only the legacy of auscultation and cautioned that it might not bring fortune.[78] The only lucrative situation that he could hope to pass on would be that of physician to the Duchesse de Berry, and not for at least a decade, during which both his health and the government would have to hold.[79] When he was not well, Laennec sometimes refused to attend rich patients, but the family maintained that he always served the poor, and after his death they discovered that he had been a generous giver of alms.[80]

Among other well known people said to have been attended by Laennec was Victor Cousin (1792–1867), philosopher, professor, and conservative liberal.[81] Cousin has been called the "*chien de garde*" (watch dog) and apologist for the Restoration. When he became popular with those opposed to ultraroyalism, however, his courses were abruptly "terminated" in 1820, and he was arrested in 1824. Politically and philosophically, he professed a middle way, which he called "eclecticism," between liberal materialism and reactionary ultraconservatism.[82] In his own teaching and in defiance of Broussais who considered "eclecticism" an insult, Laennec applied Cousin's word to what he considered the ideal medical philosophy: one that eschewed exclusive theories and embraced useful notions from the past, including the concept of a vital principle.

Cousin introduced Laennec to the musicologist, C.-C. Fauriel (1772–1844), who shared his interest in folk culture, poetry, and music. During their "exciting encounters," Laennec played the flute and Fauriel sang Breton songs. The scene was described by C. A. Sainte-Beuve (1804–1869), literary journalist and critic, who was also a doctor and a former student of Laennec: "Fauriel knew the words, but Laennec knew all the tunes, tunes learned in his childhood never to be forgotten. He brought his flute (and you have to have seen Laennec to really imagine him cast as Lycidas) and while his friend recalled the words, he tried to jot them down. . . . A touching scene the mere idea of which brings a smile, so worthy of these souls, of these hearts truly antique and pure."[83] Laennec continued his study of Breton and tried to establish contacts through Forbes with Celtic scholars in Britain.[84] While French priests were seeking to reconvert their postrevolutionary flock, the doctor speculated on the merits of a Breton-speaking clergy.[85]

Laennec's consultations could be conducted through letters, some of which have been published.[86] They include a law student with mumps involving the testis and a woman in Rennes whom he instructed to seek a stethoscopic examination from his former student, Toulmouche.[87] As in the earlier practice, they emphasize Laennec's long-standing recognition of the significant effects of psyche on soma. His old friend and medical colleague Courbon-Pérusel (1779–1839) wrote to consult about a lesion on his genitals. Laennec's suggestions did not seem to help, and the anxious doctor wrote twice more, afraid that he could pass the condition to his future wife. Laennec said he was "scandalized" to learn his friend was "still allowing the same idea to run through his head," making him ill with worry. The problem was minor, he reassured the man: "if I had a daughter or a sister to marry, your condition would not at all prevent me from giving her to you."[88]

Charles Saunier of Côte d'Or near Dijon, a *négotiant* (probably in wine), wrote at least twice. He had consulted Laennec for headache and a chest complaint; during the course of the interview, however, Laennec elicited the history of a dog bite some eight years before. Fears of rabies were aroused, either because of the doctor's queries, or because the man had been preoccupied with the idea for many years. The next day, Saunier wrote to ask eight questions about rabies, to which Laennec must have replied, for he was thanked and sent forty francs. In the second letter, the man expounded on his symptoms for three pages. Laennec brought both letters to his teaching: the first, he annotated "melancholia, fear of hydrophobia" and placed it with a lecture on rabies; the second, he labeled "rare example of unreasonable anxiety (fear of rabies) which has none of the features of vesania," and he filed it with his lectures on mental illness.[89]

In general, English observers seem to have had fewer complaints about Laennec's psychosomatic views than his younger French colleagues. James Clark wrote from Rome to discuss mutual patients, and seek the inventor's advice on a new stethoscope.[90] Clark shared Laennec's opinion about emotional disturbance as a cause of organic illness; he thought that because of the turmoil of its recent history, France suffered from such diseases more than Britain. He recounted the story of a man who died of apoplexy caused by the reversal in his fortune resulting from "late political changes" in France; Laennec's invention would help to identify the signs of such an illness at an earlier stage when it could be cured.[91] Scudamore agreed that the passions could produce "severe and dangerous disease," but, unlike Clark, he thought that those diseases were less frequent in France than in England. Suggesting his stay in Paris had been happier than Clark's, he said that the French were healthier because of their free use of light wines, drier climate, lighter diet, greater bodily exercise, and more cheerful disposition, which causes them to "constantly cultivate amusement."[92]

Being auscultated by Laennec held a special cachet and may have become a not-to-be-missed experience for a certain class of people in the tubercular Paris of the mid-1820s. After reading Laennec's book, one man, "believed he was afflicted with a terrible disease" and according to his physician, was "continually occupied with the project of submitting his chest to [Laennec's] exploration."[93] Laennec catered to these demands, but he did not shrink from calmly disagreeing with people, like Saunier and the vigorous Chateaubriand, whose illnesses seemed to have no physical basis and who should not be afraid.

Laennec and Broussais (or his students) shared other patients and their differences would emerge at the bedside, even in their absence.[94] As had been the case for Dr. Chauveau, the sickroom of a dying physician became the arena for medical debate; so, too, for the young doctor, Athanase Vorogidès. Born in Constantinople and endowed with an "excellent mind," Vorogidès had learned medicine in Vienna and Bucharest, before coming to Paris to continue studies in medicine and literature. He had adopted the practice of preventing his severe headaches by applying twenty-five leeches to his anus once a month. Having overlooked his "so to say 'monthly' evacuation," he developed a severe headache, fever, and delirium.[95] A steady stream of luminaries and their disciples flocked to the bedside. Laennec and Collin prescribed a phlebotomy, which was followed by immediate improvement. The revived patient asked to have ten leeches applied to each side. Cayol and Rostan also appeared, as did "students of the physiological doctrine" who "wanted their master's opinion." Broussais arrived in the evening and prescribed forty leeches which were allowed to flow all night; the patient deteriorated. In the following days, Laennec recommended a blister; Broussais a bag of ice to the head, mustard baths for the feet, and leeches to the nostrils. And so the parade continued and the arguments proceeded, until the man expired. On 2 March 1826, Broussais and Laennec's associates, Cayol and Collin, attended the autopsy, which, not surprisingly, revealed pallor of all the organs.[96]

Now Laennec was famous. He was named to a public commission to study mineral waters, chaired by Chaptal; he became a member of the Légion d'honneur; and was summoned to deliver his opinions in distant cities and in court.[97] He spoke as an expert witness at the 1823 trial of the medical poisoner, Dr. Castaign, who was executed for murdering two brothers with morphine after having convinced them to make him the beneficiary of their wills. Laennec's testimony, with that of M. J. B. Orfila (1787–1853) and N. L. Vauquelin (1763–1829) served to show that the victim's symptoms could have been caused either by drugs or by disease.[98] The following year, he left his vacation in Brittany and traveled to Bordeaux at the request of a rich Spaniard who had offered a thousand pistoles for a consultation. Medical coverage of the visit described Laennec's changing opinion about the rich man's diagnosis and his rounds in the women's ward of the St. André hospital where he was trailed by young men who, "after a revolutionary education, could be doctors without being humanists," and who could not understand Laennec's bedside prescriptions given in Latin. His most "notable mistake," the reporter said, was to diagnose "metallic tinkling" in the chest of a deeply religious woman, only to have one of the young nonhumanists produce a rosary from around the patient's neck.[99]

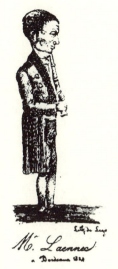

Figure 10.2. Caricature of Laennec at Bordeaux, 1824. The inventor is shown wearing his spectacles, dressed in old-fashioned clothing, and holding an elaborate cylinder as if it were a flute. The image was discovered in the shop of a Bordeaux antique dealer. Lithograph by Légé, *Journal médicale de Gironde*, 1824. Source: reproduced in Gélineau 1902, and in *Laennec, inventeur de l'auscultation*, 1981, 89. Photograph: Queen's Medical Photography Services.

The hostile coverage of Laennec's journey prompted an apology from Dr. Cazeneuve of Cadillac, but Laennec refused to have his letter published.[100] The publicity also alerted Laennec *père*, through his spy in the post office, who had reported that his son would have six thousand francs for the journey and fifty thousand francs, if the patient were cured. Laennec *père* complained to Christophe that "the man of the fifty-thousand-franc cure is back in Paris. . . . His fortune exceeds three hundred thousand" but he cannot "find the two thousand francs promised a father who will soon be an octogenarian."[101] Laennec referred to the "illusion at Bordeaux" in his lecture notes, and a flattering version of the expensive consultation, in which he was said to have made a charming lesson out of his mistake, was published a century later. A caricature of an old-fashioned, bespectacled Laennec is said represent the inventor with his stethoscope in Bordeaux (fig. 10.2).[102]

THE MARRIAGE

After almost a year of living in the Paris hotel, Laennec moved into a more comfortable, but more expensive, apartment building, with room for his cousins and a stable for his horse and carriage on the rue du Cherche Midi.[103] His old housekeeper, Angélique, had retired, and he now turned to the widowed Jacquemine Guichard Argou whom he had known since his visits to Couvrelles and had tended as a patient at least twice. When Mme Argou became the paid companion of Mme de Pompéry, she had been forced to leave her seven-year-old daughter, Clementine, in a Quimper pension, because her benefactress "did not want" the little girl being educated with her own children. Mme de Pompéry complimented the young mother for having "consented to the sacrifice," and Clementine was eventually sent to a convent in England.[104] During the war of 1814, the Pompéry family fled the chateau at Couvrelles, leaving Mme Argou alone and in charge. At least one historian scoffed at the fact that she was so terrified by the arrival of the "Cossacks" that she was sick for almost a year.[105] But a psychic-physical ailment of this sort was no laughing matter for Laennec; it corresponded precisely to many other sicknesses in family and friends, numerous cases in his treatise, and the indispositions he suffered himself. Rouxeau speculated that her postwar illness may have prompted the first attempt at mediate auscultation.[106]

Meanwhile, the protectress Mme de Pompéry returned to Quimper where she declined slowly, her vision so dim that she could no longer read music. "She died like an angel," Ollivry wrote to Laennec in 1822, and he described the autopsy findings of pus in the pelvis. Within the year, her husband was dead, too, and an annuity of six hundred francs was left to Mme Argou, who was now in her early forties, impoverished, and homeless. Here was a capable Breton woman, someone who had shared the bright days of his youth, a person experienced in the management of a much larger house than Laennec could ever hope to own. He happily engaged her as his housekeeper in September 1822.[107]

Two years later, and shortly after the trip to Bordeaux, Laennec and Mme Argou decided to marry. All Quimper was abuzz with the rumor that she was his mistress and had feigned pregnancy in order to trap him. Laennec consulted the new Bishop of Quimper, who told him to ignore the gossip and applauded the couple's "wise decision" to have their "friendship sanctified by a sacrament."[108] To the family, he expressed his surprise and pleasure at the change in his situation: "at first she said no, then yes"; the only reason he had for doubting the good sense of the decision was the fact that his "*cher papa*" heartily approved (fig. 10.3).[109] Christophe approved, too, but reported to his aunt de Miniac on the malicious gossip in Quimper and the hilarity provoked by the lovelorn figure of his aging cousin among the younger family members.[110] The civil and religious ceremonies took place on 16 December 1824 at the *mairie* of the eleventh arrondissement and at the Paris church of St. Sulpice. The handful of witnesses included Récamier, Cayol, and Mériadec.[111]

The new Mme Laennec fell gravely ill only a few months after her wedding, but she was shocked by the visit of a priest and soon recovered. Predictions that there would be no children seem to imply that she had suffered a miscarriage. Sometime during that same year, word arrived from England that her twenty-seven-year-old daughter had died. I cannot help but wonder if there was a relationship between this sad news and the incapacity in one whose physique had already been proven vulnerable to emotional stress.[112] Mme Laennec's belief in the psychic causes of physical demise is evident in several of her letters to Mériadec during her husband's last illness, especially when she begged the young cousin to solve their financial concerns: the monetary "worries contributed greatly to his illness" and he needed to be

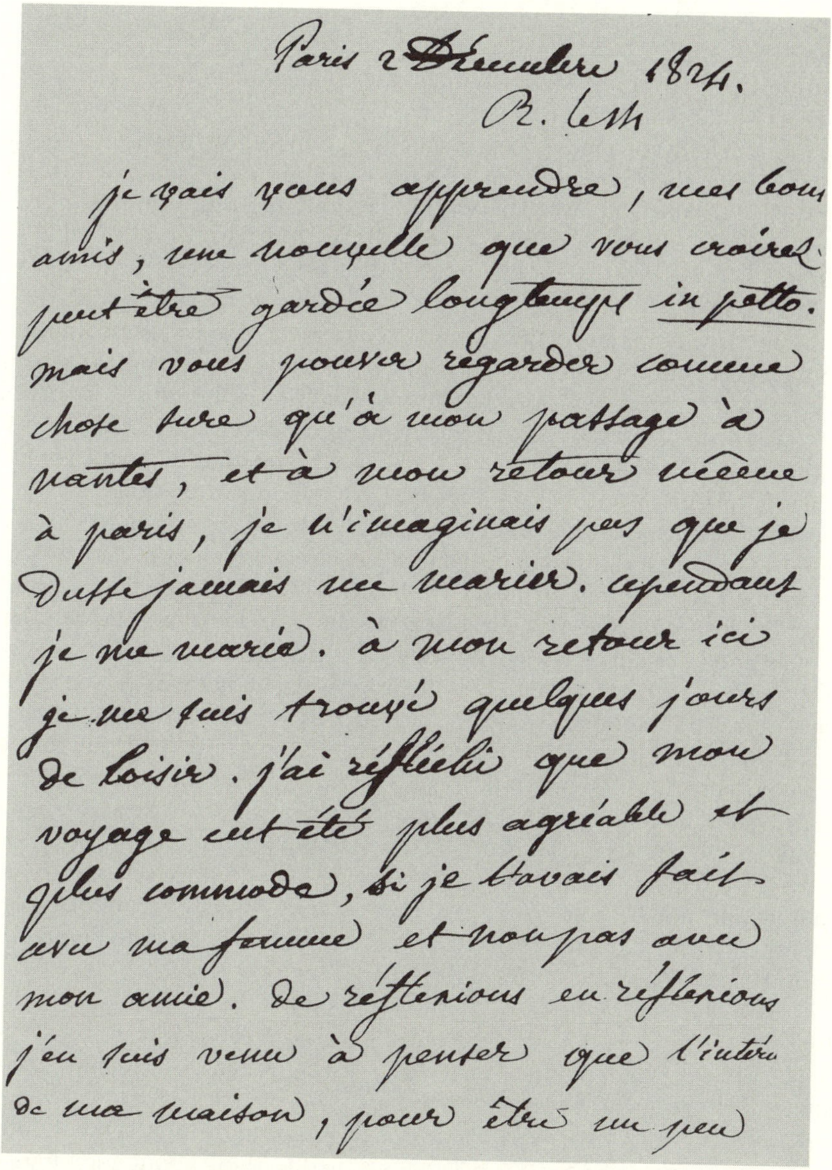

Paris 2 Décembre 1824.
R. le 14

je vais vous apprendre, mes bons
amis, une nouvelle que vous croirez
peut être gardée longtemps in petto.
mais vous pouvez regarder comme
chose sure qu'à mon passage à
nantes, et à mon retour même
à paris, je n'imaginais pas que je
dusse jamais me marier. cependant
je me marie. à mon retour ici
je me suis trouvé quelques jours
de loisir. j'ai réfléchi que mon
voyage eut été plus agréable et
plus commode, si je l'avais fait
avec ma femme et non pas avec
mon amie. de réflexions en réflexions
j'en suis venu à penser que l'intérieur
de ma maison, pour être un peu

Figure 10.3. Letter from Laennec to "my good friends" and his cousin Christophe in Nantes to announce his forthcoming marriage to Madame Argou, 2 December 1824. Source: MS Bertrand Laennec. By permission of Dr. Eric Laennec, Lyons. Photograph: Queen's Medical Photography Services from a photocopy.

"tranquilized" before he could recover. "Chagrin is worth nothing to a sick man," she said.[113]

After the recovery of Mme Laennec, the couple took a brief holiday near their old haunts in Soissonais with their friends, the Le Veyer family. They were in the midst of a move to an even more commodious apartment, in rue de St. Maur; their numerous possessions—walnut and mahogany furnishings, silk curtains and armchairs of blue, yellow, and red, paintings of religious subjects, together with Laennec's lathes and "dry wood suitable for turning"—were documented in detail for the estate auction that took place only a year later.[114]

Some have maintained that Laennec's marriage was a loveless union of convenience, but the letters testify to affection between two original personalities. As the groom explained to Christophe, "At first I tried an association pure and simple, but I found that the friendship between a man and a woman is too cold, especially if one tries not to expose oneself to that which would make it too intense [*vive*]; as a result I have found in marriage a *mezzo-termino*." Little is known of the character of Mme Laennec, but her devotion to her husband through his painful last illness pervades her letters. She was joined to "the best of men," "a husband who loves me and whom I love."[115] But some historians have portrayed her as clumsy and tactless, and they blamed her honesty with her spouse for his ultimate demise.[116]

Even as he married, Laennec was ill; professorial obligations prevented the long walks and hunting trips that he had once used to restore himself, and he made plans for a permanent retirement. He alerted Cruveilhier, the royalist Catholic student of Dupuytren, about a forthcoming academic opportunity in the vacancies that would result from his departure. Cruveilhier said that he would not forget what Laennec had chosen to tell to him "alone"; he regretted only that his arrival in Paris would coincide with Laennec's departure and they would not be able to traverse the "*pénible carrière*" (painful career) together.[117] But Laennec continued working on his Collège de France lectures because they were to form the basis of his next book.

In a few short years, Laennec's life had been completely transformed. Not only had he become a married man with a distinguished ménage, but now he also had the security of two professorships, a hospital ward for research, and a busy practice that gave him influence at court and in the government, influence that he was not shy to use. He continued to think about auscultation, but his latest discovery was a theory of disease. True to his physiological view of illness, he would consolidate his knowledge of pathological anatomy and his reservations about its universal application as he professed from the Collège de France chair of Corvisart and Hallé.

At the Collège de France: The Second Unpublished Book

If the animal organism consists in these three things, solids,
liquids, and vital principle, each of them can be altered
even in a primary fashion.

—*Laennec, Collège de France, lesson 2, 1822, f. 8v*

IN THE QUARTER CENTURY that elapsed from Laennec's first writings to his last, the focus of his interest shifted from pathological anatomy to disease. One reason for the change had been his clinical practice; a second, was his intervening research on auscultation. The stethoscope endorsed an anatomical approach to disease, but it also enhanced his appreciation of the physiological aspects of illness that defied explanation by dissection. A third reason was the corresponding change in the subjects he taught: as a student, he had concentrated on the new science of pathological anatomy, but as Professor at the Collège de France, he lectured on clinical medicine. With this reorientation, came an accompanying reconsideration of the "lesion" as it related to disease.

As professor at the prestigious Collège de France, Laennec finally had the cathartic opportunity to explain to the world in magisterial form how exactly he should be understood. He would tout the benefits of auscultation and flaunt his extensive knowledge of pathological anatomy, but, in his opinion, the topic of disease exceeded the bounds of a method based only on anatomical correlations. He would elaborate a theoretical classification of disease—not of pathological anatomy, nor of physiology alone—but a synthetic theory that accommodated evidence from the quick and the dead gathered by reputable observers from the fifth century B.C. until his own time. No longer would he simply talk about the deficiencies of the anatomical method, he would overcome them. His new classification would rely on objective identifiable changes, lesions, in either the structure *or* the function of the body. It would thereby incorporate pathological anatomy and also compensate for its limitations. As his correspondence clearly shows, the lectures were to become a comprehensive treatise on clinical medicine, which would utilize but surpass his earlier works in pathology and diagnosis.[1]

The Collège de France lectures began on 3 December 1822 and continued for one hour every Tuesday, Thursday, and Saturday for thirty weeks until the end of June.[2] The full course took two years to complete, and the two-year cycle was repeated once from winter 1824 until spring 1826. Manuscripts of all but eight of Laennec's 171 lectures have been preserved.[3] In addition, at least three incomplete sets of student notes have been traced.[4]

One student, who had attended the classes of both Laennec and Broussais, wrote this oft-cited description of Laennec's arrival and the atmosphere in the hall:

> At one o'clock, a cabriolet clattered into the courtyard of the Collège de France. From it alighted a small man, engulfed in a wide coat over a completely black suit that featured old-fashioned short pants and was topped by a broad-brimmed hat. He climbed up into his chair facing only forty listeners at most, but a select group, scholars all, whose attention never wavered . . . He began by reading the subject for the day, but often digressed to make observations, to recount a few original anecdotes, to strike a few blows at, or knock a few edges off the physiological doctrine [of Broussais] which he debated in name [and substance]. His tone quickly became acerbic and sarcastic, and his eyes shot lightning, keenly felt even through the horn-rimmed glasses, which he always wore perched in front of his eyes. His sharp words were received by a generalized smile. At the end of his charming and eminently instructive lesson, there was no applause, but all promised themselves to return.[5]

In a world that placed a high value on medical travel, Laennec attracted students from England, Scotland, Ireland, Belgium, Germany, Austria, Switzerland, Prussia, Spain, Italy, Greece, Sweden, Holland, Poland, Russia, Newfoundland, the United States, and Mexico.[6] They were eager to attend the rounds and clinics at the Necker or Charité hospitals, as Carswell and Thomson had done in 1822; but the most dedicated also followed the lectures. The French tended to neglect his course—perhaps as part of the anti-royalism that typified other students, or because they found their intellectual needs and political sympathies were satisfied elsewhere.

The foreign students appeared to have appreciated the professor, although the number of formal registrations for his course seems to have been small.[7] The Musée Laennec holds several individual letters of gratitude and a certificate signed by thirty students and doctors expressing "sincere thanks and recognition for the trouble [he had] taken to advance their education."[8] William Thomson wrote from Edinburgh in 1823 to inform Laennec that his father was already making use of the stethoscope in his lectures. H. C. Van Hall (1801–1874) sent his thesis on auscultation from Amsterdam, and Charles Scudamore presented a copy of his essay on Laennec's method of forming a diagnosis to his "kind and gentle master."[9] In return, the visitors sought his approbation in writing.[10]

The students also left vivid character portraits of their teacher. Van Hall said that Laennec was "small, but seemed to have a very penetrating mind";

he had the "look of a fox [*regard de renard*]," especially when he was making fun of Broussais.[11] Toulmouche wrote of his master's extreme sobriety at table, his conservative taste in clothing, and his restrained praise when pleased: "that will do."[12] A doctor from Strasbourg who spent 1825–1826 in Paris said that he "was a thin man who had the air of being just as sick as the bedridden individuals lying in his ward." This same visitor had been put off by the numerous Englishmen who "threw themselves" on the pitiful patients "as if they were prey."[13] When the Englishmen went home, they spoke of Laennec's "eminence" as a pathologist, his "accurate observations," and his "inventive genius," but "many" told his translator that Laennec did "not possess in a high degree the mental qualifications necessary to constitute a great and skillful practitioner."[14] Some British visitors remembered the experience quite differently. Before complaining about Laennec's lack of acoustic ability, C. J. B. Williams wrote of his "urbane and amiable deportment," the "mental abilities" that "excited our respect," his "great talents," "wonderful acuteness of perception," and "solicitous interest" in helping others to derive the "inestimable advantages" of his discovery (fig. 11.1).[15]

Laennec kept his own list of 112 foreign visitors, doctors, and students—a list that reflects his respect for the medicine of the previous century and his connections with people from the countries that had been at war with Bonaparte. He noted that a Scottish visitor, Dr. Charles Mitchell (1783–1856), had been on St. Helena with the British navy at the death of Napoleon and had witnessed the autopsy. He was pleased to have taught the "grandson" (actually the great-nephew) of William Cullen (1712–1790) and the sons of James Gregory (1753–1821) and John Thomson (1765–1846), all of Edinburgh.[16] Notwithstanding his treatment of Victor Collin, he sometimes admitted that students could provide a stimulus to research: for example, he credited Eugène Legallois with having proposed an ingenious pathophysiological mechanism for the cause of emphysema.[17]

STRUCTURE AND CONTENT OF THE LECTURES: A THEORY OF DISEASE

Most historians who have commented on Laennec's lectures have focused on the inaugural address—an ode to observation—and the only lesson to be published.[18] But the course was an overview of all medicine and all disease. It was presented under a new framework and amplified by frequent reference to predecessors and contemporaries and by examples from his twenty-five years of clinical experience. It was divided into four parts: first an introduction about medical philosophy and the nature of disease (lessons 1–3); second, a summary of pathological anatomy (lessons 4–28); third, a presentation of generalized diseases including fevers, gout, rheumatism, scurvy, scrofula, and rachialgia (lessons 29–68); and finally, a lengthy discussion of localized diseases organized around organ systems (lessons 69–82 of the first year and 2–89 of the second).

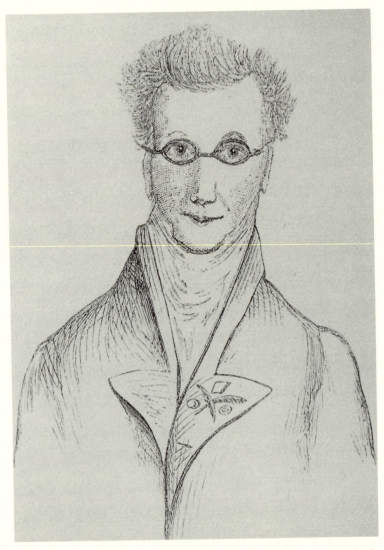

Figure 11.1. Sketch of Laennec by C. J. B. Williams. The British physician had gradu-ated from Edinburgh one year before he traveled to Paris to join Laennec's foreign students in 1825–1826. The horn-rimmed spectacles were often mentioned in word portraits, but are rarely seen in images. Source: C. J. B. Williams, 1884, 46. Photo-graph: Rob McCallum, Kingston, Ontario.

Introduction

In the introduction Laennec presented what he called his own "doctrine" (fig. 11.2)[19] It could be seen as a direct response to the physiological doctrine, but more importantly, it joined with Broussais in attacking the rigid and exclusive application of pathological anatomy to the study of disease. Elaborated for the Collège de France, Laennec's theory of disease incorporated ideas that he had long entertained, including his classification of pathological anatomy and the concept of the vital lesion. Classifications were theories, he reminded his listeners, and a theory was merely a "scaffolding," a way of seeing things, a prop for human understanding.[20]

In Laennec's doctrine, the human body was composed of solid, liquid, and vital principle; each of these components existed separately and could be altered with or without secondary changes in either of the other two. Laennec said that he was not the first to recognize the triad. Hippocrates had known of it and had given names to the three components of the organism, "that which contains, that which is contained, and the life force."[21] It had also been recognized by all other "good minds" in medicine, including Hermann Boerhaave, his nephew Abraham Kaau Boerhaave (d. 1758), Phillipe Pinel, and the Montpellier clinician-philosopher Paul-Joseph Barthez (1734–1806).[22] Although Laennec cited C. L. Dumas (1765–1813) on other matters, he did not mention Dumas's use of the same triad in his treatise on physiology, featured in the review by his deceased friend, Savary des Brulons.[23]

Next, Laennec attempted to prove the independent existence and alteration of the three components of the body, especially the liquids and vital principle.[24] Body liquids were endowed with life, independent of the organs, he said, offering the examples of blood, the embryo of an egg, the semisolid consistency of the brain, and the false membranes and adhesions that form from extravasated fluids.[25] As for the vital principle, which he knew was becoming a contentious concept, he prepared a credo-like document on why he acknowledged its existence. He did not believe in effects without causes; forces did not have to be visible in order to be recognized: "a stone does not remain suspended in air."[26] "Movement" (change) in structure or in function was evidence of the life force. He liked to use the classical words that named the life force or vital principle for the observable movement it caused: ὁρμῶντα (hormonta), *impetum faciens, "ce qui imprime le mouvement"* (fig. 11.3). Laennec's vital principle was a real but invisible force like gravity, whose existence could be known by observation of its effects in the laboratory or in the clinic. Working at the same time on revisions to the treatise on auscultation, he replaced the references to Corvisart in his preface with praise for Isaac Newton (1642–1727), the champion of an invisible but universally acknowledged force, who had been invoked frequently by the clinical physiologists of the eighteenth century, including Barthez.[27]

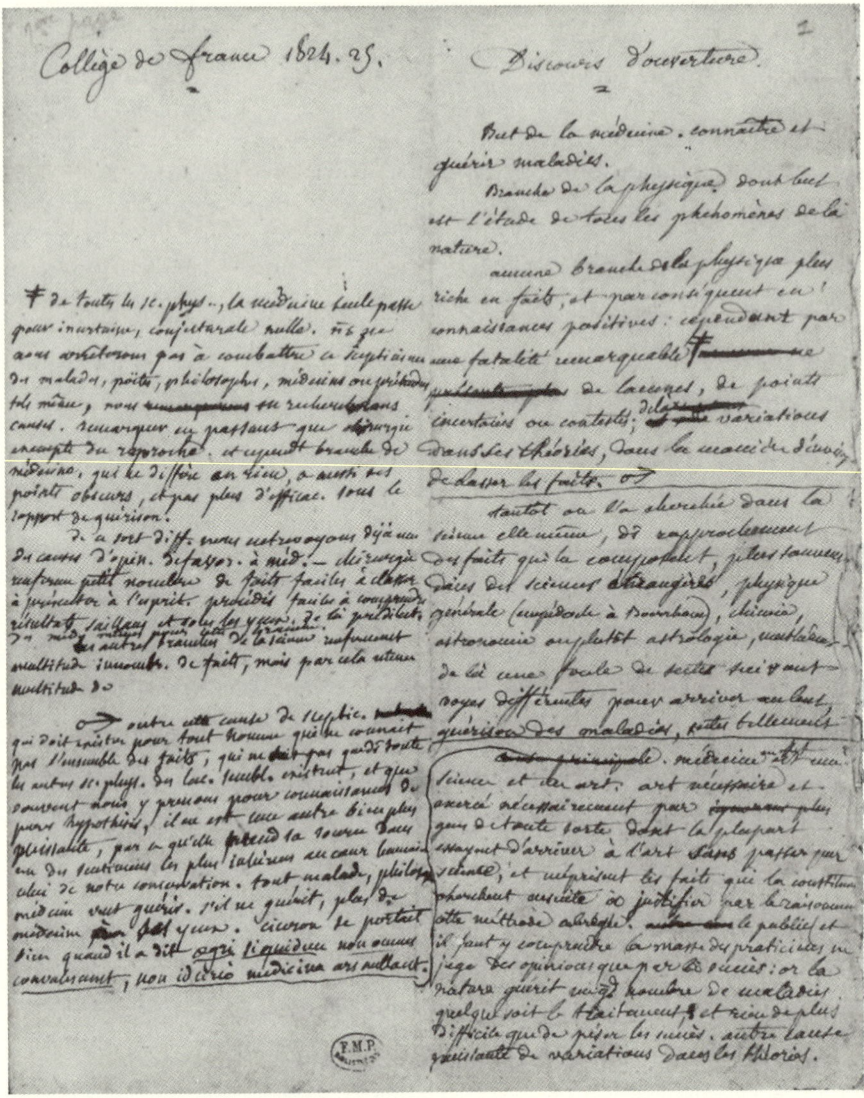
Collège de France 1824. 25.

Discours d'ouverture.

But de la médecine. connaître et guérir maladies.

Figure 11.2. Title page of Laennec's opening address at the Collège de France, December 1822. The collected lessons form a would-be treatise on disease, consisting of 1,100 pages of manuscript in abbreviated notes and references, following a structure determined by Laennec's theory of disease. Source: BIUM MS 2186 (IV), f. 1. Photograph: Bibliothèque Interuniversitaire de Médecine, Paris.

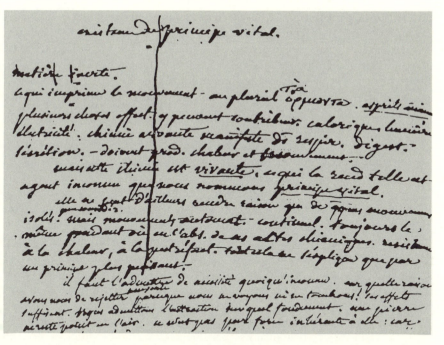

Figure 11.3. "Existence of the vital principle," undated manuscript in the hand of Laennec (detail). The first paragraph refers to the Greek word, and the concepts of electricity, light, and caloric. The last paragraph: "although unknown [the life force] must be acknowledged. What reason do we have to reject it? because we neither see it nor touch it? Its effects suffice. On what basis do we acknowledge attraction [gravity]? a stone does not remain suspended in the air." Source: BIUM, MS 5172 (III), lot 1, f. 1. Photograph: Bibliothèque Interuniversitaire de Médecine, Paris.

Again, like Barthez, Laennec said that the vital principle was not the religious soul. Diseases of the soul might occur, but they had no place in medicine; "let us avoid metaphysics," he said, "we follow only the observations of physiologists."[28] And among the modern "physiologists," he cited Barthez and J. F. Blumenbach (1752–1840) once each; the other well-known physiological vitalists, Dumas, G. Stahl (1659–1734), and J. C. Reil (1759–1813), appeared only in more specific contexts, whereas Cabanis was never mentioned.[29] Laennec drew far more from the work of those who had carried on from Bichat and are now considered the founders of experimental physiology.

Without naming Buisson, Laennec rehearsed the criticisms of Bichat's "unfortunate" definition of life, as the "ensemble of functions that resist death"; his vital "properties" were too few, and his divisions of life functions served only "to roll back the difficulty."[30] Those who strove to correct these flaws and push forward the frontiers of understanding were Chaussier with his work on thermometry, Magendie on poisons, Barry on the heart, Pierre Nysten (1771–1818) on galvanism, and J. J. C. Legallois on the spinal cord and the principle of life.[31] The treatise of Legallois in particular contained a number of ideas that seem to have been a source of inspiration for Laennec, who, in his final years, was working with "the son of the physiologist," as he always described Eugène Legallois.[32] Even the old enemy Dupuytren also figured in the list of experimental physiologists for his work on rabies and gases, although he was criticized for his anatomical discoveries.[33] Laennec included himself in the list for his research in auscultation and therapy as physiological investigation.

Having established the physical evidence in support of the separate existence of the three components of the organism, Laennec then constructed three corresponding classes of disease, each identified by the location of its lesion. The concept of "lesion" was generalized from his knowledge of pathological anatomy to be a potentially detectable, pathognomonic alteration in any of the three components of the body. Disease was defined as "a disturbance in function with or without a lesion in the organs [solids]."[34] Diseases without anatomical lesions had lesions in one of the two other body components. It would be simplistic to try to explain all diseases by relying exclusively on the observation of only one of these three components, solid, liquid, and vital principle. These errors were the narrow doctrines of solidism, humoralism, and vitalism—errors, Laennec believed, he avoided with his own variety of Cousin's "eclecticism," a word, which he used in December 1822 to describe an ideal medical philosophy open to all forms of explanations.[35]

Objective identification of the "lesion" would provide the most effective means of identifying diseases; however, medical science had yet to find methods for characterizing all lesions. Organic or solid lesions could be detected in the living patient by correlating physical examination and pathological anatomy. The diagnosis of liquid changes required clinical chemistry. Diagnosis of vital lesions depended on physiology and an understanding of the patient's experience; these vital lesions were still the most difficult to uncover, but their eventual elucidation would be a boon to the prevention of illness.

Changes associated with stress and sadness were the vital lesions. They could produce disease either directly, as in the case of Bayle's nostalgia, or indirectly by producing intermediate alterations in the liquids and the solids of the body (see fig. 9.7). Auscultation could be expected to contribute to the detection of vital lesions; it had already defined the physiological signs of puerile respiration and murmur, which indicated alterations in function. Laennec looked to electricity to provide more signs of vital change. Therapeutic successes with electricity and/or galvanism, which he mentioned at least thirty times in twenty-three different lessons, seemed to confirm the existence of connections between the psyche and the organs via some kind of psychocybernetic force not unlike electricity, heat, or light. He once referred to the human body as "a little electric machine," which, he said "did not imply the exclusion of intelligence."[36] Laennec's observations were not particularly new; eighteenth-century physicians had already made similar statements about mind and body problems.[37] His originality was in the notion of a vital lesion that could serve as an organizing principle for study and conceptualization of disease and that could be detected by physical means.

The evidence for diseases without anatomical lesions came from many clinical observations: either from patients like old *cadet Rousseau* who died of recognizable symptom patterns without changes in the cadaver, or from those in whom anatomic lesions were of "insufficient" severity to account for illness and death. Until objective definition of all the various liquid and vital lesions had been discovered, diagnosis of disease without anatomic change must continue to rely on the symptom grouping of the nosologists.

Second Part

The medical philosophy presented in the introduction determined the subsequent structure of the course. The second part of the course dealt with diseases of solids. It can best be characterized as a outline of general pathological anatomy, in which the main types of changes in organs and tissues were presented, just as they had been in 1803 and in 1812. These were hypertrophy, atrophy, inflammation, softening, congestions of blood and of lymph, disruption of continuity, and accidental productions (tumors), both analogous (benign) and nonanalogous (including malignant tumors, tubercles, cirrhosis, and foreign bodies both "animate" and "inanimate"). The lessons on "animate foreign bodies" addressed the biology and classification of the parasites that had been an object of fascination since his student days.

Third Part

In the third part, Laennec turned to the theme of liquids and their lesions, beginning with a discussion of generalized diseases. As he had done in 1804, he claimed that the classification of fevers should be simplified. He contested the myriad subdivisions of continuous fevers: they should be grouped either in a single category, or in only two categories, relating to periodicity and to accompanying rashes.[38] Liquids flowed throughout the body; if a specific alteration could be identified in a liquid, then it could be used to identify and explain a generalized disease. Some of the changes in liquids, such as urinary calculi and lentine cataract, were visible to the naked eye and could be studied by the pathologist. In the future, he said, chemistry or physiology might be able to characterize lesions of the liquids of the body with the same kind of precision that was emerging in pathological anatomy of the solids (organs). To that end, he referred to the experiments of Fourcroy, Magendie, Louis-Nicolas Vauquelin (1763–1869), Gilbert Breschet (1784–1845), and Michel-Eugène Chevreul (1786–1889).[39] For some reason that may or may not have had to do with an as-yet-to-be-discovered vendetta, he did not mention his colleague Chomel, whose 1821 essay on the controversial topic of fevers expressed similar doubt about the universality of localization and contained the same idea of lesions in the liquids.[40]

The notion of specificity held sway in the classification of disease, as it had done in the designation of stethoscopic signs. For example, Magendie had shown that there was an inoculable change in the saliva of rabid animals. Laennec conceived of this alteration as a "specific" lesion of saliva and classified rabies as a disease with an alteration in liquid.[41] Other diseases that he thought might eventually prove to be associated with specific liquid lesions included syphilis, gout, and exanthematous fevers. He was increasingly interested in "diathesis," as the disseminated manifestation of a specific type of liquid change, and he began to consider various "diatheses"—such as gout, scurvy, rheumatism, scrofula, phthisis, and cancer—as the functions of isolated specific lesions in a widely distributed body fluid. For example, a single chemical alteration in a fluid that perfused the entire body could result in multiple numbers and types of lesions in many different tissues; the liquid lesion was unique, but its effects varied depending on the tissues involved. With this idea of specificity in mind, he commented on the self-inoculation experiments of the young Legallois presented at the Académie Royale de Médecine.[42]

Fourth Part

In the fourth and longest part of his course, Laennec focused on the local diseases. It began at the end of the first year and filled the entire second year. It was organized around body systems following the order of Morgagni (head, thorax, abdomen): nervous system, including the organs of hearing, sight, and smell; respiratory system (including a lesson on auscultation); circulatory system; digestive system; urinary system; reproductive system of both men and women; and finally the skin. The possible uses of the stethoscope extended well beyond diseases of the chest to the detection of parasites, fractures, muscle spasms, digestive colic, and bladder stones.[43]

Diseases with lesions in the vital principle were discussed throughout this section of his course, each considered a manifestation of an alteration in the vital principle as it affected an anatomical system. These diseases included asthma, angina pectoris, tetanus, poisonings, epilepsy, chorea, and the mental illnesses. Small changes might be found in the cadavers of some of these patients, but, Laennec maintained, either the changes were too slight (as in the case of exanthems), or they were too inconsistent (as in the case of angina), to be the invariable cause of fatality. Reluctant to gloss over the significance of "lesionless" states, he insisted on, if not exaggerated, their importance in his philosophy of all diseases.

Here again, Laennec cautioned against exclusivity: doctors should look for organic changes as often as possible because they were accessible and observable, but they should not equate those changes with the cause of a disease. Above all, they should mistrust Broussais's desire to see all diseases as localized products of inflammation and irritation.[44] Imbued, like his colleagues, with the philosophy of the uncited Cabanis, he repeatedly stated that causes were unknown, beyond the ken of mere mortals. So deeply ingrained was the reluctance to explore causes that he sometimes forgot to refer to them at all: in several lessons, passages on etiology appear in marginal notations, as if they had been afterthoughts.[45]

Laennec's philosophy of disease and his method of pathology were rigorously applied to every organ, tissue, and liquid within each system. Thus, he spoke on the solid changes (hypertrophy, atrophy, congestions, softening, tumors, etc.), liquid changes, and changes in the vital principle of each organ and of each and every one of its myriad appendages. The same method of study was applied to the liquid secretions and excretions of the body. For example, not only did he present the lesions of such tiny, solid structures as the pia mater, eyelids, tear ducts, gingiva, glottis, pericardium, and ureters, but also those of body fluids, such as saliva, bile, milk, and semen. Some lectures pertaining to the ancillary structures may have been quite dull, but they were tenaciously faithful to his method and were spiced up with reference to contemporary debates.

Asthma and mental diseases were presented as lesions of the vital force localized in the lung or brain, respectively. The lessons on asthma reflected the physiological redefinitions made for the second edition of the treatise on auscultation; the stethoscope could be used to explore changes in the function of the body as well as its structure (see chap. 7). Those on mental diseases became a platform for Laennec's strongest criticism of the new generation of pathologists and, by curious political extrapolation, a justification for the recent changes in the faculty. In mental diseases he said that there were no consistent organic changes and physical methods of healing were not helpful; however, the new moral therapy was "very effective," implying that the cause of mental disease was also moral, a vital lesion. He followed the symptom-based diagnostic categories of Pinel and divided the vesanias into hallucinations, monomania or melancholy, mania, dementia, and idiotism. Nostalgia illustrated with the "story of Bayle" was a form of monomania.[46]

The second time Laennec read his lectures on mental disease in 1825–1826, he ranged over centuries of history, citing instances of mass insanity, which he saw as the rigid pursuit of systematic ideas and likened to the manic exclusivity of medical reductionists like Brown and Broussais. A flood of examples filled the revised pages: barbarian invasions and dictators, Caesar, Attila, prejudice against Jews, the Albigensian crusades, the crusade of St. Louis, the "convulsionaires" of St. Médard, the French Revolution, the Terror that followed, and the mob of university students, "who spilled blood within these very walls erected by King François I to honor science and letters" when they "slit the throat" of his predecessor, Ramus—Pierre de la Ramée (1515–1572)—for having pronounced the Latin words "*Quis qwa qod* [*sic*]!"[47]

In this tirade, the sentiments that he had once expressed to Lamennais about good order, good government, and good behavior loomed large; they consisted of a special blend of political philosophy and physiology that has been well described by Stephen Jacyna.[48] These ideas seemed to emerge from the philosophy of Bonald, "*mauvaise génie*" of the extreme right and long-time champion of Buisson and the other Congréganistes.[49] Bonald spoke in medically suggestive terms of the "*principe constitutif*" of society, as if its components were body parts, and its mood, a vital sign.[50] The Restoration was not simply a return to the Ancien Régime, but the creation of a sane and natural order through adaptation of the best elements of the old monarchy to the new structures of the Revolution. In terms of the once clandestine Congrégation, the 1823 royalist coup over public instruction was medically justified; Laennec's deep involvement in the interference, the work of a good doctor. The coup was seen as a responsible act of functional healing for the social organism, a therapeutic intervention intended to prevent even worse structural damage from a vital lesion of universal exclusivity.

STYLE, METHOD, AND THEMES

The four parts of the course were not mutually exclusive. Cross-references to Laennec's introductory statements and theory were frequent, and he often acknowledged the benefits of alternative methods of classification. Since alterations in the vital principle might precede all organic or liquid changes, virtually all local diseases could eventually be reclassified, if and when methods became available to define the prior changes in liquids or in the vital principle. Until science provided such methods, diseases should be studied under the most accessible rubric: pathological anatomy, or in the absence of a solid change, symptomatic nosology. Description of an organic lesion implied little or nothing about its cause.

Laennec often began his lectures with a question; then he would examine the evidence in favor of several possible answers. Like his theory, his evidence was eclectic and harkened back to Hippocrates and the other ancient writers through the works of Avicenna, Fernel, Paré, Sydenham, Boerhaave, von Haller, De Haen, Stoll, Stahl, Cullen, and Hunter to the experimental findings of his contemporaries cited above. Sometimes he would answer his opening question; sometimes he would say that no answer could yet be given.

In preparation, Laennec made extensive use of existing publications. He tended not to quote literature on the topics with which he had the greatest personal familiarity, especially diseases of the chest; instead he referred to his own experience. In other areas, for example diseases of the ear or of the generative organs, his notes are a distillation of bibliography. He relied heavily on Morgagni, the bibliography of Wilhelm Gottfried Ploucquet (1744–1814), and other dictionaries, as well as notes that he had made at different stages of his career, including his course on pathological anatomy and the preparation for his unsuccessful bid for the chair of Hippocratic medicine.[51] Approximately one-third of the way into the second year (near lesson 30), references to Ploucquet and other sources seem to become more complete, suggesting that it was in early 1824 when he began to realize that he had been building the outline of a new book—a book that he might not live to complete.

The notes are permeated with an incipient form of positivism. Laennec's native skepticism, together with his cautious respect for the difference between theory and facts (*"faits"*), kept him aware of the importance of accuracy and detail in observation and the potential need to revise a theory in the light of some future discovery that might seem passingly small. Similarly, he referred to numerical evidence and statistical probability of clinical events.[52] It was in this context that he sometimes declined to answer his own opening question. In passages reminiscent of the future work of Comte on positivism, he repeatedly defined science as *"ce que l'on sait"* (what is known). Pedagogically, he recognized what is not known, or not yet known, as hypotheses or questions. But they were theory, and for him, theory did not belong to science, it was the frame on which the facts were assembled.[53]

Laennec was aware of disease as theory. Diseases were ideas assembled from "what was known" about a group of clinical observations; the observations based on "illness" were the "facts." Running like a thread throughout the course was his preoccupation with "new" and "old" diseases, when they appeared and/or disappeared. Thucydides' account of the Plague of Athens was mentioned three times;[54] he also spoke of the vanished "English Sweate," the relatively new "Mal de la Baie St. Paul" of Canada, and the history and modifications of syphilis and leprosy.[55]

A fascinating collection of capsule histories, like those selected for the treatise on auscultation, served as evidence in support of a disease or a theory. Most were recounted in only a few words. Laennec would jog his memory with the patients' names, names that may not always have been uttered in class. We find "Bayle," "Mme de Chateaubriand," "M. de Bruno de Douarnenez," "Mme Jalis de Guincamp," "Mgsr. de Casal," the "constipated Mr. Courgeolle," and the strange case of "the man who died under the faucet."[56] Patients from Brittany seem to recall his days with his uncle Guillaume: the old woman of Nantes who died two days after a snake bite; a woman who needed to be bled on alternate days; the mysterious "drummer" who had lost his *"organe de circonspection"* and somehow ended his days with a "rupture."[57] These one-sentence stories were used to support the various disease concepts, "the scaffolding" that Laennec built around them.[58]

Other themes emerged: the vitalistic understanding of physiological processes, the use of musical ideas and metaphors,[59] a surprisingly vigorous polypharmacy (despite frequent reference to the healing power of nature), and a tolerance for galvanism. It has suited historians to emphasize Laennec's therapeutic skepticism, but the lectures show that his pharmacopoeia was typical of his period; only twice did he describe diseases as untreatable (cancer of stomach or lung; tubercles in the liver). Once he recommended a therapy for phthisis that he considered to be hopeless, because "it is always necessary to prescribe something."[60]

Laennec also criticized dead heroes, soon-to-be-dead heroes, and future leaders: Andral, Bichat, Broussais, Cruveilhier, Dupuytren, Esquirol, Lallemand, Portal, and Pinel. Not even his friends were spared: Bayle made errors in confusing tubercles with malignant tumors; and Récamier developed overly subtle distinctions in his diagnosis of arachnoiditis and misconstrued its physical signs. Although most of these remarks were simply critical, some, especially those applied to Broussais, Dupuytren, and Pinel appear to have been sarcastic. Broussais or his doctrine figured in at least one-third of the lessons. Laennec mocked his enemy, his physiological medicine, and his simplistic pathology, but once again, by their very number, these references demonstrate respect for his opponent and their common ground. Where Laennec and Broussais had most agreed was in their opposition to nascent organicism, and that was the strongest theme in Laennec's lectures. Like a testy old man, he berated the inadequacies of the young doctors of France and their exclusive mania for anatomical change.[61]

LAENNEC'S ATTACK ON THE ORGANICISTS

Organicism was a positivistic extrapolation of the anatomoclinical method that favored the characterization of all diseases by associated, localized, organic changes. The philosophy germinated within Laennec's lifetime and grew with the impact of his discovery, but it did not come into full bloom until twenty years after his death. It was expounded "almost like a religion" by Rostan, who coined the word *organicism* in 1831, but situated his earliest efforts to promote it in 1818.[62] Its advocates were dedicated pathologists and clinicians, and they included J. B. Bouillaud. The organicists were careful not to deny the existence of the soul, but because the soul was immortal and immutable, they said, it had no place in medicine.[63] Laennec agreed with their separation of the soul from physiology, but for him the as-yet-to-be-named organicism committed the theoretical error of exclusive "solidism."

The organicists refused to conceive of any disease without organic change. Convinced that anatomical lesions would eventually be found for all diseases, they maintained that, if such changes had not yet been identified, it was due to inattention or inadequate technology. Since the organic change was all that could be observed, the organicists recommended that practitioners equate the cause with its effect. Rostan admitted that lesions were often undetectable in some diseases. Although "it would be better for the regularity of science if such diseases did not occur," he said, their existence did not constitute a "reason to reject the principles of organicism, which are applicable in the majority of circumstances." He was "deeply convinced" that more organic changes would be found and obscure causes would become fewer and fewer "as our means of investigation are perfected and pathological anatomy progresses."[64]

About "cause" and "science," Rostan wrote the following, now tellingly weakened by the unfortunate pre-germ-theory example selected to illustrate his meaning:

> The anatomical lesion is not the last word in diagnosis, beyond it there is the cause . . . but it is at the lesion one must stop or risk falling into conjectures and hypotheses which are the death of all science.
>
> Pneumonia results from cold, from laborious singing, from a blow to the chest, etc. What does all this have to do with the treatment? Are not the site and extent of the alteration much more important?[65]

The hypothesized lesions came to be seen as the essence and cause of the disease, a conceptualization that would foster surgical therapies and anatomical research.

Some historians have perceived vitalistic aspects in organicist philosophy, and Duchesneau found a precursor in the work of Théophile Bordeu (1722–1776).[66] Nevertheless, organicism developed as self-conscious materialism; nineteenth-century dictionaries defined it as the positivistic opposite of vitalism.[67] Rostan proclaimed that there was no "vital principle" and that all diseases could be reduced to physical or chemical changes in the solids or liquids of the body.[68] In recounting the 1849 defense of his thesis, Paul Broca (1824–1880) indicated the extent to which organicism had come to dominate Paris medicine: "I defended the view against M. Chomel that there is no disease without a lesion, as everyone must do who knows his anatomy and physiology."[69]

The stethoscope was key to the detection of anatomical lesions, and organicists acknowledged their debt to its inventor.[70] Yet they would never see him as one of their school, nor did he wish to belong. To the consternation of younger physicians, the innovator claimed to have used his stethoscope to explore disorders in the antiquated vital principle. He even went so far as to equate some of the abnormal sounds he heard inside the bodies of his living patients as diagnoses in themselves. For Laennec, the message was clear: all sounds are absent in the cadaver; abnormal sounds, which were produced in life but not connected with a physical alteration after death, must represent manifest alterations in the vital principle. Auscultation opened a window on a clinical physiology that was beyond the reach of pathologists and discounted by fledgling organicists. Long before the doctrine of organicism had been fully enunciated, he called the project "absurd," its proponents arrogant and possessed of "an excessively high opinion of themselves." Similarly, he likened rigorous systems in medicine to a form of mass mania, one of the "most dangerous" causes of which, he said, was "excessive self-love."[71]

Laennec constantly raised doubts about the reliability of dissection, and he belabored the physical changes that occurred in all cadavers because of death. His reluctance to use the loupe or the microscope stemmed not only from technical problems, but also from his belief that a lesion had to be "sufficient" to cause disease or death before it could reasonably be linked with a disease. Many cadavers contained the surprising finding of massive physical changes that had produced no symptoms during life and could not have contributed to death. Because structural damage could be tolerated without illness, he doubted that a search for minute changes could elucidate disease. "Pathological anatomy must not be done with the loupe."[72]

Laennec devised a set of criteria by which an organic lesion could linked to a disease.[73] A year later, he revised the criteria to indicate how an organic lesion could be proven to be the cause of a disease, a sort of Koch's postulates *avant la lettre* of organic disease causation. In order to be accepted as the cause of a disease the lesion had to be:

1. Constant;
2. Anterior to, or at least concomitant with the symptoms;
3. Proportional to and sufficient to have caused the symptoms;
4. Not simultaneous with a more serious lesion or a more likely cause;
5. Productive of the same symptoms in every case.[74]

If these criteria were not met, then the disease could still be identified and classified by its associated organic lesion, but the lesion should not be mistaken for the cause.

Most organic changes were the result of some prior insult. In addition to the emotion-based changes in the vital principle, Laennec conceived of hereditary and individual predispositions, generalized alterations in body fluids, and congenital or acquired lesions that might eventually be characterized by chemistry. He reminded his listeners that perceptible disease was not so much a manifestation of an internal change, as it was the effort of nature itself to correct the alteration in the vital principle or liquids, thereby creating both the organic lesions and the symptoms. This disease process was physiological, a more elaborate version of Broussais's "irritation." It was the pathophysiology of Bayle's nostalgia; it had been decisive in many of his patients; it dominated the illness experiences of his brother, his wife, and himself.

CRITICISMS OF THE LECTURES: A PERCEIVED VITALISM

Laennec's opposition to organicism, his royalism, and his Catholic faith were combined, conflated, and criticized not only by his enemies, but also by those who are now presumed to be his intellectual heirs. One anonymous writer said that "in his lectures" he had "supported certain errors, which doctors, much less enlightened than he, would never have committed" and implied that these errors stemmed from "contamination by a partisan spirit."[75] Many had personal and political reasons for disagreement with him:

Broussais, Magendie, Rostan, and Bouillaud were politically liberal, anticlerical, and in some cases atheist. But others, like Andral and A. L. J. Bayle, were supposed admirers, if not friends, who shared his political and religious beliefs. Yet, they all found his medical philosophy to be a puzzling array of metaphysical conjectures and they attributed his "errors" to his imagination, his classification, and his philosophy, rather than to mistakes in his method or demonstrable inaccuracies in his observations. Their criticisms can be related to personal differences (in each case I will outline what these might be), but I think that the personal differences merely sensitized the critics to their primary objection: a perceived vitalism. Laennec's ideas about the vital principle were not published and have enjoyed the comparative advantage of historical anonymity. In his lifetime, however, these so-called errors were known and ridiculed by contemporaries. To them, Laennec may have been a royalist-Jesuitic-opportunist with an exaggerated notion of the importance of his invention, but his lectures were worse: they appeared to be the insignificant, or even embarrassing utterings of a mediocre clinician turned scientific crank.

François Magendie was one of the most materialist members of Laennec's generation in Paris. Notwithstanding his early references to a unitary vital force, he gradually came to the view that the properties of life were a function of physics and chemistry.[76] The frequency with which Laennec and Magendie must have encountered each other has rarely been noticed; the silence of most historians on this point seems to hint at the impossible conclusion that they occupied almost mutually exclusive worlds: one man in the morgue of the new pathology; the other in the laboratory of the new physiology. Historian Stephen Jacyna has identified problems with this possibly more apparent than real separation of medicine and physiology.[77] There were a number of reasons for animosity between Magendie and Laennec including politics, religion, and the rivalry for positions in the Académie des Sciences and the Collège de France.[78] These differences might have caused them to avoid each other, but they both belonged to medical societies, their friends conspired over elections at the Institute, Laennec read Magendie's *Journal de physiologie expérimentale et pathologique* (founded in 1821), and he cited the physiologist's work on gases, poisons, rabies, and medications in at least nine of his lectures.[79] Laennec does not seem to have left any criticisms of Magendie's work.

What Magendie may have thought of the references to his research is not known; however, his later ridicule of Laennec's interpretation of the heart sounds seems to have been based on something other than a reading of the *Treatise on Auscultation*.[80] Magendie succeeded Récamier in Laennec's old chair at the College de France in 1830. He devoted a lecture to demonstrating how his penultimate predecessor had been mistaken: he removed the chest wall from a living goose, applied the stethoscope to the still beating heart, and heard nothing. He concluded (also erroneously as it turns out) that the heart sounds were due to impact against the chest wall. He said that

Laennec's failure was the result of his "absurd convictions," "excessive self-confidence," and "blind belief in the products of his own imagination."[81] Historians E. H. Ackerknecht and John Lesch have both suggested that Magendie disputed the physiology of Broussais, but some of his criticisms may also have been aimed at the so-called armchair physiologists of the eighteenth century and their "holdover" successors in his own time who seem to have appealed to Laennec.[82]

Rostan and Laennec may have had their first encounter on the wards of the Salpêtrière, where they both served as volunteers during the typhus epidemic of 1814. The events had served the older man as evidence for the beneficial effects of native culture on lonely soldiers, but Rostan later told a different version. He described the Breton soldiers as dim-witted primitives whom no one could bear to attend except Laennec, one of their countrymen (and presumably of like intelligence). The initiative of grouping the men in a single ward he claimed as his own.[83] In his treatise, Laennec did not cite Rostan's essays relating breathlessness to mechanical derangement of the heart.[84] Rostan criticized the oversight and disputed the new notion of spontaneous cure in tuberculosis. He said that the author "seems to indulge in conjectures that someone with a less lively imagination would have immediately repressed or, at least, presented with more skepticism."[85]

Rostan's research on brain pathology was his best-known work, and by the early 1820s, he had already described a new disease entity, "softening of the brain" ("*ramollissement cérébral*").[86] Here, too, he adopted a materialistic stance regarding the causes of disease, especially diseases of affect and intelligence. Laennec was aware of these contributions. He even diagnosed Rostan's entity, "softening of the brain," in his own patients who had suffered apoplexy.[87] Rostan's name appears only once in the Laennec papers, however, as a fellow consultant in the illness of Vorogidès (see chap. 10) and his achievements do not seem to have impressed Laennec. In the first round of lectures at the Collège de France, Laennec awarded priority for the recognition of "brain softening" to others, and he mocked its application to mental illnesses.[88] Without denying its existence, he questioned the frequency with which the eager young pathologists purported to encounter it. In many cases, *ramollissement cérébral* was merely a postmortem artefact or an insignificant variation of normal tissue; when the softening could be linked to disease, it was confused by sloppy pathologists with antecedent lesions that were more important and more likely to provide reliable diagnostic criteria.[89]

In 1825, the Académie de Médecine, prompted by Esquirol, held a competition for the best essay on the organic changes associated with mental disease. The final report was written by Bouillaud, who had also published on inflammation of the brain.[90] None of the seven entries was deemed worthy of the prize, although the committee awarded a medal for "encouragement"; three essays were selected for special commentary in the report, and one was chosen not for praise, but for ridicule. With Laennec's classification of disease in full view, Bouillaud said that the ignominious essay was an attempt to prove that diseases could exist without organic lesions. It belonged "to that anonymous school of doctors, fortunately few in number, . . . who never hesitate to invoke metaphysics in medicine as if they did not know that physical and sensory phenomena are the sole basis on which all medicine must rest."[91] In short, opposition to organicism was categorically "metaphysical"; it was unscientific. The description of the ridiculed essay suggests that author may have been Laennec or someone who shared his opinion about the limitations of pathological anatomy in exploring the causes of disease.

Laennec's stormy outburst in the second round of lectures on mental illness had been provoked by Bouillaud's report. He attacked *ramollissement cérébral* and the medical materialism of Bouillaud, and he deplored the arrogance and the "prejudicial question" of the biased evaluators, who had not disguised their blatant agenda: they "wish that mental disturbances are caused by organic lesions; they even go so far as to state positively by *inflammation.*" In the medal-winning essay, epilepsy was attributed to organic lesions that were diverse in both form and position; in many cases, Laennec thought, they were nothing more than the artefacts of death. He continued, "There is no ignorance worse than believing oneself to be educated in something one does not really know."[92] By 1826, Laennec's veiled critique of Bouillaud became explicit when he chastised the younger man for undue emphasis on inflammation in Bertin's treatise on the heart.[93]

Laennec's vendetta against inflammatory causes may have had something to do with his apparent dismissal of the work of A. L. J. Bayle, the nephew of his deceased friend. The younger Bayle is generally cited as the first to link general paresis of syphilis with an organic change; his ideas were not immediately accepted, however, and Laennec is among those who appear to have rejected them. In Bayle's 1822 thesis, six patients with mental illness were found to have inflammation of the meninges (only two were said to have had venereal disease); another set of eleven patients with gastritis was presented with citation to Prost and Broussais.[94]

Included in Laennec's blanket indictment of the organic lesions supposedly responsible for mental disease, were the "brain softening" of Rostan, the encephalitis of Bouillaud, and inflammation of the meninges and stomach of A. L. J. Bayle. Without naming these men, Laennec railed against the methodological and philosophical stance that sought to reduce complex human behaviors to organic brain alterations—an echo of Buisson's attack on Bichat—especially when those alterations were defined by careless technique. The somaticist debate over mental diseases had only just begun in earnest; it would result in the eventual separation of neurology, psychiatry, and anthropology; it has still not been resolved.[95]

In turn, Bouillaud objected to Laennec's medical philosophy, his politics, and his attacks on Broussais. The shocked tone of his numerous criticisms has spilled over into the accounts of later historians. For example, he said Laennec's questioning of precordial thrill was "unworthy" of his "handsome genius;" his rejection of murmur was "really surprising" but stemmed from his "basic mistrust of the most obvious laws of physics and chemistry pushed too far"—"an unbelievable heresy" from "the immortal inventor of auscultation"; his idea of cardiac spasm was "a completely imaginary new disease."[96] Like Magendie, Bouillaud blamed Laennec's unsuccessful interpretation of the heart sounds on his "theorizing" and his propensity "to invoke the least plausible of hypotheses to explain the most simple of phenomena in pathological physics."[97] In an indirect assault on Laennec's perceived vitalism, he mocked the new references to Newton. Of the classification of disease and the physiology, he said, the inventor of the stethoscope had "imagined the most antiphysical of theories and . . . lost himself in the imaginary species of a vitalism that could not have been more inappropriate."[98] Grappling with the feisty personality behind the admirable contributions, historian Ralph Major wrote that Bouillaud ought to be revered despite his "minor shortcomings," which, in 1945, were described as "wholesale bleedings" and "rancorous criticisms."[99] It is tempting to suggest that Bouillaud's 1836 attack on surgical therapy for empyema may have been inspired by his contempt for its champion, Laennec.[100]

Unlike the other critics, Andral was also a practicing Catholic and a royalist. He has been described as one of Laennec's "eclectic" and more vitalistic followers; however, their relationship was not amicable.[101] Their disagreements cannot be reduced to religion or politics, even if they were not always intellectual. They engaged in the aforementioned priority dispute over bronchophony and its relationship to pectoriloquy (see chap. 7). In addition, in 1826, Laennec accused Andral of "bizarre" conduct because the younger man conducted independent research on auscultation, and he tried to suggest that Andral's research had taken place two years later than it actually did.[102] A reviewer of the second edition asked why Andral should have been singled out for such hostility; he excused the actions of the "hard-working, young observer," by noting that Laennec's wards were packed with "crowds of foreigners" and that he rarely arrived for rounds before noon, making it impossible for busy practitioners to follow his instruction.[103]

Andral edited the fourth edition of Laennec's treatise on auscultation and took the opportunity to distance himself from the vitalistic ideas. In reference to Laennec's tubercular nuns, he said that the idea of "sad passions" as a cause of phthisis was a "great exaggeration." He explained that Laennec had puzzled his contemporaries with a philosophical stance that seemed like a paradoxical retreat from his own achievements. "Laennec was struck so often by the weakness of the science, for which he had done so much . . . that he was sometimes led to deny it completely, precisely where it was most obviously correct. . . . This rigid, but ardent mind . . . [was] not satisfied to take from vitalism all the truth that vitalism could offer [and] refused the new teachings that had just released vitalism from its errors, restraining it in its application, but reducing it to a fraction of its truth."[104]

Among the many doctors who attacked Laennec's ideas of vital principle and vital lesion, only Broussais appeared to understand why they had been invoked. He even came close to acknowledging the similarities between Laennec's theory and his own physiological doctrine, especially in their opposition to the overemphasis of cadaver medicine, when he said, " 'Vital lesion' is certainly a physiologic term."[105]

The criticisms of Laennec's perceived vitalism struck at the very heart of his medical philosophy. Added to the royalist meddling and pious Catholicism, they constitute the intellectual reasons for his unpopularity among his immediate successors. But the criticisms are largely unknown, because the object of their attack—the perceived vitalism—is also unknown, and, as I show in the next chapter, that is probably because it was suppressed.

THE LAST TRIP TO KERLOUARNEC

Laennec knew the ideas in his lectures were being attacked even as he was delivering them, but it strengthened his conviction that his classification of disease would be an improvement over blind emphasis on pathological anatomy, the exclusive "solidism" of younger colleagues. An experienced clinician and consummate pathologist, he knew that sometimes people could sicken and die; yet, their bodies would be intact. The psyche did influence the soma—even Broussais seemed to know that. Why did these young doctors, most of whom were born after the Terror, refuse to acknowledge the extent to which living can bring about its own end? Did they not read Corvisart? Had they already forgotten the Paris of 1814? Laennec's future book on clinical medicine would set them straight, but his health had broken once again, and he had yet to finish the second edition of the treatise on auscultation.

The changes made for the second edition have been discussed in chapters 7, 8, and 9, but are summarized here. Laennec restructured the work from the physiological applications of auscultation to an outline based on diseases of the chest; he added more brief clinical cases of individuals and cohorts of patients; he introduced his new sign of bronchophony; he expanded the passages on the significance of puerile respiration in asthma; he revised the meaning of the stethoscopic sounds of the heart; he responded to Broussais's criticisms; he wrote new sections on treatments and a lengthy chapter on tartar emetic; he expanded the section on operation for empyema; he declared his ideas about the etiology of phthisis; he made explicit his opinion of the cavalier use of inflammation in the Paris school; and he proclaimed his admiration for Newton. The Latin dedication to the professors of the faculty remained, but the anonymous case history pertaining to himself was replaced with another personal observation.

In late April or early May 1826, "at the moment the final page proofs were brought for approval," Laennec was exhausted, febrile, lying in his bed; he suddenly noticed that he could hear his own heart beating without the aid of a stethoscope. He called others to witness the phenomenon. A few minutes later he passed gas, and the sound disappeared; perhaps his heart beating against an air-filled organ had created a drumlike effect. He added the observation with his speculation as an autopsy-less "P.S." to the end of his book.[106]

Once again, plans were made for a return to Brittany. If this was phthisis, Laennec was ready to die. If it was simply another "vital lesion," he needed the maritime atmosphere, the manor, woods, and fields that he loved in order to be healed. He returned a list of nosy questions about his health asked by Laennec *père* with the following message: "My dear father, may the mercy of God, before whom I will appear perhaps very soon, cover you with his benediction. For two months, I have tried to purge my soul and with the grace of God it seems to me that I want to go to him now more than at any other time."[107] The faculty and the Duchesse de Berry granted him leave.[108] Some belongings were packed up, but most were left in the new apartment.

As he prepared his escape, Laennec hoped to win lucrative honors that would strengthen his ability to retire, or, should he die, enhance his estate. When he requested leave, he asked the Duchesse de Berry to advance his petition for the Cordon St. Michel, the oldest order of France held by at least half the professors of the faculty. She interceded on his behalf through the Comtesse de Noailles and the Duc de Doudeauville.[109] He also aimed for one of the Prix Montyon of the Académie des Sciences, prizes which had been revived with an new donation in 1819 for achievements in medicine and surgery, industrial hygiene, mechanics, physiology, and statistics. The medical prize of 1826 was to be given to the "most useful discovery" that had been published by December 1825, but the second edition of the treatise on auscultation would not be released until after the deadline.[110]

In mid-May 1826, Laennec had a promotional pamphlet printed about the "new facts obtained" from the last seven years of his research. He sent it to Baron Fourier of the Académie des Sciences with a covering letter to assure the committee that in 1825 alone "at least three hundred students and doctors" had received instruction and that "all the facts" in his second edition had been published or publicized before the end of that year.[111] He also sent his pamphlet with a covering letter to the *académicien* Cuvier, a fellow professor at the Collège de France with whom he had studied parasites more than twenty years before. He told Cuvier that auscultation had allowed "the most obscure of internal lesions to enter the realm of surgical diseases"; it had "uncovered a fecund mine of positive facts."[112] The pamphlet was a summary of the inventor's perspective on the most important applications of his stethoscope in four separate but equal divisions of medicine: semiotics, pathological anatomy, pathological physiology, and therapeutics. Physiology and therapeutics were still prominent in his mind, even if his colleagues and heirs tended to diminish them.

The *Moniteur universel* reported that on 27 May 1826 after evening mass in the royal chapel at St. Cloud, Laennec presented the first copy of the second edition of his *Treatise on Auscultation* to Charles X. The author's father

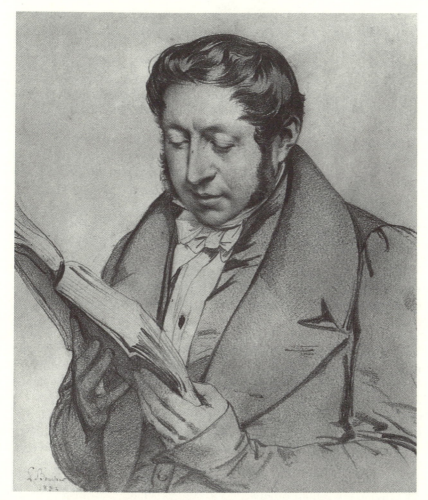

Figure 11.4. Mériadec Laennec, the young cousin, who participated in the research on auscultation as a student, a colleague, and amanuensis. He was the executor of Laennec's estate and inherited the scientific papers, including case records and lectures. Drawing by L. Boucher, 1832, Musée Laennec, Nantes. Photograph: M. Certain.

was furious and demanded to known how he was supposed to believe that his son was too sick to work, when he was hobnobbing with the King on the outskirts of Paris. Mériadec (fig. 11.4) annotated the letter "You are lying, dog, and you know that you lie," and with his older brother, he tried unsuccessfully to convince his uncle of the gravity of the cousin's condition.[113]

Laennec left Paris with his wife on 30 May 1826, two days after his new edition had been released for sale. He was weakened by fever and a chronic diarrhea that would not respond to opiates and made the trip all the more arduous. After he pulled a loose tooth, a maxillary sinus began to drain through a fistula to his mouth: "now I know the cause of that odor of pus," he wrote to his cousin back in Paris.[114] The couple declined offers to rest part way at Petit Port near Nantes and pushed on to Finistère. In unrelenting rain, the calèche had broken down only ten leagues from Paris; five days later at Vannes, it plunged down a twelve-foot ditch. Appealing to the doctor's Catholic admirers, a legend about this accident would have Laennec saying his rosary: just as the carriage turned over, he had reached the "*Ora pro nobis peccatoribus.*"[115] The travelers felt miraculously spared, but the "impression of terror" had a detrimental effect, which they remembered for weeks. "Heaven would not have allowed the accident if you had been with us," Madame Laennec wrote to Mériadec, expressing her parental feelings for him.[116] Her husband did the same: "you are my spiritual son and the heir of my stethoscope."[117] Finally they reached Kerlouarnec; Madame found the manor "charming" on the days her husband was well, and "very sad" on the days he was not.[118]

Toulmouche, Beaugendre, Ollivry, and Ambroise Laennec examined the inventor with his stethoscope and professed to find nothing wrong, but the correspondence suggests that they were uncertain of the diagnosis. Forbes later claimed that they had found a tumor in the abdomen and evidence of pulmonary tuberculosis with pectoriloquy. Ambroise reported to his brother in Paris that he suspected cavities in the apex of both lungs and possibly also at the left base.[119] Because the patient had lost his great fondness for tobacco, they allowed themselves to hope that the disease was acute.[120] Christophe joined them from Nantes and was shocked at the emaciation and weakness of his cousin, who was uncharacteristically demonstrative of his affections and wept tears of joy.[121] The invalid went out twice a day in a child's carriage pulled by two men, and he surveyed the masons and loggers working on his holdings. He ate unusually large meals, thought to be dangerous for his fever, and he stubbornly insisted on seven or eight glasses of goat's milk daily. When others tried to suggest changes to his regimen, he was petulant.

Laennec's slow decline and saintlike final moments have been told often. His affairs were put in order to the best of Mériadec's abilities: the Paris apartment relinquished with a payment of two thousand frances for nine months rent; the "leech" of a servant dismissed; and his shares in the Corrèze canals were to be sold.[122] He wrote a new will and then amended it with six codicils. The main beneficiary was his wife; Mériadec would have the scientific papers and the portrait; Ambroise would have Kerlouarnec after his wife died; the pensions for his sister and his father would be reduced.[123] Still spying through the *directrice des postes*, the father threatened to visit, but the family kept him at bay until the struggle was over; he then sent an emissary to snoop, hoping, as Rouxeau put it, to carve "a few slices off the legacy of his son" at the expense of a daughter-in-law he seemed never to have met.[124]

The investment in the Corrèze canals worried the patient greatly. Laennec had committed to purchasing fifty thousand francs worth of shares in mid-1825, possibly though his connection with Becquey; but he had paid only one quarter of the sum and, when he became ill, he wanted to sell them.[125] Keeping the shares required immediate investment, but selling them meant of loss of ten thousand francs. Laennec's cousin and his legal advisor both tried to hide the fact that they had taken over his shares: they told the dying man that they had been sold, but the money would not come for several months. A few days before his death, his wife told him the truth when she realized that he was planning to spend the nonexistent, forthcoming money on a cousin's property.[126] Her honesty has often been described as a "weakness," an unthinking "slip," a final blow that killed her husband.[127] But he appeared to take the news calmly.

Laennec's cheerful last letter was entirely in keeping with his clinical experience. It reminds us that his concept of consumption was distinguished from that of Bayle by the possibility of hope. "Calculated properly, I can only compare my case to that of Madame de Chateaubriand eight years ago. Cayol was certain she would die of phthisis in two or three months, notwithstanding the stethoscopic signs. I stood firm in my position and at the end of ten months, the huge quantity of sputum decreased by half, the fever fell, and I left for my vacation with peace of mind."[128] Nine days later, on 13 August 1826, he suddenly rose up in his bed to remove his rings, because, he said, someone else would soon be obliged to render him this service and he did not wish to cause her pain.[129] A few hours later, he was dead. There was no autopsy.

Laennec was buried in the Ploaré cemetery above the magnificent Bay of Douarnenez (fig. 11.5). Within a month, the King had instructed the ministry of the interior to provide his widow an annual pension of three thousand francs; in January 1827, the Faculty of Medicine agreed to pay Laennec's widow a lump sum of 992 francs, 44 centimes, half the salary that he would have earned from his absence in April until his death 13 August. But the royal pension was revoked with the next Revolution four years later.[130] The widow lived at Kerlouarnec until her death in 1847; she was buried with her husband. In September 1934, their bodies were exhumed for repositioning; a plaster cast was made of the doctor's skull (fig. 11.6), his bones were carefully separated from those of his wife and sealed in a "resistant" coffin, to be reinterred in the center of the cemetery.[131] During the few days that his casket reposed in the church, a line of Breton people filed into the Ploaré cemetery and took turns lowering themselves into the freshly dug grave. They believed that protection and physical well-being would be their reward for having spent a few moments within the earth that was about to receive the remains of Dr. Laennec.[132]

In the nearly two hundred years since his death, Laennec's fame has soared to mystical dimensions that extend well beyond medical hagiography to the highest religious and cultural altitudes of France. At the centennial of his

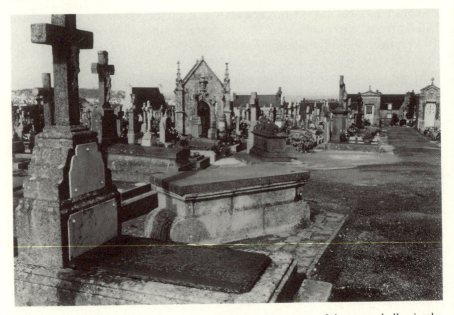

Figure 11.5. Laennec's tomb set on an angle at the corner of the central alley in the cemetery of Ploaré. Photograph: The author, 1995.

death in 1926, Ploaré witnessed a traditional religious festival, a "Pardon": the Archbishop of Quimper presided while distinguished physicians from Paris, Nantes, and Rennes paid homage to the devout medical genius; the crowd heard the tale of how Laennec's bronze statue in the town square had cured the intractable cough of the mythical King Gradlon, whose ailing granite effigy still rode high on the cathedral above. During the bicentenary of Laennec's birth in 1981, France witnessed a full year of celebrations, conferences, and displays. In the solemn opening ceremonies at the Académie Nationale de Médecine, Laennec was honored by the extraordinary presence of President of the Republic of France, Valéry Giscard d'Estaing. Back in Brittany several hundred "descendants" of the man who had no children gathered on the lawns of Kerlouarnec to trace their relationship to the great physician. Speeches were made in French and Breton praising the legacy of the stethoscope and extolling the virtues of its inventor. A speaker suggested that his remains be disinterred again and carried to the Pantheon; another called for his canonization.[133]

What did Laennec accomplish with his return to Paris in late 1821? The most important auscultatory discoveries had already been made, and his stethoscope was in the hands of enough committed users that its survival was assured. The royalist favors, the press of visitors, the second-edition revisions, and the lectures at the Collège de France probably damaged more than en-

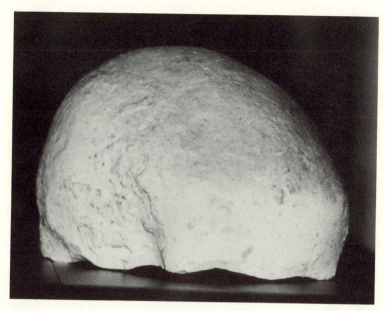

Figure 11.6. Plaster cast of the cranium of Laennec, made by Felix Graziano during the exhumation of the remains in 1934. Given by Mme Olgiati in memory of her physician husband Antoine Olgiati in 1948 to Dr. Clouard and now owned by his son, psychiatrist Dr. Paul Clouard. Photograph: Kindly provided by Dr. P. Clouard of Quimper, 1995.

hanced his reputation, and, although he enjoyed the fame and the notoriety, he believed that the return had broken his health. He died in the midst of an unsuccessful attempt to leave a full explanation of his legacy, trying to rescue his ideas from distortion and reduction. In the first century after his death, Laennec became a medical hero, but his reputation was fashioned from a skewed version of his life's work. What was retained and what was rejected were the result of winnowing—a complementary choosing and rejecting—both elements in the process of history itself.

Between the Quick and the Dead: Pathology, Physiology, and Clinical Medicine

The physician who does not unite physiology with anatomy
. . . will never become a firm and decisive practitioner,
particularly in the treatment of the organic lesions.

—*Corvisart, 1806, 17*

I fear I am not always understood even by my colleagues.

—*Laennec,* Traite d'anatomie pathologique, *ca. 1808*

IN THE MID- to late nineteenth century, as George Weisz has clearly shown, French physicians and historians were eager to promote Laennec's contributions to pathological anatomy as a way of enhancing the scientific and nationalistic claims for the discipline.[1] That special emphasis increased, and during the century after his death, French pathologists had published portions of his treatise on pathological anatomy.[2] By 1963, Foucault joined a long line of French writers who had classified the treatise on auscultation as a work of pathological anatomy, and auscultation has received considerable attention by historians of the discipline.[3] For historians of physiology, however, Laennec is almost invisible; if he is mentioned at all, it is as an anatomist who localized disease in the organs of the dead. Just as Magendie rarely figures in histories of medicine, by most historical accounts of physiology, what Laennec did was something else.[4]

But Laennec saw himself firmly rooted in the study of the living individual, and by extension, he thought that he was involved in both nascent disciplines of pathological anatomy and physiology. Because he appears in one sort of history but not in the other, we should ask if the apparent separation of these early nineteenth-century disciplines could be an anachronistic distinction, imposed by our desires to trace the genealogy of entities in our own world. Why has Laennec's physiology been ignored?

It is easy to forget that in the postrevolutionary Paris school, neither pathology nor physiology was truly separate from the clinic. Both disciplines were struggling for intellectual as well as institutional recognition, or demarcation; the boundaries were blurred. Later pathologists had no difficulty lauding the fraction of Laennec's work that his successors had chosen to venerate: the stethoscope and the pathological anatomy. Most pathologists were never aware of Laennec's clinical physiology. For the budding physiologists of the following decades, however, Laennec had come to symbolize the clinicians or the rival pathologists, who, in France at least, began to hold sway, and with whom they vied for institutional credibility. Physiologists might have been aware of Laennec's reservations about the limitations of pathology, but they had difficulties embracing his solutions for semantic and practical reasons. Laennec seemed to be allied with the style of researchers, who were perceived as, and more recently called, "holdovers."[5] He kept using the old-fashioned term, vital principle, and he emphasized the primacy of the patient—the whole illness experience with its psychic baggage. This capitulation to symptoms and feelings was a reminder of the hegemony of an uncontrollable clinical reality from which physiologists were beginning to seek their independence. As John Lesch has shown, however, the hostility toward experimentation that later physiologists projected onto clinicians of early nineteenth-century Paris is more apparent than real.[6] The example of Laennec conforms well to his thesis.

The vital principle had long provided a means of explanation and a vehicle for discussion of biological phenomena that defied reduction to physicochemical terms. Many contemporary physiologists, including the young Magendie had paid lip service to its existence, but by the time Laennec published his first edition, the term was disappearing from research vocabulary. The new physiology was growing out of anatomy through the correlation of functional abnormalities with organic change.[7] The experiments of Magendie and his pupil Claude Bernard (1813–1878) would rely heavily on surgical interventions that interfered with anatomy in order to alter and control structure as an aid to the study of function. They concentrated on localizing and measuring those life processes that lent themselves to such study.

Scholars agree that experimentation, especially vivisection, was the hallmark that demarcated physiology from pathology and from clinical medicine; by 1850, physiology had become a "rigorous experimental science" in continental Europe, and the trend was apparent elsewhere.[8] But the process of forming a distinct discipline was neither easy nor abrupt, and here again we can question Laennec's exclusion. He lived long before the structural and intellectual separation of pathology, physiology, and clinical medicine had taken place. He, too, conducted what he considered experiments in the acoustic properties of function in living beings, in clinical therapeutics, on contracting muscle, and on the properties of tissues. He could also claim to have delineated puerile respiration, a physical, even "positive" sign of altered physiology. As anatomical explanations increased and as physiologists first strove to alter artificially the organic structure of their subjects, Laennec participated in Barry's investigations on living animals and used Magendie's research to bolster his theory of disease.

Perhaps Laennec's experiments did not "count," because they did not entail the surgical alteration of his (mostly human) subjects. Nevertheless, he thought that his credentials as a physiological investigator were superior to the sloppy semantics of Broussais who had styled himself as the sole purveyor of "physiological medicine." With his connection to Bichat, Broussais is usually mentioned in histories of physiology, if only because he had monopolized the word. But Broussais also had reservations about the "artificial" animal experiments, and in the end, his medical reputation paled in contrast to that of his rival, because his simplistic theory ended up pleasing none of the experimentalists, pathologists, and clinicians who would follow.[9] I raise these points not to demand laurels for Laennec from a domain that has traditionally ignored him, but to explore the implications of his exclusion as a manifestation of how the two disciplinary histories have been constructed. The process began immediately after Laennec's death.

WHY WERE THE LECTURES NOT PUBLISHED?

Biographers have been incredulous that Laennec was not instantaneously an object of veneration: more wanton slights to be born by his long-suffering shade. The obituaries spoke of a "great loss," but they also described his "cold" personality, the "partisan spirit" that had infected him like a "sort of contagion," his severity, piety, and stubborn tenacity to opinions in which he "*believed,* so to say," opinions that "frankly speaking, did not always carry the stamp of rigorous logic."[10] One journalist suggested that in his last illness, Laennec had been a hypocrite because he did not try his own "heroic" therapy of tartar emetic, asking instead to be bled for pneumonia.[11] His supposed associates also qualified their praise in the year of his death, criticizing his total rejection of Broussais and his enthusiasm for tartar emetic.[12] In 1826, Laennec was not popular with the majority of his colleagues, and his invention, though widely thought to be clever, did not immediately enjoy the symbolic stature it would eventually attain. Despite his lobbying, Laennec was disqualified from the 1826 Prix Montyon. The 1827 prize went to Joseph Pelletier (1788–1842) and Joseph-Bienaimé Caventou (1795–1877) for their purification of quinine sulfate, and the *Treatise on Auscultation* received honorable mention and five thousand francs. Moreover, the inventor had been a political thorn in the flesh of academic medicine. The Académie de Médecine did not hear Laennec's eulogy until 1 December 1839, thirteen years after his death when Broussais and Dupuytren were both dead, too.[13] In the pre-anesthesia, pre-antisepsis world, doctors could not imagine the therapeutic benefits that might be derived from localizing chest disease, and they could not foresee the revolution that auscultation would bring in the conceptualization of all diseases. Quinine, on the other hand, was of obvious benefit.

Just before he died, Laennec had charged Mériadec with editing the Collège de France lecture notes as a treatise on clinical medicine: "You would provide a real service to instruction if you, alone or with assistance, could publish my course at the Collège de France in four volumes."[14] But the cousin did not fulfill the request. Laennec deserved recognition for the stethoscope—even his enemies conceded that point—but the idea of publishing his precious words on other topics, simply out of respect for his having written them, was far from anybody's mind.

Mériadec was devoted to his older cousin during his life and after. His letters reveal affection, reverence, and generous indulgence toward a willful personality whose drive and whims were balanced by the younger man's practicality and dedication. He made detailed annotations and amplifications for the third edition of the *Treatise on Auscultation*, which were translated separately as a short guide to auscultation.[15] He also preserved the manuscripts, leaving their safekeeping or destruction to the judgment of his own physician-nephew, Théophile-Ambroise Laennec (1830–1896), the son of Ambroise and friend of the biographer Alfred Rouxeau.[16] Mériadec was the obvious editor, and if help were necessary, it should not have been difficult to find fair copies of the lectures made by students.

Among potential editorial assistants would appear to have been A. L. Bayle. After his beginnings in clinical psychiatry, he had become a journalist and librarian with astute bibliographic reflexes. He edited the posthumous treatise on cancer of his uncle G. L. Bayle.[17] The younger Bayle was also a royalist, a member of the Congrégation, collected statistics at the Charité, and is often said to have been indebted to Laennec for special attention after his uncle's death; his mentor, Royer-Collard, had been Laennec's friend.[18] Signs of the affinity between the younger Bayle and Laennec are scarce, however; some evidence raises doubt that it ever existed. For example, he did not join in the mass exodus from the *Dictionnaire des sciences médicales* led by Laennec, who in turn had failed to cite his work on mental diseases.

Bayle knew of the Collège de France lectures. At Laennec's death, he wrote one of the few obituaries that referred to them. He praised the "original" classification of disease, which was "not confined to solids alone, but also included liquids"; however, he did not use the words "vital principle" or "vital lesions."[19] With the omission, Bayle may have been yielding to some anticipated intolerance of the vitalistic, antiorganicist notions in order to passively protect Laennec (and himself) from association with them. At the time of Laennec's death, Bayle may have been acting defensively, having just come under attack for softening his original statements about the role of anatomical change in mental diseases.[20] Or did he distort the classification out of ignorance, not having heard the lectures and begrudging Laennec's aforementioned failure to praise his achievements? If Bayle had a debt, it did not extend to active defense of unpopular theory.

Thirty years later, however, things seem to have changed. Bayle published a book on medical pathology "in the spirit of Hippocratic vitalism." It followed a debate in the Académie over the role of vitalism in medicine, and was cast as an open attack on the inadequacies of the now-named organicism. Bayle's essay bears a remarkable resemblance to Laennec's doctrine: the recognition of "solids, liquids, and vital force"; the distinction between life force and the soul; the debt to Hippocrates and all "good observers"; an attack on the "simplistic" but "seductive" doctrine of Broussais now thoroughly "discredited"; the author's admission that he had failed to appreciate the importance of "crises" in healing until later in life. Laennec, however, was barely mentioned except as someone who had once contributed to pathological anatomy.[21] Was Bayle's essay a form of revenge? Was it plagiarism? I do not know, but it seems, he was not someone to help Mériadec.

Laennec had also given his cousin the "right" to oversee new editions of the *Treatise on Auscultation* "if the need should arise."[22] In his 1831 preface, Mériadec said a third edition of the treatise on auscultation had become necessary because of discoveries in the intervening five years. This statement is peculiar, since the new "discoveries" were never clarified, and the second edition was completed only a few weeks before Laennec's death. At this time, Mériadec also announced his plan, "if circumstances allow," to publish the first two sections of the Collège de France lectures as an outline of pathological anatomy; he said that "most" of the editing was already complete.[23]

Notwithstanding his declaration, Mériadec did not edit the lectures. There are several possible reasons for his failure. First, he had his own career to develop, although his clinical activities did not inhibit his editing for auscultation—a task he had been asked to perform only "if the need should arise." Second, there may have been no obvious financial return in the collected lectures when compared to the book on auscultation. Third, he may have decided that his older cousin's good reputation depended on the stethoscope; if he could not do everything, he could at least ensure the proper reception of auscultation. Fourth, the lecture notes are written in an abbreviated format and are sometimes difficult to read. Fifth, he may have decided they should not be published.

By the mid-1830s, Mériadec was citing the fourth reason as the most serious obstacle. In a letter to Forbes, he wrote that the lecture notes were "in general very short and very disjointed, and could only be reduced to a connected form by much labor, and by someone who had heard the lessons, and was acquainted with the lecturer's method." Once again, he promised to edit the first thirty lessons and if he succeeded "so far as to produce a work not unworthy of the memory of the author" he would publish it.[24] More than six years later, however, Mériadec described the rudimentary condition of the notes to Kergaradec, but publication was no longer a possibility.[25]

Having read the lecture notes myself, I have some sympathy for Mériadec's difficulty: many pages are incomplete and tedious to read with numerous abbreviations and additions. But did Mériadec have no advantages? Had he not attended the lectures himself? Was he completely unaware of the identity or location of others, like Kitchen and Dufour, who had faithfully followed and recorded the classes in legible prose? The notes themselves may be difficult, but they are not impossible, even for a reader two centuries later. The fourth reason strikes me as an excuse.

Mériadec's own words raise suspicions that the fifth reason was more important. In the same letter to Kergaradec, he continued, "I had to fear that far from adding to the glory of my dear master, [the publication of the Collège de France lectures] would bring unfortunate consequences. I have almost always seen a cold reception given to these posthumous publications of the unfinished works of a genius, and they add nothing to the reputation of the author. Moreover full of the deepest affection [for my cousin] and having retired early from medical practice, I was no longer in a position to do the science . . . and wisely, I believe, left these unshapen manuscripts sleeping in my files."[26] Something in the notes struck Mériadec as unworthy of all the extra effort; something that menaced his cousin's slowly rising reputation; something that he may have consciously or subconsciously decided to suppress. If so, what?

Beyond the real challenge of the text, several other aspects of Laennec's lectures posed difficulties for a would-be editor in the 1830s and 1840s. First and most obvious would be the constant reminder of the royal patronage that Laennec had enjoyed by his very appointment to the chair. With the advent of the July Monarchy in 1830, those who had joined the faculty of medicine through the royalist intervention of 1823 were forced to resign. Had Laennec been alive, he, too, would have been stripped of his professorship in clinical medicine at the faculty; to keep his chair at the Collège de France he would have been obliged to swear allegiance to Louis-Philippe, something his friend and successor, Récamier, could not bring himself to do.[27] At the same time, most of Laennec's enemies came to the positions of power vacated by his ousted friends. Dupuytren continued, his security assured and his stature as a professor ever larger. Bouillaud took over Laennec's old position as clinical professor of medicine at the Charité in 1831; later he would become dean. Rostan and Bouillaud both came to preside over the Académie de Médecine, and, ironically, the latter delivered one of the formal speeches at the unveiling of Laennec's statue in Quimper in 1868 (fig. 12.1).[28] Magendie, whom Laennec had defeated in ballots for the Collège de France chair, succeeded to the same position with the resignation of Récamier. Mériadec may have looked at the layout of the post-1830 medical establishment and decided that the political, personal, and professional risks arising from reminding the medical elite of the royalist privileges and medical criticisms of his relative were simply too great.

Others who were less inimical had surpassed Laennec's contributions in pathological anatomy. Cruveilhier, protégé of Laennec but also of Dupuytren, presided over the revived Société Anatomique for four decades and in 1836 became the first occupant of the chair of pathological anatomy that was Dupuytren's legacy. Andral, a professor since 1828, was defining liquid lesions of the blood with a microscopic precision that Laennec had never

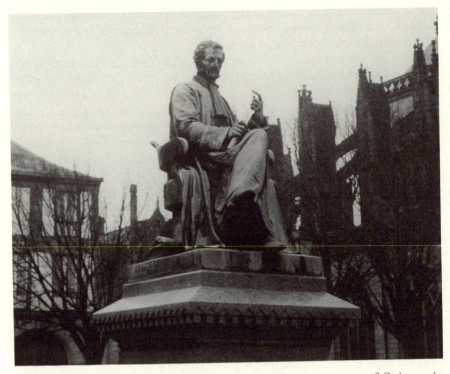

Figure 12.1. Laennec's bronze statue erected in the town square of Quimper in 1868. Photograph: François Gallouin, 1985.

known. Louis had written a clinical treatise on phthisis. Mériadec understood that Cruveilhier and Andral had raised doubts about some of Laennec's observations in pathological anatomy, while Louis took pains to distance himself from the lectures.[29] His reluctance to defend his cousin by arguing with his rivals was evident: in footnotes and addenda to his third edition, he accepted almost all their criticisms of Laennec's auscultation and pathology. If he were to become the foster parent of yet another even more controversial text on disease, he would have to confront retaliatory reviews from experts in medical science, a domain that he did not cultivate.

Second, the attack on Broussais appeared in at least a third of Laennec's lectures. In 1830, the polemicist had finally entered the faculty and for twelve years after Laennec's death, continued to hurl insults at his defunct rival. His influence may not have been overwhelming, but he had loyal supporters in high places, especially Bouillaud. Mériadec would have to wage an inherited polemic with a powerful opponent, a polemic that of necessity would become his own. His discomfort was evident when he apologized for Laennec's "futile" (*"oiseuses"*) attacks on Broussais, claiming that they were written before the "doctrine of this celebrated professor had been justly appreciated."[30] After Broussais's death in 1838, Mériadec may not have wished to stoop to the enemy's own level by attacking the dead. In any case, the battles seemed to have died of their own accord, and what people were willing to remember of Laennec no longer needed defending.

The same could be said for Mériadec's dilemma concerning Laennec's refusal to cite certain observations from the works of Bouillaud, Rostan, Collin, and the younger Bayle. Mériadec may have thought that it would be a betrayal to insert the references that his cousin had omitted on purpose; as a diligent editor, however, he knew that he probably should. Certainly, he could appreciate the danger of printing what had already been taken as an deliberate (but verbal) snub.

Moreover, the style and content of the lectures also posed difficulties: the antiquated fashion of giving priority to the ancients, the pious skepticism about "cause," and the constant reminders about the limits of pathological anatomy. These notions were not popular in the 1830s, when Rostan began to expound on organicism and the Paris faculty established its first chair in pathological anatomy. Other ideas were problematic, too: the flirtation with galvanism, soon to be the unresolved subject of two commissions in the Académie de Médecine;[31] the liberal use of high-dose tartar emetic and other treatments, which had already been condemned before Laennec died. Therapeutic aggression was not prized in 1830s Paris.[32]

The most awkward of Laennec's ideas was the perceived vitalism; implicit in the French edition of his treatise on auscultation, it pervaded the lectures. Only two years after Laennec's death, Friedrich Wöhler (1800–1882) synthesized urea, a substance that had previously been thought to occur only in living organisms. With this synthetic urea, Wöhler was considered by some historians, if not by contemporaries, to have effectively falsified vitalism as a theory of life function, and it became fashionable in some circles to say that vitalism was dead, although the topic continued to provoke debate for decades.[33] Neither pathologists nor physiologists, and only a few clinicians seemed willing to talk about vital forces as a topic for investigation; most preferred to ignore them. Laennec's attack on organicism had been cast as an epistemological justification for the existence of a vital principle; it constituted a major theme, if not the whole purpose of his lectures. Someone, possibly Mériadec, added new material on vitalism to the manuscripts, as if he found the vitalism in Laennec's lectures to require editorial justification.[34] It may have become quite apparent to the cousin that Laennec's purpose was now a "losing" battle.

With some disclaimers, the historian Elizabeth Williams published an interesting list of "winners" and "losers" in the intellectual debates of the nineteenth century.[35] Laennec appears to belong to the "winners" on all counts expect for his hesitation over the microscope and his "vitalism." With a longer life and the later technical improvements, he may have learned to appreciate the microscope; he already owned one and referred to it in his teachings. It is unlikely, however, that he would have altered his view of clinical physiology.

Mériadec's "suppression," if it happened at all, was passive, not active. He did not lie about his cousin's ideas; indeed, he even articulated a feeble, spiritualistic defense in the third edition of the *Treatise on Auscultation* as a confused retort to the charge of materialism. "How could anyone dare to accuse him of having believed that *structure* [*"organisation"*] *contained the secrets of thought and life, health and disease, . . .* he who revealed himself to be essentially *vitalist,* he whose sincere and abiding faith in Catholicism was a secret to no one." [36] Vitalism was not obvious in the earlier book, however. Why should Mériadec do so much work only to place his cousin among "losers," when all his other contributions made him a giant among "winners"? He allowed the paradoxical memory of the lectures to die with those who had attended the classes, reducing the scope of his cousin's *oeuvre* to auscultation and its applications in anatomical pathology alone. He joined the acerbic translator and Broussais in shaping the image of the inventor of the stethoscope into the form that generations of physicians and historians have made of him since.

Laennec has become a cartoonlike symbol for French medicine, Catholic physicians, pathologists, clinicians, amateurs of physical diagnosis, and various clinical specialists, including chest physicians and the few cardiologists who can pardon his "mistakes." Weisz has shown how the posthumous reputation was bolstered by the political and professional desires of French pathologists.[37] Not only was Laennec proclaimed as the hero of anatomoclinical medicine, he was also blamed for its inadequacies—curiously, the very inadequacies he had predicted. In an influential biographical dictionary, he was accused of a "repugnance" for "the application of physiology," a rigidity and narrowness in his definition of disease—the "radical solidism" that he had always deplored—and of a "therapeutic indifference" that he had never espoused.[38] Armed with this tailored version of the story, Ackerknecht saw Laennec's "empiricism" as having engineered a "dead end."[39] Few doctors or historians recalled the perceived vitalism in his work; fewer yet understood its physiological intent.[40]

British physicians were less likely to equate Laennec's perceived vitalism with his religion and royalism, possibly because they were less aware of his involvement in the right-wing meddling. Sometimes, they praised and agreed with his views on etiology, which for them seemed to represent exactly what their author had intended: clinical physiology.[41] But physiologists in early nineteenth-century France did not admire the experiments that he had conducted and/or witnessed in the name of their new discipline. Was it his antiquated vocabulary that offended? Was it because he did his research in a hospital, not in a laboratory? Or that he investigated intact humans instead of altered animals? Was it the association with men of questionable social stature who called themselves physiological investigators: a British military officer, or the son of an impoverished and nearly blind Breton amateur? Whatever the reason, Laennec was purged from the annals of physiology.

WAS LAENNEC A VITALIST?

From the foregoing, it might seem reasonable to conclude that Laennec was a vitalist and make that the surprise ending to my book. This interpretation troubles me for two reasons. First, Laennec rejected the label as well as the philosophy and did not think of himself as a vitalist. He said that he had been accused of materialism, a charge he refuted by saying that, unlike the materialists, he did not confuse the immutable soul (*"l'âme"*) with *"la force vitale, l'archée, la chimie vivante, l'électricité animale."* For Laennec, a materialist was someone who believed in the existence of vital forces but denied the existence of a soul "in the sense of philosophers and Christians."[42] His definition of a "materialist" could now be rephrased as an "atheist vitalist." I admit that Laennec may not have been the best judge of his own vitalism (or lack thereof), but I do not believe that his claims to the contrary should be ignored. If he distinguished his thought from what he perceived as vitalism, then we should at least try to understand his distinction, even we choose not to accept it.

My second reason for being concerned about the description of Laennec as a vitalist is doubt about the possibility of a consistent definition of vitalism. Reducing a philosophy to a form of vitalism simplifies and distorts the range of positions, as if any student of biology must either be a vitalist or not. Vitalism and its detection are subtle; notwithstanding the desires of historians, it is difficult to find any author, dead or living, who is purely vitalist/spiritualist or mechanist/materialist. In describing the range of eighteenth-century vitalisms and the difficulty in identifying them, G. Rousseau said that "the most successful systems of explanation . . . integrated a fundamental mechanism with a superimposed vitalism."[43] Further clouding the issue, some figures, who are now ensconced in the history of science as famous vitalists, were thought to be materialists and mechanists in their own time, whereas others, including Bichat, Cuvier, and Claude Bernard (1813–1878), have been variously classified mechanist or vitalist by different writers.[44]

For some time now, doubts about the validity of these mechanist or vitalist categories have been expressed by distinguished historians. Arthur Lovejoy and Fielding H. Garrison recommended dispensing with the imprecision, futility, "verbiage," and "unintelligible" nature of the old debate.[45] William Coleman observed that use of these terms "without full and explicit qualification . . . is usually pernicious."[46] Indeed, it would be nice to avoid what Geison has called the "hoary debate" that revolves around "large quasi-philosophical categories that have not yet been linked persuasively and concretely with evidence about the actual practice of research."[47] Whether we like it or not, however, the vitalist-mechanist debate was an active participant in the two centuries of medicine, science, history writing, and archival activity that distance us from Laennec.[48]

Laennec understood vitalism to be the *exclusive* reliance on explanations invoking the vital principle. He acknowledged that nearly all diseases could be classified in this group, but he did not think such a classification was practical.[49] For example, he suspected that the cause of phthisis lay in the realm of emotional upheaval (vital lesion), and he saw its myriad pathological forms as a manifestations of a diathesis (liquid lesion); yet, he classified it as a disease with the material, organic changes (solid lesion), because they were the most accessible and objective, even if they arose from prior liquid or vital lesions.[50] A vitalist, Laennec thought, would place the disease in the plausible but clumsy class of vital lesions.

Was there a connection between Laennec's medical philosophy and his religious and political conservatism? Indeed, what he wrote of his preferred political philosophy, similar to that of his contemporary Bonald, does have remarkable consistency with his medical philosophy. The relationship of vitalist philosophy to political and religious beliefs has been studied without finding consensus; Canguilhem criticized the inherent weakness of efforts to establish such links.[51] Nevertheless, T. Brown showed that a rise in eighteenth-century physiological vitalism can be correlated with a parallel increase in the social and institutional power of political conservatives.[52] Williams, too, related vitalism to conservatism, finding that the vitalism of Cabanis and other medical revolutionaries exerted a conservative influence, but she seemed surprised by the "tensions, paradoxes and ambiguities" that are implied by revolutionaries thinking vitalist thoughts.[53] On the other hand, Reill found an association between mechanism and royalists, whereas Pickstone argued convincingly for the links between postrevolutionary liberalism and the classifications in Bichat's so-called vitalistic physiology.[54] Others have observed that physiological vitalism can be confused with theological spiritualism through the problem of overlapping terminology, which leads to distorted agreements and conflicts.[55] It seems facile to label Laennec as a medical vitalist simply because he was a royalist and a Catholic, although those leanings may have encouraged others to do so in the past.

To understand changing perceptions of vitalism or not-vitalism in the past, it is necessary to examine the status of vitalism itself in subsequent periods. Each historian who chose to write about Laennec lived in an era that possessed its own, more or less preset attitude to vitalism and to science; the "histories" they have left reflect those views. The wish of biographers to avoid certain philosophic tags for their distant heroes complicates the task of later historians. (By making this observation, I do not presume to be immune to the influences of my own era, which has displayed a certain impatience with the whole debate.) Those who portrayed Laennec's stethoscope as a symbol of modern medicine may strive to distance the "progressive" inventor from what they think of as medical "heresy." The problem is especially evident now, when the so-called heresy in his work is not immediately apparent, and when we know that some of his papers, like the lessons pertaining to heart disease, both from his early course in pathological anatomy and from the Collège de France, have disappeared or been destroyed.

At least one of Laennec's contemporaries admitted that it was scarcely possible *not* to be a vitalist in the current state of physiology and medicine.[56] In some Restoration circles, there was an obligation to ward off charges of materialism, spawned by attempts to argue for reductionism or against vitalism, for fear of being mistaken for an antisocial atheist.[57] Nevertheless, physicochemical explanations of life and disease grew increasingly popular and powerful, whereas conscious admissions of vitalism waned with intermittent flickerings. Early in the twentieth century, in the wake of the triumph of germ theory, the biologist-turned-philosopher Hans Driesch (1867–1941) claimed to have experimentally "proven" the existence of a vital force that he called *entelechy*. His work and that of the philosopher Henri Bergson (1859–1941) encouraged a few scientists and large numbers of others to argue for vitalism.[58] The majority of scientists were skeptical of their claims.[59] The neovitalists might well have delighted in finding a figurehead in Laennec, but by then his reputation was in the hands of scientists and doctors and had been established as that of a pathological anatomist. We must remember, however, that not only did their contemporary, Rouxeau, the Nantes physiologist, write an influential biography, but he also presided over the selection, preservation, and transcription of many of Laennec's papers.

Rouxeau wrote his biography near the end of a struggle by his fellow physiologists in France and elsewhere for professional identity. In establishing themselves as members of a distinct professional discipline, physiologists conducted a kind of battle with pathologists on the one hand and clinicians on the other, highlighting their laboratory experiments as their claim to science and trying to ignore or refute the charges of practitioners who could not see useful applications for their work.[60] There were mutual accusations of arrogance. What could not be called "physiology" in a prescriptive sense that answered these social concerns, came to be called "vitalism" and was excluded. Williams has shown that holistic investigations, like Laennec's, were hounded from physiology into "the medical science of man" until the 1860s, when they were repudiated again and transformed into a rising anthropology.[61] In the early twentieth-century hagiography of the physiologist Rouxeau, Laennec was a pathologist, a clinician, and a Catholic, but he was not a vitalist, nor was he a physiologist. Laennec's claims to physiology were not acceptable to Rouxeau, but calling him a vitalist would have been even worse.

Shortly after Rouxeau's death in 1926, a few scientists said that evidence may not support the idea of vital forces, but mechanism alone would obscure "defects in knowledge" and limit possibilities for correcting them. For example, John Scott Haldane maintained that vitalism had been eliminated from the science of physiology, but doctors and surgeons would remain vitalists to a certain extent because of their experience with the sick.[62] More recently, the Medawars said that it may be impossible to think of any experiment that could falsify vitalism, but modern biologists do not find it necessary to adopt the notion of vital forces. They implied that vitalism is the opposite of science; perhaps inadvertently, they also provided a reason for its continued existence by placing it "in the limbo of that which is disregarded," because reducing life forms to material explanations has given science great success. They proposed that the equally metaphysical concept, "emergent property," be substituted for the vital force.[63] In other words, there may be more in heaven and earth than material explanations, but good science entails behaving as if there is nothing else. Whiggish authors tend to simply marvel at the incredulity of predecessors over vital forces; other more sophisticated historians have been explicit in describing vitalism as one of the famous recurring errors of biology's past. For example, Thomas S. Hall found it "interesting" that vitalism "persisted" in spite of "the successes of science"; June Goodfield-Toulmin said "no doubt the doctrine of the vital principle turned out to be wrong." As Stephen Jay Gould wryly observed, there are few, if any, self-proclaimed vitalists today.[64]

If vitalism survives in present scholarship, then its domain seems to be within the realm of mind and philosophy of mind. Psychologizing of vitalism in today's terminology is equivalent to the theologizing of the early nineteenth century. Perhaps, the shift has to do with the rising status of psychology in the aftermath of religion, reflected in the double sense of the one French word "*esprit*" conveyed by two English words, "spirit" and "mind." Is it possible that an antiphysical mind can be anything other than a metaphysical concept? Does that make its study unscientific?

In spite of the recent development of psychosomatic medicine, the possibility that emotional and spiritual conditions can translate into physical ailment is devalued in the medical context. Whenever a physical treatment can be found, psychological theorizing is discarded. For example, the advent of effective antihypertensive and antiulcer drugs closed the lively and long-standing debates about the psychological preconditions for high blood pressure and ulcer disease. Once the discussion is closed, it is as if the possibility never existed. Exemplifying the explanatory power of the medical model based on material change, a critic of modern psychiatry suggested that mental illnesses cannot be diseases, because they have no biological correlatives.[65] A similar debate surrounds the status of the new disease, chronic fatigue syndrome.[66]

The medical achievements of the preceding two centuries, including Laennec's auscultation, diminished the diagnostic credibility and significance of the patient's story. Formerly the basis of all diagnoses, symptoms became little more than unreliable signs of the objective, internal change, which had become the disease itself. Conditions without objective signs are now merely "functional," the products of a patient's imagination, insanity, or deliberate malingering. With his theory of disease—his so-called vitalism—anchored in the experience of the living patient as well as in the state of the cadaver, Laennec had anticipated the devaluing of the subjective account, and he would have sympathized with the plight of sufferers who are given no acceptable name to speak of their affliction. Functional illness for Laennec also constituted physical disease.

THE HISTORICAL DIAGNOSIS OF VITALISM

Vitalism is a word with currency in many disciplines, but its meanings are myriad and possibly meaning*less*. Vitalism is mind, free will as opposed to determinism; conversely, it has also been equated with determinism, intuition, or teleology; it is the recognition of a moral soul that influences physical being; it is holism or monism and an attack on Cartesian dualism; it is Aristotelian or Drieschian *entelechy*; it is the opposite of mechanism; the opposite of materialism; and the opposite of existentialism; it is both endorsed and refuted by Darwinian evolution; it is bioelectricity; the biological cognate of gravity; it is the opposite of scientific arrogance; it is scientific heresy.

Can vitalism be all of these things? Are there conditions under which all scholars will agree to acknowledge its existence, and can these conditions somehow be generalized? Do the typologies devised for its study really help?[67] And does vitalism exist independent of historians? Can we not correlate the discovery of vitalism or not-vitalism in the past with the political, religious, and social beliefs of individual scholars who have studied it in their times? Whether or not vitalism existed in any past philosophy, it seems we should try to clarify how it is detected by those who study it now.

The historical diagnosis of vitalism has depended on certain necessary conditions peculiar to each time and place. For Laennec, the distinguishing characteristic was "exclusivity." For Canguilhem, it was reaction to arrogance. He said that vitalism had taken on "pejorative" connotations and that "accusations" of vitalism are made to describe "the expression of mistrust . . . about the power of technology over life." If classic vitalism erred at all, he claimed, it was in the direction of too much modesty and its reticence to universalize its conception of experience.[68] His observation seems to fit the conditions under which vitalisms have been seen to arise.

For example, Rostan's confident optimism that organic lesions would eventually be found for all diseases ended discussion of diseases still awaiting their anatomic correlative: functional illness was not (yet) disease. Similar confidence arose early in the antibiotic era and again after the discovery of the structure of DNA. Ackerknecht described the enthusiastic prediction of a colleague who believed that antibiotics, hormones, and other modern drugs would soon mean that the only faculty member left in the medical school would be the historian; all other researchers would be superfluous.[69] James D. Watson expressed an equally confident sentiment with respect to molecular biology, when he said that the "mystical ideas" of the past would vanish because scientists would soon be able "to understand all of the basic features of the living state."[70] The word *nemesis,* with its implication of *hubris,* which characterizes criticisms of establishment medicine seems to conform to Canguilhem's observation.[71] Laennec had perceived this confidence in his younger colleagues, and he, too, described it as unwarranted arrogance.[72]

Recognizing "the limitations of their respective positions" has long been considered an essential step in resolving, or least retiring, the vitalist-materialist debate.[73] If ideas that come to be labeled "vitalistic" emerge in reaction to perceptions of scientific arrogance, then what is called vitalism may be a form of scientific modesty, the willingness to imagine limitations in one's own discipline. Perhaps this exaggerated, even pious "modesty," called vitalism by his peers, led a self-possessed, if not self-righteous, Laennec to accuse the medical systematists of narcissism in ignoring the reality of the patient and lessons of the past. Those who focus on areas of doubt, those who still look back, those who admit to limitations in existing methods, and especially those who insist on talking about problems that do not fit the frame and for which no words have been found, are open to the charge of antiscience and vitalism. Modern problems that evoke this kind of suspicion include the nature of control over biological organization, such as embryological differentiation and the "unzipping" of a DNA molecule.

The so-called neovitalists of the early twentieth century also conform to this pattern. They have been described as courageous because they dared to "explore the realms of experience that are neglected by science and sublimated or domesticated by myth."[74] When materialistic accounts hold sway, as they do in modern medicine, there is little room for the doubt that tempers arrogance, which has been classed by a distinguished physician as *sophrosyne*—exaggerated modesty—the equally fatal opposite of *hubris.*[75] The circle is complete: vitalists object to excessive arrogance of their so-called mechanistic colleagues; mechanists to the extreme modesty of so-called vitalists.

Scholars seem to have rejected the former definitions of vitalism long ago and presume to plow through dissimulation and verbiage to detect vitalism in many places, ignoring the claims of their subjects to the contrary. I suggest that when historians make a diagnosis of vitalism, one or more of three conditions must be met, all of which pertain to the language that frames doubt. Laennec's vitalism satisfies the first and third conditions, and a diagnosis of vitalism can be made, in our minds if not in his.

The first condition is the use of ancient, theological, or psychological language. Use of any of the old words associated with vitalism—such as vital principle or life force, *impetum faciens,* *pneuma,* ἐνορμῶντα, psyche, entelechy, anima, soul—guarantees its recognition as vitalism by late twentieth-century observers. Laennec was content to invent neologisms when he thought he had actually found some*thing* new (e.g., the stethoscopic signs and certain lesions in pathological anatomy). When he wanted to speak of the timeless clinical reality of his sick patients, a reality that had not yet been reduced to a subset of the new science, he trusted the old words of Hippocrates, even if the definition needed fine-tuning.

The second condition is the use of neologistic language. When a student of biological processes invents a new word to speak of a condition or a concept for which contemporary normal science (in the sense of Thomas Kuhn) has not yet generated conventional terminology, suspicions of vitalism are raised. If the correlative is a material thing or a physical entity, like Laennec's stethoscopic signs or his organic lesions, then the neologism is not vitalistic. If, however, the correlative is an idea, then the author is suspected of having resorted to metaphysics that falls outside the permissible bounds of science. Broussais's physiological medicine and its "irritation" would correspond to this category of vitalism. Since the middle of this century, vitalism was thought to be unscientific because it is encumbered with metaphysical entities—"the ghost in the machine"—that materialistic science can somehow avoid: "Naive" vitalisms embrace unnecessary metaphysical entities, whereas critical vitalisms do not.[76] It has been argued, however, that all language is intrinsically vitalistic and most scientific words have always contained metaphysical or metaphorical overlay.[77] Recognition of the conceptual baggage inherent in scientific language was the impetus behind the formation of nomenclature committees at research institutions and in international societies to invent labels for new viruses, enzymes, and mental diseases. Acknowledging the pervasiveness of the metaphysical baggage raises questions about the negotiation process that determines how some concepts are perceived as more metaphysical and less scientific than others.

The third condition is the subject matter itself: discussion about processes that have not been framed in physical and semantic parameters invites charges of vitalism, of arrogance, or of the "limbo of that which is disregarded." Vitalism and charges of vitalism will persist as long as people try to address the questions in life science that cannot be put in existing methodology or language, the problem that Laennec shared with Broussais. Neither managed to formulate his concerns about organicism in language that merited the approbation of "physiology" or of any other science; therefore, they were vitalists. This third condition may offer an explanation for the waxing and waning of vitalisms. Examined this way, several theories seem to have brought new waves of vitalism in their wake: mechanistic dualism, organicism, evolution, cell theory, and germ theory. Is it possible that vitalisms are found to emerge in reaction to the inadequacies of new jargon—the discourse that trails a scientific revolution—a reaction that criticizes both closure and arrogance? Do they seem to fade as the questions they seek to address are either ignored or rephrased in terminology that satisfies and can be incorporated into the new paradigm?

Laennec's apparent vitalism may have been a reaction to the materialism that his own discovery had endorsed; it represents a repudiation, or at least a mistrust, of the reductionist language that auscultation had generated. The suppression of his physiological ideas was effected by his translator, his rival, and his cousin, in response to the radical positivists of the early nineteenth century who presumed to demarcate their science from metaphysics through empirical verification. Laennec knew that the vital principle could not be falsified, because pathological anatomy would not explain all illnesses, nor could it explain the causes of those diseases that it had managed to define. There would still be another sick person, even a dead person, whose body appeared to be intact. In that, he continues to be right.

Listening to the Sick

The diagnostic possibilities introduced by the stethoscope made its inventor one of the founders of modern medicine in the conceptualization and diagnosis of disease. Laennec, however, refused to endorse the narrow extrapolation of organicism, which reduced the unknown essence and cause of disease to the physical change. Organicism was refuted by the stories of his patients and by the psychic or unknown causes of their illnesses, which were being neglected in the overenthusiastic application of his own anatomical method. In becoming a nonorganicist, he was effectively construed to be a vitalist by those who viewed that term as an insult. He recognized the existence of a "physiological something," a metaphysical entity that transcended the bounds of science to acknowledge, but not answer, the question of etiology.

The materialist counterreaction to Laennec's perceived vitalism was sufficient to blot out the memory of his lectures. His opponents were well-placed to control the praise and direct the veneration to an appreciation of only those contributions that they deemed valuable: pathology and physical diagnosis. His physiology and his therapeutics were cast aside. It is no coincidence that the resurgence of Laennec's reputation took place when the content of his unpublished lessons had been forgotten or suppressed.

Almost instantaneously, however, and long before the inventor had become a national paragon of pathology, the impact of the stethoscope was felt on both the profession and the public. Auscultation had made it possible to recast chest diseases as structural entities of the thoracic organs, instead of as the slippery, subjective patterns of symptoms that they had been. Because pulmonary diseases were considered the most frequent cause of morbidity and mortality, the revolution in thoracic diagnosis became a model for all other diseases. As a result, the explanatory power of Laennec's discovery spilled over into other domains, and medicine became preoccupied with the search for pathognomonic signs that could link gastrointestinal and psychic symptoms with lesions in the abdomen and the head. Conceptual and instrumental tools were devised to facilitate the search: phrenology, pleximeters, specula, ophthalmoscopes, and endoscopes. X-ray machines, Crosby capsules, fiberoptics, Computerized Axial Tomography (CAT scans), and Magnetic Resonance Imaging (MRI) are their direct descendants.

Finally, it was possible for physicians to prove that a person was physically sick without feeling sick. With the stethoscope, the doctor could detect a lesion before the patient had suffered any symptoms. Even people who felt completely well could no longer be certain that they were. Reiser compared Laennec's invention to Gutenberg's, as the instrument that turned the focus of medicine from sick people to disease.[78] Physicians became the custodians of knowledge that had previously belonged only to their patients. Laennec is their hero.

Soon it would become difficult for anyone to be considered sick—even in the face of debilitating, bodily symptoms—if the physician could not identify an organic "fact." This discrediting of the sufferer disturbs inhabitants of the late twentieth century, and, as Charles Rosenberg has observed, the discomfiture may have its roots in the disciplinary dilemmas of the last century: "In some ways the nineteenth century's conflicted style of thinking about physiology and pathology is still very much with us. . . . Although most of us entertain a secure faith in reductionist medicine and its credentialed practitioners, we nevertheless seek an understanding that will allow us to predict our future and impose a morally coherent meaning on individual actions."[79] Like those who praise modern medicine, critics of its paternalism and technological dependency have situated the beginning of the end of the old ways in the stethoscope.[80] Laennec could be their villain, but these critics do not know that the inventor shared their concerns. When the stethoscope told him nothing about the body of his sick patient, he continued to believe in the possibility of disease, and he listened still.

A Note on Sources: Scientific Papers and Correspondence

SCIENTIFIC PAPERS

Most papers pertaining to Laennec's professional life are kept in two archives, the Musée Laennec (ML) at the Université de Nantes and the Bibliothèque Interuniversitaire de Médecine de Paris (BIUM). The indispensable guide to the scientific papers is Boulle et al. 1982, but the excellent work of Bishop 1981 is also useful. Professeur Jackie Pigeaud of the Université de Nantes is director of a long-term project to publish the Laennec papers.

The scientific papers can be divided into four types:

I. Clinical case records of hospital and private patients
A. Hospital records (mostly but not exclusively in ML, Cl. I, II, and III). More than seven hundred case histories of patients attended between 1801 and 1826 have been preserved, but large gaps in the sequence of dates and comparison with the hospital statistics imply that the surviving records represent only a small fraction of the patients Laennec might have examined (see Tables 5.1, 5.2, 10.1). Sixty-six manuscript case reports date from the critical first phase of his work from 1816 to 1819 (in Cl. I, lot b); sixteen of these histories were published in the first two editions of the *Traité de l'ausculta-tion* (see Appendix C). Forty-three other Necker hospital cases were attended in the years following the first edition of his book. The remaining hospital histories appear to have been collected by Laennec's cousin, Mériadec, at the Hôtel Dieu and the Charité hospitals between 1819 and 1826. More than two hundred of these patients were admitted during Laennec's various absences from Paris, and their care was supervised by his friends, Cayol, Landré-Beauvais, or Récamier.

Accompanying each report are the dates of entry and of discharge or death; the hospital, ward, and bed number; the patient's name and, if a married woman, her maiden name as well; the age, occupation, and origin, if not Parisian. Problems arise in determining the exact numbers of different individuals because the students occasionally made spelling mistakes; as a result, some patients appear to have been more than one person. Records of admission and death of these same patients can be found in the Archives de l'Assistance Publique, Paris.

B. Private consultations (especially ML, MS Cl.1, Cl. 5, lot d, and Cl. 7, lot e).

II. Lecture notes used in teaching

A. The course in pathological anatomy from 1803 to 1806, divided in two parts: Laennec's own notes and those of a student (BIUM MS 2186 (I) and ML, Carnet de J. Guépin)

B. A course on Hippocratic doctrine that was never taught, ca. 1811 (ML, Cl. 1)

C. Laennec's notes for lessons at the Collège de France, 1822–1826, divided in two parts (BIUM, MS 2186 (IV) and ML, Cl. 2 lot a, parts A and B). Notes taken by three students at these lectures can be found at ML (Cl. 7, lot c), Archives of Hahneman Medical College (MS Kitchen), and College of Physicians (MS Dufour), both in Philadelphia.

III. Texts of other material intended for publication

A. The treatise on pathological anatomy, divided in two parts (BIUM, MS 2186 (III) and ML, Cl. 7, lot a)

B. Various articles scattered throughout the papers

C. Translations of classical texts (ML, especially Cl. 1, lot r [Aretaeus] and Cl. 5, lot j [Caelius Aurelianus])

IV. Loose notes, mostly citations from other authors and ideas used in preparation of other work (ML, Cl. 1, Cl. 3, and BIUM MS 5172)

The important 1818 mémoire on auscultation is held by the Académie des Sciences and several essays and reports written by Laennec for the Société de l'Ecole de Médecine can be examined in the archives of the Académie Nationale de Médecine, both in Paris.

The material at BIUM is available on microfiche. Most of the material at the ML has been microfilmed, but at the time of writing copies cannot be obtained, although scholars may make photocopies from the microfilm if they visit the ML. It is advisable to seek permission before planning a visit.

CORRESPONDENCE

Early in this century, more than one thousand letters of the Laennec family were made available to Alfred Rouxeau, professor of physiology at the Université de Nantes; approximately 350 of these letters were written by Laennec. Rouxeau transcribed the letters and published excerpts from or references to a total of 342 of the family letters (of which 196 were written by Laennec) in his authoritative two-volume biography, which became the principal source for all subsequent historians. Rouxeau's personal notes and transcriptions, with his other papers on the history of Nantes and its medical school, were donated by his widow to the Municipal Library of Nantes where they have been preserved as the "Fonds Rouxeau." Thirty-four volumes of this extensive collection pertain to Laennec.

As a source on auscultation, the letters are disappointing. Rouxeau's notes and other sources show that Laennec wrote at least 350 letters to his family and friends from 1794 to 1826, or an average of 11 letters a year (range 0 to 23). The number of originals and/or copies extant from each of the critical years from 1815 to 1820 is 23, 15, 1, 8, 22, and 18, respectively. Between January 1817 and August 1818, the period of most active research on auscultation, there are copies of three letters, only one of which I have been able to trace in the original. A similar "decline" in letters written by Laennec appears for the period 1809 to 1811, when the Laennec family was wrangling over the legal arrangement established by Michaud (see chap. 4). If they existed, letters from the important period on auscultation may have been hoarded separately long before Rouxeau asked to make his transcriptions, only to be lost or sold to unknown purchasers.

As part of the Laennec bicentenary in the early 1980s, Professeur Jean Kernéis, Dean of the Faculty of Medicine at the Université de Nantes, encouraged five medical students to undertake faithful reproduction of the Rouxeau transcriptions for their medical theses. The correspondence from 1794 to 1826 was divided into five segments, and the students' work reproduces the contents of the eleven most important volumes (*liasses*) of the Fonds Rouxeau pertaining to Laennec. They include transcriptions of a thousand letters, of which just over 300 were written by R. T. H. Laennec (see Bouvier 1980; Crochet 1982; Huybrechts 1980; Pinson 1980; Roux de Reilhac 1980). These five theses are a valuable asset to study of Laennec and the life of an entire family during the French Revolution, the First Empire, and the Restoration, but they have unavoidable limitations: being only transcriptions of transcriptions, their reliability rests on the reliability of Rouxeau.

Nearly a century later, I have been able to trace only eighty percent of the original letters by Laennec that had been copied by Rouxeau. I have found a few letters that were unknown to him, and fewer yet of the letters written by other family members. M. Hervé de Miniac of Rennes generously opened his private collection, including more than one hundred letters written by R. T. H. Laennec to his father. Dr. Eric Laennec and his brother François, on behalf of their family in Lyons, allowed me to examine the collection of more than one hundred letters written by Laennec to his uncle Guillaume and his cousins Christophe and Ambroise. Sadly, however, the Lyons Laennecs are unable to locate a manuscript of Christophe's "Souvenirs," which included an eye-witness account of the attack of Nantes, but they have carefully kept the Dubois portrait and a previously unknown, one-hundred-page manuscript, written and illustrated by Laennec on agricultural practices and architecture. The Chéguillaume family of Nantes gave permission to consult the incomplete collection of Laennec's letters to his cousin Mériadec held in the Archives Départementales of the Loire Atlantique in Nantes. Canon Jean-Louis Floc'h kindly showed me the letters from Laennec to the Bishop of Quimper held in the archives of the Eveché de Quimper. Four letters by

Laennec to the *prefet* of Finistère are held in the Archives Départementales de Finistère; and some of his correspondence with physicians, former students, and other scholars is held in the Musée Laennec. A few other letters can be found in libraries or private collections around the world. Some have been published; others have become objects of commercial interest: a three-page letter by Laennec concerning the health of a cousin was sold at public auction in the Salles Drouot Richelieu on 15 March 1995 for the sum of 40,500 French francs.

Comparison of the extant original documents with Rouxeau's copies assures us that the biographer was meticulous, his transcriptions almost complete, and the extent of his cross-referenced notes impressive. He was utterly devoted to his project and obsessive in his work; there is no reason to doubt his intellectual honesty. Nevertheless, there are the problems that result from working with copies made by human hands and minds.

First, the dating cannot be reconstructed with complete confidence, because of simple errors in copying and in converting from the Revolutionary calendar to the Gregorian calendar. There are several date discrepancies among the five Nantes theses and the Rouxeau notes. The correct dates cannot be known until the remainder of the original correspondence is made available. Usually, the dating errors are of only minor significance because the context helps to reconstruct the ordinal pattern.

Second, and more importantly, a few letters were not made available to Rouxeau for various reasons. M. Hervé de Miniac of Rennes told me that letters concerning the family's legal matters were considered too sensitive to have been loaned to Rouxeau at the beginning of this century. I am especially grateful to him for his generosity in making them available now.

Third, some of Rouxeau's original transcriptions were incomplete. One would expect that he excluded material that was not of interest to him, but we cannot know if it would have been of interest to us; nor do we know how he made his decisions, and we have reason to suspect problems here, too. When the portions of letters that he published in the biography are compared with his own transcriptions, it becomes clear that he made some omissions out of a sense of personal or professional loyalty. Always eager to portray his hero in the best light, he tended to hide what he saw as Laennec's "defects"—vindictiveness, vanity, jealousy, nonchalance, disorganization, frustration, anger—especially when it came to dealings with his father. He avoided showing similar failings in the "good" uncle Guillaume, whose profoundly disturbing five-year dismissal during the White Terror was largely ignored by Rouxeau, although it constituted a serious problem for the entire family. Conversely, Rouxeau tended not to report on the father's random and infrequent acts of generosity (a *lapsus* he confessed in 1920), nor did he belabor the genuine affection that this strange individual inspired in his brother and sons, leading them to tolerate his insults and failings. Rouxeau also minimized the student difficulties and the animosity between Laennec and his cousin Ambroise over Napoleon's defeat. The famous letter by Laennec to the Bishop of Quimper about the care given Breton soldiers in the Salpêtrière hospital was published, but the other letters to the same bishop were ignored, especially those that reveal the two men to have been engaged in furthering Laennec's prospects in the medical community through the interventionist Restoration government.

Rouxeau painted his picture of Laennec as "le bon Théophile," a quiet, bravely devout genius who waited patiently for his opportunities and used influence only when absolutely necessary. The biographer appears to have been especially uncomfortable with Laennec's well-developed royalist contacts and his readiness to use them in his Restoration society, where personal success required craft. Rouxeau also avoided the awkward moments in the past of his own faculty at Nantes. Guillaume had been denounced by men whose descendants may well have been colleagues of the biographer. Furthermore, Ambroise's son, Théophile-Ambroise Laennec, was the biographer's friend and father to Robert Laennec, whose generous donation of the scientific papers after his father's death in 1896 had been essential to Rouxeau's study and to my own. Rouxeau's own political and religious inclinations, together with his desire to avoid offending his fellow *Nantais*, operated in his selection of the published letters and perhaps also in the lacunae of more numerous transcriptions that he left uncited.

In making this criticism, I do not pretend to be immune from similar subconscious influences myself; however, the only way to avoid compounding the biases and errors of our predecessors is to ensure that the original letters, wherever they may be, are found, preserved, and made available to researchers through scholarly channels.

BRIEF DESCRIPTION OF MANUSCRIPT SOURCES BY ARCHIVE

AAP	Hospital Admission and Death Registers
AAS	Laennec's mémoire on auscultation, February 1818
ACF	Papers on Laennec's appointment to the Collège de France
	Carnet des inscriptions
ADF	Laennec's letter to the prefet of Finstère; letters by Laennec *père*
ADLA	Laennec's letters to Mériadec; material pertaining to Nantes schools
AEQ	Laennec's letters to the Bishops of Quimper
AJésuites	Laennec's Congrégation essay 1807
	Carnet des inscriptions for the Congrégation
AMN	Records of baptisms and deaths for the Laennecs of Nantes
AMP	Record of Laennec's marriage
	Record of the sale of Laennec's estate; apartment inventory
AN	Records of the Faculty of Medicine of Paris
	Records of the Ministry of the Interior

ANM-SEM   Papers of the Société de l'Ecole de Médecine
BIUM   Lectures, part of unpublished treatise on pathological
          anatomy, various notes
CPP   Dufour's notes of Laennec's lectures at the Collège de
          France, 1882
EUL   Carswell's notes on dissections, 1822.
HMCP   James Kitchen's notes on lectures of Broussais and Laennec,
          1823–1824
JHU   Letter Laennec to Cruveilhier; letter by Mériadec
ML   Patient records, lecture notes, part of unpublished treatise on
          pathological anatomy, letters, aphorisms of Corvisart, vari-
          ous essays, translations of Aretaeus and Caelius Aurelianus,
          notes on Hippocrates, notes by a student, notes of Méria-
          dec Laennec, lecture notes of Guillaume Laennec
MNFR   Papers of Alfred Rouxeau
MNQ   Baptism and Death records for the Laennecs of Quimper
NYAM   Letters of Laennec and of Broussais

Private Collections

MS Bertrand Laennec   Letters to Christophe and Guillaume Laennec
                      Will, certificates, notes on agricultural practices
MS de Miniac   Letters to Laennec *père*, other letters, will,
                      certificates
MS Puget   Petitions of Guillaume Laennec

Laennec's Finances

TABLE B.1
An Estimation of Laennec's Changing Financial Situation, 1804–1826
(in French francs)

Year	Medical Earnings	Other Income	Expenses
1804		ca. 900 father	900 fees
		600 journal	500 thesis
		300 teaching	200 clothing
1805	400	1,200 father	
		1,000 journal	
		300 teaching	
1806		6,00 father	
		1,000 journal	
		300 teaching	
1807	2,400	600 father	270 rent
		1,000 journal	508 furniture
1808	3,400–3,600		270 rent
1809	(3,000 from Fesch) +		700 clothing, etc.
			1,500 cook, servant
1810	7,000–8,000		600–1,000 father
	(3,000 from Fesch)		540 fees debt
			6,000 total costs
1811	8,000–9,000		800–1,000 father rent
	(3,000 from Fesch)		& cook
			spent 400 more than
			he earned
1812	6,000		1,200 sister
			1,500 sister's move
			1,500 legal fees
			ca. 1,000 father rent
			& cook
1813	10,000		1,200 sister
			ca. 1,000 father rent
			& cook
1814	5,400		1,200 sister
			ca. 1,000 father
			1,400 father's debt,
			rent & cook
1815	5,400		1,200 sister
			ca. 1,600 father
			rent & cook

TABLE B.1 *(cont.)*

Year	Medical Earnings	Other Income	Expenses
1816	5,400		1,200 sister
	after September Necker hospital		ca. 1,000 father
			3,000 cabriolet
1817	Necker hospital		1,200 sister
1818	Necker hospital		1,200 sister
1819	3,500 1st ed. *Traité*		1,000 scientific expense
	Necker hospital		1,200 sister
	10,000–12,000 owed from private practice (expects only 4,000 to be paid)		
1820	3,300 rent from property		900 taxes and repairs
	2,000 sale of books and furniture		3,000 to drain marsh
	10,000 still owed from practice		1,200 sister
			1,200 cost of living
1821	3,300 rent from property		300 taxes and repairs
			1,200 cost of living
			1,200 sister
1822	4,000 Duchesse de Berry		1,700 rent
	5,000 Collège de France		1,200 sister
	20,000 consultations Necker hospital		
1823	3,000 Faculty salary		1,700 rent
	5,000 Collège de France		1,200 sister
	4,000 Duchesse de Berry		
	20,000 consultations		
	10,000 rumored fee for a single consultation in Bordeaux (may have been promised 50,000 if patient was saved)		
1824	5,000 Collège de France		3,000 rent
	4,000 Duchesse de Berry		invested 12,500
	3,000 Faculty		1,200 sister
	20,000 consultations		
1825	5,000 Collège de France		3,000 rent
	4,000 Duchesse de Berry		invested 3,750
	3,000 Faculty		3,000 more in marsh
	20,000 consultations		1,200 sister
1826	3,000 Faculty		3,000 rent
	3,500 2d ed. *Traité*		invested 3,750
	Leaves Duchesse de Berry		1,200 sister
	Leaves Collège de France		

TABLE B.2
Laennec's Wills and Estate

Year	Estate
1812	Testament of 1 December 1812, executor Christophe Laennec
	Annual pension to father of 1,100F if he renounces claims on
	his children
	Annual pension of 300F to sister, but only after father's death
1824	At marriage "séparation des biens": 15,000F spouse; 40,000F himself
1826	Testament of 20 April 1826, executor Christophe Laennec
	Monetary assets 12,500F in Corrèze canals
	Anticipated 6,000F from sale of second edition of treatise
	All property and proceeds of sales to his wife, except
	books, papers, portrait, pocket watch, small property to Mériadec
	annual pension to father 1,000F; reduced to 600F/yr in a codicil
	annual pension to sister 600F; reduced to 200F in codicil
	small property and money to Emmanuel after wife's death
	books on Breton subjects to Quimper library
	Kerlouarnec to Ambroise, but not to be sold until after wife's death
	Contents of Paris apartment (5,320.75F), remainder for Mériadec after
	wife's death
1826	3,000F annual pension awarded by Crown to his widow (revoked in 1830)
	992F Faculty of Medicine paid in lump sum to widow
1827	5,000 Montyon prize honorable mention for the *Treatise on Auscultation*

Sources: Correspondence de Laennec; annual budgets in "Procès verbaux de l'assemblée des professeurs de la Faculté de Médecine," 1823–26, Archives Nationales AJ/16/6233-6; "Vente de 16 octobre 1826," AMP, D.90.E³, art. 3; testament of 1 December 1812, MS Bertrand Laennec; testament of 20 April 1826, MS de Miniac no. 129; Forbes 1834, xxivn.

Note: For comparison with other physician estates, see Weisz 1995, 273.

Patients in the Two Editions of the
Traité de l'auscultation

Case histories of Laennec's patients informed his discoveries and were used as evidence in support of his claims; in turn, the form and meaning of the records were altered by his new methodology. In this book, I have examined published and unpublished patient records to explore his development and interpretation of auscultation. Because other scholars may find new applications for these intriguing documents, this appendix is intended as a guide to the published case histories. Part I locates the fifty complete case observations in each of the first two editions of Laennec's treatise on mediate auscultation with a few features that were important to my argument. Part II locates ninety-five incomplete and often brief histories of patients or clusters of patients that peppered the text. Part III locates 124 additional histories added for the second edition. Some of these short histories do not appear to have been formally recorded: they were remembered rather than cited; others were recounted by medical authors or colleagues whose names appear in the "name" column.

Some encounters described in Part II and Part III were of greater heuristic significance than those in Part I: for example, the prototypical "*jeune personne*" who was the first to be examined with a paper stethoscope and the unnamed women in whom Laennec first recognized the phenomenon called pectoriloquy. This observation is scarcely surprising: Laennec did not realize that he had made a discovery or a small breakthrough until he had reflected on what he had seen and heard; then he would systematically examine the next patients to test his hypotheses about the new signs. Records of the discoveries might be incomplete for several reasons: the phenomenon was discounted initially and not recorded; it was recorded, but could not be found because he could not recall the name or date of the encounter; there was no vocabulary for recording it. The systematic testing and confirmation of the finding would result in a formal, complete case observation.

In Part I, the records are sorted chronologically to support the discussion in chapter 6. Patients are identified by age, sex, occupation, and name, but this information was not always complete. References and cross-references are provided for the case number, indicating the relative ordinal location in the treatise. "MS" indicates that a corresponding manuscript resides in the Musée Laennec, Nantes. As shown in chapter 6, Laennec focused on one or two new findings at a time: several complete case histories on the same topic could be collected within a few days of each other; for example, notice the occasional proximity of the ordinal case numbers in chronologically consecutive cases, especially for cases on heart signs and egophony.

In Part II, the records are ordered by their location in the first edition. The relevant diagnosis has been included. When the features of auscultation and autopsy were not indicated, then the topic of discussion usually centered on the symptoms of the illness, its cause, or its cure, that is, the pathophysiology of the disease. Laennec's debt to the work of Bayle is evident in the first edition. For the second edition, he engaged with the work of Andral, despite his criticism of the younger man in his preface. Differences between the two editions are more obvious in the presentation of the brief cases than in the complete observations. In the second edition, Laennec placed a greater emphasis on treatment and cure, with tartar emetic, magnets, and other modalities; he also conformed to a positivistic trend to include increasingly large clusters of cases to emphasize his statements. He continued to doubt the reliability of the stethoscope in the detection of aneurysms.

TABLE C.1

Complete Case Histories in the *Traité de l'auscultation médiate*, 1819 and 1826

Date	Name/Occupation	Age	Sex	Ausc.	Pm	Psych.	1819 no.	1826 no.*	MS
n.d.	M***, Mlle, piano teacher	72	f		pm	Ψ	12	2	
15 Mar 1802	C***, Marie, seamstress	41	f		pm	Ψ	18		
28 Aug 1803	Lefebvre, Philibert, farmer	65	m		pm	Ψ w	49	50	
9 Jan 1808	Anon., "un nègre"	6	m		pm		29	45	
15 Feb 1808	Lajoie, Henri Alexandre	3	m		pm		11	1	
20 July 1811	Anon., policeman	53	m		pm		14	13	
20 Dec 1811	Anon.	45	m		pm		15	14	
n.d.	Anon., lady	jeune	f				8	24	
25 Sep 1816	Gautier, Alexandrine, cook	59	f		pm	Ψ	22	30	
15 Oct 1816	Anon.	65	m		pm		30	36	MS
6 May 1817	Anon	55	f	?	pm		35		
24 May 1817	Millet, Jean, mercer	67	m	?	pm		50	51	
2 June 1817	Basset, Marie-Mélanie	40	f	a	pm		34	11	
6 Dec 1817	Potel, Marie, lingerie maker	40	f	a	pm	Ψ	47	48	
n.d. 1818	D***, M, crown prosecutor		m	a	alive		10	26	
3 Jan 1818	Bellot, Pierre	32	m	a	pm	Ψ	2	18	
9 Jan 1818	Day, servant	68	f	a	pm		1	17	
19 Jan 1818	Anon.40		f	a	pm		3	19	
8 Feb 1818	N****	40	f	a	pm		38	29	
9 Feb 1818	Anon., Polish man		m		pm		5	21	MS
14 Feb 1818	Anon., notary in Nantes	65	m	a	pm	Ψ	6	22	MS
26 Feb 1818	Potu, J. M., old soldier	30	m	a	pm	Ψ w	39	38	MS
Mar 1818	G**, English prisoner	36	m	a	alive	Ψ w	9	25	
9 Mar 1818	Anon., Basque	20	m	a	pm		40	39	MS
13 Mar 1818	Anon.	60	m	a	pm		23	31	MS
3 Apr 1818	Roussel, E., army cook	47	f	a	pm	w	32	9	
9 Apr 1818	Anon., manual laborer	62	m	a	pm		7	23	M.
24 May 1818	Anon.	37	f	a	pm		26	32	
28 June 1818	Petit (as Anon.), mason	66	m	a	pm		28	34	M!
27 July 1818	G***, Madame	48	f	a	alive		4	20	
1 Aug 1818	Hardy, Michel, day worker	42	m	a	pm		16	15	M.
12 Aug 1818	Coulon, Louis, mason	18	m	a	pm		27	33	M!
19 Oct 1818	Cocard, J. B. farmer	37	m	a	pm		19	6	M!
7 Nov 1818	Boulanger, J. metalworker	35	m	a	pm		41	40	
11 Dec 1818	Anon., butcher	40	m	a	pm		13	12	
22 Dec 1818	Anon.	50	f		pm		17	5	
5 Jan 1819	C****, carter	30	m	a	pm		20	7	
11 Jan 1819	Jolivet, Jeanne, widow	52	f	a	pm		21	8	
22 Jan 1819	Moineau, Pierre, cobbler	22	m	a	pm		43	42	M
8 Feb 1819	Dirichard, J. B., artisan	45	m	a	pm		36	49	
11 Feb 1819	Ponsard, gardener/servant	16	m	a	alive		45	46	
18 Feb 1819	Brouan, Louis F., cobbler	29	m	a	pm	Ψ w	42	43	M
18 Feb 1819	Villeneuve, J., locksmith	30	m	a	pm		48		

TABLE C.1 *(cont.)*

›ate	Name/Occupation	Age	Sex	Ausc.	Pm	Psych.	1819 no.	1826 no.*	MS
Mar 1819	Anon., enfant	12	m	a	alive	Ψ	44	44	
8 Mar 1819	Léraut, Arsène, seamstress	26	f	a	pm		31	41	MS
2 Apr 1819	Anon., manual laborer	35	m	a	pm	Ψ	46	47	
May 1819	B***, Françoise	45	f	a	pm	Ψ	33	10	
7 May 1819	Edmé, Jean, cotton factory	47	m	a	pm	w	25	35	MS
1 May 1819	Villeron, Simon, hatter	42	m	a	alive	w	24		
June 1819	Levas, Marianne, laundress	50	f	a	pm		37	28	
d. 1821–1822	Anon.		m	a	pm			3	
7 July 1822	C***[Chauveau?], physician	36	m	a	pm			37	
4 Apr 1825	Chopinet, R. M., coach driver	41	m	a	pm			4	MS
May 1825	Richard, François, weaver	22	m	a	pm			16	MS

Note: Date, applies to the date of death or autopsy; if lacking, then discharge date. MS, Correspond-ing manuscript in Musée Laennec. a, Auscultation was recorded. pm, An autopsy was performed. Ψ, psychological antecedents given in the history. w, Mention of war or the Revolution.
* No case no. 27 in 1826.

TABLE C.2
Brief Case Histories First Used in the *Traité de l'auscultation médiate*, 1819

1819	1826	Year	Patient or physician	Ausc.	Pm	Diagnosis
1:7	1:7	1816	"young" female	a		heart disease?
1:17			woman [first]	a		pectoriloquy
1:18			cluster	a		pectoriloquy, no symptoms
1:36			Bayle's case		pm	phthisis
1:37			Bayle's case		pm	phthisis
1:38	1:539		Bayle's case		pm	phthisis
1:57			Bayle's 5 cases			phthisis
1:57	1:694	1806	woman		pm	fatty liver, pthisis
1:57	1:157*		Bayle's case		pm	catarrh vs. phthisis
1:57*	1:157*		Bayle's case		pm	catarrh vs. phthisis
1:121			Bayle's case			phthisis
1:121			Bayle's case			phthisis
1:127		1817	woman	a	pm	bronchiectasis
1:148		1817	cluster 150 cases	a		pneumonia
1:161	1:395		Bayle's case		pm	pneumonia
1:163			pathology specimen		pm	hepatized lung
1:163	1:398		Anon.		pm	pneumonia
1:164	1:406		cluster 5 or 6 cases		pm	abscess in lung, pneumonia

TABLE C.2 *(cont.)*

1819	1826	Year	Patient or physician	Ausc.	Pm	Diagnosis
1:165	1:407		pathology specimen		pm	abscess in lung
1:171*	1:415*	1804	cluster			pneumonia epidemic
1:186	1:448		Bayle's 6 cases		pm	phthisis gangrenous
1:216	1:296		Taranguet's case		pm	emphysema infiltration
1:225	1:298		Magendie's case		pm	emphysema
1:273*	2:7	1804	Anon.		pm	hydatids lung
1:277	2:12	1801	Anon.			acephalocytes
1:277	2:12	1798	man		alive	hydatids
1:277	2:13		Anon.		alive	hydatids
1:278	2:13	1811	Anon.		alive	hydatids
1:285	2:23		Bayle's case			phthisis concretion
1:285	2:23		Bayle's case			phthisis concretion
1:297	2:31*		Bayle's case		pm	phthisis melanosis
1:323	2:64		Bayle's case		pm	phthisis
1:371	2:158		M*** surgeon	a	alive	retraction of chest
1:405	2:128		Anon.		pm	gangrene pleura
1:410	2:229		Morand's case			hydropsy operation cure
1:431	2:380		Richter's case			hernia diaphragmatic
1:431	2:380		Sabatier's case			hernia diaphragmatic
1:431	2:380		Boerhaave's case			hernia diaphragmatic
1:431	2:380		Grateloup's case			hernia diaphragmatic
1:433	2:242		Itard's 5 cases			pneumothorax
1:436			Bayle's case			phthisis
1:437	2:246		Littre's case		pm	pneumothorax effusion
1:437	2:247		Hewson's case		pm	pneumothorax
2:17–18	1:358		man	a	pm	pulmonary edema
2:43	1:381		man		pm	pulmonary apoplexy
2:63*			woman	a		phthisis, confused signs
2:65			old man		pm	catarrh
2:65			pathology specimen		pm	catarrh fever
2:124	2:278		man	a		Hippocratic succussion
2:181	2:332		Laennec himself		alive	accidental scalpel wound
2:249			[Laennec?]		alive	angina neurotic
2:284	2:529		published case		pm	heart partial dilatation
2:292			girl, 12 yr		alive	palpitations atrophy heart
2:292			woman, 18 yr		alive	palpitations atrophy heart
2:293	2:739		woman		pm	atrophy heart; "cholera"
2:300	2:566	1816	male law student		pm	hardening of heart
2:303	2:555		Meckel's case		pm	carditis
2:303	2:555		Benivieni's case		pm	abscess in heart
2:304			Morgagni's case		pm	abscess in heart
2:304	2:556		man		pm	abscess in heart
2:304			Anon.		pm	abscess in heart
2:306	2:558		Morand's case		pm	rupture of heart
2:306	2:558		Morgagni's case		pm	rupture of heart

TABLE C.2 *(cont.)*

19	1826	Year	Patient or physician	Ausc.	Pm	Diagnosis
18		1817	cluster 18 cases			angina of the chest
18		1812	cluster			angina of the chest
19			cluster	a		pectoriloquy disappears
25			Morgagni's case		pm	heart polyps
26			Dupuytren's case		pm	heart polyps
29			pathology specimen		pm	obstructed vena cava
29			pathology specimen		pm	obstructed carotid artery
29			pathology specimen		pm	obstructed vessels
52	2:650	1817	woman	a		heart-pulse differ
56			young woman		pm	red membrane artery
64	2:551*		man		pm	heart congenital
75	2:657		man		pm	pericarditis
76	2:658		Anon.		pm	pericarditis adherent
91			cluster		pm	pericarditis undetected
97			cluster 2 or 3		pm	tubercles in pericardium
19	2:704	1806	man		pm	aneurysm aorta
28	2:714		Zeink's case		pm	aneurysm
29	2:714		Corvisart's case		pm	false aneurysm, thoracic canal
29			pathology specimen		pm	aneurysm
31	2:717		cluster 2 or 3 cases			aneurysm aorta
31	2:716		Anon.			aneurysm aorta
34	2:720		Anon.			aneurysm aorta
36	2:722		woman			aneurysm thrill
36	2:759	1808	woman		alive	aneurysm disappears
38*			cluster 2 cases	a	pm	aneurysm aorta
38	2:723		cluster 10+ cases	a	alive	aneurysm aorta
39			woman	a	pm	aneurysm misdiagnosed
39			old man	a	pm	aneurysm misdiagnosed
40			woman	a	pm	aneurysm misdiagnosed
42	2:760		lady	a	alive	aneurysm murmur
43	2:761		lady	a	alive	aneurysm nervous origin

Note: Abbreviations are the same as those in table C.1. The 1819 reference is to the volume and page number on which the case begins. The 1826 reference is given if the case also appeared in the second edition.

Cross-reference to same case elsewhere in the edition.

TABLE C.3

Brief Case Histories First Used in the *Traité de l'auscultation médiate*, 1826

1826	Year	Patient or physician	Ausc.	Pm	Diagnosis
1:139		Andral's 2 cases		pm	catarrh
1:140	1821	man			catarrh healed
1:156		Andral's case XVII			catarrh chronic
1:165		woman, Bree's case	a?		bronchial afflux
1:168		man, politician, 70 yr			catarrh pituitous
1:168		man, politician, 60 yr			catarrh pituitous
1:169		Andral's case XIV			catarrh pituitous
1:169		Andral's case XVI		pm	catarrh pituitous
1:173		Andral's case II		pm	catarrh dry
1:173		Andral's case III		pm	catarrh dry
1:189		man	a		whooping cough
1:215		Andral's case VI	a	pm	dilatation heart, bronchial disease
1:216		Andral's case VIII	a	pm	phthisis, dilatation bronchii
1:246		child, Bretonneau's case		pm	croup, false membrane ear
1:246		Dr. Bourgeoise himself			sore throat, false membrane anus
1:246	1823	man			scarlatina, false membrane
1:264		Cayol's case		pm	ulcer bronchial
1:264		Andral's case		pm	ulcers bronchial bifurcation
1:264		Andral's case		pm	ulcers bronchial ramification
1:264		Andral's case		pm	ulcers bronchial ramification
1:265		Andral's 2 cases		pm	ulcers bronchial perforations
1:274		Guersent's case		pm	fistula into esophagus
1:275		Anon.		pm	worm hamularia lymphatica
1:286		man		pm	hypertrophy lung & retractic
1:385		young man			pulmonary apoplexy
1:409		cluster 20	a	pm	abscess in lung in pneumoni
1:410		man	a		abscess in lung
1:410		woman	a		abscess in lung
1:410	1823	Honoré's case		pm	abscess in lung
1:410		Andral's case		pm	abscess in lung
1:411	1822	young man		pm	excavation without tubercles
1:415		Andral's cases VII, IX			pneumonia rapid death
1:426		man	a		pneumonia, no stethoscopic signs
1:426*		Andral's 7 cases	a		pneumonia, no stethoscopic signs
1:436		Andral's 11 cases			pneumonia with or without sputum
1:441		Andral's 112 cases			pneumonia crises
1:485	1814	cluster soldiers			pneumonia treated
1:485		cluster			fever undertreated
1:500		cluster 28 cases			pneumonia treated

TABLE C.3 *(cont.)*

826	Year	Patient or physician	Ausc.	Pm	Diagnosis
500		cluster 34 cases			pneumonia treated
501		man			pneumonia treated, died
502	1823	man	a		pneumonia treated
502	1825	M. de C . . .	a		pneumonia treated
504	1824	cluster 40 cases			pneumonia treated
505		cluster Ellis's 47 cases			pneumonia treated
511		A. Laennec's case			tetanus cured
511*		woman			inflammation arm veins treated
539		Bayle's 4 cases		pm	phthisis
643		mortality statistic			phthisis and climate
647		community of nuns	a		phthisis
649	1806	Laennec himself			tubercle finger
650		mortality statistic			phthisis and contagion
652		Bayle's cases			phthisis and age
664	1817	man	a	pm	pectoriloquy phthisis
666		Louis's case			pneumothorax symptoms
688		man		pm	amygdales (tonsils)
698		woman			phthisis masked by hypo-chondria
701	1806	woman, 18 yr		pm	phthisis
702	1818	man	a		phthisis
716		cluster 6 cases			phthisis cure in Brittany
13	1821	lady		alive	worms in lung
87		Andral's case XX		pm	asthma, fatal suffocation
88		Guersent's 2 child cases		pm	asthma
89*		horseman			asthma
90		M. le comte H**			asthma
110		Andral's 3 cases		alive	pleurisy dry
119		Andral's case XV		pm	pleural effusion of blood
130		Andral's 2 cases		pm	gangrene pleura
130		Andral's case		pm	pleurisy acute drained
137*		Cayol's case	a		pneumothorax signs
200		Andral's case XXIV		pm	pleurisy circumscribed
201		Anon. 3 cases		pm	pleurisy circumscribed
211	1824	child	a		pleurisy effusion
230	1825	woman	a	pm	hydropsy egophony
231	1824	woman	a	pm	hydropsy
232		old woman		pm	hydropsy
283		cluster 30 cases	a		Hippocratic succussion
341		Bayle's 5 cases		pm	pneumothorax
359	1820	man	a		pneumothorax and empyema
364	1814	man		pm	pneumothorax double
364	1816	man		pm	pneumothorax double phthisis

TABLE C.3 *(cont.)*

1826	Year	Patient or physician	Ausc.	Pm	Diagnosis
2:369		Prussian man		pm	accidental production pleura tubercles
2:377		man, Dupuytren's case		pm	lung cysts
2:424	1824	lady	a		carotid bruit; hemoptysis
2:426		2 cases	a		carotid bruit
2:426		man	a		carotid bruit
2:426		lady	a		carotid bruit
2:454	1824	2 women	a		heartbeat at a distance
2:454*	1823	woman	a		heartbeat at a distance
2:455		cluster 20	a		heartbeat at a distance
2:461		Kergaradec's case	a		placental souffle
2:463		Ollivry's 4 cases	a		placenta location
2:467		nun			palpitations 8 days
2:501		Bertin & Louis's cases		pm	hypertrophy heart
2:505	1825	Anon.			hypertrophy right heart jugular vein
2:527	1826	Berard's 2 cases		pm	dilatation heart partial
2:531	1821	man		pm	hardening, hypertrophy hear
2:532		Bertin's 3 cases		pm	hardening of heart
2:547		Anon.	a	pm	perforation cardiac septum
2:550	1823	Anon.	a	pm	hypertrophy incrustations valves
2:559		Bertin's 2 cases		pm	carditis, rupture
2:570		Anon.		pm	scirrhous tumor heart
2:570	1822	Anon.		pm	cancer encephaloid heart
2:570	1822	Andral & A. Bayle's 3 cases		pm	cancer encephaloid heart
2:575		Bertin & Louis's case		pm	hardening valves
2:579		Bertin's case		pm	ossification sigmoid valve
2:604		pathology specimen		pm	red internal membrane
2:617		man, magistrate		pm	clot saphenous vein, no inflammation
2:634		girl, Tonnelier's case		pm	arsenic suicide
2:664		Corvisart's case		pm	pericarditis adherent
2:666		man		pm	pericarditis adherent
2:685		cluster 3 or 4 cases		pm	narrowing aorta
2:685		boy, 14 yr		pm	obliterated aorta
2:686		woman		pm	narrowing aorta, vegetations valves
2:715		Anon.		pm	aneurysm rupture spinal cor
2:727	1819	young woman	a	pm	aneurysm
2:729		Paré's case		pm	dilatation pulmonary artery
2:736		Scottish woman			palpitations, died of treatme

TABLE C.3 *(cont.)*

26	Year	Patient or physician	Ausc.	Pm	Diagnosis
37		notary, Corvisart's case			heart disease cured by purgatives
48		cluster several cases			angina of chest
51		woman			hiccoughs cured by magnet
51		man			paralysis cured by magnet
66		cluster	a		murmur without thrill
68		Laennec himself	a		intestinal gas, audible heatbeat

Note: 1826 reference is to volume and page number on which the case begins. Abbreviations are the
ne as those in table C.1.
Cross-references to same case elsewhere in edition.

Laennec's Network: A Glossary of Frequently Cited Names

Andral, Gabriel (1797–1876), physician, early investigator of auscultation, Laennec's rival, edited fourth French edition of the treatise on auscultation.

Argou, Jacquemine Guichard (1779–1847), widow, paid companion of Madame de Pompéry; in 1805, Laennec's friend; in 1822, his housekeeper; in 1824, his wife.

Baillie, Matthew (1761–1823), Scottish pathologist, admired by Laennec who sent him *Treatise on Auscultation* 1819.

Bayle, Antoine-Laurent-Jesse (1799–1858), nephew of G. L. Bayle, physician, Congréganist, editor, medical librarian.

Bayle, Gaspard-Laurent (1774–1816), Provençal, physician, pathologist, Congréganist, Laennec's friend.

Becquey, François-Louis (1769–1849), royalist, bureaucrat in ministry of the interior in charge of hospitals, director of office on bridges and roads, Laennec's friend and patron.

Berry, Marie-Caroline-Ferdinande-Louise, the Duchesse de (1798–1870), widowed daughter-in-law of King Charles X, mother of heir to the throne, Laennec's patient and patron.

Bichat, M. F. Xavier (1771–1802), surgeon, anatomist, physiologist, prolific author, teacher, died soon after Laennec arrived in Paris.

Bonald, Louis G.A. de (1754–1840), priest, philosopher, royalist, influenced Buisson.

Bouillaud, Jean-Baptiste (1796–1881), physician, protégé of Broussais, discoveries in pathological anatomy of the heart, mutual hostility with Laennec.

Boyer, Alexis (1757–1833), surgeon, Laennec's teacher.

Broussais, François-Joseph-Victor (1772–1838), military physician, clinician, popular teacher, later professor, founder of the "doctrine physiologique," rivalry with Laennec.

Bruté de Remur, Simon Gabriel, Breton, physician, Congréganist, later bishop in United States, Laennec's friend.

Buisson, Mathieu-François-Régis (1776–1804), physician, Congréganist, critic of Bichat, used the word "auscultation" in physiological sense in 1802, Laennec's friend.

Carswell, Robert (1793–1857) of Edinburgh, physician, pathologist, medical artist, visited Laennec in 1822, later illustrated cirrhosis of the liver.

Cayol, Jean-Bruno (1787–1856), physician, professor, Laennec's friend and colleague.

Chateaubriand, Céleste Buisson de la Vigne la Vicomtesse de (1774–1847), Breton, wife of René, Laennec's patient.

Chateaubriand, René de (1768–1848), Breton, writer, statesman, royalist, wrote early review of auscultation, Laennec's patient and friend.

Chaussier, François (1746–1828), anatomist, professor, Laennec's teacher, later his colleague and rival for chair at Collège de France.

Chomel, Auguste F. (1788–1858), clinician at Charité hospital, where he succeeded Laennec as professor in the *clinique interne.*

Clark, James (1788–1870), English physician, traveler, writer, corresponded with Laennec.

Collin, Victor (b. 1796) physician, thesis on auscultation, original descriptions in auscultation of pneumonia and pericarditis, Laennec's student and junior associate.

Corbière, Jacques-Joseph-Guillaume (1766–1853), Breton, royalist, minister of the interior, Laennec's acquaintance and patron.

Corvisart des Marets, Jean-Nicolas (1755–1821), physician to Napoleon, professor in faculty and Collège de France, clinician, revived Auenbrugger's percussion, Laennec's clinical teacher.

Courbon-Pérusel (1779–1821), Breton physician, Laennec's friend.

Cousin, Victor (1792–1867), philosopher and professor at the Sorbonne, Laennec's patient.

Cruveilhier, Jean (1791–1874), physician, anatomist and pathologist, protégé of Laennec.

Cuvier, Baron Georges (1769–1832), naturalist, professor at Collège de France, Laennec's colleague at Société de l'Ecole and at Collège de France, shared interest in parasites.

Delavau, Guy (1788–1874), royalist, Catholic, later prefect of police, Laennec's acquaintance.

Delavau, Mlle, sister of Guy, hostess of a Paris salon frequented by members of the Congrégation, Laennec's friend, cited on mesmerism in Laennec's papers.

Desgenettes, René-Nicolas (1762–1837), surgeon, professor, evaluator of *Treatise on Auscultation* for faculty, Hallé's eulogist, ousted by royalist coup in faculty, appealed to Laennec.

Dombideau de Crouseilhes, Pierre-Vincent (1751–1823), bishop of Quimper, Laennec's friend.

Duméril, Anne-Marie Constant (1774–1860), naturalist, president of the Société de l'Ecole, Laennec's colleague.

Dupuytren, Guillaume (1777–1835), surgeon, anatomist, professor, Laennec's rival.

Esquirol, J. E. D. (1772–1840), physician, alienist, Laennec's colleague.

Fauriel, C.-C. (1772–1844), musicologist, Laennec's acquaintance.

Fesch, Cardinal Joseph (b. 1763), uncle of Napoleon, Laennec's patient and patron.

Fizeau, Louis-Aimé (1776–1864), Breton, physician, Congréganist, Laennec's friend.

Forbes, John (1787–1861) of Chichester, English physician, translator of Laennec's treatise.

Fourcroy, Antoine-François (1755–1809), chemist, founding member of Ecole de Santé, Director of public education, presented prizes of 1803, Laennec's teacher.

Hallé, Jean-Noël (1754–1822), physician to royal family, professor in faculty, professor at Collège de France, Laennec's teacher, patron, and predecessor at court and Collège de France.

Itard, J. M. G. (1774–1838), physician, educator of the deaf, Laennec's colleague.

Kergaradec, Jacques-Alexandre Le Jumeau de (1788–1877), Breton, physician, Congréganist, early research on auscultation, discovered obstetrical auscultation, wrote memoirs of Laennec

Kitchen, James (1800–1894) of Philadelphia, student of Laennec and Broussais.

Lamennais, Félicité de (1782–1854), priest, philosopher, Laennec's patient.

Landré-Beauvais, Augustin-Jacob (1772–1840), physician, Laennec's colleague and friend.

Larrey, Dominique-Jean (1766–1842), military surgeon, Laennec's acquaintance and colleague at the Société de l'Ecole.

Legallois, Eugène, son of J. J. C., junior colleague of Laennec.

Legallois, Julien-Jean-César (1770–1814), Breton, physiologist, Congréganist, Laennec's acquaintance.

Leroux des Tillets, Jean-Jacques (1749–1832), physician, medical journalist, Laennec's teacher, published his first article.

Louis, P. C. A. (1787–1872), physician, Laennec's colleague.

Magendie, François (1783–1855), physiologist, physician, rival for appointments, second successor at Collège de France.

Marion de Procé, Pierre-Martin (1788–1854), Breton, physician, brother-in-law of Christophe Laennec.

Mercy, François-Christophe-Florimond de (b. 1775), physician, philologist, Laennec admired his work, possible rival for defunct chair of Hippocratic medicine.

Montmorency, Mathieu-J.-F., Duc de (1767–1826), royalist, Congréganist, Laennec's acquaintance.

Ollivry, Georges (b. 1778), Breton, physician in Quimper, studied in Paris, Laennec's friend.

Pinel, Philippe (1745–1826), physician at Salpêtrière, Laennec's teacher and colleague.

Piorry, Pierre Adolphe (1794–1870), physician, inventor of mediate percussion and pleximeter, sought advice from Laennec and dedicated his book to his memory

Pompéry, Anne-Marie Audoyn de Cosquer, Mme de (1762–1820), Breton, cousin of Laennec's mother, friend and hostess at Couvrelles.

Portal, Antoine (1742–1832), physician to royal family, anatomist, professor Collège de France, early evaluator of auscultation.

Quélen, Hyacinthe-Louis Comte de (1778–1839), priest, later archbishop of Paris, Laennec's friend.

Récamier, Joseph-Claude-Anthelme (1774–1852), physician at Hôtel Dieu, professor, early evaluator of auscultation, Laennec's friend and immediate successor at Collège de France.

Rostan, Léon-Louis (1790–1866), physician, early reviewer of auscultation, founder of organicism, hostility with Laennec.

Sainte-Beuve, C. A. (1804–1869), physician, literary critic and writer, Laennec's student.

Savary des Brulons, Charles (d. 1814), Breton, physician, Congréganist, Laennec's friend.

Scudamore, Charles (1779–1849), English physician and traveler, visited Laennec's clinic.

Staël, Germaine Necker, Mme de (1766–1817), daughter of founder of Necker hospital, writer, critic of Napoleon, patient of Portal, auscultated by Laennec in 1817.

Tesseyre, Antoine Jerome Paul (d. 1818), priest Congréganist, friend of Lamennais and Laennec.

Thomson, William (1802–1852) of Edinburgh, medical traveler, visited Laennec's clinic, early user of the stethoscope.

Toulmouche, Adolphe (1798–1876), Breton, physician, thesis on auscultation of the heart 1820, Laennec's student, his friend, and wrote memoirs of him.

Van Hall, H. C. (1801–1874), Dutch physician, thesis on auscultation 1823, visited Laennec's clinic.

Villenave, Mathieu G. F. (1762–1846), Breton from Nantes, royalist, editor, publisher, early announcement of auscultation, Laennec's former teacher and friend.

Williams, C. J. B. (1805–1889), English physician, early user of stethoscope, visitor to Laennec's clinic.

- A P P E N D I X   E -

The Family of R. T. H. Laennec

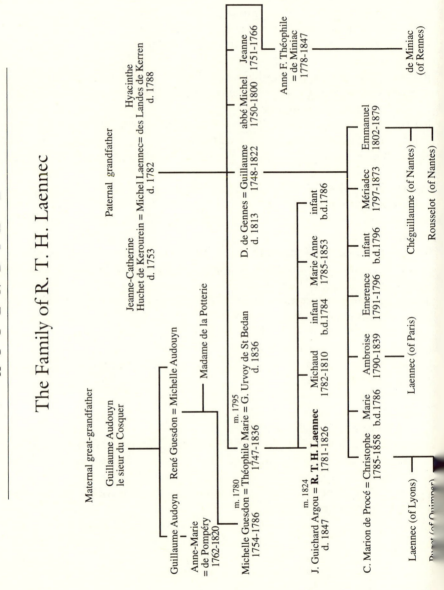

General Conventions

Laennec, used alone, always refers to R. T. H. Laennec.
Traité 1819 always refers to Laennec 1819c.
Traité 1826 always refers to Laennec 1826h.
Treatise 1821 always refers to Laennec 1821.
Treatise 1827 always refers to Laennec 1827.
[Year] A year or a date in square brackets indicates either the year in which
   a work was originally published, or the Gregorian translation of a revolu-
   tionary date.
All translations from French, unless otherwise indicated in the bibliography,
   are my own.

Archives

AAP	Archives de l'Assistance Publique, Paris
AAS	Archives de l'Académie des Sciences, Paris
ACF	Archives du Collège de France, Paris
ADF	Archives Départementales de Finistère, Quimper
ADLA	Archives Départementales de la Loire Atlantique, Nantes
AEQ	Archives de l'Eveché de Quimper
AJésuites	Archives de la Compagnie de Jésus, Vanves
AMN	Archives Municipales de Nantes
AMP	Archives Municipales de Paris
AN	Archives Nationales, Paris
ANM-SEM	Archives de la Société de l'Ecole de Médecine, Académie Nationale de Médecine, Paris
BIUM	Bibliothèque Interuniversitaire de Médecine, Paris
CPP	Library College of Physicians of Philadelphia
EUL	Edinburgh University Library
HMCP	Hahneman Medical College, Philadelphia
ML	Musée Laennec. Contents belong to the Faculté de Médecine, located in the Bibliothèque de la Faculté des Lettres, Université de Nantes.
MNFR	Médiathèque de Nantes, Section d'Histoire Locale, Fonds Rouxeau
MNQ	Archives Municipales de Quimper
NYAM	New York Academy of Medicine, Malloch Rare Book Room

PRIVATE COLLECTIONS

MS Bertrand Laennec	Bertrand Laennec and family, Lyons
MS de Miniac	Hervé de Miniac, Rennes
MS Puget	François Puget, Quimper

NAMES, JOURNALS, AND DICTIONARIES

Am. J. Card.	*American Journal of Cardiology*
Arch. anat. cytol. path.	*Archives de l'anatomie et cytologie pathologique*
BEMS	*Bulletin de l'Ecole [later "Faculté"] de Médecine de Paris et de la Société établie dans son sein,* 7 vols. (1804–1821)
Biog. UAM	*Biographie universelle ancienne et moderne (Michaud),* 45 vols. (Paris: Madame C. Desplaces, 1854–1865)
Biog. NC	*Biographie nouvelle des contemporains,* 20 vols. (Paris: Le Dentu, 1827)
Biog. UPC	*Biographie universelle et portative des contemporains,* 5 vols. (Paris: L'Editeur rue des Colombiers, 1836)
Bull. Hist. Med.	*Bulletin of the History of Medicine*
Bull. Soc. Arch. Finistère	*Bulletin de la Société Archéologique de Finistère*
Can. Med. Assoc. J.	*Canadian Medical Association Journal*
DSM	*Dictionnaire des sciences médicales par une société de médecins et de chirurgiens,* ed. Adelon, Alard, Alibert, et al., 60 vols. (Paris: C. L. F. Panckoucke, 1812–1822)
DSM: Bio méd.	*Dictionnaire des sciences médicales: Biographie Médicale,* ed. A. J. L. Jourdan, 7 vols. (Paris: Panckoucke, 1820–1825)
Hist. Refl.	*Historical Reflections/Réflexions historiques*
Hist. Sci.	*History of Science*
Hist. sci. méd.	*Histoire des sciences médicales*
Huybrechts 1980	Huybrechts-Rivière 1980
J. méd.	*Journal de médecine, chirurgie, pharmacie,* ed. Corvisart, Roux, Boyer
J. gén. méd.	*Journal général de médecine, de chirurgie, et de pharmacie françaises et etrangères, ou Recueil periodique des travaux de la Société de Médecine de Paris*
J. Hist. Biol.	*Journal of the History of Biology*

J. Hist. Med. All. Sci.	*Journal of the History of Medicine and Allied Sciences*
J. Med. Phil.	*Journal of Medicine and Philosophy*
Med. Hist.	*Medical History*
N. biog. gen.	*Nouvelle biographie générale depuis les temps les plus reculés jusqu'à 1850–60*, ed. J. C. F. Hoefer (Paris: Firmin-Didot, 1852–1866; reprint, Copenhagen: Rosenkilde-Bagger, 1969), 46 vols., in 23.
Nouv. bib. méd.	*Nouvelle bibliothèque médicale*
Nouv. j. méd.	*Nouveau journal de médecine*
Phil. Trans.	*Philosophical Transactions of the Royal Society*
Rev. d'hist. sci.	*Revue d'histoire des sciences*
Rev. méd.	*Revue médicale française et étrangère et journal de clinique de l'Hôtel Dieu, de la Charité, et des grands hôpitaux de Paris*
RPD	*Revue du Palais de la Découverte*, no. spécial 22 (août 1981): "Commémoration du bicentenaire de la naissance de Laennec, 1781–1826. Colloque organisé au Collège de France, 18–19 février 1981."
Roux 1980	Roux de Reilhac 1980
Stud. Hist. Phil. Sci.	*Studies in the History and Philosophy of Science*

• NOTES •

INTRODUCTION

1. For examples of these soaring epithets, see Ackerknecht 1967, 88; Léon Bernard, cited in Duclos 1932, 11–12; Bouillaud 1869, 3; Flint 1859, 15; Marketos 1982; Reiser 1978, 38; Sedaillan et al. 1959.

2. Vrouc'h 1958, 61–62. For nearly half a century, the periodical *Laennec: médecine, santé, éthique* has been published by the Centre Laennec of Paris.

3. *Le pardon de Laennec à Ploaré. Les fêtes du centenaire, 12 août 1926* (Quimper: Ad. Le Goaziou, 1927). See also "Giscard à l'Académie de Médecine" and other reports in *Le Quotidienne de Médecine*, no. 2372, 16 February 1981, 13–27.

4. Rouxeau [1912], [1920].

5. Laennec's life, illness, practice, and death have been used as fodder for several pieces of fiction, poetry, and at least two feature-length films. Some portrayals bear little relationship to the original. See, for example, the evil "Dr. Lasinec" of Eusèbe de Salle [1933], 307–318. See also Bernard-Luc 1949; Chausée 1981; Corlay 1981; Fosseyeux 1930, 10–11n; Holmes [1849]; Kipling 1910; Robertson and Coope 1957; poem by medical student, Jules-E. André, printed to celebrate the inauguration of the statue of Laennec, 15 August 1868 (Quimper, Kerangle, 1868), AEQ. The first film, "Dr. Laennec," 1949, was directed by Maurice Cloche for the Association Internationale Cinématographique (rereleased on VHS in 1993). The second, "La Passion de Théophile," was directed by Yvan Kovacs for the French television network, Antenne 2, on which it was aired 22 February 1981. A typescript of the latter is held by the ACF; an extensive collection of clippings about the making of the Cloche film is kept at AMQ and the screenplay was published. Bernard-Luc 1949.

6. For a recent survey of this literature, see "Introduction" in La Berge and Feingold 1994, 1–24.

7. On the patient and patient records in history, see Porter 1985a, b; Risse and Warner 1992. My approach to Laennec's patient histories has been influenced by Hunter 1991.

8. Ackerknecht 1967, 91.

9. Jacyna 1987.

10. Weisz 1995, 189–211.

CHAPTER ONE

1. Rouxeau [1912], [1920]. See also Bon 1925; Corbie 1950; Duclos 1932; Kernéis 1981a; Kervran 1960; Knegtel 1966; Malard and Malard 1959; Marketos 1982; Rist 1955; Sarradon 1949; Webb 1927, 1928. Among the secondary sources available to Rouxeau were the following accounts written by authors who claimed to have communicated either with Laennec or with persons who knew him: A. L. J. Bayle 1826, 1855; Boisseau 1822; Bouillaud 1869; Du Chatellier 1885; Forbes 1834; Granville 1854; Lallour 1892; Lecadre 1868; Pariset 1845; Saintignon 1904; Scudamore 1826; Toulmouche 1875; Villard 1927; Williams 1884.

2. On the Laennec ancestors, see Rouxeau [1912], 1–10. Laennec's baptismal certificate, signed by the priest-uncle who officiated, his father, and both grandfathers

at the parish of St. Mathieu on 18 February 1781, is in AMQ and reproduced in *Au Pays de Laennec* 1981, frontispiece.

3. At least two Quimper houses, each with a commemorative plaque, vied for recognition as the birthplace of Laennec until a 1966 urban renewal plan put an end to the quarrel by demolishing both buildings. As one journalist put it, "Two birthplaces for a single man, however celebrated he may be, is one too many." See especially R. L. M. "La seconde 'Maison natale' de Laennec," unidentified newspaper clipping, "16–17 avril 1966," Fichier Laennec, AMQ. See also note in *Bull. Soc. Arch. Finistère*, 1919, xxviii.

4. Théophile-Marie Laennec [1805]. On the poems of Laennec *père* for the restored monarch, see his letter to his son Laennec, 14 September 1819, transcribed in Pinson 1980, 177–178.

5. Another baby had died immediately after birth on 22 February 1784. Rouxeau [1912], 20; [1920], 79. Laennec *père* to Laennec, 30 October 1805, transcribed in Crochet 1982, 148. The birth and death dates for the family can be confirmed through the records of the parish of St. Matthieu, AMQ.

6. Guillaume to his son Mériadec, 19 April 1817, transcribed in Pinson 1980, 85–86.

7. Laennec to his father, 2 Ventôse An XIII (21 February 1805), MS de Miniac, no. 68, transcribed in Crochet 1982, 113–114; Rouxeau [1920], 79.

8. Guillaume to Laennec's father, 29 April 1788, cited in Rouxeau [1912], 25–26.

9. Kernéis 1981a, 14–20, 35–41; Rouxeau [1924], esp. 41 (cemeteries).

10. Bouvier 1980, 240; Kernéis 1981a, 17–18; Rouxeau [1912], 28–30; Valentin 1981. See also appeal to the municipal police signed by Guillaume Laennec and Blin, "Messieurs les juges de Police de la Ville de Nantes," 31 December 1783, AMN, FF 250, no. 2; and several manuscripts pertaining to the lawsuit written and signed by Guillaume Laennec, styling himself as "Laennec de la Renardais" [of Kerlouarnec], MS François Puget of Quimper.

11. Acte de baptême de Ambroise-François Laennec, 11 June 1790, AMN, GG 470, parish of St. Croix 1790, p. 57, no. 238 (microfilm 2 Mi EC 173).

12. Guillaume to his brother Théophile-Marie, 24 June, 22 November 1798, 11, 25 February 1800, transcribed in Bouvier 1980, 129–130, 134, 164–166.

13. Guillaume to his brother, 24 Messidor An X (13 July 1802), transcribed in Bouvier 1980, 213.

14. Guillaume to his father Michel Laennec, 14 May, 3 June 1770, cited in Rouxeau [1924], 46–48.

15. Documents in AMN, cited in *Laennec, inventeur de l'auscultation* 1981, 45; Bouvier 1980, 35. The political and religious sentiments of the Laennec family and their inclination to support a royalist escape were discussed in letters seized on 15 March 1793 from the homes of Alexandre de la Roque of Quimper and Victor de la Roque of Lorient, transcribed in Savina 1926, 85–86.

16. On the Revolution in the region of Nantes, see Hutt 1983; Konrat 1984, 257–299.

17. Rouxeau [1912], 45–46. On the location and appearance of the Laennec residences in Nantes annotations made by local historian Dr. Georges Halgan (1876–1966) on his personal copy of Pied 1906, *1*: 35 and *2*: 284, ADLA.

18. Bouvier 1980, 238. Rouxeau claimed that the house at Petit Port had belonged to Guillaume's wife, Désirée de Gennes, Rouxeau [1912], 43. The *acte de*

vente, however, shows that Guillaume acquired it in January 1793 when it was sold as a the property of the clergy. "Catalogue de la Famille Laennec," AMN.

19. Rouxeau [1912], 48–51. Rouxeau relied on the now untraceable "Souvenirs" of Christophe Laennec for this version of the story.

20. Kernéis 1981a, 20.

21. On Carrier, see Baczko 1994, 136–184, esp. 153–154; Fleury 1901; Furet 1988, 147, 154.

22. Guillaume to his wife, 4 Frimaire An III (24 November 1794), transcribed in Bouvier 1980, 17. See also Fleury 1901, 121n, 126n; Rouxeau [1912], 49–51, 56–58. Years later, Prigent, former aide of Carrier, was said to be trying to ingratiate himself with the family. Laennec *père* to his brother Guillaume, 26 Floréal An VII (15 May 1799), transcribed in Bouvier 1980, 136.

23. Deposition of 26 Frimaire An III (16 December 1794), transcribed in Bouvier 1980, 17–19. See also Bouvier 1980, 26, 36. Rouxeau [1912], 58.

24. Petition of 24 Nivôse An V (14 January 1796), transcribed in Bouvier 1980, 57.

25. Description of the courses offered to the school's ninety-five students, the names of teachers, and their salaries in "Petition aux citoyens, 19 octobre 1792, An premier," Fol. 2 ADLA, L616. On the revolutionary changes to education, see Godechot 1977, 167–176; Robiquet [1938], 84–86.

26. "Noms des élèves du Collège de Nantes," Fol. 4, Collège de Nantes, "Instruction secondaire," ADLA, L616.

27. Certificates stating that the "young citizen [Christophe or Théophile?] Laennec" had studied "very well," 19 Ventôse and 19 Germinal An II (9 March, 8 April 1794), MS Bertrand Laennec. See also Laennec to his cousin Christophe, 20 July 1819, MS Bertrand Laennec, transcribed in Pinson 1980, 162–163; Rouxeau 1912], 35.

28. Guillaume to his brother Théophile-Marie, 14 Messidor An IV (2 July 1796), transcribed in Bouvier 1980, 64–65; Laennec to his stepmother, 19 Vendémiaire An V (10 November 1796), MS de Miniac, no. 9 transcribed in Bouvier 1980, 59–70.

29. Laennec to his father, 18 Fructidor An VI (4 September 1798), MS de Miniac, no. 20, transcribed in Bouvier 1980, 131.

30. Guillaume to his brother Théophile-Marie, 14 Messidor An IV (2 July 1796), transcribed in Bouvier 1980, 64–65.

31. Laennec to his stepmother, 19 Vendémiaire An V (10 November 1796), MS de Miniac, no. 9, transcribed in Bouvier 1980, 69–70.

32. "I have a brother and a sister both with the name of Théophile," *abbé* Michel Laennec to his brother Théophile-Marie and sister Théophile-Anne-Françoise, 8 Thermidor An V (28 July 1797), transcribed in Bouvier 1980, 91. On the *abbé* Michel Laennec and his mediation of a dispute between priests and professors in 1778, see Le Floc'h 1980.

33. Guillaume to his brother Théophile-Marie, 14 Messidor An IV, 10 Fructidor An V, 3 Fructidor An VIII (2 July 1796, 27 August 1797, 21 August 1800), transcribed in Bouvier 1980, 65, 95–96, 171; information given by Jean de Bahezre to Théophile-Marie Laennec, 20 Pluviôse An XI (9 February 1803), transcribed in Bouvier 1980, 230–231.

34. Laennec to his father, 2 Ventôse An XIII (21 February 1805), MS de Miniac, no. 68, transcribed in Crochet 1982, 113–114.

35. Fourteen letters about the marriage from Laennec *père* to various correspondents between 9 Pluviôse An III and 20 Frimaire An IV (28 January and 11 December 1795) are transcribed in Bouvier 1980, 27–32.

36. The stepmother Mme Laennec to Laennec, 19 Fructidor An III (5 September 1795), transcribed in Bouvier 1980, 46–47. On another occasion she asked Guillaume to give Théophile one hundred francs on account. Mme Laennec to Guillaume Laennec, 19 Frimaire An V (9 December 1796), transcribed in Bouvier 1980, 71. In 1920, Rouxeau admitted to having omitted mention of the stepmother's gift from his 1912 volume, because he suspected it had been paid in worthless *assignats* and gave the wrong impression about the true extent of the parental generosity. Rouxeau [1920], 8.

37. The dismissals of Laennec *père* are summarized in Bouvier 1980, 42, 49, 51, 56, 119. On the end of the court battles, see Laennec to Guillaume, 16 October 1821, MS Bertrand Laennec, transcribed in Pinson 1980, 272–274.

38. Laennec, Petition "Aux citoyens professors," 4 Pluviôse An XII (25 January 1804), written and signed by R. T. H. Laennec, AN, AJ/16/886 and ML, photograph.

39. Ackerknecht 1967, 25–26; Huard and Grmek 1970, 276; Rey 1993b, 32; Weiner 1969, 51–73.

40. Certificate signed by Ulliac, chief surgeon of the military hospice in Nantes, 22 Prairial An VII (10 June 1799), transcribed in Bouvier 1980, 138–139.

41. Laennec to his father, 12 Germinal An V (1 April 1797); Guillaume to his nephew, 30 Messidor An V (19 July 1797), transcribed in Bouvier 1980, 82–83, 88–89. The Platner may have been Johann Zacharias (1694–1747) author of a 1758 Latin treatise on therapeutics or Ernestus (1744–1818) author of several works on physiology and surgery printed at Leipzig. The other books included Pinel 1797–1798 and Fourcroy 1785, 1786, or one of his many treatises on chemistry.

42. Laennec to his father, 27 Frimaire, 8 Germinal An VI (17 December 1797, 28 March 1798), the latter is MS de Miniac, no. 18, transcribed in Bouvier 1980, 115–116, 126–127. According to the autobiography of Christophe Laennec, the Greek instructor was abbé Bonnement, "exuberant man but feeble priest," who had sworn allegiance to the Civil Constitution of the Clergy, cited in Bouvier 1980, 129. Laennec did not succeed in learning English and would correspond with his translator, John Forbes, in Latin or French. Laennec to Forbes, 12 June 1824; Forbes to Laennec, 20 June 1824, ML, MS Cl. 5, ff. 65r–67v, 75r–76v.

43. Guillaume to his son Mériadec, 20 February 1821, transcribed in Pinson 1980, 255–256.

44. Procuration, 19 Frimaire An V (9 December 1796); Guillaume to his brother Théophile-Marie, 20 Pluviôse An IX (9 February 1801), transcribed in Bouvier 1980, 72, 177–179.

45. Laennec to his father, 22 Prairial, 21 Messidor, 2, 8, 18 Thermidor, 4 Fructidor An V (10 June, 9, 20, 26 July, 5, 21 August 1797), MS de Miniac, nos. 2, 4, 5 6, 7, 8, and Guillaume to his nephew, 30 Messidor An V (19 July 1797), transcribed in Bouvier 1980, 84–95.

46. Guillaume to his brother, Théophile-Marie, 10 Fructidor An V (27 August 1797), transcribed in Bouvier 1980, 95–96.

47. Poem, transcribed in Bouvier 1980, 96; Laennec *père* to his brother Guillaume, 18 Vendémiaire An VI (9 October 1797), transcribed in Bouvier 1980, 101

48. Laennec *père* to his son 11 Pluviôse An VI (30 January 1798); Laennec to his father, 16 Brumaire, 13 Frimaire, 18 Nivôse An VI, 23 Brumaire An VIII (6 Novem

ber, 3 December 1797, 7 January 1798, 14 November 1799), MS de Miniac, nos. 11, 16, 26 [18 Nivôse An VI not in de Miniac collection], transcribed in Bouvier 1980, 104, 114, 118–119, 121–122, 156–157.

49. Laennec to his father, 3, 5 Frimaire An VI (23, 25 November 1797), MS de Miniac, nos. 14, 15, transcribed in Bouvier 1980, 112–113.

50. Guillaume to his brother 10 Messidor An V (28 June 1797), Guillaume to his sister, 15 Thermidor An V (2 August 1797), transcribed in Bouvier 1980, 86–87, 92.

51. Mme Laennec to her brother-in-law Guillaume, 14 Frimaire An IX (5 December 1802), transcribed in Bouvier 1980, 228–229. See also Laennec *père* to his son, in which he asks that his letters be addressed to the local pharmacist, 11 Floréal An XII (1 May 1804), transcribed in Crochet 1982, 75–77. Another letter from Théophile-Marie to his brother Guillaume begins, "Great news! my wife is in good humor," 4 Complémentaire An VIII (21 September 1800), MS de Miniac, no. 157.

52. Laennec's father to his son, 11 Pluviôse An VI (30 January 1798), transcribed in Bouvier 1980, 121–122. See also Guillaume to his brother, 27 Thermidor An VIII (15 August 1800) in which he speaks of a "*billet doux*" from "our little sister to Théophile" brought before dawn with "all the demonstrations of a triumph," transcribed in Bouvier 1980, 170–171. See also the sarcastic remarks about Mme Laennec made by Michaud to his newly married aunt, Mme de Miniac, 28 Vendémiaire An IX (20 October 1800), transcribed in Bouvier 1980, 174.

53. Guillaume to his brother 10, 12 Prairial An VI (29, 31 May 1798); Laennec to his father, 16 Prairial An VI (4 June 1798), MS Miniac, no. 19, transcribed in Bouvier 1980, 127–128. Two years earlier, Laennec had suffered a nosebleed following the spirited chase of a donkey. Guillaume to his brother, 2 Fructidor An IV (19 August 1796), transcribed in Bouvier 1980, 67. On Laennec's delicacy, see Guillaume to his brother's wife, 4 Messidor An V (22 June 1797), transcribed in Bouvier 1980, 85.

54. Guillaume to his brother, 26 Fructidor An VII (12 September 1799), transcribed in Bouvier 1980, 143.

55. Laennec to his father, 13 Vendémiaire An VIII (5 October 1799), MS de Miniac, no. 22, transcribed in Bouvier 1980, 145. The word "Chouan" is thought to have been derived from a contraction of "*chat-huant*," the name of a nocturnal screech owl; the letter from Laennec seems to confirm the derivation. See Hutt 1983, *1*: 21.

56. Laennec to his father, 30 Vendémiaire An VIII (22 October 1799), MS de Miniac, no. 24, transcribed in Bouvier 1980, 151.

57. Notes made by Rouxeau from the autobiography of Christophe Laennec, transcribed in Bouvier 1980, 135.

58. Guillaume to his brother, 24 Prairial An VII (12 June 1799); Laennec to his father, 30 Vendémiaire An VIII and Brumaire An VIII (22 October 1799 and November 1799), in which he signed himself, "*chirurgien de 2ème classe.*" MS de Miniac, nos. 24, 25, transcribed in Bouvier 1980, 140, 152, 154.

59. The battle of the Pont du Loc had been won on 26 January 1800, but Laennec did not depart for the front until 29 January. Dupuy 1989. Guillaume to his brother Théophile-Marie, 9 Pluviôse An VIII (29 January 1800), transcribed in Bouvier 1980, 161.

60. In 1912, the manuscript of "La Guerre des Vénètes" was still missing. Before 1920, Rouxeau located it at the home of Laennec's relative, Mme Edouard Morin, and it now resides in the Musée Laennec. A century later, Dr. Paul Busquet published the seventy-three-page poem. See Laennec 1931.

61. Laennec to his father, 10 Thermidor An IX (29 July 1801), MS de Miniac, no. 32, transcribed in Bouvier 1980, 195–197; Laennec *père* to his son Théophile, 10 Nivôse An XII (1 Jan 1804), transcribed in Crochet 1982, 55–62.

62. Laennec to his father, 9 Ventôse An IX (28 February 1800), MS de Miniac, no. 28; Guillaume to his brother, 15 Ventôse An VIII (6 March 1800), transcribed in Bouvier 1980, 166–168.

63. Laennec to his father, 29 Germinal An VIII (19 April 1800), transcribed in Bouvier 1980, 169.

64. Guillaume to his brother Théophile-Marie, 22 Prairial An VIII (11 February 1800), transcribed in Bouvier 1980, 164–165.

65. Guillaume Laennec to his brother Laennec *père*, 3 Fructidor An VIII (21 August 1800), transcribed in Bouvier 1980, 171–172.

66. Guillaume to his brother Théophile-Marie, and Laennec to his father, both 29 Vendémiaire An IX (21 October 1800), the latter is MS de Miniac, no. 29, transcribed in Bouvier 1980, 175–176.

67. Laennec's father to Laennec, 2 Ventôse An IX (21 February 1801), transcribed in Bouvier 1980, 180.

68. Guillaume to his brother, 5 Germinal An IX (28 March 1801), transcribed in Bouvier 1980, 186–187.

69. Laennec to his father, 10 Thermidor IX (29 July 1801),) MS de Miniac, no. 32, transcribed in Bouvier 1980, 195–197. On the diamond, see also Laennec's father to his son Michaud, 14 Germinal An IX (4 April 1801); Laennec to his father, 20 Thermidor An X , 4 Germinal An XI (8 August 1802, 25 March 1803), MS de Miniac, nos. 33, 37, transcribed in Bouvier 1980, 187–189, 214–216, 235–236.

70. Guillaume to his brother Théophile-Marie, 4 Floréal An IX (24 April 1801), transcribed in Bouvier 1980, 191–192.

CHAPTER TWO

1. The literature on medicine and the French Revolution is voluminous. For summaries of the political, legislative, and intellectual changes, see Ackerknecht 1967, 31–44; Ramsey 1988, 71–84; Weiner 1993, 26–31. See also, Boulle 1986; Coury 1970; Huard and Grmek 1970; Imbault-Huart 1973; Lesch 1984, 31–49; Lorillot 1982; Rey 1993b, 23–57; Sournia 1989; Staum 1980; Vess 1975.

2. Gelfand 1980; Temkin 1951.

3. On the founding and resurrection of societes after the Revolution, see Ackerknecht 1967, 115–119; Lesch 1984, 55, 57; Maulitz 1987, 69–73; Ramsey 1988, 106. On journals and societies, see Huard and Grmek 1970, 255–261.

4. On disease concepts and their history, see W. Miller Brown 1985; Canguilhem 1989, 181–201; Caplan et al. 1981; Cassell 1986; Engel 1960; Grmek 1988b; Hudson 1983; Hudson 1993; King 1982; Margolis 1976; Merskey 1986; Peter 1975; Riese 1953; Risse 1978.

5. Foucault 1963, 108.

6. See Bynum 1994, 1–54; Karenberg 1994; Keel 1979; S. C. Lawrence 1985, 1988; O'Malley 1970.

7. For a table comparing six nosological classifications, see Cullen [1765], viii–x. On nosology, see King 1966; J. Martin 1990; Rey 1987, 1993a; Risse 1986, 115–117, 280–282.

8. On the history of physical diagnosis and the impact of auscultation and other diagnostic techniques, see Keele 1963; King 1976; Nicholson 1992; Porter 1993; Reiser 1979; Risse 1986, 108–114; Risse 1987; Savitt 1995, 73–98.

9. Benivieni [1507]; Bonet 1700; Morgagni [1769]. See also Jarcho 1948, 1984; Nicholson 1992.

10. Stafford 1991, 47.

11. Weiner, 1993, 181–183.

12. On clinical instruction, the Ecole Pratique, and the importance of dissection, see Gelfand 1977 and 1980, 90–92; Imbault-Huart 1973; Lesch 1984, 39; Maulitz 1987, 27, 36–37, 42–43; Warner, forthcoming; Weiner 1993, 177–183.

13. Laennec to his father, 8 Ventôse An XI (28 February 1803), MS de Miniac, no. 36, transcribed in Bouvier 1980, 231–234. Despite Laennec's statement, chairs of pathological anatomy were founded earlier in Caen (1756) and Strasbourg (1819) long before the Paris chair in 1836. Ackerknecht 1967, 34–35, 167; Maulitz 1987, 46–47; Orcel and Vetter 1976.

14. Epistemological obstacle and epistemological discontinuity (or rupture) are concepts developed by Gaston Bachelard, from whom Canguilhem claimed to have been inspired. See Canguilhem 1988, 10–11.

15. See for example, Double 1811–1822; Landré-Beauvais 1818.

16. Laennec 1804f, 1806l, 1806w, 1807b; Prost 1804. See also Foucault 1963, 186–187.

17. On the legislative changes, see Ackerknecht 1967, 38–39; Ramsey 1988, 77–85; Rey 1993b, 29–30.

18. On Hallé, see *Biog. UAM 18*:np; Dausset 1981; Desgenettes 1822; *N. biog. gén. 23*:np; Ganière [1951], 89–90, 106; Weiner 1993, 289–291.

19. Laennec to his father, 20 Messidor, 10 Thermidor An IX (9, 29 July 1801), MS de Miniac, nos. 31, 32, transcribed in Bouvier 1980, 193–197.

20. Guillaume to his brother, 10 and 24 Prairial An X (30 May and 15 June 1802), transcribed in Bouvier 1980, 207–209. On the cost of a medical education, see Ramsey 1988, 109–110.

21. For more on Corvisart, see Albury 1982; Ganière [1951]; Touche 1968.

22. Maximillian Stoll [1797], 116–117. See also Corvisart's dedication in the same volume, "A Mon Ami Le Preux," v–xiii, esp. vii.

23. Auenbrugger 1761.

24. On "tact," "gaze," and "precordial palpation," Corvisart [1806], 19–21 ("better eye" and "tact"), 185–186 ("thrill"); Corvisart, 1808, ix–x ("tact"). On the frequency of autopsies at the Charité Hospital, see Clark 1820, 130; Weiner 1993, 181.

25. "Aphorismes recueillis aux leçons du C[itoyen] Corvisart par René Théophile Hyacinthe Laennec, An X," ML, MS Cl. 8 [2], f. 1r–14v. See also Boussand-Verlingue 1977; Busquet 1929.

26. Using the clinical references in Laennec's manuscript of Corvisart's aphorisms, Boulle was able to trace eighteen of the patients whom Laennec had examined through the extant registers of the Charité hospital. Boulle 1981.

27. Antoine Michel, ML, MS Cl. 8 [I], f. 1–3.

28. Laennec 1802a; Laennec to his father, 10 Vendémiaire An XI (2 October 1802), MS de Miniac, no. 34, transcribed in Bouvier 1980, 222–225.

29. Laennec to his father, 10 Vendémiaire An XI (2 October 1802), MS de Miniac, no. 34, transcribed in Bouvier 1980, 222–225.

30. Keel 1979; Maulitz 1987, 21–26, 230–232.

31. Laennec to his father, 10 Vendémiaire An XI (2 October 1802), MS de Miniac, no. 34, transcribed in Bouvier 1980, 222–225.

32. Laennec 1802b, 1802d.

33. Laennec to his father, 10 Vendémiaire An XI (2 October 1802), MS de Miniac, no. 34, transcribed in Bouvier 1980, 222–225. Laennec did not become a member of the Société Médicale d'Emulation. For a list of members, see Rey 1987, *3*:173–200. See also Lesch 1984, 55.

34. Laennec to his father, 7 Frimaire An XI (28 November 1802), MS de Miniac, no. 35, transcribed in Bouvier 1980, 226–228. Laennec explained the inheritance of the Peyronie prizes from the old Académie de Chirugie to his uncle Guillaume, 1 Fructidor An XI (19 August 1803), MS de Miniac, no. 44, transcribed in Crochet 1982, 27–28.

35. Laennec to his father, 20 Messidor An IX (9 July 1801), MS de Miniac, no. 31, transcribed in Bouvier 1980, 193–195.

36. Laennec to his father, 10 Vendémiaire An XI (2 October 1802), MS de Miniac, no. 34, transcribed in Bouvier 1980, 222–225, esp. 225. ·

37. Laennec to his father, 19 March 1806, MS de Miniac, no. 85, transcribed in Crochet 1982, 164–166, esp. 166.

38. Laennec to his father, 13 Fructidor An XII (31 August 1804), MS de Miniac 64, transcribed in Crochet 1982, 95–98.

39. For contemporary biographies of Bayle, see A. L. J. Bayle 1833; A. L. J. Bayle and Thillaye 1855; Chomel 1816; Deleuze 1816; "S." 1820.

40. A. L. J. Bayle 1833, xv.

41. G. L. Bayle [1802]. It was reprinted together with a collection of Bayle's articles and articles by J. N. Corvisart, in Bayle and Corvisart, 1838, reprinted 1839 and 1855.

42. Rouxeau [1912], 177–179. A portion of the commentary at the defence was published in G.L. Bayle 1833–39, *1*:xix–xxxi; A. L. J. Bayle and A. Thillaye 1855, 888–892. I have been unable to trace the original manuscript, which belonged to the Cochard family around 1900; however, a fifty-one-page (possibly full) transcription is with Rouxeau's papers, "Compte rendu sténographique de la soutenence de Bayle, 23 février 1802 (4 Ventôse An X)." MNFR, liasse 2822.

43. Pinel and Bayle, cited in Bayle 1833–1839, *1*:xix–xxxi.

44. For more on Bichat, see Ackerknecht 1967, 51–58; Albury 1977; Buisson 1802a; Duchesnau 1982, 431–476; Foucault 1963, 128–35; Haigh 1975; Haigh 1984; Hall 1969, *2*:121–132; Lesch 1984, 50–79; Maulitz 1987, 19–34; Pickstone 1981; Sutton 1984.

45. Boulle 1981, 66. In studying Laennec's papers, Ackerknecht noticed that Laennec, who seems to have had a preference for lower case letters, would capitalize the "B" of Bichat. Ackerknecht 1967, 89. Laennec, however, tended to capitalize all names beginning with "L" and "B" including those less dear to him, such as Brown, Baglivi, Barthez, and Broussais. On Bichat's death and the posthumous remorse of the Paris faculty, see Garnot 1989, 80–81.

46. On Buisson, see Starobinski 1991; Grandmaison 1889, 19, 28–35; *Biog.NC* *3*:567–568; *Biog.UPC* 1:680.

47. Buisson 1802a; Maulitz 1987, 21–25.

48. *Biog.UPC* 1:680.

49. Buisson to Pierre Picot, 12 October 1802, in Starobinski 1991, 336.

50. Grandmaison 1889, 19, 28–35; "Cahier d'inscriptions de la Congrégation," AJésuites, I Pa 413, no. 1.

51. Buisson [1802b].

52. Buisson [1802b], 45.

53. Buisson [1802b], 36, 51. On Bonald, see F. Azouvi, "Introduction," in Bonald [1830]; Furet 1988, 298; Jacyna, 1987, esp. 130–133; Quinlan 1953; Reedy 1976.

54. Buisson [1802b], 45.

55. Buisson [1802b], 53n.

56. Buisson [1802b], 150–151.

57. Buisson to Picot, 12 October 1802, in Starobinski 1991, 337. For another criticism of Bichat's materialism, see Sprengel 1815–1832, 6:528–529.

58. Buisson to Picot, 12 October 1802, in Starobinski, 1991, 337.

59. Laennec 1802f, esp. 176, 180. Emphasis in the original.

60. Laennec 1804c. Laennec referred to Buisson as "*mon ami*" in a letter to his father, 8 Ventôse An XI (28 February 1803), MS de Miniac, no. 36, transcribed in Bouvier 1980, 231–233.

61. According to most accounts, Buisson died in September or October 1804, but one writer said that he died in October 1805 of a "maladie à langueur." *Biog.NC 3*:568.

62. Foucault recognized Buisson as a critic of Bichat, but grouped him with Magendie, opposed to the vitalism and the circularity in his cousin's definition of life. Foucault 1963, 147.

63. "Cahier d'inscriptions de la Congrégation," AJésuites, I Pa 413, no. 1. On the Congrégation, see Guillaume de Bertier de Sauvigny "Chevaliers de Foi" and "Congrégation," in Newman and Simpson 1987, *1*:204–205 and 241, respectively. See also Bertier de Sauvigny 1948, 1966; Grandmaison 1889.

64. Laennec to his father, 8 Ventôse An XI (27 February 1803), MS de Miniac, no. 36, transcribed in Bouvier 1980, 231–233.

65. AJésuites, I Pa 415, no. 57. The fourteen-page manuscript of Laennec's essay is in his hand, but undated and unsigned. It is bound in a volume of fifty-nine similar essays, some of which bear dates from 1804 to 1809. The topics range widely within the realm of biblical and catholic lore: confession, baptism, hell, charity and philanthropy, the transfiguration, the sacraments, the three virtues. Laennec's essay was published by Bon 1925, 71–80; the final third also appeared in Duclos 1932, 92–94. I have been unable to find a source to substantiate the oft-repeated legend that Laennec traveled with Récamier and Maisoneuve to the shrine of the medical saints, Cosmas and Damien, at Luzarches north of Paris. See Bon 1925, 81; Kervran 1960, 90; Duclos 1932, 90. For striking examples of the use of Laennec's life as an exhortation to faith, see Delassus 1902 and the Paris magazine, *Laennec; médecine, santé, éthique*, in its forty-fourth year in 1996.

66. Bon 1925, 91; Grandmaison 1889, 34 (Buisson's poems), 152–153.

67. James K. Kieswetter, "Delavau" in Newman and Simpson 1987, 308; Froment 1829.

68. Laennec, Lesson 5, Collège de France, 1823–1824, ML, MS Cl. 2 lot a (B), f. 167r.

69. Théophile-Marie Laennec [1804]; Laennec to his father, 22 Messidor An XII (11 July 1804), MS de Miniac, no. 63, transcribed in Crochet 1982, 83–86.

70. Laennec to his father, 10 March 1806, MS de Miniac, no. 84, transcribed in Crochet 1982, 162–163.

71. Laennec to his father, [13? illegible] Ventôse An XII (6 March 1804), MS de Miniac, no. 59; Guillaume to Christophe, 22 Frimaire An XIII (13 December 1804), transcribed in Crochet 1982, 73, 104. Guillaume's son, Christophe, went to St Germain l'Auxerrois to see the Pope and have his rosary blessed. Christophe to his mother, 29 Pluviôse, 21 Ventôse An XIII (12 February, 12 March 1805), transcribed in Crochet 1982, 113, 116.

72. Account in *Gazette de France*, 24 December 1804, cited in Grandmaison 1889, 51–52.

73. According to Saintignon, who was the grandson of Perdrau, Laennec was presented to the Pope together with fellow students, Fizeau, Pignié, Pidoux, and Perdrau. Saintignon 1904, 31.

74. Pickstone 1981.

75. Fizeau [1803–1804], [1804]. On Fizeau's prize in An X, see Laennec 1804h, 32n.

76. Bertier de Sauvigny has argued that the early Congrégation had little to do with the Chevaliers de Foi, the ultraright movement that became powerful after the Restoration. Others cite it as a precursor of the St. Vincent de Paul Society. Bertier de Sauvigny 1948, 312–313, 370, 403–405; Bertier de Sauvigny in Newman and Simpson 1987, 204–205, 241; Gibson 1989, 58. On the concept of "student culture" and student-faculty disagreements, see Rosner 1994.

77. Laennec and Bayle 1804a.

78. For references to "*le hasard*," see Laennec 1802h, 257. See also reference to "*une observation fortuite*," Laennec 1803b, 541, Collège de France, lesson 26, 1823–1824 ML, MS Cl. 2, lot a(B), f. 246v, 247r.

79. Laennec 1803c, 89.

80. Laennec to his father, 8 and 22 Ventôse An XI (27 February and 13 March 1803), MS de Miniac, no. 36, transcribed in Bouvier 1980, 231–233.

81. Laennec 1802h, 256–257.

82. See, for example, Laennec 1803e, 1804c, 1806f.

83. Laennec to his father, 8 Ventôse, 7 Prairial An XI (27 February, 27 May 1803), MS, Miniac, nos. 36, 40, transcribed in Bouvier 1980, 231–234, and Crochet 1982, 18–20.

84. Laennec to his father, 15 Floréal, 13 Fructidor An XII (5 May, 31 August 1804), MS de Miniac, nos. 60, 64, transcribed in Crochet 1982, 78–79, 95–98. See also Laennec to his father, 10 Nivôse, [13? illegible] Ventôse, 13 Fructidor An XII; 19 Vendémiaire An XIII (3 January, 6 March, 31 August, 11 October 1804), MS de Miniac, nos. 55, 59, 64, 65, transcribed in Crochet 1982, 68–69, 73, 95–99.

85. "That stroke of the bistoury—charming!" Laennec to his uncle Guillaume, 1 Fructidor An XI (19 August 1803), MS de Miniac, no. 44, transcribed in Crochet 1982, 27–30.

86. Laennec 1803d; Laennec to his uncle, 1 Fructidor An XI (19 August 1803), MS de Miniac, no. 44, transcribed in Crochet 1982, 27–30.

87. Laennec to his father, 21 Fructidor An XI (8 September 1803), MS de Miniac, no. 48, transcribed in Crochet 1982, 37–39. The Musée Laennec possesses the surgical instruments and book prizes, including Duret's commentary on Hippoc-

rates, two volumes of Sydenham and of Baillou, Lorry on skin diseases, and five volumes of the *Mémoires* of the Académie de Chirugie. Laennec was impressed that the elaborate bindings of each quarto volume had cost 40 livres. On Chaptal, see Weiner 1993, 110–111.

88. On the Société Anatomique and Dupuytren, see Huard and Imbault-Huart 1978; Maulitz 1987, 74–79; Orcel and Vetter 1976; Ségal 1984; Véron [1853–1855], *1*:117–120. Even Dupuytren's eulogist mentioned his notoriously jealous personality and uncharitable attitude to students. Pariset, 1845, 135–136.

89. Laennec to his father, 25 Brumaire, 7 Frimaire, 1 Nivôse An XII (17, 29 November, 23 December 1803), MS de Miniac, nos. 52, 53, 54, transcribed in Crochet 1982, 48–51, 53–55.

90. Description by the young Breton witness, F. M. C. Varsavaux, cited by Guillaume to his brother Théophile-Marie, 8 Nivôse An XII (30 December 1803), transcribed in Crochet 1982, 55. See also Rouxeau [1912], 225.

91. Christophe Laennec to his mother, 30 October 1805, transcribed in Crochet 1982, 147.

92. Laennec to his father, 15 Floréal An XII (5 May 1804), MS de Miniac, no. 60, transcribed in Crochet 1982, 78–79. The treatise on pathological anatomy has been divided in two parts held in different archives: "Traité d'anatomie pathologique," BIUM, MS 2186 (IIIa,b,c), 81 pages; and "Traité d'anatomie pathologique," ML, Cl. 7 lot a, 167 pages.

93. "Cours d'anatomie pathologique," BIUM, MS 2186 (I), f. 1–116v; "Cours d'anatomie pathologique," ML, Carnet de J. Guépin [a], f. 1–93. Comparison of these two documents makes it clear that Laennec's own notes are incomplete, and that a lesson on catarrh and all the lessons on the heart are missing. The omission appears to have be deliberate rather than accidental, since half of one page has been cut away (f. 37). The second and third lesson concerned dissection technique and were published with commentary by Letulle 1912b, 1912c.

94. Lonie 1978; Rey 1992. "Hippocrates and Modern Medicine" was the subject of a conference at the College of Physicians in Philadelphia, 4–5 May 1996; a volume is planned.

95. Boulet d'Hesdin [1804].

96. Laennec 1804h. A convincing facsimile of Laennec's personal copy, including his handwritten annotations and notes on loose pages, was published by M. Letulle in 1923. Care was taken to reproduce the tint of paper and the water marks, and the result has fooled more than one bibliophile. The original thesis, loaned by the family for preparation of the facsimile, was not returned and now appears to be lost. Grmek 1982, 4.

97. Petition "Aux citoyens professors," written and signed by R. T. H. Laennec, 4 Pluviôse An XII (25 January 1804), "Demandes d'inscription," AN, AJ 16 / 886 and ML, photograph.

98. 7 Prairial, 4 Messidor, 21 Fructidor An XI (27 May, 23 June, 8 September 1803), MS de Miniac, nos. 40, 41, 48, transcribed in Crochet 1982, 18–20, 22–23, 37–39.

99. Lonie 1978, 78. See also Finot 1960; Martiny 1975; Pigeaud 1975, 1981; Rey 1992; Robert 1981.

100. Laennec 1804h, 8. The thesis was published and sold for 1.2 francs (announcement *J. méd.* 1804 *8*:577). It is my purpose to summarize Laennec's argument, not to justify it. Those interested in comparing his assessment of Hippocratic

"doctrine" with the theory and nosological structures of ancient texts should consult Grmek 1975, 1988, 292–295; Potter 1988a, 38–51; Potter 1990.

101. Laennec 1804h, 33. In support of this statement, he cited a Hippocratic passage (*Nutriment*, 25, 26). See Littré 1861, *9*:106–109; Jones 1923, *1*:350–351.

102. Laennec 1804h, 17n; see also the chapter, "Ouvrez quelques cadavres," in Foucault 1963, 125–149, esp. 148.

103. Laennec 1804h, 32n; Broussais [1801–1802]; Fizeau [1803–1804]. See also Laennec, Lesson 30, 1822–1823, Collège de France, BIUM, MS 2186 (IV), f. 118v.

104. Laennec to his father 15 Floréal An XII (5 May 1804), MS de Miniac, no. 60, transcribed in Crochet 1982, 78–79.

105. *Ancient Medicine* 2. See Jones 1923, *1*:14–15; Littré 1839, *1*:572–573.

106. Laennec *père* to his son, 26 Nivôse An XII (17 January 1804), transcribed in Crochet 1982, 64–65; Laennec to his father, 10 Nivôse, 15 Floréal An XII (1 January, 5 May 1804), MS de Miniac, nos. 55, 60, transcribed (with an error in date) in Crochet 1982, 68–69, 78–79.

107. Rouxeau [1912], 242.

108. Laennec to his father, 23 Prairial An XII (12 June 1804), MS de Miniac, no. 61, transcribed in Crochet 1982, 80. Laennec's medical diploma was issued on 26 Prairial An XII (15 June 1804), transcribed in Crochet 1982, 81.

109. Buisson [1804], 77, 79, 80.

CHAPTER THREE

1. Laennec to his father, 13 Fructidor An XII (31 August 1804), MS de Miniac, no. 64, transcribed in Crochet 1982, 95–98. On the Société de l'Ecole, see Ackerknecht 1967, 115; Lesch 1984, 57; Maulitz 1987, 70–71; Ramsey 1988, 106; Weisz 1995, 7–14.

2. The papers of the Société de l'Ecole are in the Library of the Académie Nationale de Médecine, hereinafter ANM-SEM. The proceedings of the Société de l'Ecole and some essays were published in its journal, *Bulletin de l'Ecole de Médecine de Paris et de la Société établie dans son sein*, 7 vols. (1804–1821), hereafter *BEMS*. The title of this now rather scarce periodical altered in 1808 to recognize the change from "Ecole" to "Faculté." Volumes cover two or more years and the pagination is capricious; references must be traced using the year, issue, and page. Laennec's dispute with Duypuytren (discussed later in this chapter) suggests that issues must have appeared immediately; however, in the series at the BIUM, issues from the first eight years were published (or repinted) in 1812.

3. Bayle's long essay was based on an analysis of 88 cases and supported by five full case histories. It bears a marked similarity to the numerical method used in the later but more elaborate work of P. C. A. Louis. G. L. Bayle 1803. On this essay, see Rey 1993a, 192.

4. The sixteen new members were: Bayle, Dendrolle, Geoffroy, Husson, Laennec, Larrey, Lerminier, Louyer-Villermay, Moreau, Nysten, Peron, Roux, Royer-Collard, Schwilgue, Thenard, and Thillaye *fils*. See "Tableau des membres adjoints," on wrapper of a folder containing A. M. C. Duméril's mémoire "Sur la forme de la dernière phalange dans les mammifères." ANM-SEM, carton D, Duméril.

5. See Laennec to his father, 22 Nivôse, 23 Ventôse, 15 Floréal, 22–25 Thermidor, 13 Fructidor An XII (15 January, 14 March, 5 May, 10–13 August, 31 August

1804), MS de Miniac, nos. 56, 59, 60, 62, 64, esp. 62, 64, transcribed in Crochet 1982, 62–64, 73, 78–79, 94–95, 95–98, esp. 94 and 96.

6. See, for example, Laennec *père* to his brother Guillaume, 11, 17 April 1807, transcribed in Crochet 1982, 211, 219–220.

7. Laennec 1812a. In 1810, the Société established a commission, on which Laennec served, to oversee the publication of its proceedings and memoires. In 1812, some mémoires were finally released and the first and second volumes of its *Bulletin* were either reprinted or collated. *BEMS* 1 (1804–1808) and 2 (1809–1811). See Laennec 1810d. It appears that part of Laennec's mémoire may not have been published, because in 1822, he still referred to his "mémoire inédit sur les vers vésiculaires." Lesson 27, 1822–1823, Collège de France, BIUM, MS 2186 (IV), f. 103r. See also Laennec to his father, 19 March, 2 April, 3 September 1806, MS de Miniac, no. 85, 86, 91, transcribed in Crochet 1982, 164–168, 183–184.

8. Laennec 1805c, 1805f, 1805j, 1806x, 1807a. See also Huard and Théodoridès 1859, 1981.

9. Laennec 1811c.

10. Laennec, lesson 27, Collège de France, 1822–1823, BIUM, MS 2186 (IV), f. 105r.

11. Laennec and A.M.C. Duméril, "Rapport et observation sur un ver d'espèce inconnu, 18 Pluviôse An XIII," ANM-SEM, carton D, Duméril. Manuscript written, signed, and illustrated by Laennec. See also Laennec 1805c.

12. Huard and Théodoridès 1981, 180, 184.

13. Laennec, *Traité*, 1826, *1*:275–276.

14. For references to the microscope, see Laennec 1807a, 10; 1812a, 175–177 and plates II and IV. See also Laennec's annotations on the manuscript of Fortassin, presented to the Société on 8 Frimaire An XIII (29 November 1804), ANM-SEM, Carton 218, dossier 7, no. 1, Plate VI. After Laennec's death, his own microscope (of unidentified type) was sold at public auction for the sum of fifty-five francs to "M. Flandrin." See "Inventaire de vente de meubles après le décès de M. Laennec," 16 October 1826. AMP, Ventes, 1826–1828, D.90.E³, art 3, p. 6, item 48.

15. For more on microscopy, see Davis 1981, 87–115; Hacking 1981; La Berge 1994; Reiser 1979, 72–75.

16. Laennec 1809c.

17. Report by Cuvier and Laennec, 8 Frimaire An XIII (29 November 1804), ANM-SEM, Carton 218, dossier 7, no. 2. Fortassin had died 20 or 21 Vendémiaire An XIII (1804) at the age of thirty-seven or thirty-eight. The autopsy revealed that the right side of his chest was filled with black blood; the cause of death was said to have been a "*coup de sang*," but the unidentified author wondered what had been the effect of "*les forces vitales.*" *J. méd.* 1804–1805, *9*:132–138.

18. On Cuvier, see Appel 1987, 50; Coleman 1964, 33–37.

19. "Tous ceux que vous verrez signer [*sic*] des lettres R. ou T.L. ou R.T.L. sont également de moi," Laennec to his father, 2 April 1806, MS de Miniac, no. 86, transcribed in Crochet 1982, 167–168.

20. Laennec 1806j, 641.

21. Laennec 1806n.

22. Laennec 1806q.

23. Laennec 1806i, esp. 632.

24. Laennec 1807e.

25. Laennec 1806l, 716.

26. Laennec 1806g, esp. 443 (Pinel is not read); 1806l, 715 (Pinel as inspiration). See also Laennec 1807b.

27. Laennec 1806l, esp. 709.

28. Laennec 1806f, 1804c, esp. 567.

29. Laennec 1806i, esp. 632. The citation is from Horace, *Ars poetica*, 388. "If you ever do write anything," the passage recommends, "keep it back till the ninth year." It continues: "what you have not published you can destroy; the word once sent forth can never come back." For the text with an English translation see H. Rushton Fairclough. 1955. *Horace. Satires, Epistles, and Ars poetica*. Loeb Classical Library, London: Heinemann, 482.

30. Laennec 1804f; 1806w.

31. Laennec 1806d, esp. 363.

32. Laennec 1806e, esp. 374. See also Laennec 1806f.

33. Leroux [1803–1804]. The philosopher Etienne Bonnot de Condillac had said: "Since we give names to some things for which we have an idea, it is supposed that we have an idea for all things to which we give names. This is an error, which must be avoided." Condillac [1780], 115–116.

34. Laennec 1807n.

35. Laennec 1806h.

36. Laennec 1808d, esp. 370–371.

37. Laennec to his father, 21 Fructidor An XI (8 September 1803), 28 July 1806, MS de Miniac, nos. 48, 89, transcribed in Crochet 1982, 37–39, 179–181.

38. Laennec 1806s. See also Jarcho 1960, esp. 537–539.

39. Laennec 1806b.

40. Laennec 1806r.

41. Laennec 1807c.

42. Laennec 1805i.

43. Laennec 1805a.

44. Laennec, "Traité d'anatomie pathologique," BIUM, MS 2186 (IIIa), f. 13v–15v.

45. Laennec 1805a, 368n.

46. Dupuytren [1804], [1805a]. See also Maulitz 1987, 78; Orcel and Vetter 1976, esp. 171.

47. Laennec 1805d.

48. Dupuytren [1805b]; Note from the editors, *J. méd* Germinal An XIII [March–April 1805], *10*:102.

49. Maulitz 1987, 73–79; see also Rouxeau [1912], 252–258.

50. Boulland 1826.

51. Trousseau 1877, *3*:555; Hanot 1875.

52. For a summary of these events based on the minutes of the Société Anatomique, see Orcel and Vetter 1976. The papers of the Société Anatomique are held in the Bibliothèque Jacques Delarue, 15 rue de l'Ecole de Médecine, Paris 75006.

53. Laennec, "Discours pour la rentrée de la Société anatomique," BIUM, MS 2186 (II), f. 1r–5v; Orcel and Vetter 1976, 171. For analysis of this speech, its relationship to Bichat, and its implications for pathological anatomy, see Maulitz 1987, 72–73.

54. Magendie's presentation of 29 December 1808 was described by Laennec in his "Traité d'anatomie pathologique," ML, MS Cl. 7, lot a, Cahier R, f. 19r–20r.

55. Cruveilhier presided for nearly forty years until he was replaced by J.-M. Charcot. Orcel and Vetter 1976, 176.

56. Laennec 1812d; G. L. Bayle 1812b.

57. Laennec to his father, 18 Prairial An XIII (7 June 1805), MS de Miniac, no. 72, transcribed in Crochet 1982, 120.

58. Laennec to his cousin Christophe, 16 April 1810, MS Bertrand Laennec (copy?) and by a "succession" MS de Miniac, no. 108, transcribed in Huybrechts 1980, 69–70; Laennec to his father, 20 Thermidor An X, 28 April 1819, MS de Miniac, nos. 33, 119, transcribed in Bouvier 1980, 214–216 and Pinson 1980, 132–133. On the "painful career," see also Cruveilhier to Laennec, 13 April 1824, ML, MS Cl. 5, f. 21–22, transcribed in Roux 1980, 163–164.

59. Laennec to his father, 25 Thermidor An XI (13 August 1803), 22–25 Thermidor An XII (10–13 August 1804), MS de Miniac, no. 42, 62, transcribed in Crochet 1982, 24–25, 94–95. See also *Traité*, 1819, 2:181; *Traité* 1826, 1:649 and 2:332–333n. On Laennec's inoculation of a tubercle, see Marmelzat 1962.

60. Laennec *père* to his son Théophile, May 1806, transcribed in Crochet 1982, 170–171.

61. "Traité d'anatomie pathologique," BIUM, MS 2186 (IIIa,b,c), 81 two-sided pages; and "Traité d'anatomie pathologique," ML, MS Cl. 7, lot a, 167 two-sided pages. For a detailed description of the preface, see Boulle et al. 1982, 226–229. Parts of the introduction and the first chapter were published in four-hundred copies by Victor Cornil for "a small number of the curious, the erudite, and admirers." Laennec 1884, esp. vii–viii, xl. See also Letulle 1912a, 1912b, 1912c, 1912d.

62. Cruveilhier 1816; Andral 1829. Cruveilhier published several works on pathological anatomy beginning with his thesis in 1816 and culminating in the first volume of his monumental treatise.

63. "Traité d'anatomie pathologique," BIUM, MS 2186 (IIIc), f. 4.

64. "Traité d'anatomie pathologique," BIUM, MS 2186 (IIIa), esp. f. 11r (on Haller and Lieutaud), 12r (on Vicq d'Azyr), 14r (on Baillie). For references to the original works cited, see Baillie 1803; Lieutaud 1776–1777; Lobstein 1804; Portal 1804; Vicq d'Azyr 1790.

65. Laennec 1805h, 158.

66. Laennec, "Traité d'anatomie pathologique," BIUM, MS 2186 (IIIc), esp. f. 3r, 4r. For comparison with a twentieth-century critique of positivism, see Popper 1972, 27–35.

67. Laennec, "Traité d'anatomie pathologique," BIUM, MS 2186 (IIIc), f. 7.

68. Laennec, "Traité d'anatomie pathologique," BIUM, MS 2186 (IIIa), f. 3r–v.

69. Laennec, "Traité d'anatomie pathologique," BIUM, MS 2186 (IIIa), f. 1v–2v.

70. Laennec, "Traité d'anatomie pathologique," BIUM, MS 2186 (IIIa), f. 4v.

71. Laennec, "Traité d'anatomie pathologique," BIUM, MS 2186 (IIIa), f. 5r–5v.

72. Laennec to his uncle Guillaume, 20 July 1819, 1 January 1821 (copy), MS Bertrand Laennec, transcribed in Pinson 1980, 164–165, 251–252.

73. G. L. Bayle 1812a. On Bayle's vital lesion, see chapter 4 and Garcia Guerra 1990.

74. Rey 1993a, 195.

75. Laennec, "Traité d'anatomie pathologique," BIUM, MS 2186 (IIIa), f. 3v.

76. Laennec "Cours d'anatomie pathologique," second lesson, Collège de France, BIUM, MS 2186 (I), f. 2r–5v, esp. 4r.

77. Laennec, "Traité d'anatomie pathologique," BIUM, MS 2186 (IIIa), f. 20r.

78. Laennec 1806a, 1806b, 1815c.

79. Brown(e) 1685; Baillie [1808], 132–133.

80. Cuvi, ML, MS Cl. 7a, f. 143v–146r. See also anonymous thirty-year-old man who died in the Necker hospital, 15 June 1818, ML, MS Cl. I, lot b, f. 90r–92v.

81. Traité, 1819, 1:359–369, esp. 368–369n. On Edmé who died in May 1819, see also ML, MS. Cl. I lot b, f. 176r–177v.

82. Ferrus 1824, 1836; Erasmus 1839; Carswell 1838, "Atrophy," Plate II, np. On Carswell, see Hollman 1995; Huard and Grmek 1973; Jacyna 1991, esp. 112.

83. Hanot 1875.

84. Charcot (Prog. méd. 1877, 221–222), cited in Duffin 1987; see also Boitout 1965.

85. Mériadec's revisions are found in "Anatomie pathologique," BIUM, MS 5172 (I) and (II). There is evidence that they were written after his cousin's death and may not be an exact reflection of the ideas prior to the discovery of auscultation. Portions of the original incomplete treatise may have been filed with other papers. See, for example, essays on "elephantiasis," "pneumonia," "prostate," "animated foreign bodies," and "degenerations" in BIUM, MS 2186 (VI), lots a, b, c, d, e. Other portions may have been filed with the notes for the Collège de France lectures, but they can no longer be distinguished from the later material.

86. Dupuytren's mother wrote directly to the Emperor asking that he employ her clever twenty-six-year-old son as his surgeon on "14 Prairial An I de l'Empire" (June 1804 or 1805), cited as AN 02–815, in Ganière [1951], 413n.

87. Laennec to his father, 25 March, 30 May 1807, MS de Miniac, nos. 99, 100, transcribed in Crochet 1982, 209–211, 225–227.

88. Laennec to his uncle Guillaume, 16 November 1810, MS Bertrand Laennec, transcribed in Huybrechts 1980, 77–79.

89. See, for example, where he muses over an epigraph, Laennec 1806j; cites Pliny on honey, Laennec 1808b; reviews works on Hippocrates, Laennec 1806u, 1811e; cites Hippocrates, Laennec 1804e, 1807p. To the author of one of the Hippocratic works reviewed, Laennec signed and dedicated a copy of his thesis: "Amico suo Courbon-Pérusel, R. Th. Laennec." BMQ, cote. F.S.1341.

90. Laennec, Cours sur la doctrine d'Hippocrate, ML, MS Cl. 1 lot a (I), f. 1–40, esp. 4r–11v.

91. Laennec, Traduction d'Arétée de Cappadoce, ML, MS Cl. 1, lot r (XVIII), f. 285r–394v. Laennec worked from Hermann Boerhaave's 1730 Greek and Latin edition of Aretaeus, De causis et signis acutorum, et diuturnorum morborum, libri quatuor . . . The manuscript is not in his hand and may have been dictated or copied. It has many corrections, annotations, and alternate translations. M. Grmek has prepared a soon-to-be published edition of this translation.

92. ML, MS Cl. 1, lot r (XVIII), f. 321r. (Acute Diseases, Book II, Chap. 3, "syncope").

93. Adams 1856, xiii. For the Greek and Adams's post-stethoscopic and acoustically charged translation of the same phrase—"bruit of the heart, with violent palpitation," see Adams 1856, 30, 271.

94. *Traité*, 1826, *1*:651; Lesson 8, 1823–24, Collège de France, ML, MS Cl. 2 lot a(B), f. 177v–179v.

95. Laennec, Traduction de Caelius Aurelianus, ML, MS Cl. 5, lot j, f. 1–10v. *Acute Diseases*, book I (preface and part of chap. 1, phrenitis), book III (intestinal obstruction), *Chronic Diseases*, Preface, part of book I (headache). For the text with an English translation, see I. E. Drabkin. 1950. *On Acute Diseases and on Chronic Diseases/Caelius Aurelianus.* Chicago: University of Chicago Press, 2–11, 388–395 440–449.

96. Robert 1981, 241–242.

97. Foucault 1963, 181.

98. On the later essay, see Laennec to his uncle Guillaume, 17 December 1821, MS Bertrand Laennec, transcribed in Pinson 1980, 288–290. The proposed essay seems to have been lost.

99. Mercy 1820a, b, c. See also, "Procès verbal de la séance du 20 juillet 1809: Demercy [*sic*] addresse sa traduction des premier et troisième livres des *Epidémies* d'Hippocrate à la Société," *BEMS* 2 (1809, vi): 103. For references to letters from de Mercy (or Chaussier on his behalf) to the Faculty of Medicine, 5 March, 6 August 1812, 22 April 1813, see Procès verbal de l'assemblé des professeurs de la Faculté de Médecine de Paris, AN, AJ 16 / 6230, pp. 64, 85, 122. See also Rouxeau [1920], 112–117.

100. On de Mercy's talents, Littré said "perhaps it is not for me to give my opinion here on this work," but Daremberg bluntly declared that his work "fourmille de contre-sens [is crawling with mistakes]." Littré 1839 *1*:553; Daremberg 1855, xiv.

101. Mercy 1808; "Rapport sur un ouvrage de M. de Mercy," 9 June 1808, in the hand of Laennec and signed by Hallé, Chaussier, and Laennec. ANM-SEM, carton D.

102. For many years, Laennec was the doctor to a Madame de Mercy (née Hamar) who had connections to Nantes and was "a little related to him through her husband," but I have been unable to determine if she was the wife of the chevalier. Laennec to Christophe, 11 July 1816, MS Bertrand Laennec, transcribed in Pinson 1980, 74–76.

103. Some references are merely notations on scraps of paper, like a form of cross-referenced index made during his reading of ancient texts; they may have been kept for preparing lectures, reviews, or other publications. See especially ML, MS Cl 3, f. 1–449r. With the help of the *Catalogue* (Boulle et al. 1982), the following, probably incomplete, list of early authors cited by Laennec has been assembled: (1) early scientific and medical authors: Pythagoras (sixth century B.C.); Democritus, Empedocles, Euryphon (fifth century B.C.); Plato, Aristotle, Diocles de Carystus, Praxagoras (fourth century B.C.); Erasistratus, Herophilus, Archimedes (third century B.C.); Aesclepiades of Bithynia, Themison (first century B.C.); Archigenes, Celsus, Dioscorides, Aretaeus, Pliny the Elder (first century A.D.); Soranus, Galen (second century A.D.); (2) early medieval scientific and medical writers: Oribasius (fourth century); Caelius Aurelianus (fifth century); Aetius, Alexander of Tralles, Procopius de Caesaria (sixth century); Rhazes (ninth century); and Avicenna (tenth century); (3) nonmedical writers: Homer, Thucydides, Julius Caesar, Cicero, Virgil, Horace, Ovid, Phaedrus, Plutarch, and Juvenal.

104. Pigeaud 1981, 234; Ackerknecht 1967, 98.

105. On Aubry, see especially ML, MS Cl 3, f. 93. On Barker and Lorry, see Laennec's handwritten note in his personal copy of Barker 1768, ML. See also Aubry [1776]; Pigeaud 1975; 1981, 236; Robert 1981, 244.

106. Laennec to his uncle Guillaume, 14 June–3 July 1812, MS Bertrand Laennec, transcribed in Huybrechts 1980, 94–99. For more on the dictionary, see Rouxeau [1920], 97–99; Weiner 1993, 290–291, 310.

107. Laennec, "Traité d'anatomie pathologique," BIUM, MS 2186 (IIIc), f. 6.

CHAPTER FOUR

1. Léonard 1978, 97–100; Ramsey 1988, 110–122. On Laennec's later practice, see chapter 10; on his finances, see Appendix B.

2. On the relationship of diseases to the medical theory, see Risse 1979; Stevenson 1982.

3. Laennec to his uncle Guillaume, 14 June to 3 July 1812, 20 December 1815, both MS Bertrand Laennec, transcribed in Huybrechts 1980, 94–99, and Pinson 1980, 49–51.

4. Ambroise to Christophe, 27 July 1817, and Guillaume to Mériadec, 15 December 1817, transcribed in Pinson 1980, 94, 96.

5. Guillaume Laennec, "Cours de matière médicale élémentaire," ML, MS Cl. 4, 213 recto-verso pages; see also, Paillat-Carbonell 1984; Paillat 1984. On the 1808 legislative changes, see Coury 1970, 151.

6. "Discours d'inauguration," *J. méd.* 1808, *16*:239–240.

7. Until 1805, Laennec said that he wanted only to be a professor; by 1807, it was clear that academic positions were eluding him, and he seemed content with practice. Laennec to his father, 8 Ventôse An XI (28 February 1803), 30 May 1807, MS de Miniac, nos. 36, 100, transcribed in Bouvier 1980, 231–233 and Crochet 1982, 225–227. See also Christophe to his mother Désirée de Gennes Laennec, 5 January 1805, transcribed in Crochet 1982, 106–107.

8. On Bayle's family, see letter from R. Moutard-Martin, grandson of Bayle's brother-in-law, to Rouxeau, 23 June 1916, MNFR, liasse 2798.

9. Laennec to his father, 31 December 1806, MS de Miniac, no. 95, transcribed in Crochet 1982, 198–200.

10. Christophe to his mother, 13 January 1805, transcribed in Crochet 1982, 108–109.

11. Christophe to his father, 18 May 1805, transcribed in Crochet 1982, 119–120; Laennec to his father, 15 Messidor, 1 Thermidor An XIII (4, 21 July 1805), MS de Miniac, nos. 73, 74, transcribed in Crochet 1982, 122, 125–126.

12. On Christophe's illness, see Laennec to his aunt, 31 December 1806, Christophe to his parents, 2, 19, 29 April and 10 May 1807, transcribed in Crochet 1982, 200–201, 211, 220. On Ambroise's illness, Ambroise to Christophe, 23 March 1816, transcribed in Pinson 1980, 55. On Mériadec's illness, see Guillaume to Mériadec, 22 August 1817, transcribed in Pinson 1980, 95. On Laennec's prescribing for his stepmother, see his letters to her, 5 January, 21 March 1807, MS de Miniac, nos. 96, 98, transcribed in Crochet 1982, 202–203, 209.

13. On Laennec's habit of self-treatment, see Christophe to his mother, 29 April 1807, transcribed in Crochet 1982, 220.

14. Laennec to his father, 7 October 1809, MS de Miniac, no. 106.

15. Laennec to his father, 2 Ventôse An XIII (21 February 1805), MS de Miniac, no. 68, transcribed in Crochet 1982, 113–114.

16. Laennec to his father, 2 Ventôse, 14 Germinal, 14 Thermidor An XIII (21 February, 4 April, 2 August 1805), MS de Miniac, no. 68, 71, 76, transcribed in Crochet 1982, 113, 118, 127–128; Christophe to his mother, 2 August 1805, transcribed in Crochet 1982, 126–127; Christophe to his father Guillaume, 10 August 1805, transcribed in Crochet 1982, 128.

17. Corbie 1950 (notice the publisher, "Editions Spes"); Corlay 1981. Historians have been fond of constructing long lists of the many talented victims of tuberculosis. Earlier in this century, Havelock Ellis and A.C. Jacobson tried to establish links between the disease and genius or creativity. Jacobson 1970, 40–49; Dubos and Dubos 1952, 64–65; Sontag 1979, 20–35.

18. Laennec to his father, 10 Thermidor An IX, 7 Fructidor An XI, 7 Frimaire An XII (29 July 1801, 25 August 1803, 29 November 1803), MS de Miniac, nos. 32, 46, 53, transcribed in Bouvier 1980, 195–197 and Crochet 1982, 32, 53–54.

19. Laennec to his uncle, 20 July 1819, MS Bertrand Laennec, transcribed in Pinson 1980, 164–167.

20. Testament de R. T. H. Laennec, 1 December 1812, MS Bertrand Laennec, transcribed in Huybrechts 1980, 120–121.

21. Guillaume to Mériadec, 19 April 1817, transcribed in Pinson 1980, 85–86; Laennec to his uncle, 20 July 1819, MS Bertrand Laennec, transcribed in Pinson 1980, 164–167. On Laennec's angina see ML, MS. Cl. 7 lot e–3, f. 1r.

22. Pompéry 1884, *1*:v–xxxix. See also Rouxeau [1912], 262–277; Rouxeau [1920], 109, 128.

23. Kervran 1960, 81.

24. Laennec to his father, 7 Vendémiaire An XIV (1 October 1805), MS de Miniac, no. 81, transcribed in Crochet 1982, 130–134. The Louis XIV chateau of Madame de Pompéry with its gothic chapel is now the private *Centre International de Rencontres* of the DOSNON company at Couvrelles 02220.

25. Laennec to his father, 14 Thermidor An XIII (2 August 1805); 7 Vendémiaire An XIV (1 October 1805), 1 December 1805, 12 October, 12, 31 December 1806, 18 January 1807, MS de Miniac, nos. 76, 81, 80 [*sic*], 92, 94, 95, 97, transcribed in Crochet 1982, 127–128, 130–134, 157–159, 191–193, 196–200, 204–205.

26. See Laennec *père* to Théophile, 30 October 1805, transcribed in Crochet 1982, 147–149; Laennec to his father, 26 Ventôse An XIII (17 March 1805), MS de Miniac, no. 70, transcribed in Crochet 1982, 116–117; Laennec, "Milbee et Tytiv," dramatic poem in Breton, MS de Miniac, no. 127. According to the father's letter, Laennec may have learned some Breton as a small child, but by 1805 he seems to have forgotten what he once knew: Esnault described the early letters as those of a "neophyte." He eventually developed a reputation as a scholar of Breton and corresponded with leading experts in celtic languages, Le Gonidec, Abbé Claude-Vincent Armerye, and Eloi Johanneau. For translations and philological analysis of sixteen Breton texts, including eight letters by Laennec and loaned by the de Miniac family through Rouxeau, see Esnault (1919). The BMQ holds a manuscript of the sixteenth-century Breton physician, Etienne Gourmelin, donated by Laennec in 1818, and his 1826 bequest of Breton books bearing his bookplates.

27. Cantique sur la fausse philosophie, AEQ, MS, "Laennec," stanza 2.

28. Laennec to his father, 12 December 1806, MS de Miniac, no. 94, transcribed in Crochet 1982, 196–198. See also Laennec to Christophe, 16 October 1808, 28

September 1813, both MS Bertrand Laennec, transcribed in Huybrechts 1980, 29–30, 146–147.

29. Laennec to his uncle, 20 July 1819, MS Bertrand Laennec, transcribed in Pinson 1980, 164–167.

30. Laennec to his father, 9 December 1818, MS Bertrand Laennec, transcribed in Pinson 1980, 112–114.

31. In 1824 and 1825, Laennec went hunting in western Champagne, probably at the home of the Le Veyer family in Hourges, and at the chateau de Salsogne near Couvrelles. Laennec to Christophe, 30 August 1824, MS Bertrand Laennec, transcribed in Roux 1980, 178; Laennec to Mériadec, 12 September 1825, ADLA, MS Chéguillaume, no. 19.

32. Albury 1982.

33. Christophe to his mother, 5 January 1805, transcribed in Crochet 1982, 106–107.

34. Christophe to his parents, 15 Messidor An XIII (5 July 1805), 2 August 1805, transcribed in Crochet 1982, 123, 126.

35. Laennec to his father, 19 March 1806, MS de Miniac, no. 85, transcribed in Crochet 1982, 164–166; Laennec to his uncle, 14 April 1816, MS Bertrand Laennec, transcribed in Pinson 1980, 65–67.

36. Laennec to Christophe, 21 October to 9 November 1807, MS Bertrand Laennec, transcribed in Crochet 1982, 244–246. Christophe to his parents in Nantes, 12 July 1807, transcribed in Crochet 1982, 233.

37. Laennec to Christophe, 16 October 1808, MS Bertrand Laennec, transcribed in Huybrechts 1980, 29–31; Laennec to his father, 7 October 1809, MS de Miniac, no. 106. See also Broglie 1887, *1*:366.

38. Christophe to his mother, 2 April 1807, transcribed in Crochet 1982, 211.

39. Laennec to Christophe, 16 October 1808, MS Bertrand Laennec, transcribed in Huybrechts 1980, 29–31. On the long-standing tradition of consultation by letter, see Brockliss 1994.

40. Laennec to his father, 12 October 1806, MS de Miniac, no. 92, transcribed in Crochet 1982, 191–193. The "lady" may have been Mlle Delavau.

41. His father to Laennec, 6 December 1806, 5 March 1807, transcribed in Crochet 1982, 194–196, 206–207.

42. Helen Castelli, "Quélen," in Newman and Simpson 1987, *2*:853–856.

43. Rouxeau [1920], 123.

44. Léonard *et al.* 1977, esp. 860–861; Ramsey 1988, 62–65.

45. Laennec to his father, 7 October 1809, 11 May 1812, MS de Miniac, nos. 106, 116.

46. Laennec to his uncle Guillaume, 16 November 1810, MS Bertrand Laennec, transcribed in Huybrechts 1980, 77–79. On the gifts, see *Laennec: inventeur de l'auscultation* 1981, 52. Laennec gave the crucifix to his medical friend Bruté of Rennes who became a priest, emigrated to the United States, where he rose to Bishop. Bruté kept the crucifix at his bedside and once reported to Laennec that it was on the altar of the cathedral in Baltimore. Bruté to Laennec, 27 April, 10 July 1816, 8 July 1823, transcribed in Pinson 1980, 67–68, 74, and Roux 1980, 132. A plaster bust, valued at 18 francs (when combined with with four curtains and an old carpet), was among the unsold items at the auction of Laennec's effects following his death. "Inventaire de vente de meubles après le décès de M. Laennec," 16 October 1826, item 128. AMP, Ventes, 1826–1828, D.90.E^3, art 3.

47. ML, MS. Cl. 1, lot f(VI), B(e), f. 181–189.
48. ML, MS. Cl. 7, lot e–1(I), f. 1–17.
49. Rouxeau [1920], 101–105; Laennec 1810e. See also chapter 8.
50. *Traité* 1826, *1*:647. See also chapter 7.
51. Roussel 1893, *1*:48; Nora Hudson 1936, 126–127; Lamennais 1971, *1*:386, 390, 397, 409 (Lamennais to "Jean" (his brother), 1818); and *2*:428–429, 431–432 (letters to the Comte de Senfft, 1823).
52. Lamennais 1829, *2*:90–93n. Laennec's identity is established in a letter by Lamennais to Laennec, 26 December 1820, cited in Rouxeau [1920], 384.
53. Laennec, Collège de France, Lesson 8, 1823–1824, ML, MS Cl. 2a(B), f.172r–174v.
54. Laennec to his father, 6 July 1819, MS de Miniac, no. 121, transcribed in Pinson 1980, 151–153.
55. Weiner 1982.
56. Société philanthropique, *Rapports et comptes rendus, 1815–1845, 1* (1803–1810), esp. 1809, 63; *2*(1811–1815); *3*(1816–1819), esp. 1817, 144. A set of these reports is in the Bibliothèque Mazarin, Institute de France, 8° AA 59^M.
57. Laennec to Christophe, 8 November 1812, MS Bertrand Laennec, transcribed in Huybrechts 1980, 112–113. On the iconography of Laennec, see Finot 1966; Rouxeau [1920], 429–434.
58. Laennec to the physician Dr. Wuilhorge of Beauvais, n.d. Wuilhorge had written to Laennec 27 April and 6 November 1809 in care of the abbé Potel of St. Sulpice, the same priest who would officiate at Laennec's wedding in 1824. ML, MS., Cl. 1, lot f(VI) (A 3), f. 115–124v, esp. 115r–v.
59. Laennec re Thérèse Guillemin, 30 January 1811, ML, MS., Cl. 1, lot f(VI) (A 2), f. 110–112.
60. Laennec 1807h.
61. Laennec to his uncle 14 June to 3 July 1812, MS Bertrand Laennec, transcribed in Huybrechts 1980, 94–99.
62. Céleste de Chateaubriand 1929, 42. See also Chinard 1939; Gentil 1958; Valentin 1994. Some historians have mused on the possibility of Laennec's having encountered or treated Chateaubriand's mistress, Juliette Récamier (1777–1849). The couple supposedly met at the deathbed of their mutual friend Germaine Necker, Mme de Staël (1766–1817), whom Laennec examined briefly in her final illness (see chap. 6). No evidence can be found to support this possibility.
63. Céleste de Chateaubriand 1929, 218, 225, 260.
64. Laennec wrote, "Catarrhe muqueux chronique . . . Mme de Chateaubriand a eu," Collège de France, Lesson 29, 1823–1824, ML, MS. Cl. 2 lot a(B), f. 256v.
65. Porter 1985b, 17.
66. *Mélanges littéraires*, Décember 1819, in René de Chateaubriand n.d., *6*:557–558. A fragment of a letter suggests that Laennec may have used his influence in the right-wing crackdown of 1823 to help Chateaubriand obtain the position of minister of foreign affairs. Audoyn to his cousin Laennec, 6 January 1823, excerpted in Roux 1980, 95. For more on similarities between Bonald and Laennec, see chapter 11.
67. Laennec to his father, 3 April 1808, MS de Miniac, no. 105, transcribed in Huybrechts 1980, 10–11. Michaud to his aunt Mme de Miniac, 28 August, 23 October, 25 December 1807, 26 February 1808, transcribed in Crochet 1982, 239, 243, 246–249, 255; Michaud to his cousin Christophe, 11 October 1808, transcribed in Huybrechts 1980, 16.

68. Michaud to his aunt Mme de Miniac, 25 December 1807, transcribed in Crochet 1982, 246–249.

69. Laennec to Christophe, 16 October 1808, MS Bertrand Laennec, transcribed in Huybrechts 1980, 29–31. See also Michaud to Christophe, 11 October 1811, transcribed in Huybrechts 1980, 16, 32 (list of father's poems).

70. Laennec *père* to his brother Guillaume, 31 October 1821, transcribed in Pinson 1980, 277–278. See also Huybrechts 1980, 84, 163.

71. Michaud to his aunt Mme de Miniac, 2 September 1809; Christophe to his mother, 6 September 1809, transcribed in Huybrechts 1980, 41–43.

72. Laennec to his stepmother, 19 February 1809, transcribed in Huybrechts 1980, 52–57; Laennec to his father, 7 October 1809, MS de Miniac, no. 106.

73. Laennec to his father, 27 January 1810, MS de Miniac, no. 107, transcribed in Huybrechts 1980, 51.

74. Letters from Christophe to his aunt de Miniac, 24 October 1809, 13 February 1810, transcribed in Huybrechts 1980, 49, 58–59.

75. Laennec *père* to his son Théophile, 24 March 1810, transcribed in Huybrechts 1980, 61–68.

76. Laennec *père* finally renounced his claim on Michaud's estate 27 August 1813. Laennec to his father 11 May, 18 November 1812, MS de Miniac, nos. 116, 117, transcribed in Huybrechts 1980, 111, 136–138; Laennec *père* to his nephew Christophe, 19 June 1813, transcribed in Huybrechts 1980, 145.

77. Guillaume to his brother, 21 July 1806, transcribed in Crochet 1982, 175–179. See also Guillaume to Laennec, undated 1808; Christophe to Laennec, 13 November 1812, transcribed in Huybrechts 1980, 12–14, 114. The separation of the parents appears to have lasted from 1809 until at least 1815 or 1816. Christophe Laennec to his aunt de Miniac, 13 February 1810, transcribed in Huybrechts 1980, 58–59; Guillaume Laennec to his brother, 27 February 1815, and the reply, 4 March 1815, transcribed in Huybrechts 1980, 209–211.

78. Laennec *père* to his brother Guillaume, 21 December 1818, 13 February 1820, transcribed in Pinson 1980, 117–119, 208–210.

79. Laennec *père* to his brother Guillaume, 31 October 1821, transcribed in Pinson 1980, 277–278.

80. Laennec to his father, 15 June 1819, MS de Miniac, no. 120, transcribed in Pinson 1980, 140–142. See also, Laennec to his father, 7 October 1809, 24 July 1810, 15 September 1811, 18 November 1812, MS de Miniac, nos. 106, 109, 114, 117. Only one of these letters was transcribed by Rouxeau, and subsequently retranscribed into a Nantes thesis: 15 September 1811 (MS de Miniac, no. 114), Huybrechts 1980, 88–90.

81. See, for example, the father's letter to his nephew Christophe, 13 January 1820, transcribed in Pinson 1980, 202.

82. Laennec to his uncle Guillaume, 16 October 1821, MS Bertrand Laennec, transcribed in Pinson 1980, 272–274; Guillaume to Laennec, 12 December 1821, transcribed in Pinson 1980, 285–287.

83. Guillaume to his brother, 6 March 1800, transcribed in Bouvier 1980, 167–168.

84. Laennec to his father, 25 Brumaire An XII (17 November 1803), MS de Miniac, no. 52, transcribed in Crochet 1982, 48–51; Laennec *père* to his son, 10 Nivôse An XII (1 January 1804), transcribed in Crochet 1982, 55–62.

85. Marie-Anne's two extant letters were written to her father shortly after her physician brother's death, 29 August, 29 September 1826, MS de Miniac, both no. 135.

86. Christophe to his aunt Mme de Miniac, 24 October 1809, transcribed in Huybrechts 1980, 49.

87. Christophe to his aunt Mme de Miniac, 13 February 1810, 30 October 1820, transcribed in Huybrechts 1980, 58–59 and Pinson 1980, 250.

88. Laennec to his father, 5 May, 12 June, 1804, 1 December, 1805, MS de Miniac, nos. 60, 61, 80, transcribed in Crochet 1982, 78–79, 80, 157–159.

89. Laennec to his uncle Guillaume, 14 June to 3 July 1812, MS Bertrand Laennec, transcribed in Huybrechts 1980, 94–99; Laennec to his father, 18 August 1812, transcribed in Huybrechts 1980, 100.

90. "Note sur le partage de M. Laennec, médecin, et de Mlle Marie-Anne Laennec, sa soeur," 1–4 December 1812, transcribed in Huybrechts 1980, 119.

91. Laennec to Christophe, 10 March 1813, MS Bertrand Laennec, transcribed in Huybrechts 1980, 128–129.

92. Laennec to Christophe, 22, 29 January, 10 February 1814, all MS Bertrand Laennec, transcribed in Huybrechts 1980, 163–164, 165, 168. Laennec asked that the trunks be returned the following June; it seems that they had not been opened in the interval. Laennec to Christophe, 19 June 1814, MS Bertrand Laennec, transcribed in Huybrechts 1980, 183.

93. Grandmaison 1889, 33–34; Kernéis 1981a, 29. See also Hirsch 1883, 1:545, 586–587.

94. Laennec to Christophe, 22, 26, 28 April, 2 May 1814, all MS Bertrand Laennec, transcribed in Huybrechts 1980, 174, 175, 177. Marion de Procé had defended his medical thesis on the doctrine of temperaments in 1812.

95. Boulle 1986, 2:3, 6, 17_1.

96. Laennec to Dombideau de Crouseilhes, Bishop of Quimper, 12 June 1814, transcribed in Huybrechts 1980, 181–182; AEQ, MS Laennec, no. 1. A native of Pau, Dombideau de Crouseilhes may have met the Congréganist Laennec at his 1805 consecration in Paris. Laennec probably saw the bishop during his visit to Brittany in August–September 1814, a few weeks after sending the letter about the soldiers. In future trips to Quimper, he would sometimes stay at the Eveché. On Dombideau de Crouseilhes, Le Floc'h ca.1989, 116–117.

97. Esnault 1919.

98. "S." 1820, 77.

99. Laennec to Christophe, 20 August 1813, MS Bertrand Laennec, transcribed in Huybrechts 1980, 143–145. See also, Laennec to his uncle Guillaume, 16 November 1810, 14 June to 3 July 1812, both MS Bertrand Laennec, transcribed in Huybrechts 1980, 77–79, 94–99.

100. G. L. Bayle 1810a, 4–5; G. L. Bayle 1833–1839. See also, G. L. Bayle 1803, 1805; G. L. Bayle and Cayol 1812.

101. On Bayle's work on tuberculosis, see Ackerknecht 1967, 85–89; Dubos and Dubos 1952, 79–80; Keers 1978, 38–41; King 1982, 31–34; Rey 1993a; Temkin 1946b.

102. G. L. Bayle [1810b], 1812a, esp. 64. See also Ackerknecht 1967, 88; García Guerra, 1990.

103. G. L. Bayle 1810a, xix.

104. G. L. Bayle 1812a, 68, 74. See also, Maulitz 1987, 81–82.
105. Ackerknecht 1948; Convor 1978; Dubovsky 1975; Lomax 1977.
106. G. L. Bayle 1812a, 63–64. See also García Guerra 1990.
107. G. L. Bayle [1810b].
108. Corvisart's notes in Auenbrugger 1808, 171–180.
109. Roth 1991; Sontag 1979, 22.
110. Castelnau 1806, 10–13. The age of the patient was incorrect because Bayle was thirty-two at the time of Castelnau's defense. Castelnau's patient was identifed as Bayle, in A. L. J. Bayle and Thillaye 1855 2:893.
111. Laennec, Collège de France, Lesson 8, 1823–1824, ML, MS Cl. 2 lot a(B) f.179r. Laennec used Bayle's name in class because it also appears in the notes taken by one of his students. HMCP, MS James Kitchen, "Leçons pratiques de la médecine de Mons. Laennec," 18.
112. The poet was identified as "Gaudefroy, who died at 32 years of age in 1809," in G. L. Bayle 1833–1839, 1:l–lvii.
113. G. L. Bayle 1810a, 407–411. Bayle's identity is confirmed by Laennec's comment at case 53 in his notes on Bayle's book: "Bayle lui-meme." ML, Laennec, MS Cl. 1, lot f(VI) B(b), f. 174.
114. A. L. J. Bayle and Thillaye 1855, 2:893–894.
115. Deleuze 1816, 10. Deleuze was vice-president of the Société philanthropique in 1815–1816.
116. G. L. Bayle 1855.
117. Laennec 1816a. A "notice" about Bayle is with the Laennec papers, but there is no evidence where or when it was read, ML, MS Cl. 5 lot 3, f. 1r-v. William Osler also purchased notes made by Laennec about Bayle. See Osler 1912.
118. Laennec to Christophe, 5 June 1816, MS Bertrand Laennec, transcribed in Pinson 1980, 69–71.

CHAPTER FIVE

1. Laennec to Christophe, 10 February 1814, 20 March, 13 April, 19, 28 May, 6, 16, 21, 23, 28 June, 10 July, 17 August, 31 December 1815, all (except 20 March 1815) MS Bertrand Laennec, transcribed in Huybrechts 1980, 168, 212, 215–216, 219–232 (esp. 212 and 227) and Pinson 1980, 36–42, 52–53. Rouxeau copied these letters, but cited only one (20 March 1815). Rouxeau [1920], 143.
2. Laennec to his uncle Guillaume, 16 November 1810, 28 June 1812, MS Bertrand Laennec, transcribed in Huybrechts 1980, 77–79, 94–98. See also Christophe to his aunt de Miniac, 12 October 1812, transcribed in Huybrechts 1980, 108; Laennec to Christophe, 28 September, 5 November 1813, 7 August 1814, all MS Bertrand Laennec, transcribed in Huybrechts 1980, 146–147, 149–150, 184.
3. Ambroise to Christophe, 30 September 1815; Guillaume to Mériadec, 15 June 1818, transcribed in Pinson 1980, 44, 101–102.
4. Laennec to Christophe, 10 July 1815, MS Bertrand Laennec, transcribed in Huybrechts 1980, 229–232; Christophe to his wife, 26 October 1815, transcribed in Pinson 1980, 45–46; Ambroise to Christophe, 10 July 1815, transcribed in Huybrechts 1980, 229. Froment 1829, 2:228–230. On the social consequences of the Restoration, see Furet 1988, 273–321; Bertier de Sauvigny 1966. On the Restoration and the medical profession, see Léonard 1982; Delaunay 1932, 1949.

5. Laennec to Christophe, 19 May 1815, MS Bertrand Laennec, transcribed in Huybrechts 1980, 219–221.

6. Laennec to Christophe, 10 July 1815, MS Bertrand Laennec, transcribed in Huybrechts 1980, 229–232.

7. Dupuy 1989; La Varende 1970, 294–296.

8. *De la Féodalité.* A copy of this anonymous booklet is in the Bibliothèque Nationale, Lb 46/567. Another was given to his editor friend Villenave and now belongs to Dr. Michel Valentin. Laennec to Christophe, 10 July 1815, MS Bertrand Laennec, transcribed in Huybrechts 1980, 229–232; Ambroise to Christophe, 30 September 1815, transcribed in Pinson 1980, 44. See also Rouxeau [1920], 145; Valentin 1993.

9. Chateaubriand, *De Buonaparte et des Bourbons* [30 March 1814] in Chateaubriand n.d, 7:9–41. See also Shelby Outlaw, "Chateaubriand," in Newman and Simpson 1987 1:200–202.

10. Léonard 1982, 71; Maulitz 1987, 83–85.

11. Laennec 1815b, 3.

12. Laennec 1815b, 17.

13. Juvenal, "Moralists without Morals," *Satire 2*, 24. For the text with an English translation, see G. G. Ramsay 1930. *Juvenal and Persius.* Loeb Classical Library, London: Heinemann, 22–23.

14. Ambroise to Christophe, 5 December 1815, transcribed in Pinson 1980, 49; Laennec to Christophe, 11 April 1816, MS Bertrand Laennec, transcribed in Pinson 1980, 61–64; A. Laennec 1816.

15. Laennec to Christophe, 11 April 1816, MS Bertrand Laennec, transcribed in Pinson 1980, 61–64.

16. Laennec to Guillaume, 14 April 1816, MS Bertrand Laennec, transcribed in Pinson 1980, 64–67.

17. Kerviler [1899], 2:2–3.

18. Laennec to his cousin Christophe, 27 March 1816, transcribed in Pinson 1980, 55–57; Guillaume to Mériadec, 26 February 1818, 8 March 1819, transcribed in Pinson 1980, 99–100, 129–130.

19. Laennec to Christophe, 29 March 1816, 11 July 1816, MS Bertrand Laennec, transcribed in Pinson 1980, 58–61, 74–76.

20. See, for example, Laennec to his uncle, 19 January, 3, 10 April, 7 May, 20 December 1815, MS Bertand Laennec, transcribed in Huybrechts 1980, 206, 212–213, 214–215, 217–218, and Pinson 1980, 49–51.

21. Guillaume to Mériadec, 7 September 1818, 20 February 1819, transcribed in Pinson 1980, 108, 126–127.

22. On Becquey, see Geiger 1994, 78–80; James K. Kieswetter, "Becquey," in Newman and Simpson 1987, 1:83–84.

23. Laennec to Christophe, 5 June, 20 August 1816, MS Bertrand Laennec, transcribed in Pinson 1980, 69–71, 78–79. Rouxeau cited the 5 June letter at least twice, but assiduously avoided mention of the problems in Nantes and Laennec's attempts to have them solved through his royalist friends. Rouxeau [1920], 179, 181–182.

24. Guillaume to Mériadec, 12 January 1819, transcribed in Pinson 1980, 120–123. In another letter to his son, Guillaume said, "I was a much better royalist than all those ultras." 27 July 1818, transcribed in Pinson 1980, 102–103.

25. Guillaume assigned Mériadec to visit Etienne Pariset, General de Tilly, and one of the Royer-Collard brothers (but it is not clear which: either the physician

Antoine-Athanase (1768–1825) or his more famous statesman brother Pierre-Paul (1763–1845). He also sought help from L. M. R. de St. Aignan, F. L. Becquey, Pierre-Augustin Béclard (1785–1825), newspaperman M. G. T. Villenave, and Joseph Guyet, a bureau chief in the ministry of finance. See, for example, Guillaume to Mériadec, 26 February 1818; 2, 11, 20 February, 2 March, 28 July 1819; 22 April, 12 August 1820, transcribed in Pinson 1980, 99–100, 123–128, 173–175, 223–224, 235–237. On St. Aignan, see Kerviler [1899], *11*:449–450.

26. Mériadec to Christophe, 3 March 1819, transcribed in Pinson 1980, 128–129.

27. Léonard 1982, 75.

28. Laennec to Christophe, 5 June, 11 July, 20 August 1816, MS Bertrand Laennec, transcribed in Pinson 1980, 69–71, 74–76, 78–79; Laennec to his father, 6 July 1819, MS de Miniac, no. 121, transcribed in Pinson 1980, 151–153. On 28 June, the *Conseil général des hospices* of the ministry of the interior assigned a surprised Laennec to the Beaujon hospital, but two weeks later and for reasons unknown, the *Conseil* consented to a switch with Renauldin who had been named to the Necker hospital. Historians have been led astray because Laennec's appointment to the Beaujon hospital was announced in the *Moniteur universel*, but he never worked there. Beaujon hospital had been founded in 1785 as a hospice for the care and maintenance of twenty-four orphans, but it was temporarily transformed into a general hospital in 1795. The Necker was closer to Laennec's dwelling, but the institutions were approximately the same size with strikingly similar admission and mortality rates. By 1816, they were both operated by the Sisters of Charity. Weiner 1993, 40, 113, 134; Boulle 1986, *1*:101 and 2:15–17$_1$.

29. Tenon 1788. On Necker Hospital, see Boulle 1982; Boulle 1986, *1*:34 and 2:5–7; Hannin 1984; Risse forthcoming; Weiner 1993, 38–40. On Necker's dismissal, see Furet 1988, 83.

30. Boulle 1986, 2:6, 17$_1$. A census revealed that the number of patients remaining in hospital on 1 January of each of 1818, 1822, and 1823 was 122, 107, and 113, respectively. Registre des Entrées, Hôpital Necker, 1818, 1822, 1823, AAP, 1Q2.21, 1Q2.25, and 1Q2.26. The January census was not recorded in the intervening years.

31. La Berge 1992, 61. Ackerknecht 1967, 17. In 1790 at the Hôtel-Dieu hospital of Paris, one patient died for every 4.5 patients admitted, a mortality rate thought to have been the highest "in the world." Weiner 1993, 51. In 1814, most Paris hospitals had mortality rates of 20% to 25%. Kernéis 1981a, 26.

32. Gelfand 1977, 406.

33. For example, there are four separate accounts of the last illness of seventy-year-old Adrien Fouleux, ML, MS Cl. I, lot e, f. 4r, ML, MS Cl. III, f. 280r–v, 327–329, and 334–337. Duplicate records are often written by different hands. Boulle et al. 1982, 63.

34. The ancient doctrine of temperament was still a topic of medical interest for the postrevolutionary students of Hallé and Cabanis. For example, see the thesis by the brother-in-law of Christophe Laennec. Marion de Procé 1812.

35. Laennec to his "friend" M. Marquer at "Kerfunteun near Quimper," 29 April 1822, AEQ, MS Laennec, no. 6.

36. Laennec to Courbon-Pérusel, 22 and 29 April 1817, published in Thayer 1920; transcribed in Pinson 1980, 86–91.

37. Ambroise to Christophe, 27 July 1817, transcribed in Pinson 1980, 94.

38. Ambroise to Christophe, 27 July 1817, transcribed in Pinson 1980, 94; Mériadec to Christophe, 10 July 1817, 16 April 1818, transcribed in Pinson 1980, 91–92, 100–101; Laennec to Guillaume, 20 July 1819, MS Bertrand Laennec, transcribed in Pinson 1980, 164–167.

39. Laennec to Mériadec, 23 June 1826, ADLA, MS Cheguillaume, no. 33, transcribed in Roux 1980, 329–330.

40. Imhof 1987. See also Ramsey 1988, 67; Rey 1991b; G. Smith 1985.

41. Comiti 1981. "Pathocenosis" was coined by Grmek in 1966; see Grmek 1988a, 2–4.

42. The categories of these occupations follow Henry 1967, 46–48, and 1980, 22–24.

43. Louise Robert, 12 years, ML, MS Cl. II, f. 35r–36v; Mathieu Louvet, 16 years, ML, MS Cl. II, f. 241r; Théodore Seray, 17 years, ML, MS Cl. II, f. 73r–74v; Pierre-Léonard Clément, 18 years, ML, MS Cl. I, lot a, f. 15r; Anon., 18 years, ML, MS Cl. I, lot c, f. 27.

44. Marguerite Jobet, ML, MS Cl. I, lot c, f. 23.

45. Jean-Baptiste Gournay, ML, MS Cl. III, lot 1, f. 1–6; Louis Dupont, ML, MS Cl. II, f. 256r–v; François Lebel, ML, MS Cl. II, 526r; Jean Maillet (or Mailler), ML, MS Cl. III, lot 10, f. 474r–481v.

46. See, for example, Jean-André Vaché (or Vacher), ML, MS Cl. I lot a[I], f. 19v and ML, MS Cl. II, f. 501; Eugène Duflau, ML, MS Cl. II, f. 400r; Baptiste Dehor, ML, MS Cl. I, lot a [I] f. 19r; Etienne Guillaume Duné, ML, MS Cl. III, lot 2, f. 100r; Marie Léopold Derval (or Decerval), ML, MS Cl. III, lot 2, f. 102r–107v.

47. *Traité* 1826, 1:270–271.

48. Farge 1980; La Berge 1992, 159–177.

49. Femme Dumont, 1816, ML, MS Cl. I, lot b, f. 15r–16v.

50. Herbé, 1819, ML, MS Cl. I, lot b, f. 159r–160v.

51. Anonymous, 1819, ML, MS Cl. I, lot b, f. 167–169v.

52. Fleuret, 1824, ML, MS Cl. II, f. 250r.

53. On the narrative aspects of clinical histories, see Hunter 1991.

CHAPTER SIX

1. Grmek 1991b, 15–16; F.L. Holmes 1985, 502. For more on discovery, see Taton 1962, 79–91; Grmek 1976, 1981b, 9–42. On the relationship of sources to the historical problems of chance, preparation, and individual creativity with respect to a few specific bioscientific discoveries, see Grmek, 1991b, 67–103; Holmes 1985, 454–455, 486–502; Bliss 1982, 11–19; Geison 1995, 3–21.

2. On the possibilities and pitfalls of using patient records in the history of medicine, see Risse and Warner 1992. For an example of a collaborative statement describing the hospital as a site of research, see Anonymous 1823b.

3. *Traité* 1819, 1:7–8; *Traité* 1826, 1:7; Laennec, "Mémoire sur l'auscultation à l'aide de divers instruments d'acoustique employée comme moyen d'exploration dans les maladies des viscères thoraciques et particulièrement dans la phthisie pulmonaire," AAS, MS in two parts, part 1, f. 5.

4. *Traité* 1819, 2:119–120. For Hippocratic references to direct auscultation, Laennec directed his readers to the treatise, *Diseases II*, 59 and 61. See Littré 1851, 7:92–97; Potter 1988, 5:302–303, 306–309.

5. Keele 1973, 193. Pliny, *Natural History*, Book 16, LXXIII–184. For an English translation, see Rackham 1945, 4:506–507

6. Granville 1854, 19–24.

7. Kergaradec 1868.

8. Laennec, "Mémoire sur l'auscultation," pt 1, 5.

9. Granville 1854, 20

10. Toulmouche 1875.

11. The Laennec correspondence suggests that Mériadec and Toulmouche could not have made their journey before late fall 1816 or early 1817. As for Granville, he made the false assertions that Laennec was at the Necker hospital in 1815 and that the inventor had called his instrument, "*pectoriloque.*" If Laennec were actually working in the Necker hospital on 13 September 1816, it would have been his first week on duty—yet Granville implied that the teaching clinic was already well established.

12. Grmek 1981a, 110.

13. Double 1811–1822, 2 (1817):31. See also Finot 1972.

14. Double 1811–1822, 1 (1811):367–378 (circulation) and 2 (1817):104–128 (voice and speech), 239 (stomach).

15. *Traité* 1826, 1:5. Laennec, "Aphorismes recueillis aux leçons du Cen. Corvisart," 1801, ML, MS Cl. 8, 2, f. 4, aphorism no. 8. See also chapter 2.

16. For example, the 1900 "rediscovery" of the work of Gregor Mendel has been cited as the resolution of a later priority dispute over the laws of heredity. Bowler 1989, 112–116; Mayr 1982, 727–730.

17. Savary. 1812. Auscultation. *DSM* 2:460. See also chapter 2.

18. Wollaston 1810, 3–4; *Traité* 1826, 2: 430–433.

19. Case of D. Argou, ML MS Cl. 7, lot e3, f. 13r. Rouxeau's notes on Madame Argou, born 11 November 1779, MNFR, liasse 2817. Grmek observed that Laennec was mistaken about Mme Argou's age on at least one occasion; dating this record on the basis of the age that he assigned his future wife is problematic. Grmek 1981a, 112.

20. Laennec to his father, 12 October 1806, MS de Miniac, no. 92, transcribed in Crochet 1982, 191–193.

21. The words written were, "presque puberte." James Kitchen, "Leçons de Laennec," 1823–1824, MS HMCP, 59. Laennec's corresponding notes indicate only "découverte fortuite." ML MS Cl. 2, lot a(B), f. 247r.

22. Case XXXIV, *Traité* 1819, 2:32–37. There are no manuscripts pertaining to this case.

23. Alexandrine Gauthier, died 25 September 1816 at Hopital St Louis, case XXII, *Traité* 1819, 1:299–302; an anonymous sixty-five-year-old man who died 15 October 1816, at Necker Hospital, case XXX, *Traité* 1819, 1:439–446. The manuscript record of the sixty-five-year-old man had been preserved; it contains no mention of the stethoscope. ML, MS Cl I (b), f. 9r–12v.

24. Anon., case XXXV, and Millet, case L, *Traité* 1819, 2:49–54, 411–418.

25. Aronson 1985, 2. See also Rosenberg 1977.

26. Herold 1958, 107, 417.

27. Portal 1817.

28. Laennec later spoke of the therapeutic use of magnets in his Collège de France lectures: on the first occasions to cast doubt about it; on the latter two, to recommend it cautiously for migraine and chest pains, respectively. Lesson 51, 1822–1823, and Lessons 5, 7, and 39, 1823–1824, ML MS Cl. 2 lot a(A) f. 64r, and lot a(B), f. 167r, 170v, and 291r.

29. Broglie 1887, *1*:366.

30. Laennec, "Mémoire sur l'auscultation" AAS, part 1, f. 9. Portal's account of the death of Mme de Staël had also appeared in the *Journal des débats* as well as the *Journal universel.* See Rouxeau [1820], 190–191, 198. Laennec also cited a report in the *Bibliothèque médicale* (without precisions), and another in the *Annales politiques, morales, et littéraires,* 26 September 1817 (see note 62 below).

31. Pinson 1980, 97.

32. Laennec, "Mémoire sur l'auscultation," AAS, part 1, f. 8. Only the passage of the manuscript concerning Récamier is not in Laennec's hand. The royalist Récamier joined the Congrégation in 1817, the same year in which he demonstrated auscultation. On Récamier, see Grandmaison 1889, 331–333; Triaire 1899; Véron [1853–1855], 114–116.

33. *Traité* 1819, *1*:xi–xiv.

34. Laennec 1818c, d, e, f.

35. Laennec to his uncle Guillaume, 2 to 4 August 1818, MS Bertrand Laennec, transcribed in Pinson 1980, 104–105.

36. Laennec, "Mémoire sur l'auscultation" AAS, part 1, f. 11–13. *Traité* 1819, *1*:9–12. See also Toulmouche 1875.

37. The highest price went to a mahogany and cane couch with six armchairs. "Inventaire de vente de meubles après le décès de M. Laennec," 16 October 1826, items 71–82, especially items 80 and 81. AMP, Ventes, 1826–1828, D.90.E³, art 3.

38. Beaugendre 1818, 16.

39. *Traité* 1819, *1*:11n; Guillaume Laennec to his son Mériadec, 15 June 1818, transcribed in Pinson 1980, 101–102.

40. De Lens 1821, 586.

41. Mériadec Laennec 1821, 13n.

42. Nacquart 1819, 370; Clark 1820, 153.

43. "Dumont," ML, MS Cl. I (B), f. 15–16. See also full presentation of her case in chapter 5.

44. Amand Guérin, ML, MS Cl I (b), f. 17r–20v.

45. Jean Millet, died 24 May 1817, Case L, *Traité* 1819, *2*:411–418.

46. Marie Potel, case XLVII, *Traité* 1819, *2*:346–351.

47. Laennec, "Mémoire sur l'auscultation " part 1, f. 2; *Traité* 1819, *1*:6; *Traité* 1826, *1*:5.

48. Laennec, *Traité* 1826, *1*:xxxv.

49. Anglophone physicians debate at length over the correct terms for abnormal lung sounds. There are many variations on the conventions that I will summarize here. In English, "*râle crepitant*" has become "crepitation" or "fine rales"; "*râle muqueux*" has become simply "rales—wet, large or moist"; "*râle sonore*" has become "rhonchus"; and "*râle sibilant*" is "wheezing." In other words, *all* these sounds were "*râles*" to Laennec when he spoke French, or "*rhonchi*" when he spoke Latin. See also Robertson and Coope 1957.

50. Baume 1819, 11, 14.

51. *Traité* 1819, *1*:161.

52. Laennec, "Aphorismes recueillis aux leçons du Cen. Corvisart," ML, MS Cl. 8, 2, f. 10, 28, aphorisms nos. 31, 133.

53. *Traité* 1819, *1*:160–181. J. Duffin, "Pneumonia," in Kiple 1993, 939–942.

54. *Traité* 1819, *2*:32–39.

55. Elizabeth Roussell and Françoise B***, Cases XXXII and XXXIII, *Traité* 1819, *2*:19–26, 26–32.

56. *Traité* 1819, 2:37.

57. Rostan, 1818a, b; Laennec 1817b.

58. Grmek 1981a, 113.

59. Nacquart 1818b; Mérat 1819; Granville 1854, 22.

60. *Traité* 1819, 1:17–18.

61. Laennec, "Mémoire sur auscultation," AAS, part 2, f. 3.

62. *Annales politiques, morales, et litteraires*, 26 September 1817.

63. Laennec to Christophe, 29 February 1816, MS Bertrand Laennec, transcribed in Pinson 1980, 54–55. On Villenave, see *N. biog. gén.* 1866, 45–46:n.p., Valentin 1993.

64. "Extrait du prospectus," *Annales politiques, morales, et littéraires*, 16 December 1815.

65. Laennec, "Mémoire sur l'auscultation," AAS, part 1, f. 9.

66. Scudamore 1826, 10–11.

67. *Traité* 1819, 1:52–53n; *Traité* 1826, 1:664–665.

68. *Traité* 1819, 1:149.

69. Henri Alexandre Lajoie and Mlle M***, Cases XI and XII, *Traité* 1819 1:128–138.

70. ML, MS Cl. 2(B), f. 260r. Laennec, *Traité* 1826, 1:215.

71. Rault 1819, 21.

72. Collin 1823, 32–35; Collin 1824, 49–50.

73. *Traité* 1826, 1:63–65, 212–241.

74. Laennec, "Mémoire sur auscultation," AAS, part 2, f. 28.

75. *Traité* 1819, 1:57. In the 1821 English translation, this passage was omitted.

76. J. M. Potu, case XXXIX, *Traité* 1819, 2:128–143; J. M. Potu, ML, MS. Cl. I(b), 45–48. See also Maulitz 1987, 99–101.

77. Laennec 1818a.

78. Without specifying the edition he was using, the Hippocratic source that Laennec gave for succussion was *Internal Affections* 25. In the treatise on auscultation, Laennec gave two other Hippocratic references: *Diseases II*, 45, and *Coan Prenotions*, 432. *Traité* 1819, 2:121–126. The chapter numbers indicate that Laennec was using the 1665 edition of Vander Linden. For translations of these passages, see *Internal Affections* 23 in Potter 1988, 6:150–151 and Littré 1851, 7:226–227; *Diseases II*, 47, in Potter 1988, 5:272–275 and Littré 1851, 7:66–71; *Coan Prenotion*. 424, in Littré 1846, 5:680–681. On other references to succussion in Hippocrates see the index in Littré 1861, 10:803.

79. *Traité* 1819, 2:122–123.

80. Corvisart in Auenbrugger 1808, xviii. See also, Corvisart [1806], xviii.

81. Arsène Leraut Case XXXI, Louis Brouan Case XLII, Pierre Moineau Case XLIII, *Traité* 1819, 1:452–456, esp. 454; 2:157–167, esp. 160; 2:167–187, esp. 170.

82. *Traité* 1819, 2:118. The reference given was *Diseases II*, 59. Potter's English translation of this passage is "seethes" rather than "boils"; Littré chose "bout comme du vinaigre" as opposed to Laennec's "vinaigre bouillant." See *Diseases II*, 61. Littré 1851, 7:92–97; Potter 1988 5:306–307.

83. *Traité* 1819, 2:117–128.

84. Case XLIII, *Traité* 1819, 2:167–187, esp.173; Pierre Moineau, ML, MS. Cl. I b 137–43; 1819. The Hippocratic source given by Laennec was Physician [6] Littré 1861, 9:212–213; Potter 1995, 8:306–307.

85. Rault 1819, 23–24.

86. Sometimes the Latin record was kept with the final report. Several Latin hospital records can be found in ML, MS Cl. III.

87. Laennec, *Traité* 1819, *1*:48 and *2*:91–95, esp. 95.

88. Laennec, *Traité* 1819, *2*:94.

89. Case XXXVIII, *Traité* 1819, *2*:102–106.

90. Case XXXVII, *Traité* 1819, *2*:94–102

91. *Traité* 1819, *2*:108–110. No new cases were added to the second edition on this subject. Two manuscript records of metallic tinkling from 1824 are held at the Musée Laennec, MS Cl. II, f. 107r–113v, 156r–159v. Laennec spoke on metallic tinkling at the Collège de France, Lesson 27, 1823–1824, Ml, MS Cl.2 a(B), f. 252r.

92. *Traité* 1819, *1*:225–229. Laennec cited a French translation of Baillie 1803.

93. *Traité* 1819, *1*:plate 3; Toulmouche 1875.

94. Cases XVIII and XIX, *Traité* 1819, *1*:234–247. The manuscript record of J.B. Cocard (also "Coquard") has been preserved. ML, MS Cl. 1 (b), 113–116. The *Traité* gives 2 July 1818, as the date on which Laennec first recorded his suspicions of emphysema, but the manuscript places the moment on 5 July.

95. Case XXI, *Traité* 1819, *1*:251–260, esp. 253.

96. Laennec 1819b.

97. Laennec, "Mémoire sur l'auscultation," AAS, part 2, f. 18–19.

98. Rault 1819, 19, 22.

99. Grigy, ML, MS Cl. I (b), f. 29r–31v. Grmek 1981a, 113.

100. Dumesnil, ML, MS Cl. I(b), f. 183–188. For a detailed analysis of this case, see Risse forthcoming.

101. Edmé, Case XXV, *Traité* 1819, *1*:361.

102. Villeron, Case XXIV, *Traité* 1819, *1*:354–359.

103. *Traité* 1819, *1*:89n, 148, 392n. On Bayle's limited observation, see discussion at note 91 above.

104. In a speech read at Lille on 7 December 1854, Pasteur was said to have remarked: "In the fields of observation, chance favors only the mind that is prepared." Vallery-Radot 1927, 76. Geison has recently given a realistic new twist to this old saw by exploring Pasteur's prepared mind as one that interpreted through preconceived ideas. Geison 1995, 16, 87–89, 132–138.

105. An anonymous sixty-year-old notary from Nantes admitted 29 December 1817 and the eighteen-year-old mason, Louis Coulon, admitted 24 March 1818. *Traité* 1819, *1*:88–94 and 388–395, esp. 89n and 392n.

106. Laennec, *Traité* 1819, *1*:238n, 246–247n, 253, and *2*:194n.

107. For examples of studies that address specific problems of language and scientific ideas, see Anderson 1984; Benjamin et al., 1987; Cross 1981; Gerhart and Russell 1984; E. Martin 1990; Skoda 1988, 1–5. On more general relationships between science and language, see Knorr-Cetina 1981; Knorr-Cetina and Mulkay 1983. See also chapter 9.

108. Laennec to Courbon-Pérusel, 22 and 29 April 1817, transcribed in Pinson 1980, 86–91, and published in Thayer 1920.

109. Laennec to Christophe, 24 April 1819, MS Bertrand Laennec, transcribed in Pinson 1980, 134–135.

110. Laennec to his father, 6–16 July 1819, MS de Miniac, no. 121, transcribed in Pinson 1980, 151–157.

111. Beaugendre 1818; Collin 1823; M. Laennec 1821; Rault 1819; Toulmouche 1820.

112. Baume 1819, 11–13; Dalbant 1819, 20–21n; Mazet 1819, 13; Noverre 1820, 10–11, 37, 42, 47.

113. Toulmouche 1875, 470.

114. Dalbant 1819, 20n; Noverre 1820, 23–24; Rault 1819, 19; Toulmouche 1820, 19.

115. Bouillaud 1823, 22–24; See also, Beaubien 1822, 41–42; Kernéis 1981a, 36; V. Bouvier 1981.

116. Laennec to his father, 28 April, 6–16 July 1819, MS de Miniac, nos. 119, 121, transcribed in Pinson 1980, 132–133, 151–157; to his uncle Guillaume, MS Bertrand Laennec, 1 August 1819, transcribed in Pinson 1980, 167–172.

117. See for example, Guillaume to his brother, 15 May 1819, transcribed in Pinson 1980, 135–136; Laennec *père* to his son, 31 May 1819, and to his brother, 17 July 1819, transcribed in Pinson 1980, 136–137, 160–161; Guillaume to his son, Mériadec, 17 July, 15 September, 16 December 1819, 20 February 1821, transcribed in Pinson 1980, 157–159, 179, 198, 255–256.

118. Laennec to his uncle Guillaume, 2 August 1818, 1 August 1819, both MS Bertrand Laennec, transcribed in Pinson 1980, 105, 167–172; Laennec to his father 15 June, 6–16 July 1819, MS de Miniac, nos. 120, 121, transcribed in Pinson 1980, 140–142, 151–157.

119. Laennec to his father, 16 July 1819, transcribed in Pinson 1980, 154–157; Laennec to Christophe, 20 July 1819, MS Bertrand Laennec, transcribed in Pinson 1980, 162–163; Laennec to his uncle, 1 August, 1819, MS Bertrand Laennec, transcribed in Pinson 1980, 167–172.

120. Mériadec to Christophe, 12 June 1819, transcribed in Pinson 1980, 138–139.

121. Laennec 1819 *1*:vii–x; translated in Chauvois 1968.

122. "Procès verbaux de l'assemblé des professeurs de la Faculté de Médecine de Paris," meetings of 22 July, 5, 19 August 1819, AN, AJ 16 / 6232.

123. *Nouv. j. méd.* 1819, *6*:155; Rouxeau [1820], 216. The price of the two volumes of the larger second edition rose to twenty and twenty-five francs, with color plates for two francs extra. See announcement in *Nouv. bib. méd.* 1826, *11*:467.

124. Laennec 1819d.

125. Laennec to his father, 29 September 1819, MS de Miniac, no. 122, transcribed in Pinson 1980, 180–182.

CHAPTER SEVEN

1. Buisson 1802b, 150–151; Laennec 1802f, 176, 180.

2. *Annales politiques, morales, et littéraires,* 26 September 1817, 2; Laennec, "Mémoire sur l'auscultation," AAS, part 1, 10.

3. Albury 1982, 22.

4. *Traité* 1819, *2*:249–250.

5. Keers 1978, 49. On tuberculosis, see also Grmek 1988a, 177–197; Johnston, "Tuberculosis," in Kiple 1993, 1059–1068; King 1982, 16–69.

6. *Traité* 1819, *1*:19.

7. Hirsch 1886 *3*:174; Comiti 1981, 124–129; Dubos and Dubos 1952, 229–231; Goubert 1974, 267–269; W. D. Johnston, "Tuberculosis," in Kiple 1993,

1063–1064; Lebrun 1971, 276–279; Léonard 1977, 92; McKeown 1979, 92–96; Meindl and Meindl 1982.

8. Ackerknecht 1967, 95; Coury 1972, 27–30; Cummins 1949, 108; Dubos and Dubos 1952, 84; Keers 1978, 44; Léonard 1977, 275; Meachen 1936, 10.

9. Sylvius 1681, 526–537.

10. Morton 1694, 69–73.

11. Portal 1792.

12. Pascale 1979.

13. On attitudes to consumption in the nineteenth century, see Sontag 1979; Grellet and Kruse 1983.

14. Portal 1792, 404–405; *Traité* 1819, *1*:viii. For other references to Baglivi's lament, see Bouillaud 1836, 86–87; Capuron 1827, 427; Collin 1823, epigraph; Toulmouche 1820, aphorisms.

15. G. L. Bayle 1810a.

16. *Traité* 1819, *1*:37.

17. Cummins 1949, 109; Keers 1978, 41.

18. Laennec, "Cours d'anatomie pathologique," BIUM, MS 2186 (I), f. 10r–13v.

19. Laennec, Collège de France, lesson 10, 1822–1823, BIUM, MS 2186 (IV) f. 81v.

20. *Traité* 1826, *1*:534. Compare with the weaker version of the same idea in *Traité* 1819, *1*:22.

21. Cummins 1949, 109.

22. *Traité* 1819, *1*:32–34; *Traité* 1826, *1*:555, 562–580.

23. *Traité* 1826, *2*:147–148.

24. Laennec, Collège de France, lesson 10, 1822–1823, BIUM, MS 2186 (IV) f. 81v; Collège de France, lesson 35, 1823–24, ML, MS Cl. 2, lot a (B), f. 281v.

25. *Traité* 1819, *2*:360–361; Forbes 1821, 417–418. On the dispute with Broussais, see chapter 9.

26. *Traité* 1819, *1*:124.

27. *Traité* 1819, *1*:60, 65, 71, 111.

28. Herbé, ML, MS Cl. I, lot b, f. 159r–160v.

29. *Traité* 1819, *1*:103; *Traité* 1826, *1*:628.

30. Albury 1982, 30.

31. Louis 1825, 371–372, 503.

32. On Laennec's concept of "sufficient" lesion, see chapter 11.

33. G.L. Bayle 1810a, 411; Laennec, *Traité* 1819, *1*:62, 112–113; *Traité* 1826, *1*:638–639.

34. *Traité*, 1819, *1*:57n. On G. L. Bayle's case history, see chapter 4, near reference 115.

35. *Traité* 1819, *1*:20. Louis "agreed" with this definition. Louis 1834, 6–7.

36. *Traité* 1826, *1*:650.

37. *Traité* 1826, *1*:650–651.

38. *Traité* 1826, *1*:646.

39. *Traité* 1826, *1*:647–648.

40. *Traité* 1826, *1*:644–645.

41. *Traité* 1826, *1*:64–66.

42. *Traité* 1826, *1*:213, 420–421.

43. Rault 1819, 21.

44. *Traité* 1826, *1*:213, 215–216.

45. Andral 1823–1827, *2*(1824): 21, 24, 334–335. On Andral, see Ackerknecht 1967; Boulle 1984; Béclard 1880; Chauffard 1877; Huard and Imbault-Huard 1982.

46. *Traité* 1826, *1*:xi–xiii. Emphasis in original.

47. Cases III, *Traité* 1826, *1*:227–229.

48. Cases IV, *Traité* 1826, *1*:229–241.

49. Chopinet, ML, MS Cl. III, f. 236–243 (without annotations), 244–254 (annotated). Compare examination of 21 April on f. 238v with the same on f. 246 and *Traité* 1826 *1*:232.

50. Laennec, Collège de France, Lessons 27, 30, 32, 1823–1824, ML, MS Cl. 2 a(B), f. 248v, 249r, 261r, 269v, 270r.

51. Kitchen, "Leçons de Laennec," 1823–1824, MS HMCP, 70, 76.

52. Collin 1823, 32–35; Collin 1824, 49–50.

53. Kitchen, "Leçons de Laennec," 1823–1824, MS HMCP, 70, esp. 76.

54. Compare the words "*2e degré bronchophonie*" on f. 269v, with the crossed out words "*2e degré*" on f. 270 (emphasis in original). Laennec, Collège de France, lessons 32, 1823–1824, ML, MS Cl. 2 a(B), f. 269v, 270r.

55. *Traité* 1826, *1*:420–421.

56. On Fourcroy and respiration, see Bloch 1987; Holmes 1985, 414–415; Smeaton 1962, 136–137.

57. Compare successive editions of Major's textbook from its 1945 third edition, to more recent editions, Major 1945b, 163; Delp and Manning, 8th ed., 1975, 341; 9th ed., 1981, 212. Another recent text refers only to a potential decrease in intensity of vesicular sounds, implying that increase is not within the realm of clinical possibility. Macleod et al. 1985, 32. On the later history of "puerile respiration," see Duffin 1991.

58. *Traité* 1819, *1*:155–158; *Traité* 1826, *1*:50–53.

59. *Traité* 1826, *2*:137.

60. Collin 1823, 27–28; Collin 1824, 37–38.

61. *Traité* 1819, *2*:83–84. See also *Traité* 1826, *2*:75.

62. Heberden [1802], 62–69.

63. Rostan 1818b.

64. Floyer [1698]; Lullier-Winslow 1812; Chomel 1821a. On the history of asthma, see Gabbay 1982, 23–48; Peumery 1984, esp. 71–128.

65. On the problem of organic correlatives for fever and mental illness, see Bynum 1981, 143–144; Dowbiggin 1991, 22–32; Foucault 1963, 177–198; Goldstein 1987, 253.

66. *Traité* 1819, *1*:64, 72, 88; *2*:26.

67. Rostan 1818b; 1833, 15.

68. *Traité* 1819, *2*:81.

69. *Traité* 1819, *2*:84. See also Peumery 1984, 129–134.

70. *Traité* 1826, *2*:71–98.

71. On Mériadec's 1819 examination of Laennec, see Forbes 1827, xix; 1834, xxii.

72. *Traite* 1826, *2*:86.

73. *Traite* 1826, *2*:80. Laennec did not cite Floyer on asthma, but at the Collège de France he mentioned his work in a lecture on emphysema. Floyer [1698], 55–57. Laennec, Collège de France, lesson 31, 1823–1824, ML, MS, Cl. 2, lot a (B), f. 264r.

74. *Traité* 1826, 2:89–90. Laennec, Collège de France, lesson 31, 1823–1824, ML, MS, Cl. 2, lot a (B), f. 293r.

75. *Traité* 1826, 2:88–89. On the concept of internal and external sensations, see Locke [1694], Book II, chapter 1, 89–98; Condillac [1780], 87–89.

76. Laennec, Collège de France, lesson 39, 1823–1824, ML, MS Cl. 2, lot a (B) f. 292 r. On the discovery of morphine, see Lesch 1984, 139–140. In the present concept, asthma does not result from, but causes an increased need for oxygen: the body has not suddenly begun to consume more oxygen, but because of bronchospasm, the lungs have suddenly begun to provide less. Narcotics do not reduce the organism's "need" for oxygen; in fact, they reduce the efforts made to obtain it. Their use in asthma could have been deadly. How often Laennec used them and with what result cannot be determined from his papers.

77. On Legallois, see Lesch 1984, 87–89.

78. Andral 1824, 2 (1824):observation xx; Guersent 1821.

79. Statements pertaining to auscultation and related physiology have been confirmed in one or all of the following: Bates 1991; DeGowin 1986; Lehrer 1993.

80. Some readers may be troubled by this reasoning because they will know that physiologists no longer conceive of a "more perfect," "more complete," or more efficient respiration than the normal breath. Oxygen deficiency does not bring a healthy lung to absorb more oxygen from room air in each breath, because, in health, almost all the oxygen that can be absorbed is absorbed. In a respiratory challenge, oxygen levels are maintained, not by a change in the qualitative efficiency of each breath, but by an increase in the depth and rate of ventilation, an increase in the heart rate, and metabolic shifts in blood chemistry.

The same readers may also wonder what Laennec "heard" in those clinical situations with rapid respiration that are now thought to occur in response to the body's "need" for extra oxygen or ventilation and in the absence of lung disease—conditions such as diabetic ketoacidosis, fever, and thyrotoxicosis, in which the patient breathes deeply and rapidly and can die suddenly. In these patients, autopsy would not necessarily reveal changes in the lungs. In short, these cases could easily resemble Laennec's asthma. Perhaps his "puerile respiration" actually did reflect a "need" for increased breathing (if not oxygen), and some of what he labeled "puerile respiration" may have been the kind that we now ascribe to Adolph Kussmaul (1822–1902). Unfortunately, few of his cases are suggestive of these metabolic conditions, and the hypothesis must remain an untested speculation.

81. *Traité* 1826, 2:87.

82. Laennec 1826g, 5.

CHAPTER EIGHT

1. Bedford 1972, 1195; Bourgeois 1981, 2047; East 1958, 32–33; Herrick 1942, 88; Keele 1973, 197; McKusick 1958a, 137; Rullière 1981, 136; Willius and Dry 1948, 317. Some histories of cardiology simply ignore Laennec. See, for example, Wiggars 1960.

2. *Traité* 1819, 1:7–8; *Traité* 1826, 1:7–8.

3. Laennec, "Mémoire sur l'auscultation," AAS, pt 1, 2. The rest of the presentation dealt not with heart disease, but with the instrument and the exploration of the voice.

4. Koyré 1973, 14. On scientific errors, see also Schlich 1993.

5. On the development of cardiology, see Howell 1985; Christopher Lawrence 1985. On medical specialization in France, see Weisz 1994.

6. Jarcho 1980, vi.

7. McKusick 1960, 16.

8. According to Littré, a Hippocratic passage (*Diseases IV*, 38) was the source of a "popular notion" that the heart cannot be sick. Littré 1851, 7:554–557. See also Herrick 1941, 137; Katz and Katz 1962.

9. See, for example, Bonet 1700, 816–845; Morgagni [1769] *1*:675–708; Baillie [1808], 13–38; McDougall and Michaels 1972.

10. Vieussens 1715, 120–124.

11. Sénac 1749, 1778.

12. Sénac 1749, 2:286–287, 318; 1778, *1*:34.

13. Portal 1804 *1*:v.

14. Heberden [1802], 362–369.

15. Parry 1799; Fothergill [1776]. See also Leibowitz 1970, 73–103.

16. Baillie [1808] 83–95, esp. 94.

17. Corvisart [1806]; Auenbrugger 1808, 420–432; Laennec 1808d.

18. Corvisart [1806], 185; Soulié 1955.

19. Laennec 1808d, 370.

20. Corvisart [1806], 121, 124, 127.

21. Corvisart [1806], 315–324.

22. Corvisart [1806], 18, 26, 28–30, 117–118, 275–276.

23. Corvisart [1806], 275.

24. Albury 1982.

25. John Forbes, Laennec's translator, claimed to share this opinion of Corvisart's sentimentality with R. J. Bertin. See Forbes in Laennec, *Treatise* 1827, 584n.

26. Corvisart [1806], 276.

27. Burns [1809], 39–42, 136–152.

28. Burns [1809], 44.

29. Burns [1809], 44–46; Parry 1799, 113–114; 1815, 162.

30. Testa 1823, 143–144, 238–268. Laennec referred to the first edition of 1810

31. Kreysig 1814–1817, on classification, 2:Table I; on hypertrophy (*Verstär kung*), 2:318–330; on dilatation (*Erweiterung*), 2:330–338; on angina, *3* (i.e. 2:pt 2): 512–563. For more on these authors, see Herrick 1942, 33–34, 78, 81–83, 139

32. Corvisart [1806], 19.

33. Laennec 1802a; Laennec and G. L. Bayle 1804a.

34. Bertin 1824, 283.

35. *Traité* 1826, 2:497–498n.

36. Laennec, "Cours d'anatomie pathologique," ML, MS carnet de Guépin, 65–66. Laennec 1812b, 50.

37. Laennec 1805i.

38. *Traité* 1819, 2:281–284. For Corvisart on dilatation, see Albury 1982, 22.

39. *Traité* 1819, 2:256–257; *Traité* 1826, 2:496–497.

40. *Traité* 1819, 2:334–337; *Traité* 1826, 2:630–651. Forbes thought tha Burns had noticed the lesion earlier. Forbes 1821, 430. See also Mann and Mann 1981, 451–452. The valvular changes may be due to disseminated intravascular coag ulation and/or marantic endocarditis (Joel D. Howell, personal communication).

41. *Traité* 1819, 2:256–257; *Traité* 1826, 2:496–497. See also Forbes 1821 583–584n. Other British physicians shared this psychosomatism. See chapter 12.

42. Howell 1985; McMahon 1976; Kowal 1960; Skerrit 1983.

43. Hope [1831], 101.

44. *Traité* 1819, 2:255, 335; *Traité* 1826, 2:494, 619–620.

45. *Traité* 1819, 2:256; *Traité* 1826, 2:495–496.

46. Bertin 1824, 4–78, 239–282, 392–409.

47. *Traité* 1819, 2:251–254, 308–324, 334–353; *Traité* 1826, 2:490–494, 572–587.

48. *Traité* 1819, 2:251–252, 302.

49. Bertin 1824, 392–409, esp. 392–393. Bertin's section on cardiac hypertrophy filled nearly one hundred pages (283–375).

50. Dalbant's five cases all displayed the redness, which he claimed was present in twenty-eight of eighty-one cadavers. Dalbant 1819, 9, 12, 21, 23, 29. See also Mazet 1819, 11–12.

51. *Traité* 1826, 2:598–605. See also *Traité* 1819, 2:353–363.

52. Compare *Traité* 1819, 2:258–285 with *Traité* 1826, 2:497–531, esp. 538–539n. Bertin had dedicated his book to Corbière, the royalist minister of the interior, which may have vexed his liberal-minded assistant, Bouillaud.

53. On Bouillaud and endocarditis, see Major 1945a. For more on Laennec's unease with inflammation and Broussais, see chapter 9.

54. F. L. Holmes 1985, xvii.

55. My statements concerning cardiac auscultation rely on one or all of the following: Bates 1991; Hurst 1990; Luisada and Portaluppi 1982; Ravin 1967; Winwood 1981.

56. Harvey [1628], 26, 135; Albrecht von Haller [1786], 67–68. *Traité* 1819, 2:217–218; *Traité* 1826, 2: 384, 405–408, 417–418n, 420n.

57. Rullière 1981, 133. For other examples of "strange but true" style of history, see Bedford 1972, 1195; Keele 1973, 197; McKusick 1958a, 137.

58. *Traité* 1826, 2:420n. On Harvey and the Cartesian explanation of cardiac physiology, see French 1994, 223–224; Hall 1969, 1:257–259; Whitteridge 1971, 155.

59. *Traité* 1819, 2:217–220; *Traité* 1826, 2:405–408. See also Collège de France, lesson 44, 1823–1824, ML, MS Cl. 2 lot a(B), f. 307r–v.

60. *Traité* 1819, 2:199–200; *Traité* 1826, 2:387.

61. Laennec to his uncle Guillaume, 1 January 1821, MS Bertrand Laennec, transcribed in Pinson 1980, 251–252; Guillaume to Mériadec, 25 January 1821, transcribed in Pinson 1980, 254–255; Laennec to Mériadec, 8 June 1821, ADLA, MS Chéguillaume no. 14, transcribed in Pinson 1980, 257–260.

62. *Traité* 1826, 2:429–448, esp. 436–438.

63. François Nogry, admitted to the Charité Hospital, 23 November 1824, treated with tartar emetic and "cured." ML, MS Cl. II, f. 514r–515v.

64. Rouxeau [1920], 307–308.

65. Stokes and Blythe 1995.

66. *Traité* 1826, 2:429–433. Laennec cited Erman in Gilbert's *Annalen für Physik* 1812 1:19. See also, Laennec, Collège de France, lesson 45, 1823–1824, ML, MS Cl 2a(B), f. 308 v; James Kitchen, "Leçons de Laennec," MS HMCP, 122.

67. On Savart, Poiseuille, and others, see McKusick and Wiskind 1959.

68. Erman to Laennec, 7 February 1820, ML, MS Cl. 5(b), f. 18r–v.

69. *Traité* 1826, 2:431–433; Wollaston 1810.

70. *Traité* 1826, 2:415–420; Laennec 1825e, 1826b, c, i, j.

71. Barry 1827, 5; see also Barry 1825, 1826. On Barry, see Johnston [1917] *1*:172, no. 2601; Munk 1878, 214–216.

72. *Traité* 1826, 2:417.

73. On the northern limits of Paris, Montfaucon had been the site of the gibet where Andreas Vesalius claimed to have stolen cadavers three centuries earlier. By the early nineteenth century, it had been engulfed by the city to become "one of the most widely publicized health problems" in France. See La Berge 1992, 216–232, esp. 216.

74. Mériadec to Mme Laennec, 17 July 1826 and to Laennec, 1 August 1826, transcribed in Roux 1980, 369–370, 387–388, esp. 388.

75. Barry 1827, 9. My emphasis.

76. Stokes 1825, 137–139.

77. *Traité* 1826, 2:637. On examination of the pulse, see Keele 1963, 31–35.

78. *Traité* 1819, 2:220, 237–240; *Traité* 1826, 2:476, 492.

79. *Traité* 1819, 2:269; *Traité* 1826, 2:504. See also Corvisart [1806], 121, 129; Lancisi [1745], 309–313.

80. Laennec 1802a, 302.

81. Laennec 1826g, 2.

82. *Traité* 1819, *1*:302; 2:322, 338, 383–384. See, for example, Anon. male, admitted to Necker hospital, 29 December 1817, ML, MS Cl. I, lot b, f. 69r–72v, esp. 69r.

83. *Traité* 1819, 2:206–209; *Traité* 1826, 2:394–397.

84. Barry 1827, 20; Bertin 1824, 289.

85. *Traité* 1819, 2:268–270; *Traité* 1826, 2:512. Toulmouche 1820, 30.

86. *Traité* 1826, 2:506.

87. *Traité* 1826, 2:507.

88. Broussais 1821, 2:751. See also chapter 9 .

89. *Traité* 1819, 2:214–215, 308–324.

90. *Traité* 1819, 2:316.

91. *Traité* 1819, 2:215, 316.

92. *Traité* 1819, 2:213.

93. Rullière 1981, 134.

94. Laennec, Collège de France, lesson 45, ML, MS Cl. 2 lot a(B), f. 308v; Kitchen, "Leçons de Laennec," MS HMCP, 122.

95. Collin 1824, 61.

96. Collin 1824, 63–64.

97. *Traité* 1826, 2:421–457, 572–587, 755–756.

98. *Traité* 1826, 2:424–425. Four other "musical" patients were described in the following pages (426, 433). According to Rouxeau's notes, the first patient was Mme de Talaru. MNFR, liasse, 2823. Laennec's vivid description of this woman can be read in Chapter 10.

99. Cruveilhier to Laennec, 13 April 1824, ML, MS Cl 5 lot b, f. 21–2, transcribed in Roux 1980, 163–164.

100. *Traité* 1826, 2:429, 443, 453, 763–764.

101. Anonymous, Hôtel Dieu, ML, MS Cl. I, lot d, f. 11r–12v. The case was mostly likely recorded by Mériadec Laennec.

102. Juelle, ML, MS Cl. II, f. 80r–82v.

103. *Traité* 1826, 2:457–466. Kergaradec 1822.

104. Toulmouche 1820, 37.

105. Collin 1823, 44, 77–78; Collin 1824, 64–65, 115–116.

106. *Traité* 1826, 2:446.

107. Bouillaud 1835, *1*:196. Rullière noticed that Bouillaud had misread Laennec when he accused him not only of ignoring Collin, but also of failing to mention the friction sound at all. Rullière 1981, 135.

108. Kitchen, "Leçons de Laennec," MS HMCP, 127.

109. Most older textbooks on heart disease indicate that absence of the friction rub is usual in chronic calcific pericarditis, which may complicate tuberculosis, and in advanced states of pericardial effusion or tamponade, when fluid separates the membranes and prevents the physical production of the sound. With newer technology, the latter part of this assertion has become controversial. See Hurst 1990, 210.

110. Collin 1824, 2–3.

111. Jurine 1815, 5–25.

112. Desportes 1811, 69–83.

113. Laennec 1810e. Laennec, ML, MS Cl. 7, lot e-2; Other papers in Latin, including the consultation of Cardinal X, dated 1810, may have formed part of the final essay. ML, MS Cl. 7, lot e-1, and e-3. Another two pages from Laennec's draft manuscript on angina have slipped from the original file into the papers of Rouxeau, MNFR, liasse 2824. The coronary arteries were not mentioned in Laennec's "Cours d'anatomie pathologique," ca. 1803, ML, MS carnet de Guépin, 65–66.

114. Laennec, ML, MS Cl. 7, lot e-2, f. 9. See also Jurine 1815, 91.

115. Rouxeau [1920], 101–105, esp. 104. See also Warren [1812].

116. Laennec, ML, MS Cl. 7 lot e-2, f. 25r–26v. In keeping with current angina, Millot's pain had been brought on by effort and relieved by rest; its quality poses problems, however; the pain was "most cruel, . . . as if someone were trying to tear of his left breast [or] to kill him"; it began under his left arm, moved to the axilla, and settled, "he said, in a square the size of two playing cards overlying his heart."

117. Laennec, ML, MS Cl. 7 lot e-3, f. 1r; *Traité* 1819, 2:249–250.

118. *Traité* 1826, 2:488–487, 731–732, 745–750.

119. *Traité* 1819, 2:274–275; *Traité* 1826, 2:517–518.

120. *Traité* 1819, 2:432–445; Noverre 1820.

121. *Traité* 1826, 2:723–727; Bouillaud 1823, 22.

122. Bedford 1972, 1195.

123. *Traité* 1819, 2:321–324, 337–344, 346–353, 382–391, 398–403, 411–418.

124. *Traité* 1826, 2:582–585, 623–630, 636–642, 642–650, 675–680, 696–703.

125. *Traité* 1819, 2:54–62.

126. For the cross-references omitted in the second edition, see *Traité* 1819, 2:278.

127. Anonymous, October 1819, ML, MS Cl. I, lot d, f. 1r–3v. On this case and two others, see Duffin 1989.

128. Anonymous provençale, ML, MS Cl. I, lot d, f. 11r.

129. Moissenet, ML, MS Cl. I, lot c, f. 5–7.

130. Anonymous, ML, MS Cl. I, lot b, f. 69–72, esp. 71v, 72r. For the published version of the same case see, *Traité* 1819, *1*:307; *Traité* 1826, 2:46–47.

131. Charon, ML, MS Cl. III, f. 271; Laurent, ML, MS Cl. III, f. 261; Magdelain, ML, MS Cl. III, f. 61r–62v.

132. *Traité* 1826, *1*:518–527. Compare with Richard, ML, MS Cl. III, f. 274r–276v.

133. Compare the files ML, MS Cl. I, lot b (1816–1819) with MS Cl. III (1823–1826).

134. Forbes in *Treatise* 1827, 579n. See also *Treatise*, 1821, 429–431.

135. Compare Laennec's 1803 course notes with those taken by a student: Laennec, "Cours d'anatomie pathologique" BIUM, MS 2186 (I), f. 96v–98r; and "Cours d'anatomie pathologique," ML, MS, Carnet de J. Guépin, f. 64v–66v.

136. Compare Laennec's lectures notes, in which part of lesson 45 and lessons 46 to 53, are missing, with those taken by a student: Laennec, Collège de France lessons 44, 45 [incomplete], 1823–1824, ML, MS Cl. 2, lot a(B), f.306–308v; and Kitchen, "Leçons de Laennec," MS HMCP, 119–127.

137. Rouanet 1832. According to McKusick, Laennec's "error" in interpretation of the heart sounds was first recognized in 1829 by "John William Turner (1790–1836), Professor of Surgery (!) in Edinburgh." McKusick 1958b, 38. See also East 1958, 35; McKusick 1958a; Schott 1980; Segall 1963; D. C. Smith 1978.

138. Beau 1856, 234–314, esp. 275; Corrigan [1832]; Magendie 1838, 158, 162.

139. Williams 1835, 163n–179n.

140. On the history of cardiac auscultation and the debate over the motion and control of the heart, see Cournand 1975; Frank 1988; Geison 1978, 193–267; Huard 1981a; Keele 1973. On the role of technology in conceptual change (for myocardial infarction, or heart attack), see Fye 1985.

141. Bouillaud 1935, *1*:196. James Hope and Thomas Hodgkin recognized murmurs of aortic and pulmonic origin, and Hope described valvular insufficiency in 1831. Hope [1831]. See also East 1958, 34–36.

142. Cannon 1995; Leibowitz 1970, 106; Lie 1986, 1991; MacAlpin 1980; Weintraub and Helfant 1983.

143. Luisada and Portaluppi, 1982, 32.

144. Lie 1991, 147.

145. On the relationship between theory and the entities created through technology, see Fleck 1979; Hacking 1981.

146. Hacking 1975, 31–48; King 1976; Murphy 1981.

147. McKusick and Wiskind 1959; Keele 1973, 197.

148. On the history of the concepts of medical decision making, see Edwards 1954; Fleck 1979, 1986; Lillienfeld 1982; Reiser 1978. On "sensitivity," "specificity," "false positive," and "false negative" and their use in medical decision making, see Galen and Gambino 1975, 10–14; Kraemer 1992, 33–40, 63–95; Lusted 1968, 107–111; McNeil et al. 1975.

149. Popper 1972, 27–42.

150. Holmes 1985, 499–500.

151. *Traité* 1819, *1*:52–53n; *Traité* 1826, *1*:664–665. See also Scudamore 1826, 10–11.

152. *Traité* 1819, *1*:127; *Traité* 1826, *1*:212–215; Laennec, Collège de France, lesson 30, 1823–1824, ML, MS. Cl. 2, lot a (B), f. 261r.

153. *Traité* 1826, *1*:145–149, 158–159, 163–166, 173–179, 188, 195, 201–206.

154. Andral 1823–1827, *2* (1824):571–572; *Traité* 1826, *1*:83–84.
155. Nicolas Millot, ML, MS. Cl. 7 lot e-2, f. 25r–26v.
156. *Traité* 1826, *1*:650–651.
157. *Traité* 1819, *1*:xxi–xxii, esp. 413–414; *Traité* 1826, *2*:233–234. See epigraph at the beginning of Part Three.

CHAPTER NINE

1. *Traité* 1819 *1*:vii–viii; Kergaradec 1826a, 319; Mériadec Laennec 1821, 36. Rouxeau collected criticisms of auscultation in a special file. MNFR, liasse 2819.
2. Nacquart 1818a; Salle [1833], 307–318. See also Fosseyeux 1930, 10–11n and the report on Laennec's 1825 trip to Bordeaux, chapter 10.
3. Rostan 1819–1820.
4. Nacquart 1818a, b.
5. Nacquart 1819, esp. 370.
6. Rouzet 1820. According to Rouxeau, an anonymous reviewer in the *Gazette de Santé*, 15 Janvier 1820 (issue missing from collection at the BIUM), alluded to the ridicule, but he also recommended that doctors practice auscultation. See Rouxeau [1920], 2:231.
7. Bricheteau 1819.
8. Kergaradec 1820–1821.
9. Kergaradec 1826a, 320.
10. Orphaned and imprisoned during the Revolution, Kergaradec also had a military background and had begun his medical studies at age eleven. He came to Paris in 1802, one year after Laennec, and was admitted to the Congrégation in May 1804. Kergaradec resigned from the *Dictionnaire des sciences médicales* with Laennec in 1818. See Laennec 1818g; Rouxeau [1920], 2:319 and reference 104 below. On Kergaradec, see Pinkerton 1969; Stofft 1981.
11. Kergaradec 1821, *73*:162–164.
12. Kergaradec 1822. Forestier ca. 1822. See also Pinkerton 1969, 483; Stofft 1981, 165.
13. De Lens 1821; Mérat 1819.
14. Cloquet 1819, 350n. See also [Anonymous] 1820.
15. Rault 1819, 19.
16. Matthew Baillie to Laennec, 18 November 1819, ML, MS Cl. 5 lot b, f. 74.
17. Laennec 1821. On early English-language reviews, see Jarcho 1962a, b.
18. Forbes, in Laennec 1821, ix–x, xxvi. On the construction of Laennec as hero of pathological anatomy, see Maulitz 1987, 168–169; Weisz 1995, 189–211.
19. Forbes 1821, 423, 425, 429.
20. Compare Case IX, *Traité* 1819, *1*:109–112 or Case XXV, *Traité* 1826, *1*:635–638 with Case 9, *Treatise* 1821, 34–36.
21. Forbes to Laennec, 13 December 1823, ML, MS Cl. 5, lot b, 61r–62v. Forbes 1824, viii–ix, xiv, xxvi (emphasis in original). Forbes's in-patient and out-patient records are held in the West Sussex Record Office, Chichester, UK.
22. Forbes to Laennec, 20 June 1824, ML, MS Cl. 5, lot b, f. 65r–66v.
23. Laennec's handwritten translation and excerpt from "*London Med. and Physiol. Journal* no. 276," February 1822, ML, MS Cl. 5, lot c, f. 2r–5v; elsewhere he cited this periodical as the *London Med. and Chirur. Journal* Feb. 22, Laennec 1822b, ACF.

24. Forbes to Laennec, 13 December 1823, ML, MS Cl. 5, lot b, 61r–62v.

25. Laennec to his uncle Guillaume, 1 January 1821, MS Bertrand Laennec, transcribed in Pinson 1980, 251–252; Laennec to Mériadec, 8 June 1821, transcribed in Pinson 1980, 257–260. See also William Thomson to Laennec, 29 April 1823, ML MS Cl. 5, lot b, f. 70r–71v; handwritten excerpt from "*Revue encyclopédique* publiée à Paris avril 1822," ML, MS Cl. 5, lot c, f. 1; and Laennec's handwritten annotation that auscultation had been mentioned in December 1821 in the "new england journal of medicine and surgery no. 2 vol. x Boston" [*sic*] on a copy of Laennec [1822b], held by ACF.

26. Müller to Laennec, 30 Nov 1822, ML, MS Cl. 5, lot b, f. 63r–v, transcribed in Roux 1980, 89–91. The translator of the German edition is unknown, although some suspect it was Dr. Ludwig Friedrich von Froriep (1779–1847).

27. Knegtel 1970. See also Van Hall to Laennec, 25 June 1823, ML, MS Cl. 5, lot b, f. 72r–73v; reply, nd, transcribed in Roux 1980, 129.

28. On editions of the treatise on auscultation, see Bishop 1981; Genty 1926; Viets 1926.

29. On the dissemination of auscultation see King 1959; Knegtel 1981; Nicholson 1993; Nicolas and Kernéis 1981; Sakula 1981; Segall 1963, 1967; D. C. Smith 1978; Tuchman 1993, 64–65. See also a review of the translation of Collin's manual in *Boston Medical and Surgical Journal* 1828–1829. *1*:811–812.

30. Kernéis 1981a, 36–37; V. Bouvier 1981; Piorry 1828, 16.

31. Collin 1824; Kergaradec 1822; Lisfranc 1823; Bouillaud 1823; Andral 1823–1827, esp. his second volume of 1824; Louis 1825; Piorry 1828, esp. 15. On Laennec's hopes for auscultation in Itard's research with the deaf, see *Traité* 1819, *1*:xxxvi–xxxvii. See also Laennec 1808f; and Laennec, Hallé, and Moreau, "Rapport sur les mémoires de M. Itard relatifs aux sourds-muets," 8 July 1808, ANM-SEM, MS carton I–J–H.

32. Patients no. 191 and 200, admitted on 6 and 9 March 1816, respectively. Registre des Entrées, Hôpital Necker, 1816, AAP, 1Q2.19.

33. "Phthisie pulmonaire," patient no. 320, admitted 7 April 1821. Registre des Entrées, Hôpital Necker, 1821, AAP, 1Q2.24.

34. Anne Claude, patient no. 678, Registre des Entrées, Hôpital Necker, 1818, AAP, 1Q2.21.

35. See, for example, the entries concerning Marie Geneviève Mauchon, no. 220; Jeanne Vignesse, no. 282; Catherine Eli, no. 397; André Mercier, no. 428; Anne Cappin, no. 690, Registre des Entrées, Hôpital Necker, 1819, AAP, 1Q2.22.

36. Emphysema in Jean-François Perinelle, 48 years, patient no. 64, census of patients in hospital on 1 January 1822; pulmonary edema in Louise Salagi, 62 years, patient no. 342, admitted 2 April 1822, Registre des Entrées, Hôpital Necker, 1821, 1822, AAP, 1Q2.24–5.

37. Maulitz 1990.

38. Acute pleurisy in Louise Morin, patient no. 208, admitted 5 March 1819; Marie-Rose le Boulanger, patient no. 223, admitted 10 March 1819, Registre des Entrées, Hôpital Necker, 1816–1821, AAP, 1Q2.19–24, especially 1819, 1Q2.22.

39. "Malades restant 1 janvier 1822," Registre des Entrées, Hôpital Necker, 1822, AAP, 1Q2.25.

40. Registre des Entrées, Hôpital Necker, 1822, AAP, 1Q2.25.

41. Beaubien 1822, 22. See also Segall 1967, 415.

42. *Traité* 1826, *1*:xxv.

43. Laennec to Mériadec, 24 April 1820, transcribed in Pinson 1980, 224–226. Mérat 1819.

44. Mériadec Laennec 1821, 36. Mériadec's examiners were Desgenettes, Lallemand, Pelletan, Duméril, De Jussieu, and Richerand. His defense on 16 June 1821 was said to have been "*très satisfaisant*" as were four of his six previous examinations. See "Dossiers des étudiants," AN, AJ 6761, 1821, no. 92.

45. Clark 1820, 154–155.

46. Larrey 1820, 86.

47. Laennec to his uncle Guillaume, 16 October 1821, MS Bertrand Laennec, transcribed in Pinson 1980, 272–274.

48. Laennec to Christophe, 24 August 1821, MS Bertrand Laennec, transcribed in Pinson 1980, 267–268.

49. The Breton, Georges Ollivry, defended a Paris medical thesis on croup in 1810. He would attend Laennec in his last illness. Stofft 1981.

50. Laennec to Mériadec, 10 June, 4 July, 1821, ADLA, MS Chéguillaume nos. 15 and 16, transcribed in Pinson 1980, 260–263.

51. Weisz 1995, 167–169.

52. Laennec to Mériadec, 4 February 1820, ADLA, MS Chéguillaume no. 6, transcribed in Pinson 1980, 206–207; Laennec to his uncle Guillaume, 1 January 1821, Laennec to Christophe, 1 January 1821, both MS Bertrand Laennec, transcribed in Pinson 1980, 251–252, 252–253. See also Laennec to Mériadec, 28 March 1820, ADLA, MS Chéguillaume no. 8, transcribed in Pinson 1980, 219–220.

53. Rouxeau [1920], 2:256. Rouxeau's source for the hunting anecdote was Du Chatellier, in the Breton newspaper, *l'Océan*, 13 August 1868. See also Laennec to Christophe, 18 January 1820, MS Bertrand Laennec, transcribed in Pinson 1980, 204–205.

54. Laennec, "Observations sur les cultures, plantations, et édifices considérées comme objets de décoration et de l'utilité" (ca. 1820), MS Bertrand Laennec, bound with the family copy of Laennec's *Traité* and his *De la Féodalité*, 1815b.

55. Laennec 1820; Rouxeau [1920], 2:258.

56. Laennec to Mériadec, 28 December 1819, 10 February, 28 March, 16 May 1820, ADLA, MS Chéguillaume nos. 4, 7, 8, 10, transcribed in Pinson 1980, 198–200, 207–208, 219–220, 227–228; Laennec to Christophe, 18 January, 23 March 1820, both MS Bertrand Laennec, transcribed in Pinson 1980, 204–205, 210. I was told the anecdote about the trapdoor by M. André Halna du Frétay, the present owner of Kerlouarnec, 4 March 1995.

57. Laennec to Christophe, 26 November 1819, MS Bertrand Laennec, transcribed in Pinson 1980, 191–192; Laennec to Dombideau de Crouseilhes, the Bishop of Quimper, 24 August 1820, AEQ, no. 2, transcribed in Pinson 1980, 238; Bishop of Quimper to Laennec, 29 January 1822, transcribed in Roux 1980, 31–32.

58. Laennec to Mériadec, 15 November 1819, 7 January, 28 March 1820, ADLA, MS Chéguillaume, nos. 2, 5, 8, transcribed in Pinson 1980, 189–190, 201, 219–220.

59. Laennec to his tenant farmers, 23 November 1815, translated in Esnault 1919; Laennec 1820. A transcription of this letter is in MNFR, liasse 2825. See also Pinson 1980, 257.

60. Laennec to his father, 6 to 16 July, 29 September 1819, MS de Miniac nos. 121, 122, transcribed in Pinson 1980, 151–157, 180–182; Laennec to Mériadec, 8 June, 4, 25 July 1821, ADLA, MS Chéguillaume, nos. 14, 16, 17, transcribed in

Pinson 1980, 257–260, 262–263, 266–267. See also letters from Laennec to the Prefect of the Department of Finistère, 24 April, 6 October, 11 November 1825, 12 April 1826, "Travaux publiques" ADF, 100 J 825; Laennec to the Bishop of Quimper, 1 December 1825, AEQ, no. 9.

61. G. Monot to Rouxeau, 2 June 1919, MNFR, liasse 2825.

62. Laennec *père* to his nephew Christophe, 13 January 1820, transcribed in Pinson 1980, 202.

63. Laennec to Guillaume, 8 March 1820, MS Bertrand Laennec, transcribed in Pinson 1980, 213–217.

64. Christophe to Mme de Miniac, 20 October 1820, transcribed in Pinson 1980, 250. See also Laennec to Christophe, 18 January 1820, MS Bertrand Laennec, transcribed in Pinson 1980, 204–205.

65. Guillaume to his brother Laennec *père*, 15 May 1819, and to Mériadec, 20 February 1821, transcribed in Pinson 1980, 135–136, 255–256.

66. Guillaume to Mériadec, 30 January, 9 May 1820, transcribed in Pinson 1980, 205, 226–227.

67. Guillaume to Mériadec, 12 August, 27 September 1820, transcribed in Pinson 1980, 235–237, 248–249.

68. Ramsey 1988, 78.

69. Guillaume to Mériadec, 22 April 1820, transcribed in Pinson 1980, 223–224.

70. Guillaume to Mériadec, 5 and 18 July 1820, transcribed in Pinson 1980, 230–231, 233–235. Laennec to his uncle Guillaume, 17 December 1821, MS Bertrand Laennec, transcribed in Pinson 1980, 288–290; Ambroise Laennec 1825. On Ambroise Laennec's career, see Pinson 1980, 298–300.

71. Guillaume to Mériadec, 7 February, 13 September 1820, transcribed in Pinson 1980, 207, 243–244.

72. *Traité* 1819, title page. Library of the Yale University School of Medicine. See also Viets 1926

73. Guillaume to Mériadec, 18 April 1820, transcribed in Pinson 1980, 221–222.

74. Guillaume to Mériadec, 19 October 1820, 14 July 1821, transcribed in Pinson 1980, 249–250, 264–265.

75. Ambroise to Mériadec and Laennec, 12, 14, 15, 21 January, 4 February 1822, transcribed in Roux 1980, 19, 20–27, 39–40.

76. Guillaume to Mériadec, 28–29 November 1821; Guillaume to Laennec, 12 December 1821, transcribed in Pinson 1980, 283, 285–287.

77. Ackerknecht 1950, 53. See also Weisz 1995, 200–201.

78. Foucault 1963, 188–198, esp. 189. See also Ackerknecht 1953, 1967, 61–80, and 1981; Canguilhem 1989, 47–64.

79. On Broussais's life and work, see Braunstein 1986, 15–16, 192–195; Sigerist [1933], 267–274; Valentin 1988, 119–140, 201–203; 1994; E. Williams 1994, 166–175.

80. Laennec 1804h, 32n. Laennec to his uncle Guillaume, 28 June 1812, MS Bertrand Laennec, Huybrechts 1980, 94–99, esp. 96.

81. Broussais 1808.

82. Braunstein 1986; Williams 1994, 166–175.

83. Prost 1804. See also Laennec 1804f.

84. Broussais to his father, 1795, in Valentin 1988, 114. Prost and Broussais may have observed the erosions, now called stress ulcers (or Cushing's gastritis), or they may simply have had an unusual opportunity to observe the tissues soon after death.

Gastritis and superficial ulceration are frequent complications of any acute illness, even when no other organic lesion is present. Healthy stomach mucosa appears brilliant red in the immediate postmortem state, but fades rapidly after death. The frequency of typhoid and the use of arsenic therapy (hence arsenic poisoning) may also have added to an increased incidence of "gastritis" in the early nineteenth century. See Ackerknecht 1953, 331–332; Braunstein 1986, 37–39.

85. Comte [1828], 337–338.

86. Ackerknecht 1953, 1967, 135; Maulitz 1987, 134–157; Warner 1985, 1991, forthcoming.

87. Sigerist [1933], 273; Ackerknecht 1953, 1967, 62.

88. Bouillaud 1836, 420. See also Ramsey 1988, 48, 122.

89. Kitchen, "Notes des Leçons de Mons. Broussais," MS HMCP. Laennec's lectures will be discussed in chapter 11.

90. See, for example, Authenac 1821–1823; Caste 1824; Lesage 1823; Michu 1824. See also Ackerknecht 1950; Lesch 1984, 160–161; Maulitz 1987, 205.

91. Proposal by "L'Athenée de Médecine de Paris," *Rev. méd.* 1823, *10*:459.

92. Casimir Broussais 1823, 1827; Pons 1818; Lecadre 1827. On physiological medicine in the theses of Laennec's students, see Dalbant 1819; Mazet, 1819. See also chapter 6.

93. Broussais 1828. See also Genty 1935; Valentin 1988, 255–268.

94. Bouillaud 1836, 87–93, esp. 87.

95. Forbes 1827, xxvi; 1834, xxv.

96. Kergaradec 1826a, 320–321; Mériadec Laennec, "Avertissement," in Laennec 1831, *1*:i–viii, esp. iii.

97. Claude François Herman Pidoux, cited in *Bulletin de l'Académie Impériale de Médecine.* 1866–1867, *32*:1278 and in Lecadre 1868, 19.

98. Laennec 1802d.

99. Laennec 1804f, esp. 266, 271.

100. *Traité* 1819, *1*:167n.

101. Laennec 1812b; G. L. Bayle 1812a.

102. *Traité*, 1819, *2*:114. Broussais's criticism of Bayle was repeated in his second edition, Broussais 1821, *2*:715–716. See also Valentin 1988, 185–187.

103. *Traité*, 1819, *2*:114, 360–361.

104. Laennec 1818g. Compare title pages of volumes 23 and 24, *DSM* 1818. The names that disappeared are Alard, Bouvenot, Cayol, Geoffroy, Guilbert, Kergaradec, Landré-Beauvais, Lullier-Winslow, Mouton, and Pétroz. See also Rouxeau [1920], *2*:318–319.

105. Laennec, "De l'irritation," ML, MS Cl. 7, lot d (B), f. 57r–69v. I. Bricheteau. 1818. Inflammation. *DSM 24*:549–594; J. B. Montfalcon. 1818 Irritation. *DSM 26*:130–150.

106. *Traité* 1819, *1*:163. See the illness of Dr. Vorogidès in chapter 10.

107. *Traité* 1819, *2*:114.

108. Broussais 1821, *2*:672–761, esp. 701–761; Braunstein 1986, 40–43.

109. Laennec to his uncle Guillaume, 16 October 1821, MS Bertrand Laennec, transcribed in Pinson 1980, 272–274. See also Laennec to Mériadec, 25 July 1821, ADLA, MS Chéguillaume no. 17, transcribed in Pinson 1980, 266–267.

110. Forbes in Laennec, *Treatise* 1827, x, 103n.

111. *Traité* 1819, *1*:20–21, 36, 310–311.

112. Laennec to his uncle Guillaume, 16 October 1821, MS Bertrand Laennec,

transcribed in Pinson 1980, 272–274. See also Laennec to Mériadec, 25 July 1821, ADLA, MS Chéguillaume no. 17, transcribed in Pinson 1980, 266–267.

113. Laennec, "Matériaux d'une réponse aux attaques de Broussais," ML, MS, Cl. 7, lot d [A], f. 1–56. See also portions cited in Rouxeau [1920], 2:326.

114. Braunstein 1986, 102–109. For more on eclecticism in the Collège de France lectures, see chapter 11.

115. Braunstein 1986, 190–192; Rouxeau [1920], 2:341–357.

116. Braunstein 1986, 185; Valentin 1988, 198–203.

117. See, for example, Anonymous 1824, esp. 408. See also *Annales de la médecine physiologique*, 1825, 7:149–150; 1826, 9:198.

118. Duclos 1932, 253; Flint 1859, 16; Kergaradec 1826a, 320–321; 1826b, 15–16; Rouxeau [1920], 2:338.

119. Rouxeau [1920], 2:324, 339–340. See also MNFR, liasse no. 2820.

120. *Gazette de Santé*. February 1823, 50:37, esp. 61.

121. Broussais 1821 2:686, 700; Laennec, *Traité* 1826, 1:xxiin, 707n. See also Ackerknecht 1953, 326.

122. Gaultier de Claubry 1826, 411; Bouillaud 1836, 354–356.

123. Lecadre 1868; Kitchen, "Leçons de Laennec" and "Leçons de Broussais," 1823, both MS HMCP.

124. *Traité* 1826, 1:xx–xxxii.

125. Broussais 1821, 2:739; Laennec, *Traité* 1826, 2:228–232.

126. Broussais 1821, 2:751. See also chapter 8.

127. Broussais 1821, 1:6–39; Laennec, *Traité* 1826, 1:xxix–xxxn. On Laennec's research on ancient concepts, see chapter 10.

128. Broussais 1821, 2:710, 717; Laennec, *Traité* 1826, 1:492–516 and 2:217–220.

129. Broussais 1829–1834, 4:141–335, esp. 163, 172, 251, 299, 332.

130. Broussais 1829–1834, 4:160–162, 189.

131. Broussais 1829–1834, 4:169–175.

132. Broussais 1829–1834, 4:189–190, 205–209, 290–302, esp. 298.

133. Broussais 1829–1834, 4:165, 171, 176, 185, 189–190, 275, 298, 302, esp. 275, 298.

134. Gaultier de Claubry 1826, 411.

135. *Traité* 1819, 1:31–32; *Traité* 1826, 1:562–580; Dalbant 1819, 32n.

136. Broussais 1829–1834, 4:151, 214–218.

137. Merton 1973, 286–324, esp. 317–321. See also Hagstrom 1965, 85–98; Taton 1957, 131.

138. On scientific revolution as a shift in paradigm, see Kuhn 1962. For analysis of various specific scientific disputes over discovery, see Cranefield 1974, 44–54; Farley and Geison 1974; Grmek 1990, 60–77; Harley 1990, 138–164; Labrousse and Soman 1986, 31–45.

139. On the need for (and obstacles to) reconciliation between philosophical and sociological studies of cognitive aspects of science, see Nico Stehr, "Robert K. Merton's Sociology of Science," in Clark et al. 1990, 285–294.

140. Broussais 1821, 2:716; Laennec, "Matériaux d'une réponse aux attaques," cited in Rouxeau [1920], 2:326.

141. A. L. Bayle 1822. See also Broussais 1839 2:333–343, esp. 413–414; Laennec, *Traité* 1826, 2:538–539n, and Laennec's notes for his lecture on "vesania" with the annotation, "lésions organiques rapport du prix Esquirol," Collège de France,

lesson 8, 1823–1824, ML, MS, Cl 2, lot a (B), f.174, 183r–v. See also Braunstein 1986, 49, 52.

142. Broussais 1839, 2:504–506; Laennec said "if [you are] obliged to restrain [the patient] with a straitjacket, do not hasten to return [him] to society." Laennec, Collège de France, lesson 8, 1823–1824, ML, MS Cl. 2 lot a(B) 181v. See also Braunstein 1986, 45–52, 77–81.

143. *Traité* 1819, 2:360–361 (praise for Broussais's bloodletting); 2:292–295, 439, 443 (Valsalva). Laennec's source for the "Valsalva" treatment may have been Morgagni's laudatory description. Morgagni [1769], 1:452–453.

144. Braunstein 1986, 244–247.

145. *Traité* 1819, 1:xxi–xxii and esp. 413–414; *Traité* 1826, 2:233–234. See these same passages cited as epigraphs in chapters 7 and 11.

146. Broussais 1829–1834, 4:334.

147. Broussais 1828, 437–439. See also Williams 1994, 196.

148. Broussais 1839, 2:424–434, 433n.

149. Broussais 1829–1834, 4:142.

150. On this process, see Jewson 1976; Ziporyn 1992.

151. Comte 1828. See also Braunstein 1986, 203–226.

152. Broussais 1829–1834, 4:334–335.

153. Foucault 1963, 108.

154. The much discussed term, *anomie*, has been used to describe a multitude of settings, both cognitive and social, desirable and undesirable, by a host of authors from Thucydides to Merton. I use it here to designate an unintended social, and cognitive result of anatomoclinical medicine, a state of "normlessness" with respect to language (or discourse) and the possibilities of framing concerns about the potential failings of the new method. On anomie, see Orrù 1987; Marco Orrù, "Merton's Instrumental Theory of Anomie," in Clark, et al. 1990, 231–240. On "confusion" following new ways of perceiving and its relationship to new theory, see Fleck 1979, 26.

155. On the general relationship between language and science, see Knorr-Cetina 1981, 49–67, 94–135; Knorr-Cetina, "The Ethnographic Study of Scientific Work: Towards a Constructivist Interpretation," in Knorr-Cetina and Mulkay 1983, 115–140; Michael Mulkay, Jonathan Potter, and Steven Yearley, "Why an Analysis of Scientific Discourse is Needed," in Knorr-Cetina and Mulkay 1983, 171–203. On specific problems of science and language, see Anderson 1984; Benjamin et al., 1987; Gerhart and Russell 1984; E. Martin 1990.

156. Braunstein made a similar observation in describing Broussais's "anti-onto-logisme," Braunstein 1986, 250–252.

CHAPTER TEN

1. Laennec's correspondence suggests that he helped to promote Récamier, but his friend may not have received or needed much help, since he was quickly chosen as the first of two nominees for the chair of "clinique de perfectionnement" only ten days after Laennec's return to Paris. The appointment was confirmed one month later. Séances of 24 November, 20 December 1821, Procès verbaux de l'assemblée des professeurs de la Faculté de médecine, AN, AJ/16/6232. Laennec to Mériadec, 25 July 1821, ADLA, MS Chéguillaume no. 17, transcribed in Pinson 1980, 266–267; Laennec to Guillaume, 17 December 1821, MS Bertrand Laennec, transcribed

in Pinson 1980, 288–290; Ollivry to Laennec, 31 January 1822, ML, MS Cl. 5, lot b, f. 35r–39v, transcribed in Roux 1980, 33–35.

2. Laennec 1808d, 370–371.

3. Beach 1971, 410–413. On the Duchesse de Berry and her other physicians, especially her "*accoucheur*" Dr. Deneux, see Orczy 1936, 52–53; Cronin 1966, 23–78.

4. Laennec to the Bishop of Quimper, Dombideau de Crouseilhes, undated ca. 1 February 1822. AEQ, MS Laennec, no. 5, transcribed in Roux 1980, 37–38.

5. On physician remuneration in the eighteenth and nineteenth centuries, see Chaussinand-Nogaret 1977; Ganière [1951], 96, 100–101; Jewson 1974; Léonard et al.1977; Véron [1855], *1*:106.

6. Comte de Brissac to Laennec, 21 July 1826, transcribed in Roux 1980, 375. The Renaissance cello, dated 1562, became the property of the Quimper museum only to be destroyed by a fire in 1939. *Bull. Soc. Arch. Finistère* 1919, xxiii; 1939, xvi. For the family legends, see Rouxeau [1920], *2*:281.

7. M. Weiner 1960, 193–204.

8. Names of Laennec's noble patients include the Duc de Levis, the Duchesse d'Estissac, the Comtesse de'Arbouste, the Comte d'Hanache, the Marquise de Chavagne, the Marquis de Talaru, Mme de Mercy, Mme de Lorient, Mme de Bec de Lièvre [*sic*, possibly a satire], and the daughters of the Comtes de Kersant and de Senfft. *Traité* 1826, *2*:90–91; ML, MS Cl. 1, lot f(VI) (B), f. 169, 178–180; MS Cl. 1, lot t(XX) 396–415; MS Cl. II, f. 496r, 511r; Cl. III, lot 3, f. 176r; MS Cl. 2, lot a (B), f. 293r.

9. Laennec to the Bishop of Quimper, Dombideau de Crouseilhes, 6 March 1823 and undated (ca. 1 February 1822 or 1823?), AEQ, MS Laennec, nos. 4 and 5, transcribed in Roux 1980, 37–38, 111–112. Delavau was appointed prefect of police on 20 November 1821; Doudeauville, director-general of posts in September 1822. On Delavau and the Duc de Doudeauville, see James K. Kieswetter, "Delavau," and "Doudeauville," in Newman and Simpson 1987, 308, 335–336. On the police under Delavau, see Froment 1829.

10. On Corbière and Villèle, see Guillaume de Bertier de Sauvigny, "Corbière," and John K. Creigton, "Villèle," both in Newman and Simpson 1987, *1*:258 and *2*:1090–1091, respectively. See also Bertier de Sauvigny 1966; Furet 1988, 288, 296–298.

11. On Frayssinous, see Guillaume de Bertier de Sauvigny, "Frayssinous," in Newman and Simpson 1987, *1*:436. Hermopolis was the title given to a cleric who holds the rank of bishop but does not have a See.

12. Helen Castelli, "Quélen," in Newman and Simpson 1987, *2*:853–856.

13. On the resurrection of the *Académie Royale de Médecine*, see Weisz 1995, 3–32, esp. 10–14. For more on the Restoration, the medical profession, and the closure of the faculties, see Corlieu 1896, 222–223; Delaunay 1932, 38–80, 103; Jacyna 1987; Léonard 1982; Spitzer 1987, 43, 240, 244–247.

14. Laennec to Christophe, 1 January 1821, MS Bertrand Laennec, transcribed in Pinson 1980, 252–253; Mériadec to Guillaume, 25 December 1821, transcribed in Pinson 1980, 290–291. On the Chevaliers de la Foi, see Bertier de Sauvigny 1948; 1966, 13–16; "Chevaliers de la Foi," in Newman and Simpson 1987, 204–205.

15. Roux 1980, 96.

16. Minutes of the séances des professeurs du Collège de France, 10 March 1822 (votes for Chaussier), 17 November 1822 (ratifying Laennec's appointment), Or-

donnance du Roi, 31 July 1822 (naming Laennec), photographs of documents in other files, ACF Fichier CXII Laennec. Laennec to the Bishop of Quimper, Dombideau de Crouseilhes, 28 August 1822, AEQ, MS Laennec, no. 7, transcribed in Roux 1980, 71. See also Laporte 1981; Rouxeau [1920], 2:284–286.

17. Desgenettes 1822.

18. Léonard 1982, 76.

19. Procès verbaux de l'assemblée des professeurs de la Faculté de médecine, 27 November 1822, AN, AJ/16/6232.

20. Corbière's nomination of Laennec was signed on 17 January 1823 and at least three meetings of the commission were held in the Ministère de l'Intérieur, 20, 22, 24 January 1823, transcribed in Roux 1980, 101. See also Jacyna 1987; Rouxeau [1920], 2:288–289.

21. Kergaradec 1826a, 320; 1826b, 13; Rouxeau [1920], 2:290.

22. Kervran 1960, 173; Lallour 1892, 66.

23. Bishop of Quimper to Laennec, 15 January 1823, transcribed in Roux 1980, 97–99.

24. Desgenettes to Laennec, 6 May, 17 July 1823, ML, MS Cl. 5, lot b, f. 20r, 29r–v, transcribed in Roux 1980, 125, 134.

25. Froment 1829, 2:392–395.

26. Séances of 10, 12, 24 March 1823, Procès verbaux de l'assemblée des professeurs de la Faculté de médecine, AN, AJ/16/6233. See also, Procès verbaux, Minstère de l'Intérieur, Instruction publique, séance no. 209, 23 November 1823 (text of royal order to close faculty of medicine signed by Corbière); séance no. 228, 8 February 1823 (text of royal order concerning reorganization of faculty of medicine, signed by Corbière), AN, F 17/13631.

27. Laennec read the new questions at a meeting of the professors on 19 November 1824. They were printed and distributed again 16 February 1826. Procès verbaux de l'assemblée des professeurs de la Faculté de médecine, AN, AJ/16/6234 and AJ/16/6237. Laennec's questions are kept with his papers, "*Quaestiones pathologicae et medico-practicae pro secundâ et quintâ medicinae candidatorum periclitatione, in Academia Parisiensi, solvendae*," ML, MS, Cl. 6, lot b, f. 1r–22v.

28. On Carswell and Thomson, see Hollman 1995; Jacyna 1991; Maulitz 1987, 147–148.

29. Jacyna 1991, 117. The notes of Carswell and Thomson on French and Italian hospitals are in Gen. 590–592, EUL. More than a thousand of Carswell's color drawings are in the Library of University College London; some were reproduced in his *Atlas* 1838. Carswell used a numbering system to refer to drawings in his Paris notes, but the drawings are no longer with his notes and the system does not obviously connect with the London drawings.

30. Postmortem examinations by Laennec 28 August, two undated cases, 7, 16 October 1822. Cross-reference to drawings nos. 4, 24, 34, 28, 29. EUL, Carswell's Notes, I Gen. 590, 120–122, 123–124, 127–130, 130–132, 132–135.

31. Cicatrix of lung, case seen in Necker hospital, nd 1822. Cross-reference to drawing no. 33. EUL Carswell's Notes, I Gen. 590, 139–140.

32. Cases seen on 27 August, 7 and 16, 18 September 1822. Cross-references to drawings nos. 2, 3, 11, 12. EUL, Carswell's Notes, I Gen. 590, pages 90, 97–98, 105–106, 117–118. See also Carswell 1838, Atrophy, discussion re: Plate II.

33. Clark 1820, 170–173.

34. Scudamore 1826, 9, 82–87; Ambroise Laennec 1825; Toulmouche 1825.

35. Mériadec Laennec 1824a,b; 1825a,b; Vyau de Lagarde 1826. On the Charité in the years immediately following Laennec, see Jacyna 1989; Ratier 1827.

36. Louis 1825, 1835. On Louis and the numerical method in medicine, see Ackerknecht 1967, 9, 104; Bynum 1994, 42–44; Murphy 1981; Thébaud 1981; E. Williams 1994, 155, 159, 168.

37. *Traité* 1826, *1*:666; *2*:501, 575; Louis 1834, 4–5.

38. "Diagnostics des six espèces de phthisies pulmonaires établies d'après Bayle dans ses observations," and "Pronostics pour la phthisie pulmonaire établis par Mr [*sic*] le professeur Laennec," ML, MS Cl. 6 lot a [1] and [2].

39. His cousin also noted the date discrepancy, Mériadec Laennec, in Laennec 1831, *2*:495n.

40. Haller 1975.

41. Guillaume Laennec, "Cours de matière médicale élémentaire," 1809, ML, MS Cl. 4, f. 82r–87v.

42. *Traité* 1826, *1*:492–518, esp. 511 (on Ambroise); Laennec, "Mémoire sur l'emploi du tartre stibié à hautes doses," ML, MS Cl. 1 lot c [III], 45r–58v; François Nogry, cured of tetanus, 1824, ML, MS, Cl. II, 514–515.

43. Scudamore 1833, 89; Toulmouche 1838; Vyau de la Garde 1824. On James Kitchen's 1828 publication and his use of antimony, see Haller 1975, 246–247.

44. Usé, 1822, ML, MS, Cl. I, lot c, f. 78r–79r.

45. *Traité* 1826, *2*:263–272, esp. 264, 268.

46. Gaultier de Claubry 1826, 410–411. There is no evidence that Laennec had cared directly for Royer-Collard whose illness endured at least four months. Procès verbaux de l'assemblée des professeurs, de la Faculté de médecine de Paris, séance de 1 July 1825, AN AJ/16/6235.

47. See, for example, *Annales de médecine physiologique* 1823, *4*:208–289; 1825, *7*:149–150; 1826, *9*:198; Broussais 1829–1834, *4*:171, 176, 185, 189–190; Gaultier de Claubry 1826, 415–419; Ratier 1827, 168, 176–177.

48. Mériadec Laennec 1825a.

49. Bouillaud 1836, 353–355; Kergaradec 1826b, 16; Mériadec Laennec in Laennec 1831, *2*:495–517; Pariset 1845, 273.

50. Duffin and René 1991.

51. *Traité* 1826, *2*:732–743, esp. 735. Laennec used the word "heroic" without pejorative connations in his treatise and his lectures at the Collège de France to denote therapy in the face of devastating disease. See, for example, Laennec, Collège de France, Lessons 37, 38, 40, 60, 65, 72, MS Cl. 2 lot a (A), ff. 18r, 21r, 25v, 93r, 104v, 128v. On use of the word "heroic" in therapeutics, see Sullivan 1994.

52. William Withering, "An Account of the Foxglove" (1785), reprinted in Aronson 1985, 184.

53. Vicéra, ML, MS Cl. II, f. 161 r–v. Vicéra left the hospital with her symptoms unchanged. Digitalis was also prescribed and discontinued in the case of Florentin Taguel, a forty-year-old tailor whose clinical diagnosis of cardiac hypertrophy was confirmed at autopsy in late November 1824. ML, MS Cl. II, f. 466r–468v.

54. Laennec, Collège de France, lesson 11, 1823–1824, ML, MS Cl. 2, lot a (B), f. 191v.

55. Laennec, Collège de France, lesson 5, 1823–1824, ML, MS Cl. 2, lot a (B), f. 166v–168v; Rouxeau [1920], *2*:308–309.

56. *Traité* 1826, *1*:644, 716–717. See also Rouxeau [1920], *2*:313–314.

57. Forbes in Laennec, *Treatise*, 1827, 369n. Broussais 1829–1834, *4*:251.

58. *Traité* 1826, 1:647–648; Later, his cousin would liken the hapless nuns to animals dying in the King's zoo. Mériadec Laennec in Laennec 1831, 2:120n.

59. Laennec to his father, 6 July 1819, MS de Miniac no. 121, transcribed in Pinson 1980, 151–153.

60. Laennec referred to "*nature médicatrice*" often in his lessons at the Collège de France, sometimes but not always in conjunction with Hippocrates. This notion was implicit rather than explicit in the Hippocratic texts and came to be read in later by Galen and other commentators. On the origin and use of the concept of the healing power of nature, see Neuburger 1934.

61. Laennec 1804h, 15–16.

62. Laennec 1823a, xvii.

63. Laennec had spoken of his sick friend Marion de Procé as having a salutory crisis on the fourteenth day, Laennec to Christophe, 28 April 1814, MS Bertrand Laennec, transcribed in Huybrechts, 177.

64. Laennec 1808d, 370–371.

65. Pigeaud, "L'Hippocrate de Laennec," 232.

66. Laennec to Guillaume, 17 December 1821, MS Bertrand Laennec, transcribed in Pinson 1980, 288–289. The essay was never finished and has apparently been lost.

67. Mériadec to his father, 25 December 1821, transcribed in Pinson 1980, 290–291.

68. Laennec, Collège de France, lessons 34 and 35, 1822–1823, BIUM, MS 2186 (IV), f. 129r–133r, esp. 132v.

69. Louis Chapelier, gardener, 38 years, March 1824, ML, MS Cl. I, lot a, f. 31v.

70. Auguste Lelong, stonecutter, 23 years, April 1824, ML, MS Cl. I, lot a, f.45v.

71. Jean-Baptiste Boucher, locksmith, 25 years, April 1824, ML, MS Cl. I, lot a, f. 46v.

72. Mathias Fouquié, cabinetmaker, 22 years, November 1824, ML, MS Cl. II, f. 83.

73. Jean Legrand, mason, 20 years, December, 1824, ML, MS Cl. III, 24r–34v (three versions).

74. See, for example, the following cases labeled "fièvre continue":

Pierre Léonard Clement, mason 18 years, December 1823, ML, MS Cl. I, lot a, f. 15;

Pierre Petitpas, pastrychef, 18 years, January 1824, ML, MS Cl. I, lot a, f. 19v;

Ferdinand Duret, cabinetmaker, 18 years, January 1824, ML, MS Cl. I, lot a, f. 27r;

Edouard-Joseph Verneuil, 23 years, June, 1823, ML, MS Cl. II, f. 21–22r–v;

Louise Garin, dressmaker, 18 years, ML, MS Cl. II, f. 92–95r–v.

75. Sometime after November 1826, Mériadec annotated a patient history: "This, too, if I am not deluding myself, is a case of misplaced crisis." ML, MS Cl. II, f. 151.

76. Laennec to Mériadec, 12 September 1820, ADLA, MS Chéguillaume no. 13, transcribed in Pinson 1980, 240–243. See also Laennec to Guillaume, 12 September 1820, MS Bertrand Laennec, transcribed in Pinson 1980, 239.

77. Laennec to Mériadec, 12, 18 September 1825, ADLA, MS Chéguillaume nos. 19, 20.

78. Christophe to Laennec, ca. 1 February 1823, transcribed in Roux 1980, 107.

79. Laennec to Mériadec, 12 September 1825, ADLA MS Chéguillaume no. 19.

80. Forbes 1834, xxv; A. L. J. Bayle 1826.

81. Dédéyan 1981.

82. On Cousin, see Bertier de Sauvigny 1966, 348–349; Eisenstein 1968, 21–52, esp. 30–31; Goldstein 1994; Spitzer 1971; 1976; 1987, 72–96; E. Williams 1994, 120–121.

83. Sainte-Beuve 1847, 2:565–566n.

84. Laennec to Forbes, 12 June 1824, ML, MS Cl. 5 lot b, f. 75r–v; Forbes to Laennec, 20 June 1824, ML, MS Cl. 5, f. 65r–66v; Eloi Johanneau to Laennec, 7 November 1825, Rouxeau [1920], 2:382; Laennec to Johanneau, 6 May 1826 [original said to belong to J. M. Charcot], transcribed in Roux 1980, 257–258. Laennec read Lloyd and corresponded with Le Gonidec who made use of the observation, sent by the man whom he called "a good philologist as well as a great doctor." Le Gonidec 1850, vi. On Le Gonidec and Breton-speaking clergy, see Esnault 1919.

85. On the missionary ventures of the Restoration, see Furet 1988, 302–307.

86. Cilleuls 1956; Kernéis 1981b; Laignel-Lavastine 1914; Valléry-Radot 1952.

87. Charles Chauvelot, 7 January 1822, ML, MS Cl. 1, lot n(XIV), f. 262–263; Laennec to Mlle Similienne Arthur de la Gauthraye, 10 March 1825, text reproduced in catalogue of Laurin-Guilloux-Buffetaud-Tailleur, for auction at the Salles Drouot-Richelieu. On 15 March 1995, this letter sold for 40,500 French francs to an unidentified buyer.

88. Laennec to Courbon-Pérusel, 22 April 1817, 16 August 1819, 18 January 1820, transcribed in Pinson 1980, 86–91, 175–177, 203, and in Thayer 1920. Courbon-Pérusel had worked with Laennec on the *Journal de médecine*, but left Paris for a practice at Carhaix in Brittany.

89. Saunier to Laennec, 8 June 1825, ML, MS Cl. 2, lot a(A), f. 65–66r–v; Saunier to Laennec, 10 July 1825, ML, MS Cl. 2, lot a(B), f. 175r–176r. The first letter came from a Parisian hotel. Saunier may have come to the city to visit a relative, since Perrine Saunier, a twenty-five-year-old seamstress, was in Laennec's hospital at the same time. ML, MS Cl., II, f. 506–507. His own temperate habits, notwithstanding, Laennec may have been doing business with the *négotiant*; his estate sale disposed of 132 bottles of ordinary red and white wine, 47 bottles of Bordeaux (at one franc each), 17 bottles of Chablis, and other spirits. AMP, Vente de meubles, 16 October 1826, D.90.E^3, art. 3., items 129 to 132.

90. Clark (in Rome) to Laennec, 8 April, 12 May 1823, ML, MS Cl. 5, lot b, f. 52r–56v.

91. Clark 1820, 157; Scudamore 1826, 63.

92. Scudamore 1826, 63.

93. Letter re "Gillibert" from Hourdin [? illegible] physician at Angoulême to Laennec, 1 April 1825, ML, MS Cl. 5, 43r–v. Laennec annotated the letter: "I believe that this letter should not come to the attention of Mr. Gillibert."

94. See for example *Traité* 1826, 2:263–272; Louise Boisot, 45 years, servant ML, MS, Cl. III, f. 156–158. See also the description of Laennec's inaccurate diagnosis in a young lady with phthisis by a disciple of Broussais. Capuron 1827, 426–427. Rouxeau described one other encounter with Broussais that I have been unable to trace. Rouxeau [1920], 2:317–320.

95. The coy formulation "monthly evacuation" invites consideration of the gendered uses of bloodletting. See Carter 1982.

96. Vorogidès ML, MS Cl. 1, lot j (X), f. 238–246. See also Rouxeau [1920], 2:317–320.

97. Laennec was named to the *Légion d'honneur* in 1824, and may have been promoted in 1825, but there are varying reports about the date. See Roux 1980, 174, 177; Ambroise to Laennec, 8 June 1825, transcribed in Roux 1980, 217–218. On the mineral water commission, see Weisz 1995, 137–158.

98. Taylor 1848, 494–497, esp. 495.

99. Excerpts from letters 28 October 1824 and 28 November 1824, *J. de médecine de la Gironde*, 1824, *11*:351, 418–419, reprinted in *La Chronique Médicale*. 1902–1903, *9*:421 and *10*:557, 559, transcribed by Rouxeau, MNFR, liasse nos. 2799, 2823.

100. After Laennec's death, Cazenave sent his letter to Kergaradec who read it at the Académie de Médecine on 12 February 1827. In his notes on the Cazenave letter, Rouxeau cited "*Rev. méd.* 1827 and *Archives générales* XIII 441," MNFR, liasse 2799.

101. Directrice de la poste to Laennec *père*, 6 October 1824; Laennec *père* to Christophe, 11 November 1824, transcribed in Roux 1980, 183, 193.

102. Laennec, Collège de France, lesson 25, 1823–1824, ML MS Cl. 2, lot a(B), f. 246r. *La Chronique Médicale* 1925, *32*:10. See also transcription in Roux 1980, 185–191. The famous caricature was discovered by Dr. Gélineau in the shop of a Bordeaux antique dealer. Letter from Dr Gélineau to *La Chronique Médicale* 1902, *9*: 420–421, transcribed in Roux 1980, 185–186.

103. The move took place in October 1822. Laennec to Christophe, 15 July 1822, MS Bertrand Laennec, transcribed in Roux 1980, 60–61.

104. Madame de Pompéry to her cousin, 14 May 1805, cited in Pompéry 1884, 2:327–328; Villard 1927.

105. Mme Argou was "so impressed with the scenes of violence that she was sick for more than a year," Rouxeau's note citing Edouard de Pompéry, 2 December 1887, MNFR, liasse 2817. Laennec's Latin notes on her case also describe her terrified reaction to the invasion by the "*Cosacis.*" ML MS Cl. 7, lot e3, f. 13r.

106. Rouxeau's notes on Mme Argou, MNFR, liasse 2817.

107. Ollivry to Laennec, 31 January 1822, transcribed in Roux 1980, 33–35; Laennec to Christophe, 17 September 1822, MS Bertrand Laennec, transcribed in Roux 1980, 76–78. Pompéry 1884, *1*:xx, 2:329.

108. Bishop of Quimper, Jean-Dominique Poulpiquet de Brescanel, to Laennec, 21 December 1824, transcribed in Roux 1980, 201.

109. Laennec to "*chers amis*" (Christophe), 2 December 1824, MS Bertrand Laennec, transcribed in Roux 1980, 194–195

110. Christophe to Mme de Miniac, 10 December 1824, transcribed in Roux 1980, 196. The gossip won out in certain sectors: Villard, who was the nephew of Mme Laennec's dressmaker, complained that Rouxeau did not accept his tale of the doctor's lack of tenderness for his wife, which, he thought, was exemplified by his demand that she pray for her sins every time they passed the Chapelle de la Ste. Croix at Kerlouarnec. Villard 1927. Rouxeau's impatience with Villard's unflattering version of Laennec's marriage is apparent in his papers. MNFR, liasse 2817.

111. Laennec-Guichard, 16 December 1824, Registre des mariages, AMP, adj. F3704, 5MI2 microfilm, number 151; also Extrait du Registre des Actes de Mariages de l'Eglise paroissiale St. Sulpice, 16 December 1824, transcribed for Rouxeau on 19 November 1913, photocopy in Roux 1980, 197.

112. Rouxeau [1912], *1*:267. Ambroise to Laennec, 8 June 1825; Christophe to Mériadec, 8 July 1825; Mériadec to Christophe, 23 July 1825, transcribed in Roux 1980, 217, 220, 222. I have been unable to trace Rouxeau's source for the death of Clementine Argou.

113. Mme Laennec to Mériadec, 15, 18 July 1826, transcribed in Roux 1980, 367–368, 371–372.

114. Vente de meubles, 16 October 1826, AMP, D.90.E³, art. 3. See also the far less legible "*état de lieu*," the description and inventory conducted on the day the apartment was sealed by municipal officials in the presence of Mériadec. AMP, D.10.U¹, Inventaire, 28 August 1826. See also, Ribault 1981.

115. Mme Laennec to Mériadec, 19 June 1826, ADLA, MS Chéguillaume no. 31, transcribed in Roux 1980, 319–321. According to Villard, who had clearly believed the tale about a simulated pregnancy, Laennec's wife was said to have a long nose and worn her hair in trailing grey ringlets under a straw hat. She was a heavy user of tobacco, partial to fried pork brains and cooked chestnuts, and fond of animals, especially parrots, chickens, and donkeys, while the famous spaniels, Kiss and Moustache, accompanied her to church. Villard 1927.

116. Rouxeau [1920], *2*:421; Kervran 1960, 112, 208; Duclos 1932, 171, 278. See also chapter 11.

117. Cruveilhier to Laennec, 13 April 1824, ML, MS Cl. 5, lot b, f. 21–22. See also, Cruveilhier to Laennec [in Latin], 8 February 1824, ML, MS Cl. 5, lot b, f. 46r–v; Laennec to Cruveilhier, 19 June 1824, Johns Hopkins University, Library of the Institute of the History of Medicine.

CHAPTER ELEVEN

1. Laennec to Mériadec, 19 June 1826, ADLA, MS Chéguillaume, no. 31, transcribed in Roux 1980, 319–321.

2. "Collège Royal de France," *Moniteur universel*, 5 December 1822.

3. Laennec's Collège de France lessons 1–35, 1822–1823, are in BIUM, MS 2186 (IV); lessons 36–81, 1822–1823, and lessons 1–89, 1823–1824, are kept in ML, MS Cl. 2, lot a (A) and (B), respectively. Lessons 45–53, 1823–1824, on heart disease, are missing. On the Collège de France lectures, see Ackerknecht 1962, 1964; 1967, 96–98; Laporte 1981.

4. Dufour, "Cours de Médecine de M. Laennec, premère année," (encompassing lessons 5–82, 1822–1823 and lessons 1–7, 1823–1824), CPP, Z10, no. 96; James Kitchen, "Leçons pratiques de la médecine de Mons. Laennec, délivrées dans le Collège de France à Paris dans l'Année 1823," (encompassing part of lesson 82, 1822–1823, which Laennec may not have read until the following year and lesson 2–53, 1823–1824, and including at least some of the missing lessons on heart disease), HMCP; Anonymous, "Extraits du discours prononcé par Mr Laennec au Collège de France," 15 June 1825 and 28 November 1825 (encompassing lessons 73–82, 1824–1825 and 2–15, 1825–1826), ML, MS Cl. 2, lot b, f. 2r–30v and lot c, 2r–20v.

5. Lecadre 1868, cited in Rouxeau [1920], 327. Kitchen also attended Broussais's classes. James Kitchen, "Notes des leçons de Mons. Broussais," 17 November 1823, MS, HMCP.

6. On foreign students in Paris, see Jacyna 1991; Logan 1972; Maulitz 1987, 134–157; Warner 1985, 1991, forthcoming.

7. During period of Laennec's lessons from 1823 to 1826, the number of students who appear to have enrolled each year was 13, 7, 37, and 3, respectively. However, these figures are probably unreliable. The slim Register for inscriptions at the Collège de France was kept in a desultory fashion, beginning with Hallé in 1808, ending with Magendie in 1840, with some years missed entirely. "Registre des inscriptions pour le cours de médecine par M. Hallé, commencé 29 novembre 1808," ACF.

8. Magnus Chrétien Retzius with twenty-nine others, "MM les médecins et élèves étrangers ['et français': annotation in hand of tenth signatory, Ribail]" to Laennec 1824, ML, MS Cl. 5 lot b, f. 7; for a transcription, see Huard and Grmek 1973.

9. William Thomson to Laennec, 29 April 1823; Van Hall to Laennec, 25 June 1823; C. Scudamore to Laennec, 2 May 1826, ML, MS Cl. 5, lot b., f. 70r–71v, 72r–73r, 79r.

10. Logan 1972; Mériadec to Laennec, 1 August 1826, transcribed in Roux 1980, 387–388.

11. A. Knegtel 1970.

12. Toulmouche 1875.

13. Victor Stoeber (1803–1871) cited in Huard and Grmek 1973, 317.

14. Forbes 1834, xxvi–xxvii.

15. C. J. B. Williams 1834, vii.

16. Laennec, "Liste des élèves étrangers qui ont suivi mes cours, et dont j'ai connu les noms," ML, MS Cl. 5 lot b, f. 2r–5v. Laennec may have been inspired by Retzius to keep the list, because the names follow the order of the signatures in the letter. See n. 8, above.

17. *Traité* 1826, *1*:303n.

18. Laennec 1823a. See also Ackerknecht 1964; Dausset 1981; Laporte 1981.

19. Laennec, Collège de France, lesson 2, 1822–1823, BIUM, MS 2186 (IV), f. 8r. See also "Doctrine de Laennec," ML, MS Adversaria, 4 unnumbered pages following page 51. These latter notes are partly in Laennec's hand and partly in the hand of his cousin who wrote that they had been faithfully copied from originals. With this particular meaning, the word "doctrine" appears only in the hand of Mériadec Laennec.

20. Laennec, Collège de France, lesson 1, 1822–1823, BIUM, MS 2186 (IV), f. 5v; Laennec 1823a, xv–xvi. For Magendie's similar use of "scaffolding" in 1809, see Albury 1977, 115.

21. Laennec wrote, "τὰ ἴσχοντα, ἢ τὰ ὁρμῶντα, ἢ τὰ ἐνισχόμενα." He attributed these words to the Hippocratic treatise *Epidemics VI* [8, 7], which he cited in an undated fragment BIUM, MS 5172 (III), k, f. 1r. He had probably been influenced by Galen's commentary on this passage as the three "elements" of the body, as *"continentia, contenta, et impetum facientia"* (see C. G. Kühn, *Claudii Galeni Opera Omnia 14*:696). See also, Hippocrates, *Epidemics VI*, 8, 7, in W. D. Smith 1994, *7*:280–281; Littré 1846, 5:346–347.

22. Laennec cited the younger Boerhaave in 1803: "τὰ ὁρμῶντα, hipp[ocrate] *impetum faciens*, Kaw [*sic*] Boerhaave." Laennec, "Traité d'anatomie pathologique," BIUM, MS 2186 (IIIa), f. 3v. He was referring to Abraham Kaau Boerhaave, *Impetum faciens dictum Hippocrati. . .* (Leiden: Luchtmans, 1745). On Barthez's use of the triad, see Thivel 1989. On Barthez, see also Duchesneau 1982, 384–430; 1985, 259–295; Haigh 1977; E. Williams, 1994, 46–50.

23. Savary des Brulons 1808, esp. 166, 173. Dumas's brand of physiology has been described as a "holdover." Lesch 1984, 83, 85.

24. Laennec, Collège de France, lesson 2, 1822–1823, BIUM, MS 2186 (IV) f. 8r–v. See also "Doctrine de Laennec," MS Adversaria, unnumbered f. 55.

25. Laennec, Collège de France, lesson 2, BIUM, MS 2186 (IV), f. 9r. On body liquids endowed with life in Bichat, see Albury 1977, 105.

26. Laennec, Collège de France, lesson 2, BIUM, MS 2186 (IV), 8r–9v; Laennec, "Existens du principe vital," BIUM, MS 5172 (III), lot l, f. 1–2.

27. Traité 1826, 1:viii; Barthez 1806, 2:8–9. On Newton and physiological vitalism, see Duchesneau 1982, 447–449; Goodfield-Toulmin 1969, 285–307; Lesch 1984, 95–96; E. Williams 1994, 49.

28. Laennec, Collège de France, lesson 3, BIUM, MS 2186 (IV), f. 13v; "Doctrine de Laennec," ML, MS Adversaria, f. 55. For Barthez's distinction between the soul and the vital principle, see Barthez 1806, 1:20, 85.

29. Laennec, Collège de France, lesson 3, 6, 29, 1822–1823, BIUM, MS 2186 (IV), f. 13v (Barthez), 24r (Dumas), 113v (Stahl); lessons, 57, 75, 87, 1823–1824, ML, MS Cl. 2, lot a (B), f. 323r, 371r, 407r (Reil on digestion and reproduction); lessons 3, 56, 71, 1823–1824, ML, MS Cl. 2, lot a (B), f. 162v, 315r, 352v (Stahl on fevers and digestions); ML, "Du principe de la vie," MS Adversaria, f. 36 (Blumenbach on the "force de formation").

30. Laennec, Collège de France, lesson 2, 1822–1823, BIUM, MS 2186 (IV), f. 8r. See also, Laennec, "Du principe de la vie," ML, MS Adversaria, f. 35–36.

31. See, for example, Laennec, Collège de France, lesson 52, 1822–1823, ML, MS Cl. 2, lot a (A), f. 70r (Magendie on poisons); lesson 1, 1823–1824, ML, MS Cl. 2, lot a (B), f. 156r (Bichat); ML, MS Adversaria, f. 35–36 (Bichat, Chaussier), f. 46 (Legallois). On these early experimental physiologists, see Lesch 1984, 80–98.

32. J. J. C. Legallois [1812].

33. On Dupuytren, see Laennec, Collège de France, lesson 51, 1822–1823, ML, MS Cl. 2, lot a (A), f. 63v; lessons 11, 1823–1824, ML, MS Cl. 2, lot a (B), f. 193r.

34. Laennec, Collège de France, lesson 2, 1822–23, BIUM, MS 2186 (IV), f. 8r; Laennec 1823a, xvi.

35. Laennec, Collège de France, lesson 3, 1822–1823, BIUM, MS 2186 (IV), f. 13r–v. On Cousin and eclecticism, see Ackerknecht 1967, 101–113; Goldstein 1994, 101–107; Spitzer 1971, 1976; E. Williams, 120–121, 140–151.

36. Laennec, ML, MS Adversaria, 55. In the same passage, Laennec described the body as the tool of the mind, like the instrument of a talented artist. This passage is reminiscent of Bonald's definition of a human: "an intelligence served by organs," cited by both Buisson and Laennec in 1802. Buisson 1820b, 36, 51; Laennec 1802f, 173.

37. Wright 1989.

38. Laennec, Collège de France, lessons 30, 33, 1822–1823, BIUM, MS 2186 (IV), f. 116v, 118v, 126v.

39. See for example, the discussions of tumors and fevers, Laennec, Collège de France, lessons 22, 30–32, 1822–1823, BIUM, MS 2186 (IV), f. 90v, 118–127.

40. Chomel 1821b, 5, 7, 9. Laennec may not have accepted Chomel's statistic that three-quarters of all febrile patients have ulcers in the intestines. Chomel was at the Charité Hospital before Laennec's arrival, succeeded him as professor,

and shared his abhorrence of Broussais's doctrine, but I have found his name only once in the Laennec papers. ML, MS Cl. 1 lot f, B, f. 205r. On Chomel, see Jacyna 1989.

41. Magendie 1821; Laennec, Collège de France, lesson 51, 1822–1823, ML, MS Cl. 2, lot a (A), f. 63v.

42. Laennec, Collège de France, lesson 29, 1822–1823, BIUM, MS 2186 (IV), f. 111r–v; Laennec 1825d.

43. On the extrathoracic uses of auscultation, see Laennec, Collège de France, lesson 27, 1822–23, BIUM, MS 2186 (IV), f. 106r; lessons 9, 65, 69, 80, 1823–1824, ML, MS Cl. 2, lot a (B), f. 187r, 347r, 356v, 389r.

44. Laennec, Collège de France, lesson 69, 1822–1823, ML, MS Cl. 2, lot a (A), f. 118r–v.

45. For cause of disease added to the margins as an afterthought, see Laennec, Collège de France, lessons 33, 1822–1823, BIUM, MS 2186 (IV), f. 126v; lesson 78, 1822–1823, ML, MS Cl. 2, lot a (A), f. 142v; lessons 28, 35, 74, 79, 1823–1824, ML, MS Cl. 2, lot a (B), f. 256r, 279v, 370v, 384v.

46. Laennec, Collège de France, lessons 8, 9, 1823–1824, ML, MS Cl. 2, lot a (B), f. 171v–186r, esp. 179r (nostalgia). Kitchen, "Leçons de Laennec," MS HMCP, 18. For lengthy citations from these lectures, see Ackerknecht 1962.

47. Laennec, Collège de France, lesson 8, 1823–1824, ML, MS Cl. 2, lot a (B), f. 171v–177r, esp. 173r, 174v. The reference to the "Prix Esquirol, 1825" and the fact that the examples of mass insanity do not figure in the notes of Kitchen, who was in Paris in 1823–1824, confirm the impression that the political digression was part of a revision for the second cycle of lectures. Professor of Greek and Latin, the protestant Pierre de la Ramée (or Ramus) was murdered in a politically charged dispute over (among other things) the pronounciation of classical languages.

48. Laennec 1829; Jacyna 1991. On parallels between political philosophy and Bichat's physiology, see Pickstone 1981.

49. On Bonald's politico-theological philosophy in Restoration France, see Furet 1988, esp. 298; N. Hudson 1936, 181–182.

50. See for example, Bonald [1796], *1*: 9–32; [1830].

51. Ploucquet 1808–1809. Classeur 3 of the Nantes collection of manuscripts contains many excerpts from medical writers, in the same (but neater and possibly younger) hand than the one that jotted the Collège de France notes. A few of these pages have been placed with the lecture notes, suggesting they were transferred by Laennec himself from the older files. See for example, Laennec, Collège de France, lessons 14 and 23, 1823–24, MS ML, MS Cl. 2, lot a (B), f. 204r, 238r.

52. For references to statistics, see, for example, Laennec, Collège de France, lesson 46, 1822–1823, ML, MS Cl. 2 lot a (A), f. 45v; lessons 30, 36, 66, 60, 1823–1824, ML, MS Cl. 2, lot a(B), f. 263v, 282r, 349v, 389r.

53. See, for example, Laennec, Collège de France, lesson 1, 1822–1823, BIUM, MS 2186 (IV), f. 6v; lessons 68, 81, 1822–1823, ML, MS Cl. 2, lot a (A), f. 114v, 154r; lessons 1, 81, 1823–1824, ML, MS Cl. 2, lot a (B), f. 157v, 390v.

54. Laennec, Collège de France, lessons 36, 44, 64 , 1822–1823, ML, MS Cl. 2, lot a (A), f. 15r, 39r, 102r.

55. On "Mal de la Baie," see Laennec, Collège de France, lesson 53, 1822–1823, ML, MS Cl. 2, lot a (A), f. 72r. On "English sweat" together with "history of syphilis," see lesson 36, 1822–1823, ML, MS Cl. 2, lot a (A), 16r and lesson 13, 1823–

1824, ML, MS Cl. 2, lot a (B), f. 200r. On "history of leprosy," see lesson 88, 1823–1824, ML, MS Cl. 2, lot a (B), f. 413.

56. Laennec, Collège de France, lesson 37, 1822–1823, ML, MS Cl. 2, lot a (A), f. 17v.

57. Laennec, Collège de France, lessons 50, 66, 70, 1822–1823, ML, MS Cl. 2, lot a (A), f. 59r, 108r, 122r, respectively.

58. On medical retelling of patient stories, see Hunter 1991.

59. On references to music, see Laennec, Collège de France, 1823–1824, ML, MS Cl. 2, lot a (B) lesson 8, f. 179v (music therapy for melancholy); lesson 15, f. 209r (hearing, Itard and the musician Vandermonde); lesson 24, f. 242r (voice and cultural differences among European peoples [Kitchen, "Leçon de Laennec," MS HMCP, 55: "Bretons are the best musicians in France"]); lesson 25, f. 245r (percussion, harp); lesson 27, f. 249v (egophony and oboe), 250v (sonorous rales and bass violin); lesson 40, f. 295r (egophony and oboe).

60. Laennec, Collège de France, lesson 37, 1823–1824, ML, MS Cl. 2, lot a (B), f. 286v. Laennec cited in Kitchen, "Leçons de Laennec," MS HMCP, 100.

61. For criticisms of tendencies "*toute recente*," see, for example, Laennec, Collège de France, lessons 61, 74, 1822–1823, ML, MS Cl. 2, lot a (A), f. 94r, 131r; lessons 1, 85, 1823–1824, ML, MS Cl. 2, lot a (B), f. 159v, 401r.

62. Rostan 1820, 1846. On the organicism of Rostan, see Grmek and Rousseau 1966, esp. 37; Hall 1969, 2:251–254.

63. Bouillaud 1860, esp. 1162. See also Hall 1969, 2:252.

64. Rostan 1833, 15.

65. Rostan 1864, "Aphorisme XLII," 385–387.

66. Duchesneau 1982, 36. See also Corlieu 1896; Rey 1991a; Temkin 1946b; E. Williams 1994, 196.

67. Dunglison 1874, 732; Power and Sedgwick 1892.

68. Rostan 1832, ii.

69. Paul Broca, cited in Schiller 1979, 78. On Broca's antivitalism, see E. Williams 1994, 258–262.

70. Rostan 1826, *1*:137–138.

71. Laennec 1823b, x; Laennec, Collège de France, lesson 2, BIUM, MS 2186 (IV), f. 8r. See also Laennec, Collège de France, lesson 9, 1823–1824, ML, MS. Cl. 2 lot a (B), f. 181v; Kitchen "Leçons de Laennec," MS HMCP, 20.

72. Laennec, Collège de France, lessons 3, 31, 1822–1823, BIUM, MS 2186 (IV), f. 14v, 119r; lesson 69, 1822–1823, ML, MS Cl. 2, lot a (A), f. 119v. See also *Traité* 1826, 1:280. On medical microscopy in early nineteenth-century France, see La Berge 1994.

73. Laennec, Collège de France, lesson 4, 1822–1823, BIUM, MS 2186 (IV), f. 14 r–v.

74. Laennec, Collège de France, lesson 1, 1823–1824, ML, MS Cl. 2, lot a (B), f. 159 r–v. See also ML, MS Adversaria, f. 39–41.

75. Anonymous 1827, esp. 623.

76. On Magendie and Laennec, see Olmstead 1944, 21, 30, 202–203, 208–210. On Magendie, see also Albury 1977; Lesch 1994, 92–98; Temkin 1946a.

77. Jacyna 1991, 137.

78. Rouxeau [1920] 2:284–286. See also chapter 10.

79. For references to Magendie, see Laennec, Collège de France, lessons 7, 32,

51, 52, 80, 1822–1823 and lessons 10, 31, 1823–1824, BIUM MS 2186 (IV), f. 31r–v, 121v; ML Cl. 2 lot a (A) 61r, 63r, 63v, 70r, 149r and lot a (B) f. 191r, 264r.

80. *Traité* 1826, *2*: 404–405.

81. Magendie also rejected the hypothesis of J. Rouanet saying it was "*physiologiquement inadmissible.*" Magendie 1838, esp. 158, 162. See also Olmstead 1944, 208–209.

82. Braunstein, 1986, 60–61; Ackerknecht 1953, 333; Lesch, 1984, 160–161.

83. Rostan 1832, 46.

84. Rostan 1818a, b; 1820.

85. Rostan 1819–1820, esp. 1820, 310, 320, 328.

86. Rostan 1823.

87. For examples of Laennec's patients diagnosed with brain softening, see Edmé Butte, 5 March 1824, ML, MS Cl. I, lot a, f. 37v, no. 114; Claude Ansillon femme Chevalié, 12 March 1824, ML, MS Cl. I, lot a, f. 40r, no. 127 and also ML, MS Cl. II, f. 174r–177v; Pierre Piot, 7 December 1821, ML, MS Cl I, lot c, f. 8r–10v; Pierre Bonnafoux, 26 February 1822, ML, MS Cl. I, lot c, 41r–43v; Catherine Lallemand, 16 March 1822, ML, MS Cl I, lot c, f. 54r–55v; Joseph Jacquemin, 17 November 1825, ML, MS CL. III, f. 444r–447v. Rostan's name appears only once in the Laennec manuscripts, as a fellow consultant at the bedside of the dying physician, Athanase Vorogidès, February 1826, ML, MS Cl. 1, lot j(X), f. 238–248, esp. f. 245v.

88. On brain softening, Laennec recognized Morgagni, G. L. Bayle, Récamier, I. Bricheteau and C. F. Lallemand of Montpellier. Laennec, Collège de France, lesson 8, first year, 1822–1823, BIUM MS 2186 (IV), f. 39v (especially addendum in margin likely from 1824–1825); lesson 73, 1822–23, ML, MS Cl. 2, lot a (A), f. 128v–130v.

89. Laennec, Collège de France, lesson 8, 1823–1824, ML, MS Cl. 2, lot a (B), f. 183r–v.

90. Bouillaud 1825a,b. On the Prix Esquirol, see Goldstein 1987, 140–141, 253.

91. Bouillaud 1825a, 197–199.

92. Laennec, Collège de France, lesson 8, 1823–1824, ML, MS Cl. 2, lot a (B), esp. f. 174v, 183r. Emphasis in original. The medal essay by Bouchet and Casavieilh on epilepsy and mental illness was published in *Arch. gén. méd.* 1825, *9*:510–542 and 1826, *10*:5–50. The essays submitted for the 1825 Prix Esquirol are no longer in the archives of the Académie Nationale de Médecine.

93. *Traité* 1826, 2:538–541, esp 538n. See also chapter 8.

94. A. L. Bayle 1822, 1826. A. L. Bayle published several articles on similar subjects in *Rév. méd.* 1824–1825, culminating in his treatise of 1826. On A. L. J. Bayle, see Ackerknecht 1967, 170; E. Brown 1994; Müller 1965.

95. On the somaticist debate in psychiatry, see E. Brown 1994; Dowbiggin 1991, 31; Goldstein 1987, 250–254; Kirkby 1992; E. Williams 1994.

96. Bouillaud 1835, *1*:157, 172; *2*:493.

97. Bouillaud 1836, 87n, 88–91.

98. Bouillaud 1836, 92, 161–162.

99. Major 1945a.

100. Weisz 1995, 167–169.

101. Ackerknecht 1967, 98, 105–106.

102. Andral 1823–1827, esp. 1824, *2*:344; *Traité* 1826, *1*:x–xvii, esp. xii. On bronchophony, see also chapter 7.

103. Gaultier de Claubry 1826, esp. 410–411.

104. Andral in Laennec 1837, *1*:viii, *2*:176–177n.

105. Broussais 1828, 437–439. See also chapter 9.

106. *Traité* 1826, *2*:768–769. Laennec had once written about the possibility of audible heart beat in the eighth of Corvisart's collected aphorisms, but he later claimed never to have noticed the phenomenon until 1823. By 1826, he had encountered twenty patients who displayed it. *Traité* 1826, *2*:454–455; "Aphorismes recueillis aux leçons du C[itoyen] Corvisart par René Théophile Hyacinthe Laennec, An X," ML, MS Cl. 8 [2], p. 4, f. 2v.

107. Laennec to his father, 28 June 1826, handwritten copy, MS Miniac no. 126, transcribed in Roux 1980, 349.

108. Procès verbaux de l'assemblée des professeurs de la Faculté de médecine de Paris, séance du 19 May 1826. AN AJ/16/6236. Laennec to his father, 15 May 1826, MS Miniac no. 125, transcribed in Roux 1980, 263–264.

109. Duc de Doudeauville to the Comtesse de Noailles, 12 June 1825, transcribed in Roux 1980, 307.

110. On the Prix Montyon, see Crosland 1992, 164, 270–271, 276–277; Morand 1972.

111. Laennec 1826g.

112. Laennec to Cuvier, 18 May 1826, transcribed in Roux 1980, 268–269. See also letters from Laennec to Fourier, president of the Académie des Sciences, 19, 22, 27 May 1826, transcribed in Roux 1980, 270, 274, 278–279. The letter to Cuvier has been published many times, the most intriguing example being a bound facsimile printed by the mineral water concern, Vichy-Celestins, 5 September 1939, a copy of which is held at the NYAM, Malloch Rare Book Room.

113. *Moniteur universel*, 28 May 1826; Christophe to Laennec *père*, 21 May 1826; Mériadec to Laennec *père*, ca. 27 May 1826; Laennec *père* to his son, 25 June 1826, later annotated by Mériadec, transcribed in Roux 1980, 273, 275–276, 333–334.

114. Laennec to Mériadec, 2 June 1826, ADLA, MS Chéguillaume no. 23, transcribed in Roux 1980, 289.

115. Legend attributed to Laennec's widow by her friends. Lallour, 1892, 72.

116. Mme Laennec to Mériadec, 22 June 1826, transcribed in Roux 1980, 327–328.

117. Laennec to Mériadec, 23 June 1826, ADLA MS Chéguillaume no. 33, transcribed in Roux 1980, 329–330.

118. Mme Laennec to Mériadec, 19 June 1826, ADLA, MS Chéguillaume no. 31, transcribed in Roux 1980, 319–321.

119. Forbes 1834, xxiii–xxiv; Ambroise to Mériadec, 27 June 1826, transcribed in Roux 1980, 346–347

120. Mme Laennec to Mériadec, 19 June 1826, ADLA, MS Chéguillaume no. 31, transcribed in Roux 1980, 319–321.

121. Christophe to his wife Claire Marion de Procé Laennec, 25–26 June 1825, transcribed in Roux 1980, 339–341.

122. Mme Laennec to Mériadec, 18, 25 July 1826, transcribed in Roux 1980, 371–372, 381–382. The "leech" of a servant was a Mme Prépaud, whom Mériadec

was instructed to pay and dismiss. Mme Laennec to Mériadec, 18 July 1826, transcribed in Roux 1980, 371–372.

123. Laennec, Testament, 20 April 1826, MS Miniac no. 129; MS of François Puget, transciptions with codicils dated 10, 21, 25, 26 June 1826 in Roux 1980, 246–248, 302, 323, 332, 343. See also Kervran 1960, 197. Another copy was found in the files of the Quimper notary Dr. Damey during the celebrations for the centenary of Laennec's death. "Le centenaire de Laennec à Ploaré," *La Bretagne touristique*, 15 September 1926, 197. Laennec estimated an income of four thousand francs from the twenty-five different properties in his estate, ca. July 1826, see Roux 1980, 352–353.

124. Rouxeau [1920], 2:417. Mme Brunot to Laennec *père*, 20, 22, 29 June 1826; Christophe to Mme Laennec, 13 July 1826, transcribed in Roux 1980, 322, 325, 350–351, 365.

125. Mériadec to Christophe 23 July 1826, transcribed in Roux 1980, 379–380. On Becquey's role in the French canals, see Geiger 1994.

126. Mme Laennec to Mériadec, 9 August 1826, transcribed in Roux 1980, 394–395.

127. Duclos 1932, 278; Kervran 1960, 208; Rouxeau [1920] 2:421.

128. Laennec to Mériadec, 4 August 1826, ADLA, MS Chéguillaume no. 44, transcribed in Roux 1980, 389–391.

129. This story was attributed to the widow by her friends who were interviewed by Lallour in the 1860s. Lallour 1892, 85.

130. Procès verbaux de l'assemblée des professeurs de la Faculté de médecine de Paris, 5 January, 16 February 1826. AN AJ/16/6237. "Notice historique," *Rev. méd.* 1826, 4:83–100. Rouxeau [1920], 2:425.

131. "Exhumation des restes de Laennec a eu lieu le 14 septembre 1934," meeting of 25 October 1934, *Bull. Soc. Arch. Finistère* 1934, p. xxxix. I am grateful to Dr. Paul Clouard of Quimper for photographs of the cast of Laennec's cranium made by Felix Graziano and given to Dr. Clouard's father in 1948 by Mme Olgiati in memory of her husband Dr. Antoine Olgiati (1870–1948). According to M. A. Halna du Frétay, who also owns "le crâne de Laennec," many casts were made.

132. Story told to me by M. A. Halna du Frétay, who heard it from a Ploaré gravedigger who had witnessed the procession as a nine-year-old boy.

133. Stories told to me by witnesses MM. Halna du Frétay; Hervé Glorennec, archivist of the town of Quimper; and Laennec descendant François Puget.

CHAPTER TWELVE

1. Weisz 1995, 189–211.

2. Laennec 1884; Laennec 1926; Letulle 1912a, b, c, d.

3. Foucault 1963, 212.

4. On Magendie in medical history, see Jacyna 1987, 137.

5. Lesch 1984, 85.

6. Lesch 1988, esp. 132.

7. Albury 1977; Haigh 1984; Lesch 1984, 92–96, 172–173; Temkin 1946a.

8. Coleman and Holmes 1988, 8; Fye 1987, 10–11; Geison 1978, 4; 1979; 1987b, esp. 3–5; Lesch 1984, 1, 18–19, 197–224; Maulitz 1987a; Weisz 1995, 161–163; Williams 1994, 132–133.

394   • *NOTES TO CHAPTER 12* •

9. For examples of Broussaisist criticisms of animal experimentation, see *Annales de médecine physiologique* 1824, 6;110–112; Gaultier de Claubry 1826, esp. 414. See also Weisz 1995, 162–163.

10. Anonymous 1827, 622–623. Emphasis in original.

11. Gaultier de Claubry 1826, 419. During his last illness, Laennec did indeed ask to be bled (from the foot), but it is doubtful that he or anyone else thought that his disease was pneumonia. *Traité* 2:768.

12. A. L. Bayle 1826a; Kergaradec 1826b.

13. Pariset 1845. On Pariset's éloges see, Weisz 1995, 194, 215–236.

14. Laennec to Mériadec, 19 June 1826, ADLA, MS Chéguillaume, no. 31, transcribed in Roux 1980, 319–321.

15. Mériadec Laennec, notes and summaries in Laennec 1831; Mériadec Laennec 1832.

16. Grmek, "Introduction," in Boulle et al. 1982, 5

17. G. L. Bayle 1833–1839.

18. Bishop 1981, 191; E. Brown 1994; Grandmaison 1889, 390; Müller 1965, 14.

19. A. L. Bayle 1826, 12–13. With Récamier, Bayle had been a founder of *Revue médicale*, which was pro-royalist and anti-Broussais and he published Mériadec's twice yearly descriptions of Laennec's clinics.

20. E. Brown 1994.

21. A. L. J. Bayle 1856, ii–iii, 8, 9, 16, 17, 42; E. Williams 1994, 47n107.

22. Laennec testament, 20 April 1826, MS de Miniac no. 129, transcribed in Roux 1980, 246–248 and in Kervran 1960, 197.

23. Mériadec Laennec in Laennec 1831, *1*:i, viii.

24. Forbes 1834, xxix.

25. Unsigned, undated letter probably by Mériadec Laennec to Kergaradec, after 1840, ML, MS. Cl. 5, lot i, f. 9v.

26. Unsigned, undated letter probably by Mériadec Laennec to Kergaradec, after 1840, ML, MS, Cl. 5, lot i, f. 9v.

27. Delaunay 1949, 103.

28. Bouillaud 1869. See also Weisz 1995, 199.

29. Mériadec Laennec in Laennec 1831, *1*:iii; Louis 1834, 5.

30. Mériadec Laennec in Laennec 1831, *1*:ii. See also Forbes 1834, xxv.

31. Ackerknecht 1967, 138.

32. On American views of French therapeutic indifference, see Warner 1985, 1991, forthcoming. On Laennec's therapeutic practice, see chapter 10.

33. Coleman 1977, 146–147; J. Schiller 1967.

34. See, for example, the transcription of a passage concerning Barthez labeled "Andral, *J. hébdomadaire*, octobre, 1828." BIUM, MS 5172 (III) (e), f. 1 r–v.

35. E. Williams 1994, 21.

36. Mériadec Laennec in Laennec 1831, *1*:iv–v. Emphasis in original.

37. Weisz 1995, 189–211, esp. 198.

38. Boisseau 1822, 471–473.

39. Ackerknecht 1967, 122–123. See also Boulle 1984.

40. For an exceptional view that Laennec had been wrongly blamed for the empiricism of which he was accused, see Chauffard 1865.

41. Forbes, in *Treatise* 1827, 583–584n; Clark 1820, 157–158; Scudamore 1826, 63. See also chapter 10.

42. Laennec, ML, MS Adversaria, unnumbered f. 55. For a similar argument, see Laennec 1806r discussed in chapter 3.
43. Rousseau 1992, esp. 27. See also Gould 1985, 370–380.
44. On Bichat and materialism, Rey 1987, *1*:8–9, *2*:56–74; Goodfield-Toulmin 1969, 318–319. On the problem describing materialism in Claude Bernard, see Grmek 1991a, esp. 119–120. On differing assessments of Cuvier, compare Appel 1987, 50 and Coleman 1964, 33–37. For differing assessments of William Lawrence (1783–1867), compare Goodfield-Toulmin 1969 and Hall 1969 *2*:220, 228–231.
45. Lovejoy and Garrison cited in Haller 1986, 87.
46. Coleman 1977, 12.
47. Geison 1978, 348.
48. On the history of vitalism, see Coleman 1977, 11–13, 145–150; Haller 1986; Hein 1972; Temkin 1946b.
49. Laennec, Collège de France, lesson 2, BIUM, MS. 2186(IV) f. 11 recto.
50. *Traité* 1826, 1:534, 646. Also Laennec, Collège de France, lessons 10, 29, 1822–1823, BIUM, MS. 2186(IV), f. 81v, 111r–v.
51. Canguilhem [1965], 86, 99. See also Pickstone 1981; Rousseau 1992, 44, 45.
52. T. M. Brown 1974.
53. E. Williams 1994, 104–105, 176. On catholic-vitalists opposed to heretical-experimentalists, see Goldstein 1987, 359.
54. Reill 1989; Pickstone 1981.
55. Cunningham 1988; Goodfield-Toulmin 1969, 284–285; Hall 1969 *2*: 254–257.
56. Mérat 1822, 280.
57. Goodfield-Toulmin 1969, 299–300; Rey 1987, *1*:5.
58. Driesch 1914. See also, for example, Cournot 1923; Windle 1920; Joad 1923.
59. On the reception of Driesch's vitalism within the scientific community, see Freyhofer 1982, 141–143.
60. Geison 1978, 24–31; Geison 1979; Maulitz 1987a; Lesch 1984, 223–224; Lesch 1988; Schlich 1993, 435.
61. Williams 1994, 133–134, 258–272.
62. Haldane 1932, 11, 15, 17, 36.
63. Medawar and Medawar 1983, 227–232, 275–277, esp. 277.
64. Goodfield-Toulmin 1969, 305; Gould 1985, 379; Hall 1969, *2*:219.
65. Szasz 1974, 1–13.
66. Shorter 1992, 305–323; Ziporyn 1992, 81–98.
67. On typologies of vitalisms, see Benton 1974, 17–48; Coleman, 1977, 11–12; Goodfield 1960.
68. Canguilhem [1965], 86, 95, 99.
69. Ackerknecht 1973, 2.
70. Watson 1970, 33, 69.
71. Illich 1975; Horrobin 1978.
72. Laennec 1823a, x; Laennec, Collège de France, lesson 9, 1823–1824, ML, MS. Cl. 2 lot a (B), f. 181v; Kitchen "Leçons de Laennec," MS HMCP, 20. See also Chapter 11.
73. Haller 1986, 87.

74. Weinstein 1979, 39–40. See also Haller 1986; Hein 1972; Wolsky and Wolsky 1992.

75. Inglefinger 1980.

76. On the "ghost in the machine," see Ryle 1949, 15–24.

77. Rousseau 1992, 26. See also Anderson 1984; Benjamin et al. 1987; Burwick and Douglas 1992, 1–12; Cross 1981; Gerhart and Russell 1984; Knorr-Cetina 1981; Knorr-Cetina and Mulkay 1983; E. Martin 1990; Skoda 1988, 1–5.

78. Reiser 1979, 38, 100.

79. Rosenberg 1995, esp. 197.

80. Jewson, 1976; Illich 1975, 109–121, esp. 113; Lock 1995; Postman 1992, 97–100; Shorter 1985, 83–84; Ziporyn 1992, 131.

Publications, Reviews, and Other Professional Activities

For further information, see also Bishop 1981, Mettling 1926, and Viets 1926.

1802a. Observation d'une maladie du coeur. *J. méd. 4* (Messidor An X [Jun–Jul]):295–307.

1802b. I. Histoires d'inflammations du péritoine recueillies à la clinique interne de l'école de médecine de Paris sous les yeux des professeurs Corvisart et J. J. Leroux. *J. méd. 4* (Fructidor An X [Aug–Sep]):499–547.

1802c. Extrait de Benjamin Bell, "Traité de la gonorhée virulente et de la maladie vénérienne," 2e édition, traduit par E. Bosquillon. *J. méd. 4* (Fructidor An X [Aug–Sep]):565–575.

1802d. II. Histoires d'inflammations du péritoine recueillies à la clinique interne de l'école de médecine de Paris sous les yeux des professeurs Corvisart et J. J. Leroux. *J. méd. 5* (Vendémiaire An XI [Sep–Oct]):3–59.

1802e. With Tonnelier. Sur un suicide commis avec un rasoir. *J. méd. 5* (Brumaire An XI [Oct–Nov]):131–139.

1802f. Extrait de M. R. Buisson, "De la division la plus naturelle des phénomènes physiologiques considérés chez l'homme." *J. méd. 5* (Brumaire An XI [Oct–Nov]):169–180.

1802g. Extrait de A. A. Royer-Collard, "Sur l'aménorhée, ou suppression du flux menstruel." *J. méd. 5* (Brumaire An XI [Oct–Nov]):181–185.

1802h. Note sur l'arachnoïde intérieure, ou sur la portion de cette membrane qui tapisse les ventricules du cerveau. *J. méd. 5* (Frimaire An XI [Nov–Dec]):254–263.

1803a. Note sur une capsule synoviale située entre l'apophyse acromion et l'humerus. *J. méd. 5* (Pluviôse An XI [Jan–Feb]):422–427.

1803b. Lettre sur les tuniques qui enveloppent certains viscères, et fournissent des gaines membraneuses à leurs vaisseaux, adressée au cit[oyen] Dupuytren. *J. méd. 5* (Ventôse An XI [Feb–Mar]):539–575.

1803c. Suite de la lettre sur les tuniques propres, adressée au citoyen Dupuytren. *J. méd. 6* (Germinal An XI [Mar–Apr]):73–89.

1803d. Laennec takes two of four first prizes in medicine and surgery, Distribution des prix, 30 Fructidor An XI [17 Sep]. *J. méd. 7* (Vendémiaire An XII [Sep–Oct]):93–94.

1803e. Extrait de F. Herpin, "Meningitis ou l'inflammation des membranes de l'encéphale." *J. méd. 7* (Frimaire An XII [Nov–Dec]):273–276.

1804a. With G. L. Bayle. Observation sur une maladie du coeur, épaississement et dilatation du ventricule gauche, ossification aux valvules sigmoïdes et mithrales. *J. méd. 7* (Nivôse An XII [Dec 1803–Jan]):291–304.

1804b. Extrait de Larrey, "Expédition de l'Armée d'Orient." *J. méd. 7* (Nivôse An XII [Dec 1803– Jan]):367–373.

1804c. As "M.T.L." Extrait de Xavier Bichat, "Traité d'anatomie descriptive." *J. méd. 7* (Nivôse An XII [Dec 1803–Jan]):558–569.

1804d. As "M.R." Extrait de Ph. J. Desault, "Cours théorique et pratique de clinique externe." *J. méd. 7* (Ventôse An XII [Feb–Mar]):552–558.

1804e. As "M.T.L." Remarques sur les abstinences prolongées. *J. méd. 8* (Germinal An XII [Mar–Apr]):15–23.

1804f. Extrait sur P. A. Prost, "La médecine éclairée par l'ouverture des corps." *J. méd. 8* (Prairial An XII [May–Jun]):260–272.

1804g. As "M.T.L." Extrait de A. M. Constant Duméril, "Traité élémentaire d'histoire naturelle." *J. méd. 8* (Prairial An XII [May–Jun]):279–285.

1804h. *Propositions sur la doctrine d'Hippocrate relativement à la médecine pratique.* Paris: thèse méd. no. 241, Didot; also unidentified, undated facsimile of 1923.

1804i. Extrait de J. L. Alibert, "Nouveaux éléments de thérapeutique et de matière médicale." *J. méd. 9* (Vendémiaire An XIII [Sep–Oct]):81–83.

1804j. Procès verbal de la séance du 11 Brumaire An XIII [2 Nov 1804]: Laennec et Bayle deviennent membres adjoints. *BEMS 1* (iii):25.

1805a. Note sur l'anatomie pathologique, lu à la séance de la Société de l'Ecole de Médecine 6 Nivôse An XIII [27 Dec 1804]. *J. méd. 9* (Pluviôse An XIII [Jan–Feb]):360–378.

1805b. Procès verbal de la séance du 20 Nivôse An XIII [11 Jan 1805]: Laennec a lu des observations sur les vers ascarides lombricaux qui remplissaient les voies biliaires d'un enfant de deux ans et demi. *BEMS 1* (v):53–55.

1805c. Procès verbal de la séance du 18 Pluviôse An XIII [7 Feb 1805]: Laennec a fait la description d'un ver communiqué par Chartier chirurgien à Lorris. *BEMS 1* (vi):68–69.

1805d. Réponse aux observations, etc. de M. Dupuytren. *J. méd. 10* (Germinal An XIII [Mar–Apr]):89–95.

1805e. La lecture d'un mémoire sur les vers vésiculaires par M. Laennec a été remise à la séance du 22 Germinal An XIII [12 Apr]. *BEMS 1* (x):131–136.

1805f. Procès verbal de la séance du 6 Thermidor An XIII [25 Jul]: Laennec a lu un mémoire sur une nouvelle espèce de ver cysticerque à double vessie (cyst. dycistus). *BEMS 1*:162.

1805g. With L. Fizeau. Procès verbal de la séance du 4 Fructidor An XIII (23 Aug 1805): Laennec et Fizeau présentent une observation de dilatation de la valvule mithrale, dessin de Laennec. *BEMS 1* (xiii):183.

1805h. Extrait sur J. F. Lobstein, "Sur les travaux exécutés à l'amphithéâtre de Strasbourg." *J. méd. 11* (Vendémiaire An XIV [Sep–Oct]):152–158.

1805i. As "L." Extrait sur Brown, "Eléments de médecine," traduit par R. J. Bertin. *J. méd. 11* (Frimaire An XIV [Nov–Dec]):214–31.

1805j. Procès verbal de la séance du 21 Frimaire An XIV [11 Dec]: Laennec a lu une note sur le taenia visceralis de quelques auteurs, tendant à établir que cette espèce n'existe pas. *BEMS 1* (i):3.

1806a. Procès verbal de la séance du 23 janvier 1806: Laennec a lu un mémoire sur un genre d'altération morbifique de différens organes auquel il donne le nom de mélanose. *BEMS 1* (ii):19.

1806b. Sur les mélanoses, extrait du mémoire de Laennec. *BEMS 1* (ii):24–26.

1806c. As "M.T.L." Extrait sur P.J. Amoureux, "Essai historique et littéraire sur la médecine des arabes." *J. méd. 11* (Jan):289–296.

1806d. As "M.R." Extrait sur Baumes, "De la première dentition." *J. méd. 11* (Feb):357–364.

1806e. Extrait sur Barthez, "Nouveaux élémens de la science de l'homme." *J. méd.* 11 (Feb):364–375.

1806f. As "M.T.L." Extrait sur A. M. Constant-Duméril, "Zoologie analytique." *J. méd.* 11 (Feb):392–395.

1806g. As "M.T.L." Extrait sur Michel Sarcone, "Histoire raisonnée des maladies observées à Naples pendant le cours entier de l'année 1764," traduit par F. Ph. Bellay. *J. méd.* 11 (Mar):442–460.

1806h. As "M.R." Extrait sur "Mémoires de la Société Médicale d'Emulation," Paris 1806. *J. méd.* 11 (Mar):460–470.

1806i. Extrait sur Caillau, "Tableau de la médecine hippocratique," 1806. *J. méd.* 11 (May):624–632.

1806j. Extrait sur Lassus, "Pathologie chirurgicale." *J. méd.* 11 (May):633–642.

1806k. Réflexions sur les observations précédentes [C. M. A. Matthey "Recherches sur les caractères distinctifs et sur le traitement de l'hydrocéphale interne," 651–666]. *J. méd.* 11 (Jun):666–678.

1806l. Extrait sur Roederer et Wagler, "Traité de la maladie muqueuse," ed. H. A. Wrisberg, traduit par J. L. Leprieur, 1806. *J. méd.* 11 (Jun):704–706.

1806m. As "M.R." Extrait sur J. B. Davis, "Projet de Règlement concernant des décès," 1806. *J. méd.* 11 (Jun):716–717.

1806n. As "M.R." Extrait sur L. Laforgue, "De la séméiologie buccale." *J. méd.* 11 (Jun):717–721.

1806o. As Anonymous. Extrait de "Recueil de mémoires concernant la chimie," 1806. *J. méd.* 11 (Jun):725–726.

1806p. Procès verbal de la séance du 26 juin 1806: Laennec présente un cas de compression du canal thoracique par tumeur anévrismale de l'aorte. *BEMS 1* (vii):104.

1806q. As "T.L." Extrait de M***, D.M., "Alchianisme animal contenant l'alchianologie et l'alchianosologie de l'homme . . ." *J. méd.* 12 (Jul):385–386.

1806r. Exposition et examen de la doctrine du Docteur Gall [3 parts]. *J. méd.* 12 (Aug, Sep, Oct):135–150, 202–211, 284–301.

1806s. Sur un anévrisme de l'aorte qui avait produit la compression du canal thoracique, lu à la Société de l'Ecole de Médecine. *J. méd.* 12 (Sep):284–301.

1806t. As "M.T.L." Extrait sur abbé Desmonceau, "Traité des maladies des yeux et des oreilles." *J. méd.* 12 (Nov):382–383.

1806u. As "M.T.L." Extrait sur Duméril-Lesueur, "Hippocratis aphorismi cum loci parallelis Celsi." *J. méd.* 12 (Nov):383.

1806v. As "M.R." Extrait de G.J. docteur en médecine, "Des monstruosités et bizzareries de la nature." *J. méd.* 12 (Nov):384–385.

1806w. Extrait de P. A. Prost, "Coup d'oeil physiologique sur la folie." *J. méd.* 12 (Nov):385–386.

1806x. Procès verbal de la séance du 13 novembre 1806: Laennec a lu un mémoire sur une espèce de ver intestinal non encore décrite, accompagné de figures et dessins par l'auteur. *BEMS 1* (x):156–157.

1807a. Sur le Distomus intersectus nouveau genre de vers intestins, extrait du mémoire. *BEMS 1* (i):9–12.

1807b. Extrait de Roederer et Wagler, "Traité de l'épidémie qui régna à Gottingue en 1760, 1761, et 1762," traduit par Poulin, 1806. *J. méd.* 13 (Mar):202–203.

1807c. As "M.T.L." Extrait de J. B. Demangeon, "Physiologie intellectuelle ou développement de la doctrine du Pr Gall." *J. méd.* 13 (Mar):228–229.

1807d. Extrait de E. M. Itard, "Rapport fait à S. E. le Ministre de l'Intérieur sur les nouveaux développemens et l'état actuel du Sauvage de l'Aveyron." *J. méd. 13* (Mar):230–231.

1807e. Extrait de J. L. F. Terr, "Hygie ou l'art de se bien porter." *J. méd. 13* (Apr):283–308.

1807f. Procès verbal de la séance du 16 avril 1807: Laennec a lu un mémoire sur une nouvelle espèce de hernie qu'il désigne sous le nom "intrapelvienne." *BEMS 1* (v):64.

1807g. As "M.T.L." Extrait de Alphonse Leroy, "Manuel de la saignée." *J. méd. 13* (May):368–370.

1807h. Observation sur des fièvres intermittentes pernicieuses, survenues pendant la convalescence à la suite d'autres maladies. *J. méd. 14*:3–26.

1807i. Extrait de Simon Morelot, ed., "Nouveau dictionnaire général des drogues, simples et composées de Lemery." *J. méd. 14*:71–77.

1807j. With G. L. Bayle and L. A. Fizeau. Constitution médicale observée à Paris pendant les six premiers mois de 1807. *J. méd. 14*:124–136.

1807k. Extrait de Joseph Quarin, "Observations pratiques sur les maladies chroniques," traduit par E. Sainte-Marie. *J. méd. 14*:146–152.

1807l. As "M.T.L." Extrait de M. Jourdan et Mazziolo, "Le Manuel de l'art du dentiste," 1807. *J. méd. 14*:153–155.

1807m. As "M.T.L." Extrait de Paul Godofredi Van Hoorn, "Dissertatio de iis, quae in partibus membri praesertim osseis, amputatione vulneratis . . ." *J. méd. 14*:155–157.

1807n. As "M.T.L." Réflexions sur l'observation précédente [Garnier, "Observation sur un tumeur salivaire survenu à la suite de la section du canal de Stenon" 273–8]. *J. méd 14*:279–289.

1807o. As "M.T.L." Réflexions sur l'observation précédente [Cayol, "Observation sur un calcul des reins," 331–430]. *J. méd. 14*:341–345.

1807p. Réflexions sur l'observation précédente [Matussière, "Observations sur le tétanos']. *J. méd. 14*:465–483.

1808a. With G. L. Bayle, L. Fizeau, and J. J. Leroux. Constitution médicale à Paris, pour les 6 derniers mois de 1807. *Bib. méd. 20*:91–94.

1808b. Extrait sur Parmentier, "Instructions sur les moyens de suppléer le sucre dans les principaux usages qu'on en fait pour la médecine et l'économie domestique." *J. méd. 16*:155–159.

1808c. Extrait sur J. P. Maygrier, "Manuel de l'anatomie." *J. méd. 15*:223–231.

1808d. Extrait sur Corvisart, "Nouvelle méthode pour reconnaître les maladies de la poitrine par la percussion de cette cavité," par Auenbrugger. *J. méd. 15*:360–371.

1808e. Procès verbal de la séance du 12 mai 1808: Laennec lit un rapport sur des tableaux relatifs à la constitution médicale observée à Lyon, 1807, par M. Bellay. *BEMS 1* (v):64.

1808f. As Anonymous. Extrait de deux mémoires de M. Itard [rapport avec Hallé et Moreau]. *BEMS 1* (v):72–79.

1808g. Procès verbal de la séance du 24 novembre 1808: Laennec fait successivement trois rapports: 1. avec Hallé sur les maladies qui régnent par M. Gendron; 2. sur l'emploi des gouttes arsénicales par M. Colombo; 3. sur les tableaux des symptômes de M. Latour. *BEMS 1* (ix):130.

1809a. Procès verbal de la séance du 16 février 1809: Laennec communique une observation de M. Gallot sur une extirpation de la matrice. *BEMS 2* (ii):15.

1809b. Procès verbal de la séance du 2 mars 1809; Laennec communique une observation sur une extirpation de la matrice insérée dans la Gazette des Petites Antilles, 16 avril 1776. *BEMS 2* (iii):15.

1809c. Procès verbal de la séance du 31 août 1809. Laennec et Thillaye sont nommés commissaires auprès de l'Institut de France pour assister à ses séances et en rendre compte. *BEMS 2* (viii):121.

1809d. Procès verbal de la séance du 23 novembre 1809: M. Laennec et Huzard font un rapport sur une observation de Raseri relative à une hernie congénitale. *BEMS 2* (xi):171.

1810a. Procès verbal de la séance du 19 juillet 1810: Laennec et Pinel font un rapport sur un mémoire de M. Esquirol. *BEMS 2* (vii–viii):100.

1810b. Procès verbal de la séance du 8 novembre 1810: Laennec et Chaussier font un rapport sur Duval dentist, "Consomption dentaire." *BEMS 2* (x):132.

1810c. Procès verbal de la séance du 23 novembre 1810: Laennec fait un rapport sur un mémoire de M. Chaumeton, "Recherches et observations sur la plique polonaise." *BEMS 2* (x):133.

1810d. Procès verbal de la séance du 6 décembre 1810: Laennec fait partie de la commission pour la rédaction des mémoires de la Société. *BEMS 2* (x): 134.

1810e. Procès verbal de la séance du 19 décembre 1810: M. Laennec lit un mémoire latin sous le titre "De angina pectoris commentarius." *BEMS 2* (x):135.

1811a. With G. L. Bayle and A. C. Savary. Constitution médicale observée à Paris. *Bib. méd. 23*:93–95.

1811b.With G. L. Bayle and A. C. Savary. Observation sur une affection aphtheuse in Laennec, Bayle, and Savary, "Constitution médicale observée à Paris." *J. méd. 22*:113–132, esp. 118–123.

1811c. With D. Larrey. Extrait du rapport fait le 25 avril 1811 sur Alard, "Elephantiases des arabes." *BEMS 2* (iii–iv):44, 71, 87–88.

1811d. Procès verbal de la séance du 20 juin 1811: Laennec fait un rapport sur le "Traité de l'angine de poitrine" de Desportes. *BEMS 2* (vi):113.

1811e. Procès verbal de la séance du 20 juin 1811: Laennec est chargé de faire un rapport sur le travail de Courbon-Pérusel à Carhaix tiré de sa pratique avec référence aux aphorismes d'Hippocrate. *BEMS 2* (vi):113.

1811f. Procès verbal de la séance du 1 août 1811, Laennec et Chaussier sont priés d'examiner le travail de Cayol sur les hydatides ou les vers vésiculaires. *BEMS 2* (viii):151.

1811g. Procès verbal de la séance du 19 décembre 1811: Laennec présente une pièce d'anatomie pathologique sur laquelle il se propose de lire un mémoire . . . c'est une matrice dont la partie antérieure avait été extirpée pour cause de maladie suivant la méthode d'Osiander. *BEMS 2* (x):195–196.

1812a. Mémoire sur les vers vésiculaires et principalement sur ceux qui se trouvent dans le corps humain, lu à la séance du 26 Pluviôse XII [16 Feb 1804]. In *Mémoires de la Faculté de Médecine de Paris et de la Société établie dans son sein*. Paris: Didot, 1–178, 4 plates.

1812b. Anatomie pathologique. In *DSM* 2:46–61.

1812c. Ascarides. In *DSM* 2:339–352.

1812d. IV Observation: oedème de la glotte produit par un abcès placé dans les parois du larynx. In G. L. Bayle, "Mémoire sur une maladie à laquelle on peut donner le nom d'oedème de la glotte ou d'angine laryngée oedémateuse, lu à la séance du 18 aôut 1808." *Mémoires de la Faculté de Médecine de Paris et de la Société établie dans son sein.* Paris: Didot, 357–362.

1813a. Procès verbal de la séance du 18 février 1813: Laennec présente une vessie de veau très volumineuse au milieu de laquelle on observe un profond étranglement qui la divise . . . en deux portions. *BEMS 3* (ii):300.

1813b. Procès verbal de la séance du 5 août 1813: Laennec, avec Leroux, fait un rapport sur Savary "Compte rendu des maladies traitées dans la division de l'Observatoire pendant 1811." *BEMS 3* (viii):453.

1813c. Procès verbal de la séance du 25 novembre 1813: Chaussier et Laennec chargés de faire un rapport sur Duval dans les ulcères des gencives. *BEMS 3* (ix):479–480.

1813d. With Leroux. Rapport sur le mémoire de Savary, "Compte rendu des maladies traitées dans la division de l'Observatoire, pendant l'année 1811." *BEMS 3* (x):501–504.

1813e. Cartilages accidentels. In *DSM 4*:123–133.

1813f. Crinon. In *DSM 7*:365–369.

1813g. Curcurbitans. In *DSM 7*:526–527.

1814a. Dégénération. In *DSM 8*:201–208.

1814b. Dégénérescence. In *DSM 8*:208.

1814c. Diathrachyeros. In *DSM. 10*:43–45.

1815a. Procès verbal de la séance du 19 janvier 1815: Laennec est nommé commissaire, et il fera un rapport sur Arvers, "Une observation d'une tumeur du crâne." *BEMS 4* (i):260–267, 272.

1815b. As Anonymous. *De la Féodalité, ou mémoire sur cette question, le rétablissement de la féodalité étoit-il plus à craindre sous le gouvernement du Roi que sur l'Empire de Buonaparte?* Ghent: l'Imprimerie Royale.

1815c. Encéphaloïdes. In *DSM 12*:165–178.

1816a. Procès verbal de la séance du 16 mai 1816: la perte douleureuse de Bayle; Laennec promet de donner quelques détails sur les recherches auxquelles sa maladie a pu donner lieu s'il peut les obtenir des personnes qui se proposent de les faire. *BEMS 5* (iii):133.

1816b. Fibreux accidentel (tissu). In *DSM 15*:194–202.

1816c. Fibro-cartilage. In *DSM 15*:204–215.

1816d. Filiaire. In *DSM 15*:493–495.

1816e. Furie infernale. In *DSM 17*:162–163.

1817a. Procès verbal de la séance du 20 février 1817: Laennec et Percy nommés commissionaires à fin d'étudier la note par M. Savée de l'Orient [*sic*] sur des vers rendus par les urines. *BEMS 5* (ii):314.

1817b. Procès verbal de la séance du 1 mai 1817: Laennec et Percy sont nommés rapporteurs sur observation du Rostang [*sic*] sur l'asthme des vieillards dit périodique. *BEMS 5* (v):405.

1817c. Laennec ausculte Madame de Staël, in A. Portal "Sur la maladie et la mort de Madame la Baronne de Staël." *Annales politiques, morales, et littéraires*, 2 Aug, 3–4.

1817d. Procès verbal de la séance du 7 août 1817: Laennec présente une matière analogue aux perles artificielles qui provient de la tunique vaginale du testicule. *BEMS 5* (viii):492.

1817e. M. Villenave, ed. "On a rendu compte à l'une des sociétés savantes . . . d'un moyen d'investigation physiologique [avec] un rouleau de plusieurs feuilles de papier." *Annales politiques morales et littéraires,* 26 Sep, 2.

1818a. Procès verbal de la séance du 5 février 1818: Laennec annonce qu'il a en ce moment à l'hôpital Necker un malade qui présente le signe indiqué par Hippocrate [succussion]. *BEMS* 6:51.

1818b. M. Laennec lit un mémoire sur l'auscultation par des moyens acoustiques dans la pratique de la médecine, 23 février 1818. *Procès verbaux des séances de l'Académie des sciences* 4:286–287.

1818c. Procès verbal de la séance du 1 mai 1818: Laennec commence la lecture d'un mémoire ou ouvrage sur l'auscultation. *BEMS* 6 (v):129.

1818d. Procès verbal de la séance du 14 mai 1818: Laennec présente une femme qui offre, par l'application d'un cylindre de bois creux sur l'épaule droite, les signes d'une resonance particulière que M. Laennec designe sous le nom pectoriloquie. Ensuite le même M. Laennec continue la lecture de son travail sur l'auscultation. *BEMS* 6 (v):129.

1818e. Procès verbal de la séance du 11 juin 1818: Laennec continue la lecture d'un mémoire ou ouvrage sur l'auscultation. *BEMS* 6 (vi):156.

1818f. Procès verbal de la séance du 9 juillet 1818: Laennec continue sa lecture sur l'auscultation et la pectoriloquie. *BEMS* 6 (vii):171.

1818g. With Alard, Cayol, DeLens, Esquirol, Gardier, Geoffroy, Guersent, Guilbert, Landré-Beauvais, Lullier-Winslow, Marjolin, Pinel, Richerand and Royer-Collard. Lettre au sujet du *Dictionnaire des sciences médicales. Bib. méd.* 59:265–267.

1819a. "IV Observation: oedème de la glotte produit par un abcès placé dans les parois du larynx." in G. L. Bayle, "Mémoire sur l'oedème de la glotte ou angine laryngée oedémateuse." *Nouv. j. méd.* 4 (Jan):3–56, esp. 37–43.

1819b. Procès verbal de la séance du 3 juin 1819: Laennec soumet des portions des poumons provenant d'un individu qui avait été sujet à une sorte d'emphysème et dont il propose de parler dans un ouvrage qu'il fait actuellement imprimer. *BEMS* 6:413.

1819c. *De l'auscultation médiate ou traité du diagnostique des poumons et du coeur.* 2 vols. Paris: Brosson and Chaudé; also facsimile Paris: Cercle du Livre Précieux, 1965.

1819d. Procès verbal de la séance du 16 octobre 1819: la faculté charge le secrétaire de remercier M. Laennec des pièces anatomiques qu'il a déposés dans les cabinets de l'Ecole de Médecine. *BEMS* 6 (ix):484.

1820. As Anonymous. *Avis d'al labourien ha d'ar cultivaorien an arrondissement el Kemper.* Quimper: Simon Blot et Société d'Agriculture du Finistère.

1821. *A Treatise on the Diseases of the Chest in which They are Described according to Their Anatomical Characters and Their Diagnosis Established on a New Principle by Means of Acoustick Instruments.* Trans. John Forbes. London: Underwood; also facsimile New York: Hafner and the New York Academy of Medicine, 1962.

1822a. *Die mittelbare Auskultation (das Hören mittelst des Stethoscops) oder Abhandlung über die Diagnostik der Krankheiten der Lunge und des Nerzens, auf das neue Erforschungsmittel gegründet.* 1st German ed. from 1st French ed. Weimar: Landes-Industrie Comptoirs.

1822b [n.d.] *Notice sur les travaux de R. T. H. Laennec.* Paris: Feugueray.

1823a. Extrait du discours prononcé par M. Laennec à l'ouverture de son cours de médecine au Collège Royale de France. *Arch. gén. méd.* 1:v–xx.

1823b. *A Treatise on the Diseases of the Chest in which They are Described according to Their Anatomical Characters and Their Diagnosis Established on a New Principle by Means of Acoustick Instruments.* 1st American ed. Trans. John Forbes. Philadelphia: James Webster.

1824. "Les cirrhoses," in Ferrus 1824, 210–212.

1825a. Académie royale de médecine, 24 novembre 1824, Legallois présente au nom de Laennec une veine cave. *Rev. méd. 1*:150.

1825b. Académie royale de médecine, 25 janvier 1825, Adelon lit au nom de Laennec un rapport sur Velpeau: les maladies cancéreuses. *Rev. méd. 1*:471.

1825c. Académie royale de médecine, 23 août 1825, Laennec fait un commentaire sur Lassis, exposé des expériences sur la peste et la fièvre jaune. *Gazette de santé 52* (no. 25, 5 Sep):193–196.

1825d. Académie royale de médecine, 11 octobre 1825, Laennec fait un commentaire sur les expériences sur l'inoculation de Legallois. *Gazette de santé 52* (no. 32, 15 Oct):268.

1825e. Rapport sur les expériences de M. Barry, lu par Adelon aux noms de Laennec et Orfila. *Arch. gén. méd. 9*:605–608.

1826a. Académie royale de médecine, 22 novembre 1825, Laennec, Rullier et Mestivier font un rapport sur la note de M. Noble de Versailles sur la cautérisation dans la variole. *Rev. méd. 1*:157.

1826b. Académie royale de médecine, 22 novembre, 3 décembre 1825, Adelon en nom de lui, Laennec, et Orfila fait un rapport sur les expériences de M. Barry. *Rev. méd. 1*:157–162, 320–321.

1826c. Académie royale de médecine, 27 décembre 1825, Laennec présente un poumon dans lequel se trouve la matière cérébriforme. *Rev. méd. 1*:324.

1826d. Académie royale de médecine, 10 janvier 1826, Laennec parle de ses vingt ans d'études personelles sur le magnétisme animal. *Rev. méd. 1*:494, 498–499.

1826e. Académie royale de médecine, 24 janvier 1826, Laennec exprime son opinion sur le magnétisme animal. *Arch. gén. méd. 10*:306–315, esp. 309.

1826f. Académie royale de médecine, 28 [?] février 1826, Laennec nommé à la commission d'étudier le magnétisme animal. *Arch. gén. méd. 10.*

1826g. *Notice des faits nouveaux obtenus par suite des recherches de M. Laennec 18 mai 1826.* Paris: Feugueray.

1826h. *Traité de l'auscultation médiate et des maladies des poumons et du coeur.* 2d ed. 2 vols. Paris: Chaudé.

1826i. With Adelon and Orfila. Rapport sur les expériences de M. Barry. *Arch. gén. méd. 10*:129.

1826j. Report of Laennec, Adelon, and Orfila to the Académie Royale de Médecine. In *Experimental Researches on the Influence exercised by Atmospheric Pressure upon the Progression of the Blood in the Veins* . . . London: Underwood, 174–175.

1827. *A Treatise on the Diseases of the Chest and on Mediate Auscultation.* 2d ed. Trans. John Forbes. London: Underwood.

1829. As Anonymous. Letter to Félicité de Lamennais ca. 1820. In F. de Lamennais, *Essai sur l'indifférence en matière de religion.* 8th ed. Paris: Belin-Mandar-Devaux, 2:90–93n.

1831. *Traité de l'auscultation médiate et des maladies des poumons et du coeur.* 3d ed. 3 vols. ed. M. Laennec. Paris: Chaudé.

1833–1836. *Trattato della ascoltazione mediata e delle malattie dei polmoni e del cuore.* 1st Italian ed. from 3d French. 4 vols. Trans. Angiolo Modigliani. Livorno: Bertani, Antonelli.

1834. *A Treatise on the Diseases of the Chest and on Mediate Auscultation.* 4th English ed. Trans. John Forbes. London: Longman, Rees, Orme, Brown, Green and Longman.

1836. "Les cirrhoses." In Ferrus 1836.

1837. *Traité de l'auscultation médiate et des maladies des poumons et du coeur.* 4th French ed. 3 vols. Ed. G. Andral. Paris: Chaudé.

1839. "Les cirrhoses." In Erasmus 1839.

1846. *Treatise on Diseases of the Chest, with Notes by Andral and by F. H. Ramadge.* Trans. from the 4th French ed. by a member of the College of Physicians. Ed. T. Herbert. London: Baillière.

1884. *Traité inédit sur l'anatomie pathologique.* Ed. V. Cornil. Paris: Alcan.

1912. See Letulle 1912a, 1912b, 1912c, 1912d.

1926. *Documents inédits.* Ed. M. Letulle. Paris: Masson.

1931. *La Guerre des Vénètes.* Ed. P. Busquet. Paris: Masson.

Ackerknecht, Erwin H. 1948. "Anticontagionism between 1821 and 1867." *Bull. Hist. Med.* 22:562–593.

———. 1950. "Elisha Bartlett and the Philosophy of the Paris Clinical School." *Bull. Hist. Med.* 24:43–60.

———. 1953. "Broussais, or a Forgotten Medical Revolution." *Bull. Hist. Med.* 27:320–343.

———. 1962. "Laennec und die Psychiatrie." *Gesnerus* 19:93–100.

———. 1964. "Laennec und sein Vorlesungsmanuskript von 1822." *Gesnerus* 21:142–154.

———. 1967. *Medicine at the Paris Hospital, 1794–1848.* Baltimore: Johns Hopkins University Press.

———. 1973. *Therapeutics from the Primitives to the Twentieth Century.* New York: Hafner.

———. 1981. "Laennec and Broussais." In *RPD,* 208–212.

Adams, Francis. 1856. *The Extant Works of Aretaeus the Cappadocian.* London: Sydenham Society.

Adelon, Béclard, Biett, Breschet et al. 1821–28. *Dictionnaire de médecine.* 21 vols. Paris: Béchet jeune.

Albury, William Randall. 1977. "Experiment and Explanation in the Physiology of Bichat and Magendie." *Stud. Hist. Biol.* 1:47–132.

———. 1982. "Heart of Darkness: J. N. Corvisart and the Medicalization of Life." *Hist. Refl.* 9:17–31.

Anderson, Wilda C. 1984. *Between the Library and the Laboratory: The Language of Chemistry in Eighteenth-Century France.* Baltimore: Johns Hopkins University Press.

Andral, Gabriel. 1823–1827. *Clinique médicale ou choix d'observations recueillies à la clinique de M. Lerminier.* 5 vols. Paris: Gabon.

———. 1829. *Précis d'anatomie pathologique.* 2 vols. Paris: Gabon.

[Anonymous]. 1820. "[Review of Rault 1819]." *Nouv. j. méd.* 8:67–68.

[Anonymous]. 1823a. "Review des journaux de médecine." *Gazette de Santé; Journal de médecine et des sciences accessoires par une société de médecins* 50: 37, 61.

[Anonymous]. 1823b. "Prospectus." *Bib. méd.* 12 4e année:1–10.

[Anonymous]. 1824. "Catechisme de la médecine physiologique, ou Dialogue entre un savant et un jeune médecine élève du professeur Broussais." *Annales de la médecine physiologique* 5:402–408.

[Anonymous]. 1827. "Notice sur M. René-Théophile Laennec." *Arch. gén. méd.* 13:620–623.

Appel, Toby A. 1987. *The Cuvier-Geoffroy Debate: French Biology in the Decades before Darwin.* New York: Oxford University Press.

Aronson, J. K. 1985. *An Account of the Foxglove and its Medicinal Uses, 1785–1985.* London: Oxford University Press.

Au pays de Laennec: Quimper et Cornouaille. 1981. Quimper: Le Berre.

Aubry, J. F. [1776] 1810. *Oracles de Cos.* Montpellier: J. G. Tournell.

Auenbrugger, Leopold. 1761. *Inventum novum ex percussione thoracis humani ut signi abstrusos interni pectoris morbus detegendi.* Vienna: J. T. Trattner.

———. 1808. *Nouvelle méthode pour reconnaître les maladies internes de la poitrine par la percussion de cette cavité.* Trans. J. N. Corvisart. Paris: Migneret.

Authenac, S.P. 1821–1823. *Defense des médecins français contre la doctrine de M. Broussais.* 3 vols. in 1. Paris: Bechet et Gabon.

Baczko, Bronislaw. 1994. *Ending the Terror: The French Revolution after Robespierre.* Trans. Michel Petheram. Cambridge: Cambridge University Press.

Baillie, Matthew. 1803. *Traité d'anatomie pathologique du corps humain.* Trans. M. Ferrall. Paris: Samson.

———. [1808] 1977. *Morbid Anatomy of Some of the Most Important Parts of the Human Body.* Reprint of 2d American ed. Walpole, N.H.: G. W. Nichols for Thomas and Thomas.

Barker, John. 1747. *An Essay on the Agreement betwixt Ancient and Modern Physicians.* London: Hawkins.

———. 1768. *Essai sur la conformité de la médecine ancienne et moderne.* Trans. A. C. Lorry. Paris: Cavelier.

Barry, David. 1825. *Recherches expérimentales sur les causes du mouvement du sang dans les veines.* Paris: Crevot.

———. 1826. *Experimental Researches on the Influence Exercised by Atmospheric Pressure upon Absorption, etc. with Reports of Cuvier, Duméril, Legallois, Laennec, Adelon, and Orfila.* Trans. of 1825 French ed. London: Underwood.

———. 1827. "Discours pour le passage du sang à travers le coeur." Thèse méd. no. 117, Paris.

Barthez, Paul Joseph. 1806. *Nouveaux éléments de la science de l'homme.* 2d ed. 2 vols. Montpellier: Goujon et Brunot.

Bates, Barbara. 1991. *A Guide to Physical Examination and History Taking.* 5th ed. Philadelphia: J. B. Lippincott.

Baume, Jean-Joseph. 1819. "Recherches sur l'hydropneumonie." Thèse méd. no. 159, Paris.

Bayle, A. L. J. 1822. "Recherches sur les maladies mentales." Thèse méd. no. 247, Paris.

———. 1826a. "Notice historique sur M. Laennec." *Rev. méd.* 4:83–100.

———. 1826b. *Traité des maladies du cerveau et de ses membranes.* Paris: Gabon.

———, ed. 1833. "Biographie de G. L. Bayle." In G. L. Bayle, *Traité des maladies cancéreuses.* 2 vols., *1*:i–lviii. Paris: Laurent.

———. 1856. *Eléments de pathologie médicale ou précis théorique et pratique écrit dans l'esprit du vitalisme hippocratique.* Paris: Baillière.

Bayle, A. L. J., and Auguste Thillaye. 1855. *Biographie médicale par ordre chronologique.* 2 vols. Paris: Delahaye.

Bayle, G. L. 1802. "Considérations sur la nosologie, la médecine d'observation et la médecine pratique." Thèse méd. no. 70, Paris.

———. 1803. "Remarques sur les tubercules, lu à la Société de l'Ecole de Médecine, 12 Ventôse An XI." *J. méd.* 6:3–72.

———. 1805. "Dégénérescence tuberculeuse non enkystée du tissu des organes, sous la direction de M. Dupuytren." *J. méd.* 9 (Ventôse [Feb.–Mar.]):427–441, *10* (Germinal [Mar–Apr.]):32–76.

———. 1810a. *Recherches sur la phthisie pulmonaire.* Paris: Gabon.

———.[1810b] 1855. " 'Idée générale de la thérapeutique,' reprinted from *Bibliothèque Médicale*, 1810." In Bayle and Corvisart 1855, 604–608.

———. 1812a. "Considérations sur l'anatomie pathologique." In *DSM*, 2:61–78.

———. 1812b. "Mémoire sur une maladie à laquelle on peut donner le nom d'oedème de la glotte ou d'angine laryngée oedémateuse, lu à la séance du 18 août 1808." In *Mémoires de la Faculté de Médecine de Paris et de la Société établie dans son sein*. Paris: Didot. Reprinted in *Nouv. j. méd.* 4 (1819):3–56.

———. 1833–1839. *Traité des maladies cancéreuses*. 2 vols. Ed. A. L. Bayle. Paris: Laurent.

———. 1855. "Phthisie pulmonaire, article inédit." In Bayle and Corvisart 1855, 645.

Bayle, G. L., and Jean-Bruno Cayol. 1812. "Cancer." In *DSM*, 3:537–568.

Bayle, G. L., and J. N. Corvisart. 1855. *Recueil de mémoires et de travaux divers*. Paris: Bureau de l'Encyclopédie des sciences médicales, 7e division, t. 13.

Beach, Vincent W. 1971. *Charles X of France. His Life and Times*. Boulder, Colo.: Pruett.

Beau, J. 1856. *Traité expérimentale et clinique d'auscultation appliqué à l'étude des maladies du poumon et du coeur*. Paris: Baillière.

Beaubien, Pierre. 1822. "Dissertation sur le rhumatisme articulaire." Thèse méd. no. 191, Paris.

Beaugendre, François-Marie. 1818. "Dissertation sur l'apoplexie." Thèse méd. no. 111, Paris.

Béclard, J. 1880. "Eloge d'Andral." In *Mémoires de l'Académie de Médecine*. Paris: Masson, 20:1–20.

Bedford, Evan. 1972. "Cardiology in the Days of Laennec." *British Heart Journal* 34:1193–1198.

Benivieni, Antonio. [1507] 1954. *De abditis nonnullis ac mirandis morborum et sanatorum causis*. Facsimile with English trans. Charles Singer. Springfield, Ill.: Charles C. Thomas.

Benjamin, Andres E., Geoffrey N. Cantor, and John R. R. Christie, eds. 1987. *The Figural and the Literal: Problems of Language in the History of Science and Philosophy, 1630–1800*. Manchester: Manchester University Press.

Benton, E. 1974. "Vitalism in Nineteenth-Century Scientific Thought: A Typology and Reassessment." *Stud. Hist. Phil. Sci.* 5:17–48.

Bernard-Luc, Jean. 1949. *Docteur Laënnec: récit du film de Maurice Cloche*. Paris: Editions de Flore.

Bertier de Sauvigny, Guillaume de. 1948. *Le Comte Ferdinand de Bertier (1782–1864) et l'énigme de la Congrégation*. Paris: Les Presses Contintentales.

———. 1966. *The Bourbon Restoration*. Trans. Lynn M. Case. Philadelphia: Pennsylvania University Press.

———. 1981. "Le congréganiste, le chrétien." In *RPD*, 225–231.

Bertin, René-Joseph-Hyacinthe. 1824. *Traité des maladies du coeur et des gros vaisseaux*, 3 vols. Ed. J. B. Bouillaud. Paris: Baillière.

Bishop, James Patrick. 1981. *A Bibliography of R. T. H. Laennec (1781–1826). An Attempt to List All the Publications by or about Him, Together with a List of Manuscripts, Letters, and Other Related Material*. Brompton, London: privately printed. (Microfiche copies available from the Royal Australasian College of Physicians.)

Bliss, Michael. 1982. *The Discovery of Insulin*. Toronto: McClelland and Stewart.

Bloch, Harry. 1987. "Phenomena of Respiration: Overview to the Twentieth Century." *Heart and Lung* 16:419–423.

Boisseau, F. G. 1822. "Laennec." In *DSM: Biog. méd.* 5:471–473.

Boitout, Heide. 1965. "Die 'productions cirrhoses' des R. Th. H. Laennec." *Medizinische Welt* 27:1537–1540.

Bon, Henri. 1925. *Laennec, 1781–1826.* "Les grand catholiques". Dijon: Lumière.

Bonald, L.G.A. de. [1796]. *Théorie du pouvoir politique et religieux dans la société civile.* 4th ed. 2 vols. General editor Ch. J. de Mat. Brussels: Société nationale pour la propagation des bons livres.

―――. [1830] 1985. *Démonstration philosophique du principe constitutif de la société.* Ed. F. Azouvi. Paris: Vrin.

Bonet, Théophile. 1700. *Sepulchretum sive anatomia pratica ex cadaveribus morbo denatus*, 2d ed. Lugduni [Lyons]: Cramer et Peruchon.

Bouchet and Casavieilh. 1825–1826. "[Sur l'épilepsie et l'alienation mentale] 'mémoire qui a emporté le prix du 2 septembre 1825.' " *Arch. gén. méd.* 9:510–542, 10:5–50.

Bouillaud, J. B. 1823. "Essai sur le diagnostic des anévrismes de l'aorte et spécialement sur les signes que fournit l'auscultation." Thèse méd. no. 146, Paris.

―――. 1825a. "Extrait du rapport sur les mémoires relatifs à l'aliénation mentale." *Arch. gén. méd.* 9:197–199.

―――. 1825b. *Traité clinique et physiologique de l'encéphalite ou inflammation du cerveau, et de ses suites.* Paris: Baillière.

―――. 1835. *Traité clinique des maladies du coeur*, 2 vols. Paris: Baillière.

―――. 1836. *Essai sur la philosophie médicale et sur les généralités de la clinique médicale.* Paris: Rouvier et Bouvier.

―――. 1860. "Discours sur le vitalisme et l'organicisme." *Bulletin de l'Académie Nationale de Médecine* 25:1156–1201.

―――. 1869. *Eloge de Laennec. Discours prononcé à l'occasion de l'érection de sa statue à Quimper.* Paris: Malteste.

Boulet d'Hesdin, J. B. J. [1804.] An XII. "Dubitationes de Hippocratis vita, patria, genealogia, forsan mythologicis, et de quibusdam eius libris multo antiquioribus quam vulgo creditur." Thèse méd. no. 153, Paris.

Boulland, A. 1826. "Considérations pathologiques sur le foie." *Mémoires de la Société Médicale d'Émulation* 9:170–193.

Boulle, Lydie. 1981. "Les aphorismes cliniques de Corvisart recueillis par Laennec." In *RPD*, 65–78.

―――. 1982. "La médicalisation des hôpitaux parisiens dans la première moitié du XIXème siècle." *Hist. Refl.* 9:33–44.

―――. 1984. "Gabriel Andral." In Pecker 1984, 418.

―――. 1986. "Hôpitaux parisiens: malades et maladies à l'heure des Révolutions." 2 vols. in 3. Thèse, Ecole Pratique des Hautes Etudes.

Boulle, Lydie, Mirko D. Grmek, Catherine Lupovici, and Janine Samion-Contet. 1982. *Laennec: catalogue des manuscrits scientifique.* Paris: Masson.

Bourgeois, Pierre. 1981. "Laennec et son temps." *La Semaine des hôpitaux de Paris* 57:2047–2056.

Boussand-Verlingue, C. 1977. "Les aphorismes de Corvisart recueillis par Laennec." Thèse méd. no. 197, Paris.

Bouvier, Jean-Paul. 1980. "La famille Laennec de 1794 à 1803 d'après le fonds Rouxeau." Thèse méd. no. 2547, Nantes.

Bouvier, Véronique. 1981. "La diffusion de l'auscultation parisienne, provinciale, et étrangère à travers les thèses soutenues à Paris sur la pneumonie et la pleurésie de 1820 à 1831." Thèse méd. no. 2704, Nantes.

Bowler, Peter. 1989. *The Mendelian Revolution: The Emergence of Hereditarian Concepts in Modern Science and Society.* London: Athlone Press.

Braunstein, Jean-François. 1986. *Broussais et le matérialisme: médecine et philosophie au XIXe siècle.* Paris: Meridiens Klincksieck.

Bricheteau, Isidore. 1819–1820. "De l'auscultation médiate." *Journal complémentaire* 5:50–61, 6:245–255.

Brockliss, Laurence. 1994. "Consultation by Letter in Early Eighteenth-Century Paris: The Medical Practice of Etienne-François Geoffroy." In La Berge and Feingold 1994, 79–117.

Broglie, Achille-Charles-Léonce-Victor le Duc de. 1887. *Personal Recollections.* 2 vols. Ed. and trans. Raphael Ledos de Beaufort. London: Ward and Downey.

Broussais, Casimir. 1823. "Sur la duodénite chronique." Thèse méd. no. 59, Paris.

———. 1827. "Critique d'un dissertation ayant pour titre 'De l'ontologie considérée comme cause d'erreur en médecine' de M. Vaillant." *Annales de la médecine physiologique* 12:477–507.

Broussais, F. J. V. [1801–1802] An X. "Recherches sur la fièvre hectique sans désorganisation des viscères." Thèse méd., Paris.

———. 1808. *Histoires des phlegmasies ou inflammations chroniques.* 2 vols. Paris.

———. 1821. *Examen des doctrines médicales et des systèmes de nosologie.* 2d ed. 2 vols. Paris: Méquignon-Marvis.

———. 1828. *De l'irritation et de la folie.* Brussels: Dr. K. Comet.

———. 1829–1834. *Examen des doctrines médicales.* 3d ed. 4 vols. Paris: Delaunay, Librairie médicale française.

———. 1839. *De l'irritation et de la folie.* 2d ed. 2 vols. Paris: Baillière.

Brown, Edward M. 1994. "French Psychiatry's Initial Reception of Bayle's Discovery of General Paresis of the Insane." *Bull. Hist. Med.* 68:235–253.

Brown, Theodore M. 1974. "From Mechanism to Vitalism in Eighteenth-Century English Physiology." *J. Hist. Biol.* 7:179–216.

Brown, W. Miller. 1985. "On Defining 'Disease.'" *J. Med. Phil.* 10:311–328.

Brown(e), John. 1685. "A Remarkable Account of a Liver Appearing Glandulous to the Eye." *Phil. Trans.* 15:1266–1268.

Buikstra, Jane E., ed. 1981. *Prehistoric Tuberculosis in the Americas.* Evanston, Ill.: Northwestern University Archeological Program no. 5.

Buisson, M. F. R. 1802a. "Précis historique sur Marie-François-Xavier Bichat." In M. F. X. Bichat, *Traité d'anatomie descriptive.* 5 vols. Paris: Gabon, vol. 3, vii–xxviii.

———. [1802b] An X. "Essai sur la division la plus naturelle des phénomènes physiologiques considérées chez l'homme." Thèse méd. no. 130, Paris.

———. [1804] Vendémiaire An XIII. "Extrait et réflexions [on the thesis of Laennec]." *J. méd.* 9:72–80.

Burns, Allan. [1809] 1964. *Observations of Some of the Most Frequent and Important Diseases of the Heart.* Facsimile of the 1809 Edinburgh ed. under auspices of the New York Academy of Medicine. New York: Hafner.

Burwick, Frederick, and Paul Douglas, eds. 1992. *The Crisis in Modernism: Bergson and the Vitalist Controversy.* Cambridge: Cambridge University Press.

Busquet, Paul, ed. 1929. *Aphorismes de Corvisart recueillis par F-V Mérat.* Paris: Masson.

Bynum, W. F. 1981. "Cullen and the Study of Fevers in Britain." In W. F. Bynum and V. Nutton, eds. *Theories of Fever from Antiquity to the Enlightenment. Med. Hist.* suppl. no. 1. London: Wellcome Institute, 135–147.

————. 1994. *Science and the Practice of Medicine in the Nineteenth Century*. Cambridge: Cambridge University Press.

Bynum, W. F., and Roy Porter, eds. 1993. *Medicine and the Five Senses*. Cambridge: Cambridge University Press.

Bynum, W. F., C. Lawrence, and V. Nutton, eds. 1985. *The Emergence of Modern Cardiology. Med. Hist.* suppl. no. 5. London: Wellcome Institute of the History of Medicine.

Cabanis, P. J. G. [1798] 1956. "Du degré de certitude de la médecine." In Claude Lehec and Jean Cazeneuve, eds., *Oeuvres philosophiques*. 2 vols., Paris: Presses Universitaires de France, *1*:33–104.

Canguilhem, Georges. [1965] 1980. *La Connaissance de la Vie*. 2d ed. Paris: Vrin.

————. 1988. *Ideology and Rationality in the History of the Life Sciences*. Trans. Arthur Goldhammer. Cambridge, Mass.: MIT Press.

————. 1989. *The Normal and the Pathological*. Trans. Carolyn R. Fawcett and Robert S. Cohen. New York: Zone Books.

Cannon, Richard O. 1995. "The Sensitive Heart: A Syndrome of Abnormal Cardiac Pain." *J.A.M.A. 273*:883–887.

Caplan, Arthur L., H. Tristram Englehardt, Jr., and James McCartney, eds. 1981. *Concepts of Health and Disease: Interdisciplinary Perspectives*. Reading, Mass: Addison-Wesley.

Capuron. 1827. [Review of] "Elie Gintrac, 'Mémoires sur le diagnostic des affections aiguës et chroniques.' " *Annales de la médecine physiologique* 11:423–432.

Carswell, Robert. 1838. *Pathological Anatomy: Illustrations of the Elementary Forms of Disease*. London: Longman.

Carter, K. Codell. 1982. "On the Decline of Bloodletting in Nineteenth-Century Medicine." *Journal of Psychoanalytic Anthropology* 5:219–234.

Cassell, Eric. 1986. "Ideas in Conflict: The Rise and Fall (and Rise and Fall) of New Views of Disease." *Daedalus* 115:19–41.

Caste, L. 1824. *Réfutation de la doctrine médicale de M. le docteur Broussais et nouvelle analyse des phénomènes de la fièvre*. Paris: Gabon.

Castelnau, C. 1806. "Considérations sur la nostalgie." Thèse méd. no. 130, Paris.

Chateaubriand, Céleste Buisson de la Vigne la Vicomtesse de. 1929. *Mémoires et lettres de Madame de Chateaubriand*. Ed. Joseph Le Gras, Paris: Jonquières.

Chateaubriand, René de. n.d. *Oeuvres complètes de Chateaubriand*. 12 vols. Ed. C. A. Sainte-Beuve. Paris: Garnier.

Chauffard, P. E. 1865. *Laennec. Conferences historiques de la Faculté de la médecine: leçon faite 3 avril 1865*. Paris: Baillière.

————. 1877. *Andral. La médecine française de 1820 à 1830*. Paris: Baillière.

Chausée, Alain. 1981. "La passion de Théophile." Thèse méd. no. 2745, Nantes.

Chaussinand-Nogaret, Guy. 1977. "Nobles médecins et médecins du cour au XVIIIe siècle." *Annales ESC* 32:851–857.

Chauvois, M. L. 1968. "Traduction serée de la préface latine au *Traité de l'auscultation médiate* (t. I 1819) de R. T. H. Laennec, médecin de l'Hôpital Necker." *Phlébologie* 21:7–10.

Chevalier, Alfred. 1933. "L'esprit d'observation de Laennec dans son cours de 1824–1825 au Collège de France." Thèse méd. no. 60, Université de Paris.

Chinard, Gilbert. 1939. "Laennec and Chateaubriand." *Bull. Hist. Med.* 7:95–96.

Chomel, A. F. 1816. "G. L. Bayle." *J. méd.* 37:179.

———. 1821a. "Asthme." In Béclard, Chomel and Cloquet, eds., *Nouveau dictionnaire de médecine, chirurgie, pharmacie, physique, chimie et histoire naturelle.* 2 vols. (1821–1822). Paris: Méquignon-Marvis Crochard Gabon, *1*: 205–207.

———. 1821b. *Des fièvres et des maladies pestilentielles.* Paris: Cochard.

Cilleuls, Jean des. 1956. "Une consultation donnée par Laennec en 1805." *Hist. de la méd.* 6:15–18.

Clark, James. 1820. *Medical Notes on Climate, Disease, Hospitals, and Medical Schools, in France, Italy, and Switzerland.* London: T. & G. Underwood.

Clark, Jon, Celia Modgil, and Sohan Modgil, eds. 1990. *Robert K. Merton. Controversy and Consensus.* London: Falmer Press.

Cloquet, Jules. 1819. "De l'influence des efforts sur les organes renfermés dans la cavité thoracique." *Nouv. j. méd.* 6:307–373.

Coleman, William. 1964. *Georges Cuvier, Zoologist: A Study in the History of Evolution Theory.* Cambridge, Mass.: Harvard University Press.

———. 1977. *Biology in the Nineteenth Century.* London: Cambridge University Press.

Coleman, William, and Frederic L. Holmes, eds. 1988. *The Investigative Enterprise: Experimental Physiology in Nineteenth-Century Medicine.* Berkeley and Los Angeles: University of California Press.

Collin, Victor. 1823. "Des diverses méthodes de l'exploration de la poitrine." Thèse méd. no. 172, Paris.

———. 1824. *Des diverses méthodes de l'exploration de la poitrine.* Paris: Baillière.

Comiti, V. P. 1981. "Incidence et prévalence de la pathologie pulmonaire au temps de Laennec." In *RPD*, 124–129.

Comte, Auguste. [1828] 1911. "Examination of Broussais' Treatise on Irritation." In Frederick Harrison, ed. *Early Essays on Social Philosophy.* Trans. Henry Dix Hutton. London: Routledge, 333–352.

Condillac, Etienne Bonnot de. [1780] 1980. *La logique.* Trans. W. R. Albury. New York: Abaris.

Convor, J. H. 1978. "The Cause of Tuberculosis." *American Review of Respiratory Diseases* 117:137–143.

Corbie, Arnauld de. 1950. *La vie ardente de Laennec.* Paris: Editions Spes.

Corlay, Janig. 1981. *Laennec face à l'Ankou.* St. Malo: N.C.A. Edition.

Corlieu, Auguste. 1896. *Centenaire de la Faculté de Médecine de Paris, 1794–1894.* Paris: Imprimerie Nationale.

Corrigan, D. [1832] 1945. "On Permanent Patency of the Mouth of the Aorta." In Ralph H. Major, ed. *Classic Descriptions of Disease.* Springfield, Ill.: Charles C. Thomas, 354–357.

Corvisart, J.N. [1806] 1962. *An Essay on the Organic Diseases and Lesions of the Heart and Great Vessels.* Ed. C. E. Horeau and trans. Jacob Gates. Facsimile of the 1812 Boston edition under the auspices of the New York Academy of Medicine. New York: Hafner.

Corvisart, J. N. 1808. "Préface du traducteur." In Auenbrugger 1808, vii–xviii.

Cournand, André. 1975. "Cardiac Catheterization —Development of the Technique, Its Contributions to Experimental Medicine, and Its Initial Applications in Man." *Acta Medica Scandinavia Suppl.* 579:1–32.

Cournot, A. A. 1923. *Matérialisme, vitalisme, rationalisme: études des données de la science en philosophie*. Paris: Hachette.

Coury, Charles. 1970. "The Teaching of Medicine in France from the Beginning of the Seventeenth Century." In O'Malley 1970, 121–172.

Coury, Charles. 1972. *Grandeur et déclin d'une maladie: la tuberculose au cours des âges*. Suresnes: Lepetit.

Cranefield, Paul. 1974. *The Way In and the Way Out*. Mount Kisco, N.Y.: Futura.

Crochet, Guy. 1982. "La correspondance de René Théophile Laennec de 1803 à 1808 d'après le Fonds Rouxeau." Thèse méd. no. 2894, Nantes.

Cronin, Vincent. 1966. *The Romantic Way*. Boston: Houghton Mifflin.

Crosland, Maurice. 1992. *Science under Control: The French Academy of Sciences, 1795–1914*. Cambridge: Cambridge University Press.

Cross, Stephen. 1981. "John Hunter, the Animal Oeconomy and Late Eighteenth-Century Physiology Discourse." *Studies in the History of Biology* 5:1–110.

Cruveilhier, Jean. 1816. "Essai sur l'anatomie pathologique." Thèse méd. no. 18, Paris.

———. 1829–1842. *Anatomie pathologique du corps humain*, 2 vols. Paris: Baillière.

Cullen, William. [1765] 1785. *Synopsis nosologicae methodicae*, 4th ed. Edinburgh: Creech.

Cummins, S. Lyle. 1949. *Tuberculosis in History*. London: Baillière, Tindall, and Cox.

Cunningham, Andrew. 1988. "Getting the Game Right: Some Plain Words on the Identity and Invention of Science." *Stud. Hist. Phil. Sci.* 19:365–389.

Cunningham, Andrew, and Roger French, eds. 1990. *The Medical Enlightenment of the Eighteenth Century*. Cambridge: Cambridge University Press.

Dalbant, Eloi. 1819. "Quelques observations pour servir à l'histoire de l'artérite ou l'inflammation des artères." Thèse méd. no. 202, Paris.

Daremberg, Charles. 1855. *Oeuvres choisies d'Hippocrate*. 2d ed. Paris: Labé.

Dausset, Jean. 1981. "Laennec au Collège de France." In *RPD*, 22–30.

Davis, Audrey B. 1981. *Medicine and its Technology. An Introduction to the History of Medical Instrumentation*. Westport, Conn.: Greenwood.

Dédéyan, Charles. 1981. "Laennec et les écrivains de son temps." In *RPD*, 245–259.

DeGowin, Richard L. 1986. *Degowin and Degowin's Bedside Diagnostic Examination*, 5th ed. New York: Macmillan.

Delassus, Agile. 1902. *Laennec, médecine et religion*. Extrait de la *Revue de Lille*. Paris: Sueur-Charruey.

Delaunay, Paul. 1932. *Les Médecins, la Restauration, et la Révolution de 1830*. Extrait de *La Médecine Internationale Illustrée*. Paris: Imprimerie Tourangelle.

———. 1949. *D'une révolution à l'autre, 1789–1848. L'évolution des théories et de la pratique médicales*. Paris: Editions Hippocrate.

De Lens, A. J. 1821. "Stéthoscope." In *DSM* 52:586–590.

Deleuze, J. P. F. 1816. *Biographie de G. L. Bayle*. Paris: Belin.

Delp, Mahlon H., and Robert T. Manning. 1975. *Major's Physical Diagnosis: An Introduction to the Clinical Process*. 8th ed. Philadelphia: W. B. Saunders; 9th ed., 1981.

Desgenettes, M. le Baron. 1822. *Eloge de M. Hallé*. Paris: Didot.

Desportes, E. H. 1811. *Traité de l'angine de poitrine*. Paris: Méquignon.

Double, François. 1811–1822. *Séméiologie générale ou traité des signes*. 3 vols. Paris: Croulebois.

Dowbiggin, Ian. 1991. *Inheriting Madness: Professionalization and Psychiatric Knowledge in Nineteenth-Century France.* Berkeley and Los Angeles: University of California Press.

Driesch, H. 1914. *The Problem of Individuality.* London: Macmillan.

Du Chatellier, Armand René Maufra. 1885. *Les Laennec sous l'ancien et le nouveau régime de 1763 à 1836.* Vannes: Imprimerie Galles.

Dubos, René, and Jean Dubos. 1952. *The White Plague, Tuberculosis, Man and Society.* 1st ed. Boston: Little, Brown, 2d ed., 1953.

Dubovsky, H. 1975. "An Historical Basis for Modern Concepts of the Pathogenesis of Tuberculosis." *South African Medical Journal* 49:1105–1110.

Duchesneau, François. 1982. *La physiologie des lumières: empirisme, modèles, et théories.* The Hague: Martinus Nijhoff.

———. 1985. "Vitalism in Late Eighteenth-Century Physiology: The Cases of Barthez, Blumenbach, and John Hunter." In W.F. Bynum and Roy Porter, eds. *William Hunter and the Eighteenth-Century Medical World.* Cambridge: Cambridge University Press, 259–295.

Duclos, Henri. 1932. *Laennec.* Paris: Flammarion.

Duffin, Jacalyn. 1987. "Why Does Cirrhosis Belong to Laennec?" *Can. Med. Assoc. J.* 137:393–396.

———. 1989. "The Cardiology of R. T. H. Laennec." *Med. Hist.* 33:42–71.

———. 1991. "Puerile Respiration: Laennec's Stethoscope and the Physiology of Breathing." *Transactions and Studies of the College of Physicians of Philadelphia Ser. 5* 13:125–145.

Duffin, Jacalyn, and Pierre René. 1991. " 'Anti-moine, Anti-biotique': the Public Fortunes of the Secret Properties of Antimony Potassium Tartrate (Tartar Emetic)." *J. Hist. Med. All. Sci.* 46:440–456.

Dufour, Léon. 1888. *A travers un siècle, 1780–1865: science et histoire: souvenirs d'un savant français.* Paris: J. Rothschild.

Dunglison, Robley. 1874. *Medical Lexicon: a Dictionary of Medical Science.* Philadelphia: Lea.

Dupuy, R. 1989. "Cadoudal." In Jean-René Suratteau and François Gendron, eds. 1989. *Dictionnaire historique de la Révolution française.* Paris: Presses Universitaires de France, 172–174.

Dupuytren, G. [1804] An XIII. "Anatomie pathologique." *BEMS* 2:13–24.

———. [1805a] An XIII. "Observation sur la note relative aux altérations organiques publiée par M. Laennec." *J. méd.* 9:441–446.

———. [1805b] An XIII. "Nouvelles observations de M. Dupuytren sur la note de M. Laennec." *J. méd.* 10:96–102.

East, Terence. 1958. *The Story of Heart Disease.* London: Wm. Dawson.

Edwards, Ward. 1954. "The Theory of Decision Making." *Psychol. Bull.* 51:380–417.

Eisenstein, Hester. 1968. "Victor Cousin and the War on the University of France." Ph.D. diss., Yale University, New Haven, Conn.

Engel, George L. 1960. "A Unified Concept of Health and Disease." *Persp. Biol. Med.* 3:459–485.

Erasmus, W. J. 1839. "Liver." In R. B. Todd, ed. *Cyclopaedia of Anatomy and Physiology.* London: Longman, 3:188–189.

Esnault, G. 1919. "Laennec bretonnant." *Bull. Soc. Arch. Finistère* 98–132.

Farge, Arlette. 1980. "Work-Related Diseases of Artisans in Eighteenth-Century France." In Robert Forster and Orest Ranum, eds., *Medicine and Society in France,*

Selections from the Annales, Economies, Sociétiés, Civilisations. Trans. Elborg Forster and Patricia M. Ranum, Baltimore: Johns Hopkins University Press, 89–103.

Farley, John, and Gerald Geison. 1974. "Science, Politics, and Spontaneous Generation in Nineteenth-Century France." *Bull. Hist. Med.* 48:161–198.

Ferrus, G. 1824. "Foie." In Adelon et al. 1821–1828, 9:201–214.

——. "Foie." In Adelon et al., eds. *Dictionnaire de médecine.* 30 vols. (1832–46), Paris: Béchet, 13:210–213.

Finot, A. 1960. "Laennec helléniste." In *XVIIe Congrès International d'Histoire de la Médecine, Athènes.* 1:176–181.

——. 1966. "R. T. H. Laennec—R. Finot: Deux erreurs d'identification dans les collections de la Faculté de Médecine." *L'hôpital et l'aide sociale à Paris* 42:735–740.

——. 1972. "François-Joseph Double, inventeur de l'auscultation en 1817." *Hist. sci. méd.* 6:14–21.

Fizeau, Louis-Aimé. [1803–1804] An XI. "Recherches et observations pour servir à l'histoire des fièvres intérmittentes." Thèse méd., Paris.

——. [1804] An XI. "Recherches et observations pour servir à l'histoire des fièvres intérmittentes [extraits]." *J. méd.* 6:184–188, 437–442.

Fleck, Ludwik. 1979. *Genesis and Development of a Scientific Fact.* Trans. Fred Bradley and Thaddeus J. Trenn. Chicago: University of Chicago Press.

——. 1986. "To Look, To See, To Know." In Robert S. Cohen and Thomas Schnelle, eds., *Cognition and Fact: Materials on Ludwik Fleck.* Dordrecht: D. Reidel, 129–151.

Fleury, Le Comte Maurice. 1901. *Un Grand Terroriste: Carrier à Nantes.* 2d ed. Paris: Plon.

Flint, Austin. 1856. *Physical Exploration and Diagnosis of Diseases Affecting the Respiratory Organs.* Philadelphia: Blanchard and Lea.

——. 1859. *The Life and Labor of Laennec: An Introductory Address, New Orleans School of Medicine, 14 November 1859.* New Orleans: Bulletin, Book and Job Office.

Floyer, John. [1698] 1785. *Traité de l'asthme.* Trans. Jault. Paris: Servière.

Forbes, John. 1821. "Notes." In Laennec 1821, 417–432.

——. 1824. *Original Cases with Dissections and Observations Illustrating the Use of the Stethoscope and Percussion in the Diagnosis of Diseases of the Chest.* London: Underwood.

——. 1827. "Translator's Preface." In Laennec 1827.

——. 1834. "Life of the Author." In Laennec 1834, xvii–xxix.

Forestier, membre du ci-devant Collège et Académie Royale de Chirurgie. n.d. ca. 1822. *Lettre à M. Lejumeau de Kergaradec.* Paris: Chaigneau-Jeune.

Fosseyeux, Marcel. 1930. *Paris médical en 1830.* Paris: Librarie Le François.

Fothergill, John. [1776] 1945. "Farther Account of the Angina Pectoris." In Ralph Major, ed. *Classic Descriptions of Disease.* Springfield, Ill.: Charles C. Thomas, 422–423.

Foucault, Michel. 1963. *Naissance de la clinique.* Paris: Presses Universitaires de France.

Fourcroy, A. F. de. 1785. *L'art de connoître et d'employer les médicamens.* 2 vols. Paris: Serpente.

——. 1786. *Elemens d'histoire naturelle et de chimie.* 2d ed. 4 vols. Paris: Cuchet.

――――. [1800–1801] An IX–X. *Système de connaissances chimiques*, 10 vols. Paris: Baudoin.

Frank, Robert G. 1988. "The Telltale Heart: Physiological Instruments, Graphic Method, and Clinical Hopes, 1854–1914." In Coleman and Holmes 1988, 211–290.

French, Roger. 1994. *William Harvey's Natural Philosophy.* Cambridge: Cambridge University Press.

Freyhofer, H. H. 1982. *The Vitalism of Hans Driesch.* Frankfurt: P. Lang.

Froment, M. 1829. *La police dévoilée depuis la Restauration et notamment sous messieurs Franchet et Delavau.* 3 vols. Paris: Lemonnier.

Furet, François. 1988. *La Révolution de Turgot à Jules Ferry.* Paris: Hachette.

Fye, W. Bruce. 1985. "The Delayed Recognition of Myocardial Infarction: It Took Half a Century." *Circulation* 72:262–271.

――――. 1987. *The Development of American Physiology: Scientific Medicine in the Nineteenth Century.* Baltimore: Johns Hopkins University Press.

Gabbay, John. 1982. "Asthma Attacked? Tactics for the Reconstruction of a Disease Concept." In Peter Wright and Andrew Treacher, eds. *The Problem of Medical Knowledge: Examining the Social Construction of Medicine.* Edinburgh: Edinburgh University Press, 23–48.

Galen, Robert S., and S. Raymond Gambino. 1975. *Beyond Normality: the Predictive Value and Efficiency of Medical Diagnosis.* New York: John Wiley & Sons.

Ganière, Paul. [1951] 1981. *Corvisart: médecin de l'Empereur.* Paris: Librairie Académique Perrin.

García Guerra, Delfín. 1990. "La lesión vital en el pensamiento nosologico de G. L. Bayle." *Asclepio* 42:237–251.

Garnot, Nicolas Sainte Fare, ed. 1989. *La Révolution française et les hôpitaux parisiens. Catalogue de l'exposition.* Paris: Musée de l'Assistance Publique.

Gaultier de Claubry [signed "EGC"], C. E. S. 1826. "*Traité de l'auscultation médiate* [review]." *J. gén. méd. XCVII [or vol. XXXVI 2d series]*:407–420.

Geiger, Reed G. 1994. *Planning the French Canals: Bureaucracy, Politics, and Enterprise under the Restoration.* Newark, N.J.: University of Delaware Press; London: Associated University Presses.

Geison, Gerald L. 1978. *Michael Foster and the Cambridge School of Physiology: The Scientific Enterprise in Late Victorian Society.* Princeton, N.J.: Princeton University Press.

――――. 1979. "Divided We Stand: Physiologists and Clinicians in the American Context." In Morris Vogel and Charles E. Rosenberg, eds. *The Therapeutic Revolution: Essays in the Social History of American Medicine.* Philadelphia: University of Pennsylvania Press, 67–90.

――――, ed. 1987a. *Physiology in the American Context, 1850–1940.* Bethesda, Md.: American Physiological Society.

――――. 1987b. "Toward a History of American Physiology." In Geison 1987a, 1–10.

――――. 1995. *The Private Science of Louis Pasteur.* Princeton, N.J.: Princeton University Press.

Gelfand, Toby. 1977. "A Clinical Ideal: Paris 1789." *Bull. Hist. Med. 51*: 397–411.

――――. 1980. *Professionalizing Modern Medicine: Paris Surgeons and Medical Science and Institutions in the 18th Century.* Westport, Conn.: Greenwood.

Gélineau. 1902. "Un portrait inconnu de Laennec et son premier stéthoscope." *Chronique médicale* 9:420–421.

Gentil, Maurice. 1958. "Laennec médecin de Chateaubriand" and "Laennec à l'Académie de Médecine." *Histoire de la médecine* 8:47–47, 58–63.

Genty, Maurice. 1926. "Les éditions du *Traité de l'auscultation.*" *Progrès médical no. 51 (11 Dec.)*:1968–1970.

———. 1935. "Le cerveau de Dupuytren." *Progrès médical Suppl.* 2:16.

Gerhart, Mary, and Allan Russell. 1984. *Metaphoric Process: The Creation of Scientific and Religious Understanding.* Fort Worth: Texas Christian University Press.

Gibson, Ralph. 1989. *A Social History of French Catholicism.* London: Routledge.

Godechot, Jacques. 1977. *La vie quotidienne en France sous le Directoire.* Paris: Hachette.

Goldstein, Jan. 1987. *Console and Classify. The French Psychiatric Profession in the Nineteenth Century.* Cambridge: Cambridge University Press.

———. 1994. "Foucault and the Post-Revolutionary Self: The Uses of Cousinian Pedagogy in Ninteteenth-Century France." In Jan Goldstein, ed. *Foucault and the Writing of History.* Oxford and Cambridge: Blackwell, 99–115.

Goodfield, G. J. 1960. *The Growth of Scientific Physiology.* London: Hutchinson.

Goodfield-Toulmin, June. 1969. "Some Aspects of English Physiology: 1780–1840." *J. Hist. Biol.* 2:283–320.

Goubert, J. P. 1974. *Malades et médecins en Bretagne, 1770–1790.* Rennes: C. Klincksieck.

Gould, S. J. 1985. *The Flamingo's Smile: Reflections in Natural History.* New York, London: W. W. Norton.

Grandmaison, Charles Alexandre Geoffroy de. 1889. *La Congrégation, 1801–1830.* Paris: Plon.

Granville, A. Bozzi. 1854. *Sudden Death.* London: Churchill.

Grellet, I., and C. Kruse. 1983. *Histoires de la tuberculose: les fièvres de l'âme, 1800–1940.* Paris: Editions Ramsay.

Grmek, Mirko D. 1975. "La réalité nosologique au temps d'Hippocrate." In L. Bourgey and J. Jouanna, eds. *La collection Hippocratique et son rôle dans l'histoire de la médecine. Colloque de Strasbourg, 1972.* Leiden: Brill, 237–255.

———. 1976. "Le rôle du hasard dans le genèse des découvertes scientifiques." *Medicina nei secolo* 13:277–305.

———. 1981a. "L'invention de l'auscultation médiate, retouches à un cliché historique." In *RPD*, 107–116.

———. 1981b. "A Plea for Freeing the History of Scientific Discoveries from Myth." In M.D. Grmek, Robert S. Cohen and Guido Cimino, eds., *On Scientific Discovery. The Erice Lectures.* Trans. Margaret Roussel, Dordrecht: Reidel, 9–42.

———. 1982. "Introduction." In Boulle et al. 1982, 1–8.

———. 1988a. *Diseases in the Ancient Greek World.* Trans. Mireille Muellner and Leonard Muellner. Baltimore: Johns Hopkins University Press.

———. 1988b. "Médecine et épistémologie: transformation du savoir sur la santé et la maladie." *Hist. Phil. Life Sci.* 10 suppl.:3–6.

———. 1990. *History of AIDS.* Trans. Russell C. Maulitz and Jacalyn Duffin. Princeton, N.J.: Princeton University Press.

———. 1991a. "Claude Bernard: entre le matérialisme et le vitalisme: la nécessité et la liberté dans les phénomènes de la vie." In J. Michel, ed. *La Nécessité de Claude Bernard. Actes du Colloque de Saint-Julien-en-Beaujolais, 1989.* Paris: Meridens Klincksieck, 117–139.

———. 1991b. *Claude Bernard et la méthode expérimentale.* Paris: Payot.

Grmek, Mirko D., and A. Rousseau. 1966. "L'oeuvre cardiologique de Léon Rostan." *Rev. d'hist. sci.* *19*:33–52.

Guersent, L. B. 1821. "Asthme." In Adelon et al. 1821–1828, *3*:126.

Hacking, Ian. 1975. *The Emergence of Probability.* London: Cambridge University Press.

———. 1981. "Do We See Through a Microscope?" *Pacific Philosophical Quarterly* *62*:305–322.

Hagstrom, Warren O. 1965. *The Scientific Community.* New York: Basic Books.

Haigh, Elizabeth. 1975. "The Roots of the Vitalism of Xavier Bichat." *Bull. Hist. Med.* *49*:72–86.

Haigh, Elizabeth. 1977. "The vital principle of Paul Josepth Barthez: the clash between monism and dualism." *Med. Hist.* *21*:1–14.

———. 1984. *Xavier Bichat and the Medical Theory of the Eighteenth Century. Med. Hist.* suppl. no. 4. London: Wellcome Institute of the History of Medicine.

Haldane, J. S. 1932. *Materialism.* London: Hodder and Stoughton.

Hall, Thomas S. 1969. *Ideas of Life and Matter: Studies in the History of General Physiology, 600 B.C.–1900 A.D.,* 2 vols. Chicago: University of Chicago Press.

Haller, Albrecht von. [1786] 1966. *First Lines of Physiology.* Trans. William Cullen. New York: Johnson Reprint.

Haller, John S. 1975. "The Use and Abuse of Tartar Emetic in the 19th-Century Materia Medica." *Bull. Hist. Med.* *49*:235–257.

———. 1986. "The Great Biologic Problem: Vitalism, Materialism, and the Philosophy of Organism." *New York State Journal of Medicine* *86*:81–88.

Hannin, Valérie. 1984. "Une expérience médicale au temps du rationalisme expérimental: L'Hospice de Charité." *Revue d'histoire moderne et contemporaine* *31*:116–130.

Hanot, V. 1875. "Etude sur une forme de cirrhose." Thèse méd. no. 465, Paris.

Harley, David. 1990. "Honour and Property: The Structure of Professional Disputes in Eighteenth-Century English Medicine." In Cunningham and French 1990, 138–164.

Harvey, William. [1628] 1957. *De motu cordis.* Trans. Kenneth J. Franklin. Springfield, Ill.: Charles C. Thomas.

Heberden, William. [1802] 1962. *Commentaries on the History and Cure of Diseases.* Trans. Wm. Heberden the younger. Facsimile of the 1802 London ed. New York: Library of the New York Academy of Medicine and Hafner.

Hein, Hilde. 1972. "The Endurance of the Mechanism-Vitalism Controversy." *J. Hist. Biol.* *5*:159–188.

Henry, Louis. 1967. *Manuel de démographie historique.* Paris and Geneva: Droz.

———. 1980. *Techniques d'analyse en démographie historique.* Paris: Institut National d'Etudes Démographiques.

Herold, Jean Christopher. 1958. *Mistress to an Age. A Life of Madame de Staël.* Indianapolis: Bobbs Merrill.

Herrick, James B. 1941. "Certain Textbooks on Heart Disease of the Early Nineteenth Century." *Bull. Hist. Med.* *10*:136–147.

———. 1942. *A Short History of Cardiology.* Springfield, Mass.: Charles C. Thomas.

Hirsch, August. 1883–1886. *Handbook of Geographical and Historical Pathology.* 3 vols. Trans. Charles Creighton. London: New Sydenham Society.

Hollman, Arthur. 1995. "The Paintings of Pathological Anatomy by Sir Robert Carswell." *British Heart J.* *74*:566–570.

Holmes, Frederic Lawrence. 1985. *Lavoisier and the Chemistry of Life: an Exploration of Scientific Creativity.* Madison: University of Wisconsin Press.

Holmes, Oliver W. [1849] 1896. "The Stethoscope Song. A Professional Ballad." In *The Poetical Works of Oliver Wendell Holmes.* London: Routledge, 64–66.

Hope, James. [1831] 1842. *Treatise of Diseases of the Heart and the Great Vessels,* 1st American ed. based on 3d London ed. Philadelphia: Lea and Blanchard.

Horrobin, David F. 1978. *Medical Hubris: A Reply to Ivan Illich.* Sherbrooke, Que.: Eden Press.

Howell, Joel D. 1985. " 'Soldier's Heart': the Redefinition of Heart Disease and Specialty Formation in Early Twentieth-Century Britain." In Bynum et al. 1985, 34–52.

Huard, Pierre. 1981a. "L'auscultation cardio-pulmonaire depuis Laennec." *RPD,* 170–175.

———. 1981b. "Les facettes multiples de René Théophile Hyacinthe Laennec (1781–1826)." *Bulletin de l'Académie Nationale de Médecine* 165:249–254.

Huard, Pierre, and Mirko D. Grmek. 1970. *Sciences, médecine et pharmacie de la Révolution à l'Empire.* Paris: Les Editions Roger Dacosta.

———. 1973. "Les élèves étrangers de Laennec." *Rev. d'hist. sci.* 26:315–337.

Huard, Pierre and Marie-José Imbault-Huart. 1978. "La formation et l'oeuvre scientifique de Dupuytren (1777–1835)." *Hist. sci. méd.* 12:217–231.

———. 1982. "Gabriel Andral, 1797–1876." *Rev. d'hist. sci.* 35:131–153.

Huard, Pierre, and Jean Théodoridès. 1959. "Cinq parasitologistes méconnus: Laennec parasitologiste." *Biologie Médicale 48 (no. spéc. April 1959)*:i–xci.

———. 1981. "Laennec et la parasitologie (nouveaux documents)." In *RPD,* 176–188.

Hudson, Nora E. 1936. *Ultra-Royalism and the French Restoration.* Cambridge: Cambridge University Press.

Hudson, Robert P. 1983. *Disease and Its Control: the Shaping of Modern Thought.* Westport, Conn.: Greenwood.

Hudson, Robert P. 1993. "Concepts of Disease in the West." In Kiple 1993, 45–52.

Hunter, Kathryn Montgomery. 1991. *Doctors' Stories: The Narrative Structure of Medical Knowledge.* Princeton, N.J.: Princeton University Press.

Hurst, J. Willis, ed. 1990. *The Heart, Arteries, and Veins.* 7th ed. New York: McGraw-Hill.

Hutt, Maurice. 1983. *Chouannerie and the Counter-Revolution: Puissaye, the Princes, and the British Government in the 1790s,* 2 vols. Cambridge: Cambridge University Press.

Huybrechts-Rivière, C. 1980. "Correspondance des Laennec des années 1808 à 1815 d'après le Fonds Rouxeau de Nantes." Thèse méd. no. 2463, Nantes.

Illich, Ivan. 1975. *Medical Nemesis: the Expropriation of Health.* London: Calder and Boyars.

Imbault-Huart, Marie-José. 1973. "L'école pratique de dissection de Paris de 1750 à 1822, ou l'influence du concept de médecine pratique et chirurgicale au XVIIIème siècle et au début du XIXème siècle." Thèse Doctorat ès Lettres, Paris.

Imhof, Arthur E. 1987. "Methodological Problems in Modern Urban History Writing: Graphic Representations of Urban Mortality 1750–1850." In Roy Porter and Andrew Wear, eds. *Problems and Methods in the History of Medicine.* London: Croom Helm, 101–132.

Inglefinger, F. J. 1980. "Arrogance." *N. Engl. J. Med.* 303:1507–1511.

Jacobson, Arthur C. [1926] 1970. *Genius: Some Reevaluations.* New York: Kennikat Press.

Jacyna, L. S. 1987. "Medical Science and Moral Science: The Cultural Relations of Physiology in Restoration France." *History of Science 25*:111–146.

———. 1989. "*Au lit des malades*: A. F. Chomel's Clinic at the Charité, 1828–9." *Med. Hist. 33*:420–449.

———. 1991. "Robert Carswell and William Thomson at the Hôtel-Dieu of Lyons: Scottish Views on French Medicine." In Roger French and Andrew Wear, eds. *British Medicine in an Age of Reform.* London: Routledge, 110–135.

Jarcho, Saul. 1948. "Giovanni Battista Morgagni: His Interests, Ideas, and Achievement." *Bull. Hist. Med. 22*:503–524.

———. 1960. "Historical Milestones: Obstruction of the Thoracic Duct by Aortic Aneurysm." *Am. J. Cardiology 5*:537–539.

———. 1962a. "Historical Milestones: An Early Review of Laennec's Treatise." *Am. J. Cardiology 9*:962–969.

———. 1962b. "Historical Milestones: A Review of John Forbes' Translation of Laennec." *Am. J. Cardiology 10*:859–863.

———. 1980. *The Concept of Heart Failure from Avicenna to Albertini.* Cambridge, Mass.: Harvard University Press.

———, ed. and trans. 1984. *The Clinical Consultations of Giambattista Morgagni. The Edition of Enrico Benassi (1935).* Boston: Francis A. Countaway Library of Medicine and University of Virginia Press.

Jewson, N. D. 1974. "Medical Knowledge and the Patronage System in 18th-Century England." *Sociology 8*:369–385.

———. 1976. "The Disappearance of the Sick Man from Medical Cosmology." *Sociology 10*:225–244.

Joad, C. E. M. 1923. *The Future of Life: A Theory of Vitalism.* London: Putnam.

Johnston, William. [1917] 1968. "Roll of the Commissioned Officers in the Medical Service of the British Army, 1727–1898." In Robert Drew, ed. *Commissioned Officers in the Medical Services of the British Army (1660–1960).* Vol. 1. London: Wellcome Historical Medical Library.

Jones, W. H. S., ed. and trans. 1923. *Hippocrates.* Loeb Classical Library. Vol. 1. London: Heinemann.

Jurine, L. 1815. *Mémoire sur l'angine de poitrine.* Paris and Geneva: Paschoud.

Karenberg, Axel. 1994. "Students at the Bedside in German Universities, 1770–1830." *Caduceus 10*:87–100.

Katz, Arnold M., and Phyllis B. Katz. 1962. "Diseases of the Heart in the Works of Hippocrates." *British Heart J. 24*:257–264.

Kawakita, Yosio, Shizu Sakai, and Yasuo Otsuka, eds. 1995. *History of the Doctor-Patient Relationship. Tanaguchi Foundation 14th International Symposium.* Tokyo and St. Louis: Ishiyaku EuroAmerica.

Keel, Othmar. 1979. *Philippe Pinel, lecteur discret de J. C. Smyth (1741–1821). La généalogie de l'histopathologie: une révision déchirante.* Paris: Vrin.

Keele, Kenneth D. 1963. *The Evolution of Clinical Methods in Medicine Being the Fitzpatrick Lectures Delivered before the Royal College of Physicians, 1960–61.* London: Pitman Medical Publishing.

———. 1973. "The Application of the Physics of Sound to 19th-Century Cardiology with Particular Reference to the Part Played by C. J. B. Williams and James Hope." *Clio Medica 8*:191–221.

Keers, R. Y. 1978. *Pulmonary Tuberculosis: A Journey Down the Centuries*. London: Baillière Tindall.

Kergaradec, J. A. Lejumeau de. 1820–1821. "Extraits de 'De l'auscultation médiate.'" *Nouv. bib. méd.* *68*:289–315, *69*:190–224; *70*:145–70; *71*:321–56; *73*:151–164.

———. 1822. *Mémoire sur l'auscultation appliquée à l'étude de la grossesse*. Paris: Méquignon-Marvis.

———. 1826a. "Notice sur le Professeur Laennec." *Nouv. bib. méd.* *3*:316–325.

———. 1826b. *Notice sur le Professeur Laennec*. Paris: Gueffier.

———. 1868. "Discours de Laennec sur l'inauguration de la statue à Quimper le 15 août 1868." *Bulletin de l'Académie Impériale de Médecine 33*:807–816.

Kernéis, Jean-Pierre. 1981a. "Les échelons de la gloire." In *Laennec inventeur de l'auscultation. Catalogue 1981*, 14–38.

———. 1981b. "Postface pour des documents inédits." In *RPD*, 329–343.

Kerviler, René, ed. [1899] 1978. *Répertoire général de bio-bibliographie bretonne*. Reprinted ed. Mayenne: Joseph Floc'h.

Kervran, Roger. 1960. *Laennec: His Life and Times*. Trans. from 1955 French ed. by D. C. Abrahams-Curiel. Oxford: Pergamon Press.

King, Lester S. 1959. "Auscultation in England, 1821–1837." *Bull. Hist. Med.* *33*:446–453.

———. 1966. "Boissier de Sauvages and 18th-Century Nosology." *Bull. Hist. Med.* *40*:43–51.

———. 1976. "Evidence and Its Evaluation in Eighteenth-Century Medicine." *Bull. Hist. Med. 50*:174–190.

———. 1982. *Medical Thinking: A Historical Preface*. Princeton, N.J.: Princeton University Press.

Kiple, Kenneth F., ed. 1993. *The Cambridge World History of Human Disease*. Cambridge: Cambridge University Press.

Kipling, Rudyard. 1910. "The Marklake Witches." In *Rewards and Fairies*. London: Macmillan, 85–114.

Kirkby, Kenneth Clifford. 1992. "Proving the Somaticist Position: J. B. Friedreich on the Nature and Seat of Mental Disease." *History of Psychiatry 3*:237–251.

Kligfield, Paul. 1981. "Laennec and the Discovery of Mediate Auscultation." *Am. J. Med. 70*:275–278.

Knegtel, A. P. C. H. 1966. *Laennec* [in Dutch]. Assen: Van Grocum.

———. 1970. "Extrait du Journal de Van Hall. A propos d'un voyage à Paris en 1822." *Hist. sci. méd. 4*:143–144.

———. 1981. "Le rayonnement de Laennec aux Pays-Bas." In *RPD*, 312–330.

Knorr-Cetina, Karin D. 1981. *The Manufacture of Knowledge. An Essay on the Constructivist and Contextual Nature of Science*. Oxford: Pergamon.

Knorr-Cetina, Karin D., and Michael Mulkay, eds. 1983. *Science Observed. Perspectives on the Social Study of Science*. London: Sage.

Konrat, Michel. 1984. "Le temps des bouleversements: Révolution et Empire." In Fabrice Abbad, ed. *La Loire-Atlantique des origines à nos jours*. Saint-Jean-d'Angley: Editions Bordesoules, 257–299.

Kowal, Samuel J. 1960. "Emotions and Angina Pectoris." *Am. J. Cardiology 5*: 421–427.

Koyré, Alexander. 1973. *Etudes d'histoire de la pensée scientifique*. Paris: Gallimard.

Kraemer, Helena Chmura. 1992. *Evaluating Medical Tests: Objective and Quantitative Guidelines.* Newbury Park, Calif.: Sage.

Kreysig, Friedrich Ludwig. 1814–1817. *Die Krankheiten des Herzens.* 3 vols. Berlin: Mauererschen Buchandlung.

Kuhn, Thomas S. 1962. *The Structure of Scientific Revolutions.* Chicago: University of Chicago Press.

La Berge, Ann F. 1992. *Mission and Method: The Early Nineteenth-Century French Public Health Movement.* Cambridge: Cambridge University Press.

———. 1994. "Medical Microscopy in Paris, 1830–1855." In La Berge and Feingold 1994, 296–326.

La Berge, Ann F., and Mordechai Feingold, eds. 1994. *French Medical Culture in the Nineteenth Century.* Amsterdam: Rodopi *Clio Medica* 25/The Wellcome Institute Series in the History of Medicine.

Labrousse, Elizabeth, and Alfred Soman. 1986. "La querelle de l'antimoine. Guy Patin sur la sellette." *Histoire, économie et société* 5:31–45.

Laennec, Ambroise. 1816. "Considérations générales sur les épidémies." Thèse méd. no. 70, Paris.

———. 1825. "Observation d'hydrophobie traumatique avec pustule sublinguale ou lyssès." *Rev. méd. 1*:257–265.

Laennec: inventeur de l'auscultation, 1781–1826. Catalogue de l'Exposition organisée par la Délégation à l'Action Artistique, la Société Française d'Histoire de la Médecine, l'Académie Nationale de Médecine, et la Délégation aux Célébrations Nationales. 1981. Alençon: Firmin-Didot.

Laennec, Mériadec. 1821. "L'auscultation médiate: peut-elle servir aux progrès de la médecine pratique?" Thèse méd. no. 92, Paris.

———. 1824a. "Observations de la clinique de M. le Professeur Laennec, recueillies à l'Hôpital de la Charité par M. Laennec, chef de clinique." *Rev. méd. 1*:379–392.

———. 1824b. "Tableau des maladies observées à la Charité dans les salles de Clinique de M. le Professeur Laennec." *Rev. méd. 2*:161–184.

———. 1825a. "Tableau des maladies observées à la Charité dans les salles de Clinique de M. le Professeur Laennec." *Rev. méd. 2*:337–364.

———. 1825b. "Tableau des maladies observées à la Charité dans les salles de Clinique de M. le Professeur Laennec." *Rev. méd. 4*:365–393.

———. 1832. *A Manual of Percussion and Auscultation.* Trans. James Birch Sharpe. New York: S. Wood and Sons.

Laennec, Théophile-Marie. [1804] 30 Floréal An XII. *L'Hommage d'un père de famille, ou mes votes pour Napoléon Bonaparte, consul, empereur, monarque héréditaire.* Brest: Binard.

Laignel-Lavastine, M. 1914. "Une ordonnance de Laennec." *Bulletin de la Société Française d'Histoire de la Médecine 13*:17–21.

Lallour, Emmanuel. 1892. *Laennec: notice historique.* 2d ed. Ed. Dr. Guermonprez. Lille: Brouwer.

Lamennais, Félicité de. 1829. *Essai sur l'indifférence en matière de religion.* 8th ed. 2 vols. Paris: Belin-Mandar et Devaux.

———. 1971. *Correspondance générale.* 9 vols. Ed. Louis Le Guillou. Paris: Colin.

Lancisi, Giovanni Maria. [1745] 1952. *De aneurysmatibus: opus posthumus.* Trans. Wilmer Cave Wright. New York: Macmillan.

Landré-Beauvais, A. J. 1818. *Séméiotique ou traité des signes des maladies.* 3d ed. Paris: Brosson.

Laporte, Yves. 1981. "Allocution d'ouverture." In *RPD*, 12–21.

Larrey, M. le Baron. 1820. "Sur les plaies pénétrantes de la poitrine." *BEMS 7*: 85–88.

La Varende, Jean de. 1970. *Cadoudal.* Paris: Nouvelles Editions Latines.

Lawrence, Christopher. 1985. "Modern and Ancients: the 'New Cardiology' in Britain 1880–1930." In Bynum et al. 1985, 1–33.

Lawrence, Susan C. 1985. " 'Desirous of Improvements in Medicine': Pupils and Practitioners in the Medical Societies at Guy's and at St. Bartholomew's Hospitals 1795–1815." *Bull. Hist. Med. 59*:89–104.

———. 1988. "Entrepreneurs and Private Enterprise: The Development of Medical Lecturing in London." *Bull. Hist. Med. 62*:171–192.

Lebrun, F. 1971. *Les hommes et la mort en Anjou aux XVIIe et XVIIIe siècles.* Paris: Mouton.

Lecadre, A. 1827. "Dissertation sur le siège et la nature de l'hypochondrie." Thèse méd. no. 93, Paris.

———. 1868. *Etude comparative: Laennec et Broussais.* Le Havre: Le Pelletier.

Le Floc'h, Jean Louis. 1980. "Conflits entre Denis Berardier et l'évêque de Quimper." *Bull. Soc. Arch. Finistère 108*:225–234.

———. ca. 1989. "Dombideau de Crouseilhes." In Jean-Marie Mayeur and Yves-Marie Hilaire, eds. *Dictionnaire du monde religieux dans la France contemporaine: 3. La Bretagne.* Paris et Rennes: Beauchesne; Institut Culturel de Bretagne, 116–117.

Legallois, Jean-Julien-César. [1812] 1830. "Expériences sur le principe de la vie notamment celui des mouvements du coeur et le siège de ce principe." In J. Pariset, ed. *Oeuvres de Jean-Julien-César Legallois.* 2 vols. Paris: Le Rouge.

Le Gonidec, J. F. M. M. A. 1850. *Dictionnaire breton-français précédé de sa grammaire celto-bretonne.* Ed. Hersart de la Villemarqué. Saint-Brieuc: Prud'homme.

Lehrer, Steven. 1993. *Understanding Lung Sounds.* 2d ed. Philadelphia: W. B. Saunders.

Leibowitz, Joshua O. 1970. *The History of Coronary Heart Disease.* London: Wellcome Institute for the History of Medicine.

Léonard, Jacques. 1977. *La vie quotidienne du médecin de province au XIXe siècle.* Paris: Hachette.

———. 1978. *La France médicale. Médecins et malades au XIXe siècle.* Paris: Gallimard.

———. 1982. "La Restauration et la profession médicale." *Hist. Refl. 9*:69–81.

Léonard, Jacques, Roger Darquenne, and Louis Bergeron. 1977. "Médecins et notables sous le Consulat et l'Empire." *Annales ESC 32*:858–865.

Leroux, J. J. [1803–1804] An XII. "Sur la valeur des noms donnés aux maladies et les raisons qui nous empêchent de renoncer aux noms anciens." *J. méd. 8*:208–229.

Lesage, Louis Antoine. 1823. *Danger et absurdité de la doctrine physiologique du Docteur Broussais.* Paris: Gabon.

Lesch, John E. 1984. *Science and Medicine in France: The Emergence of Experimental Physiology, 1790–1855.* Cambridge, Mass: Harvard University Press.

———. 1988. "The Paris Academy of Medicine and Experimental Science, 1820–1848." In Coleman and Holmes 1988, 100–138.

Letulle, M. 1912a. "Oeuvre inédit de Laennec pensées et maximes scientifiques." *La presse médicale 2 (*3 July):721–722.

———. 1912b. "Notes inédites de Laennec sur la pratique des autopsies." *La presse médicale* 2 (17 July):765–767.

———. 1912c. "Notes inédites de Laennec. I. L'autopsie." *Bull. soc. fr. d'hist. méd.* 11:304–312.

———. 1912d. "Notes inédites de Laennec. II. Anatomie pathologique." *Bull. soc. fr. d'hist. méd.* 11:339–346.

Lie, Reidar K. 1986. "The Borderzone Zone Controversy: A Study of Theory Structure in Biomedicine." *Theoretical Medicine* 7:243–258.

———. 1991. "The Angina Pectoris Controversy during the 1920s." *Acta Physiologica Scandinavia suppl.* 599:135–147.

Lieutaud, Joseph. 1776–1777. *Anatomie historique et pratique.* 2 vols. Trans. A. Portal. Paris: Vicent d'Houry and Didot.

Lillienfeld, Abraham. 1982. "*Ceteris Paribus:* The Evolution of the Clinical Trial." *Bull. Hist. Med* 56:1–18.

Lisfranc, J. 1823. *Mémoire sur les nouvelles applications du stéthoscope de M. le Professeur Laennec.* Paris: Gabon.

Littré, Emile. 1839–1861. *Oeuvres complètes d'Hippocrate.* 10 vols. Paris: Baillière.

Lobstein, J. F. 1804. *Rapport sur les travaux exécutés à l'amphithéâtre de Strasbourg pendant l'An XII.* Strasbourg: Levrault.

Lock, Margaret. 1995. "The Return of the Patient as a Person: Contemporary Attitudes Towards the Alleviation of Suffering in North America." In Kawakita et al. 1995, 99–130.

Locke, John. [1694] 1981. *An Essay Concerning Human Understanding.* Ed. A. D. Woolzey. Glasgow: Collins.

Logan, J. S. 1972. "An Autograph Letter of Laennec." *Ulster Medical J. 41*: 108–110.

Lomax, Elizabeth. 1977. "Hereditary or Acquired Disease? Early Nineteenth-Century Debates on the Cause of Infantile Scrofula and Tuberculosis." *J. Hist. Med. All. Sci.* 32:356–374.

Lonie, Iain M. 1978. "Cos versus Cnidus and the Historians." *Hist. Sci. 16*:42–75, 77–92.

Lorillot, Dominique. 1982. "1789: Les médecins ont la parole." *Hist. Refl. 9*: 103–130.

Louis, P. C. A. 1825. *Recherches anatomico-pathologiques sur la phthisie pulmonaire.* Paris: Gabon.

Louis, P. C. A. 1834. *Examen de l'Examen de M. Broussais relativement à la phthisie et l'affection typhoïde.* Paris: Baillière.

———. 1835. *Recherches sur les effets de la saignée dans plusieurs maladies inflammatoires.* Paris: de Migneret.

Luisada, Aldo A., and Francesco Portaluppi. 1982. *The Heart Sounds: New Facts and Their Clinical Implications.* New York: Praeger Scientific.

Lullier-Winslow, A. L. M. 1812. "Asthme." In *DSM* 2:406–412.

Lusted, Lee B. 1968. *Introduction to Medical Decision Making.* Springfield: Charles C. Thomas.

MacAlpin, Rex N. 1980. "Coronary Arterial Spasm: A Historical Perspective." *J. Hist. Med. All. Sci.* 35:288–311.

Macleod, John, E. B. French, and J. F. Munro. 1985. *Introduction to Clinical Examination,* 4th ed. Edinburgh: Churchill Livingston.

Magendie, François. 1821. "Expérience sur la rage." *Journal de physiologie expérimentale 1*:40–46.

———. 1838. "Mémoire sur l'origine des bruits normaux du coeur [read 3 February 1834]." *Mémoires de l'Académie Royale des Sciences 14*:154–184.

Major, Ralph H. 1945a. "Notes on the History of Endocarditis." *Bull. Hist. Med. 17*:351–359.

———. 1945b. *Physical Diagnosis.* Philadelphia: W. B. Saunders.

Malard, Cita, and Suzanne Malard. 1959. *Laennec: génie français.* Paris: Letouzy et Ainé.

Mann, Frank D., and Ruth J. Mann. 1981. "Laennec as a Critical Pathologist." *J. Hist. Med. All. Sci. 36*:446–454.

Margolis, Joseph. 1976. "The Concept of Disease." *J. Med. Phil. 1*:238–253.

Marion de Procé, P. M. 1812. "Quelques vues générales sur les doctrines des tempéramens et sur le tempérament lymphatique en particulier." Thèse méd. no. 135, Paris.

Marketos, Spyros. 1982. *René Laennec:* Γαλλος Ιπποκρατης [The French Hippocrates]. Athens: Kedros.

Marmelzat, Willard L. 1962. "Laennec and the Prosector's Wart: Historical Note on Classic Descriptions of Inoculation Tuberculosis of the Skin." *Archives of Dermatology 86*:74–76.

Martin, Emily. 1990. "Toward an Anthropology of Immunology: The Body as Nation-State." *Medical Anthropology Quarterly 4*:410–426.

Martin, Julian. 1990. "Sauvages's Nosology: Medical Enlightenment in Montpellier." In Cunningham and French 1990, 111–137.

Martiny, M. 1975. "Laennec et la pensée hippocratique." In L. Bourgey and J. Jouanna, eds. *La collection hippocratique et son rôle dans l'histoire de la médecine, Colloque international hippocratique de Strasbourg, 1972.* Leiden: Brill, 97–105.

Maulitz, Russell C. 1987. *Morbid Appearances. The Anatomy of Pathology in the Early Nineteenth Century.* Cambridge: Cambridge University Press.

———. 1987a. "Pathologists, Clinicians, and the Role of Pathophysiology." In Geison 1987, 209–236.

———. 1990. "In the Clinic: Framing Disease at the Paris Hospital." *Annals of Science 47*:127–137.

Mayr, Ernst. 1982. *The Growth of Biological Thought, Diversity, Evolution, and Inheritance.* Cambridge, Mass.: Harvard University Press, Belknap Press.

Mazet, A. 1819. "Observations d'une phthisie tuberculeuse avec ulcérations intestinales et emphysème sous-muqueux mort survenue au 9e jour d'une hydrocéphale aiguë." Thèse méd. no. 157, Paris.

McDougall, J. Ian, and Leon Michaels. 1972. "Cardiovascular Causes of Sudden Death in *De Subitaneis Morbibus* by Giovanni Maria Lancisi." *Bull. Hist. Med. 44*:486–494.

McKeown, Thomas. 1979. *Role of Medicine: Dream, Mirage, or Nemesis?* Oxford: Basil Blackwell.

McKusick, Victor A. 1958a. "Rouanet of Paris and New Orleans: Experiments on the Valvular Origin of the Heart Sounds." *Bull. Hist. Med. 32*:137–151.

———. 1958b. "The History of Cardiovascular Sound." In Victor A. McKusick, ed. *Cardiovascular Sound in Health and Disease.* Baltimore: Williams and Wilkins, 3–54.

————. 1960. "The History of Methods for the Diagnosis of Heart Disease." *Bull. Hist. Med. 34*:16–18.

McKusick, Victor A., and H. Kenneth Wiskind. 1959. "Félix Savart (1791–1841), Physician-Physicist: Early Studies Pertinent to the Understanding of Murmurs." *J. Hist. Med. All. Sci. 14*:411–423.

McMahon, Carol E. 1976. "The Psychosomatic Approach to Heart Disease: a Study in Premodern Medicine." *Chest 69*:531–537.

McNeil, Barbara J., Emmett Keller, and S. James Adelstein. 1975. "Primer on Certain Elements of Medical Decision Making." *N. Engl. J. Med. 293*:211–221.

Meachen, G. Norman. 1936. *A Short History of Tuberculosis.* London: John Bale and Sons and Danielsson.

Medawar, P. B., and J. S. Medawar. 1983. *From Aristotle to Zoos: A Philosophical Dictionary of Biology.* Cambridge, Mass.: Harvard University Press.

Meindl, J., and C. O. Meindl. 1982. "Tuberculosis Meningitis in the 1830s." *Lancet 1*:554–555.

Mérat, F. V. 1819. "Pectoriloque." In *DSM 40*:9–35.

————. 1822. "Vitalisme." In *DSM 58*:280–281.

Mercier, Louis Sebastien. [ca. 1788] 1929. *The Picture of Paris Before and After the Revolution.* 2 vols. Trans. Wilfrid and Emilie Jackson. London: George Routledge.

Mercy, F. C. F. de. 1808. *Conspectus febrium.* Paris: Valade.

————. 1820a. *Au Roi: considérations sur le rapport de la Faculté de Médecine pour le maintien de la Chaire d'Hippocrate.* Paris: Veuve Agasse.

————. 1820b. *Mémoire à la Chambre des Députés des Départemens. Demande d'encouragemens pour la continuation de la traduction française de l'édition grecque complète des Oeuvres d'Hippocrate.* Paris: n.p.

————. 1820c. *Mémoire à la Chambre des Députés: Demande de l'exécution de la loi du 14 Frimaire An III pour le rétablissement d'une Chaire d'Hippocrate.* Paris: n.p.

Merskey, Harold. 1986. "Variable Meanings for the Definition of Disease." *J. Med. Phil. 11*:215–232.

Merton, Robert K. 1973. *The Sociology of Science: Theoretical and Empirical Investigation.* Ed. Norman W. Storer. Chicago: University of Chicago Press.

Mettling, Ch. 1926. "Index bibliographique par ordre chronologique de l'oeuvre de René Théophile Hyacinthe Laennec." *La presse médicale 103*:1624–1626.

Michu, J. L. 1824. *Doctrine médicale expliquée d'après les théories enseignées depuis Hippocrate jusqu'à M. Broussais.* Paris: Bechet et Compère.

Morand, Paul. 1972. *Un lésineur bienfaisant (M. de Montyon).* Paris: Gallimard.

Morgagni, Giovanni Battista. [1769] 1960. *The Seats and Causes of Disease Investigated by Anatomy.* Facsimile of the 1769 edition under the auspices of the Library of the New York Academy of Medicine. 3 vols. Trans. Benjamin Alexander. New York: Hafner.

Morton, Richard. 1694. *Phthisiologia, or Treatise of Consumptions.* London: S. Smith and B. Walford.

Müller, Stefan. 1965. "Antoine-Laurent Bayle, sein grandlegender Beitrag zur Enforschung der progressiven Paralyse." Thesis med., Zurich.

Munk, William. 1878. *Roll of the Royal College of Physicians of London. Vol. 3 (1808–1825).* London: Royal College of Physicians.

Murphy, Terence D. 1981. "Medical Knowledge and Statistical Methods in Early Nineteenth-Century France." *Med. Hist. 25*:301–319.

Nacquart, J. B. 1818a. [Editorial]. *J. gén. méd. 64* [or III, 2nd series]:133.

Nacquart, J. B. 1818b. "Des instrumens en médecine." *J. gén. méd.* *64* [or III, 2nd series]:135–136.

———. 1819. "De l'auscultation médiate . . . par R. T. H. Laennec." *J. gén. méd. 69* [or VIII, 2d series]:367–378.

Neuburger, Max. 1934. "An Historical Survey of the Concept of Nature from a Medical Viewpoint." *Isis 35*:16–28.

Newman, Edgar Leon, and Robert Lawrence Simpson, eds. 1987. *Historical Dictionary of France from the 1815 Restoration to the Second Empire*. 2 vols. New York: Greenwood.

Nicholson, Malcolm. 1992. "Giovanni Battista Morgagni and Eighteenth-Century Physical Examination." In Christopher Lawrence, ed. *Medical Theory, Surgical Practice*. London: Wellcome Institute for the History of Medicine and Routledge.

———. 1993. "Introduction of Percussion and Stethoscopy to Early Nineteenth-Century Edinburgh." In Bynum and Porter 1993, 134–153.

Nicolas, G. and J. P. Kernéis. 1981. "La diffusion américaine de la cardiologie de Laennec." In *RPD*, 299–303.

Noverre, George-Pierre. 1820. "Dissertation sur les anévrysmes de l'aorte." Thèse méd. no. 13, Paris.

Olmstead, J. M. D. 1944. *François Magendie: Pioneer in Experimental Physiology and Scientific Medicine in Nineteenth-Century France*. New York: Schuman.

O'Malley, C. D., ed. 1970. *The History of Medical Education. An International Symposium, February 1968*. Berkeley and Los Angeles: University of California Press.

Orcel, L., and Th. Vetter. 1976. "Dupuytren, Cruveilhier, et la Société Anatomique." *Arch. anat. cytol. path.* 24:167–179.

Orczy, Baronness. 1936. *The Turbulent Duchess*. New York: Putnam.

Orrù, Marco. 1987. *Anomie. History and Meanings*. Boston: Allen and Unwin.

Osler, W. 1912. "Men and Books: VII. Letters of Laennec." *Can. Med. Assoc. J.* 2:247–248.

Paillat, Serge. 1984. "Un manuscrit de Guillaume Laennec: son cours nantais de matière médicale en 1808: 2e Partie en 2 vols." Thèse méd., Nantes.

Paillat-Carbonell, Michèle. 1984. "Un manuscrit de Guillaume Laennec: son cours nantais de matière médicale en 1808: 1ère Partie." Thèse méd., Nantes.

Pancoucke, C. L. F., ed. 1812–1822. *Dictionnaire des sciences médicales par une société de médecins et de chirurgiens*. 60 vols. Paris: Panckoucke.

Pariset, E. 1845. "Eloge de Dupuytren" and "Eloge de Laennec." *Histoire des Membres de l'Académie Royale de Médecine ou Recueil des Eloges*. Vol. 2. Paris: Baillière, 103–148, 240–275.

Parry, C. H. 1799. *An Inquiry into the Symptoms and the Causes of the Syncope Anginosa*. London: Cadell and Davis.

———. 1815. *Elements of Pathology and Therapeutics*. London: Underwood.

Pascale, J. N. 1979. "Bordeu, Bouvart et Rostan: trois médecins face à la tuberculose en 1772." In J. Proust, ed. *Recherches nouvelles sur quelques écrivains des lumières*. Montpellier: Université Paul Valéry, 2:63–71.

Pecker, André, ed. 1984. *La Médecine à Paris du XIIIe au XXe siècle*. Paris: Editions Hervas and Fondation Singer-Polignac.

Peter, J. P. 1975. "Disease and the Sick at the End of the Eighteenth Century." In *Biology of Man in History. Selections from the Annales*. Ed. Robert Forster and Orest Ranum and trans. Elborg Forster and Patricia M. Ranum, 81–124. Baltimore: Johns Hopkins University Press.

Peumery, J. J. 1984. *Histoire illustrée de l'asthme de l'antiquité à nos jours.* Paris: Dacosta.

Pickstone, John V. 1981. "Bureaucracy, Liberalism and the Body in Post-Revolutionary France: Bichat's Physiology and the Paris School of Medicine." *Hist. Sci.* *19*:115–142.

Pidoux, Claude-François-Herman. 1866–1867. *Bulletin de l'Académie Impériale de Médecine 32*:1278.

Pied, Edouard. 1906. *Notice sur les rues, ruelles, quais, ponts, boulevards, places, et promenades de la ville de Nantes.* Nantes: A. Dugat.

Pigeaud, Jackie. 1975. "L'hippocratisme de Laennec." *Bulletin de l'Association Guillaume Budé 4e série no. 3*:357–363.

———. 1981. "L'Hippocrate de Laennec." In *RPD*, 232–238.

———. 1992. "La médecine et ses origines." *Can. Bull. Med. Hist. 9*:219–240.

Pinel, Philippe. [1797–1798] An VI. *Nosographie philosophique, ou de la méthode de l'analyse appliquée à la médecine.* 2 vols. Paris: Maradon.

Pinkerton, J. H. M. 1969. "Kergaradec, Friend of Laennec and Pioneer of Foetal Auscultation." *Proc. Roy. Soc. Med. 62*:477–483.

Pinson, Caroline. 1980. "La correspondance de la famille Laennec de 1815 à 1821 d'après le Fonds Rouxeau." Thèse méd. no. 2489, Nantes.

Piorry, P. A. 1828. *De la percussion médiate et des signes obtenus à l'aide de ce nouveau moyen d'exploration dans les maladies des organes thoraciques et abdominaux.* Paris: Chaudé.

Ploucquet, W.G. 1808–1809. *Literatura Medica Digesta.* 4 vols. in 2. Tubingen: J. G. Cotta.

Pompéry, E. de, ed. 1884. *Un coin de la Bretagne pendant la Révolution: Correspondance de Madame Audouyn de Pompéry.* 2 vols. Paris: Alphonse Lemerre.

Pons, P. 1818. "Essai sur les sympathies considérées sur le rapport de la médecine." Thèse méd. no. 112, Paris.

Popper, Karl. 1972. *The Logic of Scientific Discovery.* London: Hutchinson.

Portal, A. 1792. *Observations sur la nature et le traitement de la phthisie.* Paris: Du Pont.

———. 1804. *Cours d'anatomie médicale.* 5 vols. Paris: Baudoin.

———. 1817. "Sur la maladie et la mort de Madame la Baronne de Staël." *Annales politiques morales et littéraires,* August 2, 3–4.

Porter, Roy. 1985a. "The Patient's View: Doing Medical History from Below." *Theory and Society 14*:175–198.

———, ed. 1985b. *Patients and Practitioners. Lay Perceptions of Medicine in Pre-Industrial Society.* Cambridge: Cambridge University Press.

———. 1993. "The Rise of the Physical Examination." In Bynum and Porter 1993, 179–197.

Postman, Neil. 1992. *Technopoly: the Surrender of Culture to Technology.* New York: Alfred A. Knopf.

Potter, Paul., ed. and trans. 1988. *Hippocrates.* Loeb Classical Library. Vols. 5, 6. Cambridge, Mass.: Harvard University Press.

———. 1988a. *A Short Handbook of Hippocratic Medicine.* Quebec: Sphinx.

———. 1990. "Some Principles of Hippocratic Medicine." In Paul Potter, Gilles Maloney, and Jacques Desautels, eds., *La maladie et les maladies dans la collection hippocratique. Actes du VIe colloque international hippocratique.* Quebec: Sphinx, 237–253.

Power, Henry, and Leonard Sedgwick. 1892. *The New Sydenham Society's Lexicon of Medicine and the Allied Sciences.* 5 vols. London: New Sydenham Society.

Prost, P. A. 1804. *La médecine éclairée par l'observation et l'ouverture des corps.* 2 vols. Paris: Demonville.

Quinlan, Mary Hall. 1953. *The Historical Thought of the Vicomte de Bonald.* Washington: Catholic University of America.

Rackham, H. 1945. *Pliny, Natural History.* Loeb Classical Library. 10 vols. London: Heinemann; Cambridge, Mass.: Harvard University Press.

Ramsey, Matthew. 1988. *Professional and Popular Medicine in France, 1770–1830.* Cambridge: Cambridge University Press.

Ratier, F. S. 1827. "Coup d'oeil sur les cliniques de la Faculté de Médecine et des hôpitaux de Paris." *Arch. gén. méd.* 5:161–185.

Rault, René-Marie. 1819. "Considérations générales sur les signes diagnostiques des maladies du poumon." Thèse méd. no. 198, Paris.

Ravin, Abe. 1967. *Auscultation of the Heart.* 2d ed. Chicago: Year Book Medical.

Reedy, Walter J. 1976. "The Metaphysics of Authority: Louis de Bonald's Conservative World View." Ph.D. diss., Univerity of California, Santa Barbara.

Reill, P. H. 1989. "Anti-Mechanism, Vitalism, and their Political Implications in Late Enlightened Scientific Thought." *Francia* 16:195–212.

Reiser, Stanley Joel. 1978. "The Emergence of the Concept of Screening for Disease." *Milbank Quarterly* 56:403–425.

———. 1979. *Medicine and the Reign of Technology.* Cambridge: Cambridge University Press.

Rey, Roselyne. 1987. "Naissance et développement du vitalisme en France." 3 vols. Thèse Doctorat d'Etat en Histoire, Paris-I-Sorbonne.

———. 1991a. "La théorie de la sécrétion chez Bordeu, modèle de la physiologie et de la pathologie vitalistes." *Dix-Huitième Siècle* 23:45–58.

———. 1991b. "La vulgarisation médicale au XVIIIe siècle: le cas des dictionnaires portatifs de santé." *Rev. d'hist. sci.* 44:413–433.

———. 1992. "Anamorphoses d'Hippocrate au XVIIIe siècle." In D. Gourevitch, ed. *Maladie et maladies: Mélanges en hommage de M. D. Grmek.* Geneva: Droz, 257–276.

———. 1993a. "Diagnostic différentiel et espèces nosologiques: le cas de la phtisie pulmonaire de Morgagni à Bayle." In F. O. Touati, ed. *Maladies, médecines et sociétés: approches historiques pour le présent, Actes du VIe colloque d'histoire au présent.* 2 vols. Paris: L'Harmattan, 1:185–199.

———. 1993b. "L'Ecole de Santé de Paris sous la Révolution: transformations et innovations." *Histoire de l'éducation* 57:23–57.

Ribault, Jean-Yves. 1981. "Le dernier domicile de Laennec." In *RPD*, 260–273.

Riese, Walter. 1953. *The Conception of Disease, Its History, Its Versions and Its Nature.* New York: Philosophical Library.

Risse, Guenter B. 1978. "Health and disease: I. History of the concepts." In W. T. Reich, ed. *Encyclopedia of Bioethics.* 4 vols. New York and London: Free Press and Collier Macmillan, 2:579–585.

———. 1979. "Epidemics and Disease: the Influence of Disease on Medical Thought and Practice." *Bull. Hist. Med.* 53:505–519.

———. 1986. *Hospital Life in Enlightenment Scotland: Care and Teaching at the Royal Infirmary of Edinburgh.* Cambridge: Cambridge University Press.

———. 1987. "A Shift in Medical Epistemology: Clinical Diagnosis, 1770–1828."

In Yosio Kawakita and Yasuo Otasuka, eds. *History of Diagnostics. Tanaguchi Foundation 9th International Symposium.* Tokyo: Ishiyaku EuroAmerica. 115–147.

———. Forthcoming. *Hospitals from Antiquity to Contemporary America.*

Risse, Guenter B., and J. H. Warner. 1992. "Reconstructing Clinical Activities: Patient Records in Medical History." *Social History of Medicine* 5:183–205.

Rist, Edouard. 1955. La jeunesse de Laennec. Paris: Gallimard.

Robert, Fernand. 1981. "Laennec helléniste." In *RPD*, 239–244.

Robertson, A. John, and Robert Coope. 1957. "Râles, Rhonchi, and Laennec." *Lancet* 2:417–423.

Robiquet, Jean. [1938] 1964. *Daily Life in the French Revolution.* Trans. James Kirkup. London: Weidenfield and Nicholson.

Rosenberg, Charles E. 1977. "And Heal the Sick: Hospital and Patient in the Nineteenth Century." *Journal of Social History* 4:428–471.

———. 1995. "Catechisms of Health: The Body in the Prebellum Classroom." *Bull. Hist. Med. 69.*

Rosner, Lisa. 1994. "Student Culture at the Turn of the Nineteenth Century: Edinburgh and Philadelphia." *Caduceus 10*:65–86.

Rostan, L. L. 1818a. "Mémoire sur la distinction des anévrysmes du coeur en actifs et passifs." *Nouv. j. méd. 1*:307–323.

———. 1818b. "Mémoire sur cette question: l'asthme des veillards est-il une affection nerveuse?" *Nouv. j. méd. 3*:3–30.

———. 1819–1820. "Extrait 'De l'auscultation médiaté,' par M. Laennec." *Nouv. j. méd. 6*:154–184, *7*:308–318.

———. 1820. "Mémoire sur les ruptures du coeur." *Nouv. j. méd. 7*:265–280.

———. 1823. *Recherches sur le ramollissement du cerveau.* 2d ed. Paris: Béchet.

———. 1826. *Traité élémentaire de diagnostic, de pronostic, et d'indications thérapeutiques, ou Cours de médecine clinique.* 3 vols. Paris: Béchet.

———. 1830. *Cours de médecine clinique où sont exposés les principes de la médecine organique . . .* 2d ed. 3 vols. Paris: Bechet.

———. 1832. *Cours de médecine clinique où sont exposés les principes de la médecine organique . . .* 3d ed. Brussels: Dumont.

———. 1833. *Jusqu'à quel point l'anatomie pathologique peut-elle éclairer la thérapeutique des maladies?* Paris [contribution to a competition].

———. 1846. *Exposition des principes de l'organicisme.* 2d ed. Paris: L'Abbé.

———. 1864. *De l'Organicisme précédé de réflexions sur l'incredulité en matiére de médecine et suivi de commentaire et d'aphorismes.* 3d ed. Paris: Asselin.

Roth, Michael S. 1991. "Dying of the Past: Medical Studies of Nostalgia in Nineteenth-Century France." *History and Memory 3*:5–29.

Rouanet, J. 1832. "Analyse des bruits du coeur." Thèse méd. no. 252, Paris.

Rousseau, George. 1992. "The Perpetual Crisis of Modernism and the Traditions of Enlightenment Vitalism with a Note on Mikhail Bakhtin." In Burwick and Douglas 1992, 15–75.

Roussel, Alfred. 1893. *Lamennais d'après des documents inédits.* 2 vols. Rennes: Caillière.

Roux de Reilhac, Pia Gourdon. 1980. "La correspondance de Laennec de 1822 à 1826." Thèse méd. no. 2462, Nantes.

Rouxeau, Alfred. [1912] 1978. *Laennec avant 1806.* Facsimile ed. Vol. 1. Quimper: Editions de Cornouaille.

Rouxeau, Alfred. [1920] 1978. *Laennec après 1806.* Facsimile ed. Vol. 2. Quimper: Editions de Cornouaille.

———. [1924] 1978. "Un étudiant en médecine quimpérois (Guillaume-François Laënnec) aux derniers jours de l'Ancien Régime." In Rouxeau [1912] 1978.

Rouzet, L. 1820. "De l'auscultation médiate [review]." *Rev. méd.* 2:3–65.

Rullière, Roger. 1981. "Laennec cardiologue: le bon grain et l'ivraie." In *RPD*, 130–137.

Ryle, G. 1949. *The Concept of Mind.* London: Hutchinson.

"S." 1820. "Bayle." In *DSM: Biog Méd.* 2:75–79.

Sainte-Beuve, C. A. 1847. *Portraits contemporains.* 3 vols. Paris: Didier.

Saintignon, Henri. 1904. *Laennec: sa vie, son oeuvre.* Paris: Baillière.

Sakula, Alex. 1981. "Accueil du livre 'De l'auscultation médiate' et du stéthoscope par les médecins de Grande Bretagne." In *RPD*, 280–290.

Salle, Eusèbe François de. [1833] 1973. *Sakontala à Paris: roman de moeurs contemporains.* Facsimile of 1833 Paris ed. Genève: Slatkine.

Sarradon, Paul. 1949. Le docteur Laennec. Paris: Laffont.

Savary, A. C. 1808. " 'Principes de physiologie ou introduction à la science expérimentale philosophique et médicale' par L. C. Dumas [review]." *Bib. méd.* 20:17–26, 161–179, 289–308.

Savina, J. 1926. "Autour de R.T.H. Laennec: quelques lettres inédites de son père et de ses oncles." *Bull. Soc. Arch. Finistère* 73–107.

Savitt, Todd L. 1995. "Self-Reliance and the Changing Physician-Patient Relationship in Nineteenth and Early Twentieth-Century America." In Kawakita et al. 1995, 73–98.

Schiller, Francis. 1979. *Paul Broca, Founder of French Anthropology, Explorer of the Brain.* Berkeley and Los Angeles: University of California Press.

Schiller, J. 1967. "Wöhler, l'urée, et le vitalisme." *Sudhoffs Archiv* 51:229–243.

Schlich, Thomas. 1993. "Making Mistakes in Science: Eduard Pflüger, His Scientific and Professional Concept of Physiology and his Unsuccessful Theory of Diabetes (1903–1910)." *Stud. Hist. Phil. Sci.* 24:411–441.

Schott, A. 1980. "Historical Notes on the Mechanism of Closure of the Aterioventricular Valves." *Med. Hist.* 24:163–184.

Scudamore, Charles. 1826. *Observations on M. Laennec's Method of Forming a Diagnosis of the Diseases of the Chest by Means of the Stethoscope and of Percussion and Upon Some Points of the French Practice of Medicine.* London: Longman, Rees, Orme, Brown & Green.

———. 1833. *A Further Examination of the Principles of the Treatment of Gout with Observations on the Use and Abuse of Colchichiam.* London: Longman, Rees, Orme.

Sedaillan, Marcel, André Soubiran, and Anne Argela. 1959. *Princes de médecine.* Paris: Le livre contemporain.

Ségal, Allain. 1984. "Baron Guillaume Dupuytren, 1777–1835." In Pecker 1984, 401–402.

Segall, Harold N. 1963. "Cardiovascular Sound and the Stethoscope." *Can. Med. Assoc. J.* 88:308–318.

———. 1967. "Notes and Events: The Introduction of the Stethoscope and Clinical Auscultation in Canada." *J. Hist. Med. All. Sci.* 22:414–417.

Sénac, Jean-Baptiste. 1749. *Traité de la structure du coeur, de son action, et de ses maladies.* 2 vols. Paris: J. Vincent.

———. 1778. *Traité des maladies du coeur.* 2 vols. Reprint of pt. 6 of 1774 2d ed. Paris: Barbou.

Shorter, Edward. 1985. *Bedside Manners: The Troubled History of Doctors and Patients.* New York: Simon and Schuster.

———. 1992. *From Paralysis to Fatigue: A History of Psychosomatic Illness in the Modern Era.* New York: Free Press.

Sigerist, Henry E. [1933] 1958. *The Great Doctors.* Garden City, N.Y.: Doubleday.

Skerrit, Paul W. 1983. "Anxiety and the Heart: a Historical Review." *Psychological Medicine* 13:17–25.

Skoda, F. 1988. *Médecine ancienne et métaphore: Le vocabulaire de l'anatomie et de la pathologie en grec ancien.* Paris: Peeters/Selaf.

Smeaton, W. A. 1962. *Fourcroy, Chemist and Revolutionary, 1755–1809.* Cambridge: Heffer.

Smith, Dale C. 1978. "Austin Flint and Auscultation in America." *J. Hist. Med. All. Sci.* 33:129–149.

Smith, Ginnie. 1985. "Prescribing the Rules of Health: Self-Help and Advice in the Late Eighteenth Century." In Porter 1985b, 249–282.

Smith, W. D., ed. and trans. 1994. *Hippocrates.* Loeb Classical Library. Vol. 7. Cambridge, Mass.: Harvard University Press.

Sontag, S. 1979. *Illness as Metaphor.* New York: Vintage Random House.

Soulié, P. 1955. "Corvisart et le diagnostic clinique du rétrécissement mitral." *Hist. de la méd.* 5:55–64.

Sournia, Jean-Charles. 1989. *La médecine révolutionnaire, 1789–1799.* Paris: Payot.

Spitzer, Alan B. 1971. *Old Hatreds and Young Hopes: The French Carbonari against the Bourbon Restoration.* Cambridge, Mass.: Harvard University Press.

———. 1976. "Victor Cousin and the French Generation of 1820." In Dora B. Weiner and William R. Keylor, eds. *From Parnassus. Essays in Honour of Jacques Barzun.* New York: Harper Row, 177–194.

———. 1987. *The French Generation of 1820.* Princeton, N.J.: Princeton University Press.

Sprengel, K. 1815. *Histoire de la médecine.* 9 vols. Trans. A. J. L. Jourdan. Paris: Deterville.

Stafford, Barbara. 1991. *Body Criticism: Imaging the Unseen in Enlightenment Art and Medicine.* Cambridge, Mass.: MIT Press.

Starobinski, Jean. 1991. "Le 'médecin croyant' et le théologien genevois: une lettre écrite en 1802 par M. F. R. Buisson à Pierre Picot." *Gesnerus* 48:333–342.

Staum, Martin. 1980. *Cabanis: Enlightenment and Medical Philosophy in the French Revolution.* Princeton, N.J.: Princeton University Press.

Stevenson, Lloyd G. 1982. "Exemplary Disease: the Typhoid Pattern." *J. Hist. Med All. Sci.* 37:159–181.

Stofft, Henri. 1981. "Laennec et Kergaradec, une amitié féconde. Application à l'obstétrique de l'auscultation." In *RPD*, 152–169.

Stokes, Maria, and Max Blythe. 1995. "Muscle Sounds Rediscovered [letter]." *Lancet* 346:779.

Stokes, W. 1825. *An Introduction to the Use of the Stethoscope.* Edinburgh: Maclachlan and Stewart.

Stoll, Maximilian. [1797] An V. *Aphorismes sur la connaissance et la curation des fièvres.* Trans. J. N. Corvisart. Paris: Régent et Bernard, Méquignon.

Sullivan, Robert B. 1994. "Sanguine Practices: A Historical and Historiographic Reconsideration of Heroic Therapy in the Age of Rush." *Bull. Hist. Med.* 68: 211–234.

Sutton, Geoffrey. 1984. "The Physical and Chemical Path to Vitalism: Xavier Bichat's Physiological Researches on Life and Death." *Bull. Hist. Med.* 58:53–71.

Sylvius, Franciscus de la Boe. 1681. "Appendix tractatus IV." In *Opera medica.* Genevae: Samuelem de Tournes, 526–537.

Szasz, T. 1974. *The Myth of Mental Illness: Foundations of a Theory of Personal Conduct.* New York: Harper Row.

Taton, René. 1962. *Reason and Chance in Scientific Discovery.* Trans. A. J. Pomerans. New York: Science Editions.

Taylor, Alfred S. 1848. *On Poisons in Relation to Medical Jurisprudence and Medicine.* Ed. R. Eglesfeld Griffith. Philadelphia: Lea and Blanchard.

Temkin, Oswei. 1946a. "The Philosophical Background of Magendie's Physiology." *Bull. Hist. Med.* 20:10–35.

————. 1946b. "Materialism in French and German Physiology of the Early Nineteenth Century." *Bull. Hist. Med.* 20:322–327.

————. 1951. "The Role of Surgery in Modern Medical Thought." *Bull. Hist. Med.* 25:248–259.

Tenon, Jacques. 1788. *Mémoire sur les hôpitaux de Paris.* Paris: D. Pierres.

Testa, Antonio Giuseppi. 1823. *Della malattie del cuore.* 2d ed. 3 vols. Firenze: Gugliemo Piatti.

Thayer, William S. 1920. "On Some Unpublished Letters of Laennec." *Bulletin of the Johns Hopkins Hospital* 31:425–435.

Thébaud, Dominique. 1981. "Laennec: précurseur de la méthode numérique." Thèse méd. no. 2572, Nantes.

Thivel, Antoine. 1989. "Peut-on parler d'un vitalisme d'Hippocrate, notamment dans les Epidémies?" In G. Baader and R. Winau, eds., *Die hippokratischen Epidemien.* Stuttgart: Steiner, 88–104.

Touche, Marcel. 1968. *J. N. Corvisart, praticien célèbre, grand maître de la médecine.* Paris: Baillière.

Toulmouche, A. 1820. "Considérations sur les signes diagnostiques des maladies du coeur." Thèse méd. no. 36, Paris.

————. 1825. "D'un empoisonement par l'acide hydro-cyanique." *Rev. méd. 1:* 265–274.

————. 1838. "Expériences cliniques sur le kermès minéral." *Gazette méd. de Paris* ns 6:724–729, 7:217–220.

————. 1875. "Souvenirs relatifs à Laennec (extrait des *Arch. gén. méd.,* May 1875, 25:626–635)." *Gazette des hopitaux civils et militaires* (May), 469–470, 478–479.

Triaire, Paul. 1899. *Récamier et ses contemporains, 1774–1852: étude d'histoire de la médecine au XVIII et XIX siècles.* Paris: J. B. Baillière.

Trousseau, A. 1877. *Clinique médicale de l'Hôtel Dieu.* 5th ed. Paris: Baillière.

Tuchman, Arleen Marcia. 1993. *Science, Medicine, and the State in Germany: The Case of Baden, 1815–1817.* New York: Oxford University Press.

Valentin, Michel. 1981. "L'oncle bien aimé, le professeur Guillaume Laennec de Nantes, 1748–1822." *RPD,* 32–41.

————. 1988. *François Broussais, empereur de la médecine: jeunesse, correspondance, vie et oeuvre.* Cesson-Sévingé: Association des Amis du Musée du Pays de Dinard.

———. 1993. "De Laennec à Chateaubriand: un pamphlet royaliste anonyme de René-Théophile Laennec pendant les Cent-Jours." *Hist. sci. méd.* 27:131–135.

———. 1994. "Broussais, Laennec et Chateaubriand." *Annales de la Société d'histoire et d'archéologie de l'arrondissement de Saint-Malo*, 177–185.

Vallery-Radot, René. 1927. *Life of Pasteur.* Trans. R. I. Devonshire. Garden City, N.Y.: Garden City Publishing.

———. 1952. "Trois lettres inédites de Laennec." *Hist. de la méd.* 2:31–37.

Véron, Louis-Désiré. [1853–1855] 1945. *Mémoires d'un bourgeois de Paris, textes choisis par Pierre Josserand.* 2 vols. Paris: Le Prat.

Vess, David. 1975. *Medical Revolution in France.* Gainesville, Fla.: Florida State University Press.

Vicq d'Azyr, Félix. 1790. "Anatomie pathologique." In F. Vicq d'Ayzr, ed. [to vol. 6 only]. *Encyclopédie méthodique par une société de médecins.* 13 vols. Paris: Panckoucke, 2:237–612.

Viets, Henry R. 1926. "Some Editions of Laennec's Work on Mediate Auscultation." *Boston Medical and Surgical Journal* 195:298–317.

Vieussens, Raymond. 1715. *Traité nouveau de la structure du coeur et des causes du mouvement naturel.* Toulouse: Guillmette.

Villard, René. 1927. "Le mariage de Laennec." *Gazette médicale du centre 32*: 101–103.

Vrouc'h, A. 1958. "Comment Laennec guérit le Roi Gradlon." *Histoire de la médecine 8*:61–62.

Vyau de Lagarde, L. 1824. "Du tartrate de potasse antimoinié employé à haute dose comme moyen curatif." Thèse méd. no. 48, Paris.

———. 1826. "Tableau des maladies observées à la Charité dans les salles de Clinique de M. le Professeur Laennec." *Rev. méd.* 3:177–210.

Warner, John Harley. 1985. "The Selective Transport of Medical Knowledge: Antebellum Physicians and Parisian Medical Therapeutics." *Bull. Hist. Med.* 59:213–231.

———. 1991. "Remembering Paris: Memory and the American Disciples of French Medicine in the Nineteenth Century." *Bull. Hist. Med.* 65:301–325.

———. Forthcoming. *Against the Spirit of System: The French Impulse in Nineteenth-Century American Medicine.* Princeton, N.J.: Princeton University Press.

Warren, John. [1812] 1962. "Remarks on Angina Pectoris [1812]." *N. Engl. J. Med.* 266:3–7.

Watson, James D. 1970. *Molecular Biology of the Gene.* 2d ed. New York: W. A. Benjamin.

Webb, Gerald B. 1927. "René Théophile Hyacinthe Laennec." *Annals of Medical History* 9:27–59.

———. 1928. *René Théophile Hyacinthe Laennec, a Memoir.* New York: Paul B. Hoeber.

Weiner, Dora B. 1969. "French Doctors Face War, 1792–1815." In C. K. Warner, ed. *From the Ancien Regime to the Popular Front. Essays in the History of Modern France in Honor of Shepard B. Clough.* New York: Columbia University Press, 51–73.

———. 1982. "The Role of the Doctor in Welfare Work: The Philanthropic Society of Paris, 1780–1815." *Hist. Refl.* 9:279–304.

———. 1993. *The Citizen-Patient in Revolutionary and Imperial Paris.* Baltimore: Johns Hopkins University Press.

Weiner, Margery. 1960. *The French Exiles, 1789–1815.* London: John Murray.

Weinstein, Michael A. 1979. *Structure of Human Life: A Vitalist Ontology.* New York: New York University Press.

Weintraub, William S., and Richard H. Helfant. 1983. "Coronary Artery Spasm: Historic Aspects." *Cardiovascular Clinics 14*:1–5.

Weisz, George. 1994. "The Development of Medical Specialization in Nineteenth-Century Paris." In La Berge and Feingold 1994, 149–188.

————. 1995. *The Medical Mandarins—The French Academy of Medicine in the Nineteenth and Early Twentieth Centuries.* New York: Oxford University Press.

Whitteridge, Gweneth. 1971. *William Harvey and the Circulation of the Blood.* London: American Elsevier.

Wiggars, Carl J. 1960. "Some Significant Advances in Cardiac Physiology." *Bull. Hist. Med. 34*:1–15.

Williams, C. J. B. 1834. *A Rational Exposition of the Physical Signs of the Diseases of the Lungs and Pleura Illustrating Their Pathology and Facilitating their Diagnosis.* 2d ed. Philadelphia: Lea and Blanchard.

————. 1835. *Pathology and Diagnosis of Diseases of the Chest.* 3d ed. London: Churchill.

Williams, Elizabeth A. 1994. *The Physical and the Moral: Anthropology, Physiology, and Philosophical Medicine in France, 1750–1850.* Cambridge: Cambridge University Press.

Willius, F. A., and T. J. Dry. 1948. *A History of the Heart and the Circulation.* Philadelphia: W. B. Saunders.

Wintrobe, Maxwell. 1985. *Hematology: the Blossoming of a Science.* Philadelphia: Lea and Febiger.

Winwood, Robert S. 1981. *Essentials of Clinical Diagnosis.* London: Edward Arnold.

Wollaston, W. H. 1810. "On the Duration of Muscular Action [pt. 1 of the Croonian Lecture, read 16 November 1809]." *Phil. Trans. 100*:2–5.

Wolsky, Maria de Issekutz, and Alexander A. Wolsky. 1992. "Bergson's Vitalism in the Light of Modern Biology." In Burwick and Douglas 1992, 153–170.

Wright, John P. 1989. "Metaphysics and Physiology: Mind, Body, and the Animal Economy in Eighteenth-Century Scotland." In M. A. Stewart, ed. *Studies in the Philosophy of the Scottish Enlightenment. Oxford Studies in the History of Philosophy.* Vol. 1. Oxford: Clarendon; New York: Oxford University Press, 251–301.

Ziporyn, Terra Diane. 1992. *Nameless Diseases.* New Brunswick, N.J.: Rutgers University Press.

Académie de Chirurgie, 25, 37, 55
Académie de Médecine, 55, 57, 129, 185,
 229, 230, 243, 268, 276, 284, 290, 293,
 385n.100; eulogy of Laennec at, 288;
 Laennec at, 175
Académie des Sciences, 58, 280; Laennec
 on auscultation at, 122, 127, *128*, 132,
 136, 137–138, 145; rivalry for positions
 in, 275
accidental productions, 61–64, 70, 267
acephalocystides, 56, *57*
Ackerknecht, Erwin H., 7, 75, 225, 276,
 294, 299
acoustics, 122–123, 185, 201
Adams, Francis, 74
admission diagnoses, 238; change in,
 214–216
agriculture, Laennec's notes on, 219,
 375n.54
Albury, W. R., 82, 154, 179
anatomical diagnosis, utility of, 38, 218. *See
 also* organic lesions
anatomoclinical medicine, 6, 28–29, 74, 152,
 169, 199, 272, 294
anatomy, 24, 69; and disease, 27–29. *See also*
 pathological anatomy
ancient authors, 35, 38, 58, 73, 74–75, 224,
 270; cited by Laennec, 349n.103. *See also*
 Galen, Hippocrates
Andral, Gabriel, 67, 324; on auscultation,
 164–166, 214, 235, 240; on blood, 291;
 criticism of Laennec; 292; Laennec's attack
 on, 164, 166, 272; Laennec's debt to, 315;
 politics and religion of, 275, 278
anemia, 193
aneurysm: of aorta, 148, 196–197, 315;
 Bouillaud on, 196, 214; of heart, 178,
 180, 216. *See also* dilatation of heart,
 hypertrophy
Angélique, 83, 255
angina pectoris, 69, 178–179, 180, 201,
 205, 237, 371n.116; Laennec's Latin
 essay on, 194–196, *195*; Laennec's own,
 79, 196
Angoulême, Duchesse d', 106
animal magnetism, 249
Annales de médecine physiologique, 248
Annales politiques, morales, et littéraires, 136
Anne G., patient, 36

anomie, 238, 379n.154
Ansiaux, J. J., 175
anthropology, 277
antimony. *See* tartar emetic
Aretaeus of Cappadocia, 56, 74, 306
Argou, Clementine, 255, 256, 386n.112
Argou, Mme Jacquemine Guichard
 (Laennec's wife), 80, 94, 281–283, 324,
 360n.19, 385nn. 105, 110, 386n.115;
 auscultation of, 125; faculty pension to,
 283, 313; marriage of, 255–258
Aristotle, 49, 299
army. *See* hospitals, military service of
 doctors, war
arrogance, scientific, 273, 299–300
arsenic, 377n.84
arterial redness, 183
Assistance Publique, 107; archives of, 108
asthma, 69, 97, 152, 166–173; with vital
 lesion, 168, 237, 269; diagnosis of, 169;
 Laennec's own, 79, 82, 149
Aubry, J. F., 75
Auenbrugger, Leopold, 32, 60, 149
auscultation: Aretaeus on, 74; Buisson on,
 42, 121; as a new cachet, 253; criticism of,
 218; direct, 122, *135*; extra-thoracic applications, 214, 268; of heart, 183–201;
 Hippocrates on, 122, 124; impact of,
 213–218, 302–303; impact on hospital
 diagnosis, 213–217; Laennec's first use of
 the word, 43; of lungs, 152–173; and physiology, 7, 43, 121, 206, 259; rapid dissemination of, 209–213, 238; and tuberculosis,
 158. *See also* discovery of auscultation, disease, heart sounds, stethoscope, *and specific
 signs by name*
autopsy, 87, 108, 141, 154; Bichat's method
 of, 70; Broussais's method of, 231; of cardinals, 84, 87; Corvisart's method of, 33;
 of Fortassin, 58; Laennec's method of, 70,
 141. *See also* anatomy, dissection, pathological anatomy, *and individual cases and
 diseases by name*
Avicenna, 270

Baffos, surgeon, 139
Baglivi, Giorgio, 157
Baillie, Matthew, 67, 143, 177, 324
Barker, John, 75

Barry, David, 186–187, 189, 247, 265, 287
Barthez, Paul-Joseph, 13, 60, 185, 263, 265
Bartlett, Elisha, 229
Basset, Marie-Mélanie, patient, 125–126, 131, 133, 147
Bastille, 108
Baudeloque, J. L., 53
Baume, Jean-Joseph, 132, 148
Bayle, Antoine-Laurent-Jesse, 231, 235, 275, 277, 289–290, 293, 324, 394n.19
Bayle, Gaspard-Laurent, 6, *39*, 50, 57, 63, 65, 82, 85, 115, 237, 245, 271, 283, 324; and auscultation, 124; Broussais's criticism of, 232; on cancer, 289; classification of disease of, 97–98; and Congrégation, 44, 46; death of, 100, 108; early career of, 37–38; health of, 96–101, 105; Laennec's debt to, 69, 96, 99, 315; marriage of, 78; nostalgia of, 154, 162, 163; obituary of, 356n.117; on pathological anatomy, 48, 49; on pneumothorax, 142; poem about, 98; publications of, 96–98, 99; thesis of, 37, 38–40, 51, 68, 166, 340n.42; on tuberculosis, 55, 96–100, 142, 157, 162, 247, 344n.3; and vital lesion, 69. *See also* nostalgia
Beau, Joseph, 200
Beaubien, Pierre de, 217
Beaugendre, François-Marie, 148, 282
Beaujon hospital, 358n.28
Béclard, Pierre-Augustin, 243, 244, 245
Becquey, François-Louis, 107, 283, 324, 358n.25
Benivieni, Antonio, 28
Bergson, Henri, 297
Bernard, Claude, 200, 295
Berry, Duchesse de, 241, 242, 252, 280, 324; cello of, 380n.6; retainer of, 312
Bertier de Sauvigny, 342n.76; cited, 3
Bertin, René-Joseph-Hyacinthe, 61, 180, 183, 189, 244, 277, 368n.25, 369n.52
"better eye," vii, 33, 130, 173, 217
Bibliothèque Interuniversitaire de Médecine (BIUM), 305–306
Bibliothèque médicale, 232
Bichat, M. F. X., 7, 36, 46–47, 51, 58, 59, 61, 65, 272, 324; *Anatomie générale* of, 67, 70, 148; and Broussais, 227, 288; Buisson's criticisms of, 40–43, 277; death of, 40–41; imputed materialism of, 41, 45; imputed vitalism of, 295, 286; Laennec's supposed reverence for, 40, 340n.45; physiology of, 227, 265, 288
Billerey, 47

Bishop of Quimper, 241, 243, 244, 256, 307, 309. *See also* Dombideau de Crousheilhes
Bishop, James Patrick, 305
Blin, P. F., 14–15, 105
blood pressure, 182
bloodletting, 95, 229, 248, 254, 278, 394n.11; by Laennec, 236
Blumenbach, J. F., 265
Boerhaave, Abraham Kaau, 69, 263, 387n.22
Boerhaave, Hermann, 263, 270, 348n.91
Bohan, le sieur de, 222
Bonald, Louis G. A. de, 7, 42–43, 90, 105, 270, 296, 324, 388n.36
Bonet, Théophile, 61, 177
Bordeau, Théophile, 273
Bordeaux "illusion," 255
Bouillaud, Jean-Baptiste, 291, 324; on aneurysms, 148, 214; on bloodletting, 229; and Broussais, 230, 292; criticisms of Laennec, 193, 196–197, 201, 249, 276–277, 371n.107; on heart disease, 183, 201; Laennec's attacks on, 183, 277, 293; and organicism, 272, 276–277; politics of, 275, 369n.52. *See also* inflammation
boulimia, 115
Boulle, Lydie, 108, 305
Bourbon administration, 243. *See also* Restoration
Bourdier, Isidore, 53
Boyer, Alexis, 30, 32, 43, 53, 244, 324
brain softening, 276–277
Breschet, Gilbert, 267
Breton enclave, 30, 32, 59, 80, 87, 100, 211
Breton language, 81, 219, 221, 252, 276, 351n.26; Laennec on, 94–96
Breton soldiers, 94–96, 308
Bricheteau, Isidore, 210
British physicians: on heart, 177, 188; Laennec ignores priority of, 212; on psychosomatic medicine, 253, 294
Broca, Paul, 273
Broglie, Duc de, 127; cited, 83
bronchiectasis, 89, 137, 152, 164–165, 204
bronchitis, 204–205, 235. *See also* catarrh, rales
bronchophony, 137, 152, 154, 163–166, 194, 247, 279; enhances specificity of pectoriloquy, 204
Broussais, François-Joseph-Victor, 6, 7, 51, 63, 160, 183, 209, 217, 225–239, *226*, 236, 240, 248, 254, 260, 261, 272, 276, 277, 288, 291, 292, 301, 324, 376n.84; agreement with Laennec, 235–239, 278–

279; attack on Bayle, 231; criticism of Louis, 247; defended by Laennec's colleagues, 230; early career of, 226–227; *Histoires des phlegmasies*, 227, 230, 232; influence on Laennec's treatise, 233–234; insults of, 233, 234; Laennec's attack on, 232, 233–234, 268–269; meets Laennec at bedside, 248, 254, 384n.94; on pathologists, 232; physiological doctrine of, 227–230; politics of, 275; rejection of ancients, 250; therapeutics of, 228–229

Broussais, Casimir, 229

Brown, John, 61, 269

Brown, Theodore, 296

bruit: of carotid, 174, 192; in hemorrhage, 193

Brune, General, 22

Bruté de Remur, S. G., 44, 324, 352n.46

Buisson, Mathieu-Françis-Régis, 6–7, 37, 68, 277, 324, 388n.36; attack on medical materialism, 42; and "auscultation," 42, 121, 124–125, 154; on Bichat 42, 63; and Bonald, 42, 90, 270; career of, 41; and Congrégation, 44, 46, 85, 245, 270; Foucault on, 341n.62; on Laennec, 53, 60; Laennec ignores, 124–125; Laennec on, 42–43; poetry of, 44; thesis of, 42–43, 49, 51, 152, 154; on words, 225

Bulletin de l'Ecole de Médecine (*BEMS*), 55, 63, 70, 344n.2, 345n.7

Burns, Allan, 179, 180, 182, 188, 200, 368n.40

Burserius, 180

C***, Marie, patient, 143

Cabanis, P. J. G., 25, 30, 108, 227, 265, 269, 296

cadet Rousseau (Antoine Michel), patient, *34*, 35, 51, 97, 173, 236

Cadoudal, Georges, 22, 104

Caelius Aurelianus, 74, 306

cancer, 97, 156, 157, 268, 272

Canguilhem, Georges, 225, 296, 299

Carbonari movement, 243

Cardinal X, 84. *See also* Eriskin, Fesch, Vincenti

cardiology, 176

caricature of Laennec, *255*, 385n.102

Carrier, Jean-Baptiste, 16, 105, 106, 335n.22

Carswell, Robert, 71, 245–246, 260, 324; papers of, 381n.29

Cartesian dualism, 299

Cartesian view of heart, 184

case histories. *See* patient records, patients

Castaign, Dr., trial of, 254

Castelnau, C., 98

catalépsie, 185

cataract of eye, 267

catarrh, 132, 204–205, 214, 215, 216, 235

Catholicism, 38. *See also* Congrégation, religion and medicine

cause of disease: Laennec's neglect of, 269; Laennec's reticence about, 25, 293; Rostan on, 273. *See also* heredity, lesion, concept of, liquid lesion, organic lesions, psychic causes of disease, vital lesion

Caventou, Joseph-Bienaimé, 288

cavity of lung, 160–161; Laennec's detection of, 137; signs of, 141–142. *See also* pectoriloquy

Cayol, Jean-Bruno, 137, 139, 168, 200, 218, 219, 254, 256, 305, 325

Cazeneuve, Dr., 255, 385n.100

Chaptal, Jean-Antoine, 47, 53, 254

Charcot, Jean-Martin, 73

Charité hospital, 32, 33, 35, 38, 113, 116, 138, 143, 201, 245, 247, 249, 289, 305, 388n.40; *clinique interne* of, 246–247, 291; impact of auscultation at, 216–217; mortality in, 94, 217, 246, 249

Charles X, 241, 280–281

Charon, patient, 199

Chartier, surgeon, 57

Chartran, Théobald, 135

Chateaubriand, Mme de, 87–90, *89*, 271, 283, 325

Chateaubriand, René de, 7, 87–90, *88*, 226, 241, 242, 254, 325, 353nn. 62, 66; review of Laennec, 90

Chaussier, François, 28, 30, 44, 53, 55, 75, 227, 244, 265, 325

Chauveau, Dr., 248, 254

Chauveau, J. B. A., 200

Chéguillaume family, 307, 328

chemistry, 69, 237, 267, 274, 278

Chevaliers de la Foi, 243, 342n.76

Chevreul, Michel-Eugène, 267

children, breath sounds in, 167. *See also* puerile respiration

Chomel, Auguste F., 201, 243, 246, 267, 273, 325, 388n.40

Chopinet, R. M., patient, 165

chorea, 268

Chouans, 16, 21, 22, 104, 226

circulation, as physiology, 154. *See also* Harvey, William

cirrhosis, 62, 63, 70–73, *72*, 246, 267
Clark, James, 218, 246, 253, 325
classification: of chest diseases, 166; of disease, 27, 29, 37, 39–40, 60, 97–98, 259, 279; on Gall's, 61; Laennec on, 24; of organic lesions, 49, 54, 61, 62, 70, 230–231, 267; of parasites, 56; of physiological functions, 37, 42, 45, 64; as theory, 61
clergy, 16, 83–85, 94–96, 336n.42; Bishops of Quimper, 85, 94–96, 221, 222; Breton-speaking, 252; consultation of Cardinals, 84; Msgr. Casal, 271
clinical reasoning, 5, 176, 201–206
Cloche, Maurice, 123, 333n.5
Clouard, Dr. Paul, 285, 393n.131
coarctation of aorta, 182
Cocard, J. B., patient, 143
Cochin hospital, 70
coction, 234, 238, 247
Coleman, William, 295
colique métallique, 112
Collège de France, chair of anatomy, 28
Collège de France, chair of natural history, 58
Collège de France, chair of practical medicine: Corvisart in, 31, 32; Hallé in, 31; Laennec named to, 243; Laennec's salary in, 312; Magendie in, 275–276, 291; Récamier in, 275, 291
Collège de France, lessons at, 6, 74, 85, 137, 158, 165, 185, 245, 249, 258, 259–279, *264*, 284–285; criticism of, 274–279; failure to publish, 288–294; foreign students at, 259–260; on heart missing, 191, 200; papers of, 306; perceived vitalism in, 274–279, 293–294; schedule of, 260; structure of, 261–270; style of, 293; themes of, 271–274
Collin, Victor, 137, 148, 214, 240, 254, 261, 293, 325; on bronchophony, 164–166; experiments of, 191, 193; Laennec ignores, 166, 371n.107; on murmurs 191–194; on stethoscopy, 194
competition: on angina, 194; for entry to Ecole Pratique, 36–37; of Esquirol on organic causes of mental disease, 276–277; on gastrointestinal disease, 229; on organic causes of disease, 74; for student prizes, 47
Comte, Auguste, 227, 238
Condillac, E. B. de, on words, 346n.33
Congrégation, 7, 41, 44–46, 51, 53, 61, 83, 127, 211, 231, 243, 245, 270, 289, 342n.76, 361n.32, 373n.10
constitutions médicales, 33

consultation by letter, 83, 253
consumption. *See* tuberculosis
Cope, Henry, 74, 75
Corbière, J. J. G., 224, 243, 244, 325, 369n.52
Cornil, Victor, 347n.61
coronary artery theory of angina, 177–178, 179, 194–196, 201, 371n.113; falsified by clinical evidence, 205
Corrèze canals, 282–283
Corrigan, Dominic, 200
Corvisart des Marets, J. N., 6, 25, *26*, 31, 35, 36, 37, 38, 40, 46, 47, 53, 149, 195, 217, 258, 279, 325; and auscultation, 124; on the "better eye," vii; commentator on Bertin, 180; death of, 240; on heart disease, 177, 178–179, 182–183; on heart sounds, 393n.106; Laennec's opinion of, 37; Laennec's review of, 60; on lesionless disease, 161; on life force, 82; on nostalgia, 98; on percussion, 32–33; on pneumonia, 133; psychosomatism of, 154, 178–179, 368n.25; rejection of ancients, 32, 49, 60, 140, 240, 250; rejection of jugular sign, 188
Courbon-Pérusel, Dr., 253, 325, 384n.88
Cousin, Victor, 252, 325
Couvrelles, 80–82, *81*, 125, 256, 351n.24
crisis, 234, 238, 247, 290, 383n.75
critical days, 60, 247, 250; Laennec's rule for counting of, 251
Cruveilhier, Jean, 65, 67, 192, 258, 272, 291, 292, 325, 347n.62
Cullen, William, 27, 261, 261
Cuvi, F., patient, 70
Cuvier, Georges, 55, 58, 93, 244, 280, 295, 325, 392n.112
cylinder, 127, 128. *See also* auscultation, stethoscope
"cylindromaniac," 197

Dalbant, Eloi, 148, 183
Darbefeuille, J. B. A., 106
Daremberg, Charles, 75, 349n.100
Darwin, Erasmus, 27
death: as diagnostic sign of tuberculosis, 97, 157; sudden, 97; without organic lesions, 35, 168, 302
decision-making priorities, 202–205
degenerations, 348n.85
Delavau, Guy, 44, 242, 325, 380n.9
Delavau, Mlle, 44, 242, 325
De Lens, Jacques-Adrian, 211, 218, 229
Delpuits, J. B. B., 42, 44

dementia, 269
Desault, Pierre-Joseph, 40
Desgenettes, René-Nicolas, 25, 30, 103, 105, 149, 325; dismissal of, 245; éloge to Hallé, 244
Deslon, C., 45
Desportes, Eugène-Henri, 194
Deyeux, 53
diabetes, 115, 367n.80
diagnosis, 5; as detection of solid, liquid, or vital lesions, 266; by organic lesions, 38, 273; by symptoms, 27, 38, 50–51, 68–69, 97, 152, 155, 156, 247, 298. *See also* physical diagnosis
diathesis, 268
Dictionnaire des sciences médicales, 70, 75, 211, 230, 289, 373n.10; Laennec's resignation from, 231
Diderot, Denis, 38
digitalis, 126, 249, 382n.51
dilatation of heart, 131, 178–180, 182, 216; stethoscopic signs of, 189–190
Dirichard, patient, 197
discourse. *See* words
discovery, in general, 6, 121, 235; and chance, 46, 121; classification as, 61. *See also* priority disputes, Laennec, R. T. H.
discovery of auscultation, 121–150; breakthroughs in, 134–147; date of, 124–127; influences on, 76, 101, 111, 116–117; Laennec's account of, 122; stages in, 131–147
disease, 6, 151; Bouillaud's attack on lesionless disease, 277; causes of, 68, 162; equivalent to organic lesions, 302–303; Laennec's attention turns to, 259; Laennec's definition of, 266; names of, 152, 155, 215–217, 238; new and old, 271; as product of altered physiology, 29, 236; with vital lesions, 237; without organic lesions, 161, 168–173, 193, 196, 205–206, 237, 266, 268, 302; without symptoms, 161, 302–303
disease concepts, 6, 24–29, 50–51, 68, 151–152, 288; of Bayle, 37–40, 97–99; of heart, 176–177; impact of auscultation on, 209; of Laennec, 263–267; of Rostan, 272–273. *See also* theory
dissection, 28, 48, 65, 76; dangers of, 67, 79. *See also* anatomy, autopsy, pathological anatomy
doctrine: of Hippocrates, 50, 73–74, 250–251; of Laennec, 228, 233, 262, 290, 387nn. 19, 21

doctrine physiologique. See Broussais, François-Joseph-Victor
Dombideau de Crouseilhes, bishop, 94–96, 95, 244, 325, 355n.96
Double, François, 124
Doudeauville, Duc de, 242, 243, 280, 380n.9
Driesch, Hans, 297, 299
Dubois, Antoine, 47, 57
Dubois[-Drahonnet], A. artist, 86, 307
Duchesnau, François, 273
Dufour, student, 290, 306
Dumas, Charles-Louis, 263, 265
Duméril, A.-M. Constant, 30, 55, 57, 59, 149, 325
Dumesnil, J., patient, 145
Dumont, *femme*, patient, 114, 131
Dupuytren, Guillaume, 28, 36, 46–49, 54, 57, 58, 67, 68, 73, 76, 158, 183, 272, 288, 291, 325; Laennec's priority dispute with, 61–65; removed as examiner, 148; treatise on pathological anatomy of, 47

eclecticism, 6, 7, 233
Ecole Pratique de Dissection, 25, 36, 65
Edmé, J., patient, 71–72, 145
egophony, 131, 145–147, *146*, 315; specificity and sensitivity of, 204, 205
electricity, 266, 295
elephantiasis, 348n.85
emotions. *See* psychic causes of disease
emphysema, 131, 143–144, *144*, 152, 168, 216, 246, 261, 366n.73; as admission diagnosis, 214, 215
Empire, First, 3, 4, 105, 106, 126, 307. *See also* Napoleon Bonaparte
empyema, 279. *See also* thoracentesis
encephalitis, 277
encephaloid, 62, 63, 70, 246
English Sweate, 271
epidemics, 105
epilepsy, 97, 268, 277, 391n.92
epistemological obstacle, 29, 152, 339n.14
epistemology, medical. *See* clinical reasoning, diagnosis, disease concepts, signs, theory
Eriskin, Cardinal, 84
Erman (also Hermann) of Berlin, 185–186, 191, 219
errors: of Bayle, 97, 142, 157, 232; Condillac on, 346n.33; of exclusivity, 266, 268, 272, 296, 299; of Hippocrates, 140, 250; Laennec on, 60; of Laennec, 274–275; of Laennec on friction rub, 193; of Laennec on heart murmurs, 190; of Laennec on heart

errors *(cont.)*
  sounds, 174–176, 184, 187, 372n.137,
    384n.94; of Laennec on parasite, 58; of
    Laennec at Staël's autopsy, 127; of
    Magendie, 275; of Mériadec, 197–198; of
    organicists, 207
Esnault, 351n.26
Esquirol, J. E. D., 55, 272, 276, 325,
  389n.47, 391n.92
etiology. *See* disease: causes of
Examen des doctrines médicales, 225, 230,
  232; Laennec's reaction to, 231
exclusivity. *See* errors
experiments: of Barry, 186–187; of Collin,
  191, 193; as demarcation of physiology,
  287; of Erman, 191; of Laennec, 126, 183,
  249–250, 287–288; of E. Legallois, 268;
  of Magendie, 237, 267–268; on muscle
  contraction, 185–186, 191; in physics,
  122; of physiologists, 267–268, 270; of
  Pliny, 122–123; with seaweed, 249–250;
  therapeutic, 247, 249–250; of Withering,
  126; of Wollaston, 125
exploration, 119, 129–130

"facts," 53, 64, 68, 152, 163, 173, 233, 271,
  280
faculty of medicine, Nantes, 16–17, 78, 106,
  309
faculty of medicine, Paris, 24–30; chair in
  pathological anatomy, 293; closure of,
  244, 291; closure of, as therapeutic act,
  270; domino effect in, 73, 100, 108; Laennec dedicates book to, 149, 279; Laennec
  professor in, 244; leave granted to Laennec
  by, 280; pension granted to widow by,
  283; salary in, 312. *See also* Hippocratic
  medicine, chair of
falsification, 203, 205
Fauriel, C. C., 252, 325
Fernal, Jean, 270
Fesch, Cardinal, 83–84, 87, 241, 270, 326;
  bust of, 352n.46; retainer paid to Laennec,
  311
feudalism, Laennec's pamphlet on, 104–105,
  357n.8
fever, 29, 50–51, 97, 156, 169, 193, 214–
  216, 267–268, 388n.40; according to
  Hippocrates, 50, 251; apparent decline
  in, 214–216; Broussais's thesis on, 227;
  Fizeau on, 51, 139; Laennec's classification
  of, 51, 59, 267; Marion de Procé's own,
  94; as problem for anatomoclinical medicine, 74

Fizeau, L. A., 44, 46, 51, 63, 74, 85, 139,
  326, 342n.73
Fleuret, patient, 116
Floyer, 366n.73
Forbes, John, 200, 211–213, 230, 235, 252,
  282, 290, 326, 368nn; criticisms of Laen-
  nec, 200, 212, 249–250; Laennec's first
  edition altered by, 211–213; Laennec's
  second edition translated by, 213; national-
  ism of, 212–213; papers of, 373n.21
Fortassin, doctor, 58, 345n.17
Fothergill, John, 177
Foucault, Michel, 26, 225, 238, 286,
  341n.62
Fourcroy, Antoine-François, 19, 25, 47, 166,
  267, 326
Fouré, Julien, 106
Fragonard, Honoré, 73
Frayssinous, Denis, 243, 244
frémissement cataire. See thrill
French Revolution. *See* Revolution
Fréron, Elie, 11
friction rub, 152, 193–194, 201; as specific
  but not sensitive sign, 204

Galen, 25, 49, 56, 70, 382n.60, 387n.21
Gall, F. J., 60–61, 237
Gallot, doctor, 139
galvanism, 266, 271, 293
Garnier, surgeon, 60
Garrison, Fielding H., 295
gastroenteritis, 29, 59, 217, 227, 238, 248,
  277, 376n.84; statistics on, 388n.40
"gaze," 6, 26, 33, 38, 129, 180, 238
Gazette de santé, 229
Geison, Gerald, 295
Gelfand, Toby, 108
Gélineau, Dr., 385n.102
Gennes, Mme de (uncle's mother-in-law),
  15, 16, 21, 107
Gillibert, patient, 384n.93
Giscard d'Estaing, Valéry, 284
Goodfield-Toulmin, June, 298
Gould, Stephen Jay, 298
gout, 87, 196, 268; Laennec's own, 79–
  80, 82
Granville, A. Bozzi, 123, 124, 360n.11
gravity, 263
Greek language and medicine: derivatives
  from, 70, 129, 387nn. 21, 22; Laennec's
  studies of, 19, 32, 49–52, 73–75, 140,
  336n.42
Gregory, James, 261
Grigy, M. patient, 145–146, *146*

Grmek, Mirko Drazen, 121, 124, 134, 359n.41, 360n.19
Guérin, A., patient, 131
Guillio, Françoise, patient, 200
Gutenberg, 303

Haen, Anton de, 270
Haldane, John Scott, 297
Hall, Thomas S., 298
Hallé, Jean Noël, 30, *31*, 32, 36, 64, 258, 326; and ancient medicine, 31, 32, 49, 75; death of, 243; as hygienist, 31, 92, 112; as patron of Laennec, 48, 241
Haller, Albrecht von, 67, 184, 187, 188, 270; cited, 9
hallucinations, 269
Halna du Frétay, André, 131, 132, 133, 393nn.
Hanache, comte de, patient, 170
Hanot, V., 64
Harvey, William, 68, 184, 186, 187, 188
heart: aneurysm of (enlargement), 178; auscultation of, 131–132, 175–176, 183–201; disease of, 33, 35, 46, 115, 143; importance of hypertrophy and dilatation of, 178–180; size of, 182, 199. *See also* angina pectoris, murmurs, "organic heart disease," pericarditis, pulmonary edema, valves of heart
heart sounds, 33, 131–132, 315; amplitude of, 189, 201; Aretaeus on, 74; audible without stethoscope, 33, 74, 279–280, 393n.106; Barry's interpretation of, 186, 187; controversy over, 200–201; in disease, Laennec's interpretation of, 189–190; duration of, 184–185, 189; in health, 183–188; in health, Laennec's interpretation of, 184–185; Laennec's initial confidence in, 189–190; Laennec's loss of confidence in, 200; and music, 174, 189, 192, 370n.98; patient records on, 197–200; Stokes's interpretation of, 188
heat, 167, 266
Heberden, William, 168, 177
Helvetius, 38
hepatization of lung, 133, 154, 163, 165, 204
Herbé, N., patient, 115, 160
heredity, 162; of tuberculosis, falsified, 205
Hippocrates, 25, 31, 59, 60, 69, 74, 119, 229, 237, 250–251, 301, 382n.60; on auscultation, 122, 124; error of, 140, 250; on hats, 93; imputed empiricism of, 232–233; imputed vitalism of, 263, 289; Laennec

surpasses, 148, 211; Laennec's thesis on, 49–53, 343nn. 96, 100; and pathological anatomy, 74; on succussion, 140; on surgery, 141; theories of justified by Laennec's research, 234, 240, 247, 250–251
Hippocratic facies, 116, 224
Hippocratic medicine, chair of, 49, 73–75, 84, 271; Laennec's planned course in, 73–74, 306
history, 4, 285, 286–288; and biography, 3, 4; "diagnosis" of vitalism in, 299–302; effect of vitalist-mechanist debate on, 295–299; and Laennec, 294; of physiology and pathology, 7, 286–288
Hodgkin, Thomas, 229, 372n.141
Holmes, F. L., 121
Hope, James, 201, 372n.141
Hôpital des Enfans Malades, 137
Horace, 59
Horeau, C. E., 47
horse: experiments on, 186–187; rider of, as patient, 170
hospitals, 111; as laboratories, 122, 294; military, 18, 94, 103. *See also by name*
Hôtel Dieu: mortality in, 358n.31; of Nantes, 16, 18, 103, 106–107, 223; of Paris, 28, 41, 48, 127, 138, 211, 218, 305
Hôtel du Bon Lafontaine, 240
Huard, Pierre, 58
hubris, 300
humoralism, 266
Hunter, John, 177, 270
hydropsy, 159. *See also* pleural effusion
hypertrophy: auscultation in, 189–190, 201; in general, 62, 267; of heart, 131, 178–182, 216; missed diagnosis of, 197–198
hyperventilation, 171
hypochondria, 79, 192, 196
H[anache], le comte d', patient, 241

Idéologues, 25
idiotism, 269
illness: falsified as sign of organic lesions, 205; as sign of disease, 205–206; versus disease, 25. *See also* disease, stories of patients
Imhof, Arthur, 111
inflammation: absence of, in tuberculosis, 158–160; Broussais's view of, *228*, 229, 231; falsified as cause of lesions, 205; of intestine in fever, 29, 51; of heart, 183; Laennec's rejection of, 73, 234–235, 236, 269, 277; of lungs, 133; as organic lesion, 62, 267; of peritoneum, 36; tartar emetic for, 248

Institut de France, 58, 240, 243
irritation, 160, 238, 274, 301; Comte on, 227–228; Laennec's essay on, 231; as vital lesion, 237. *See also* inflammation
Itard, Jean-Marie-Gaspard, 55, 214, 326

Jacyna, Stephen, 7, 245, 270, 275
Jansenism, 15
Jarcho, Saul, 177
Jardinet, rue de, 37, 78
Jenner, Edward, 31, 149, 177, 194, 195
jeune personne, 122, 123, 124, 125, 165, 314
Jolivet, Jeanne, patient, 143, 147
Journal de médecine (of Corvisart), 33, 35, 36, 42, 54, 64, 67, 73, 75, 82; Laennec as editor for, 48, 58–61
Journal de physiologie expérimentale, 275
journals, 25
Juelle, Jean, patient, 192, 199
jugular vein, as sign, 33, 35, 105, 114, 139, 188
Juvenal, cited, 105

Keele, Kenneth, 122
Kergaradec, J. A Lejumeau de, 214, 230, 245, 290, 291, 326, 385n.100; placental murmur of, 193, 211, 214; on Laennec's discovery, 123, 125; reviews treatise on auscultation, 211; life of, 211, 373n.10; as biographer of Laennec, 244
Kerlouarnec, 11, 12, 96, 149, 166, *220*, 282, 283, 284, 313, 385n.110; repairs to, 219–221
Kernéis, Jean-Pierre, 94, 213–214, 307
Kitchen, James, 233, 229, 290, 326, 389n.47; cited 125, 165, 181; papers of, 306
Koch, Robert, 155
Kovacs, Yvan, 333n.5
Koyré, Alexandre, 176
Kreysig, Friedrich L., 179, 180
Kuhn, Thomas S., 235, 301
Kussmaul, Adolph, 367n.80

La Berge, Ann, 112–113
Laennec, abbé Michel (uncle), 13, 17–18
Laennec, Ambroise (cousin), 15, 77–78, 93, 248, 308, 328; as student, 103–105, 106, 107; tends his father, 224–225; tends Laennec, 282; works on auscultation, 110, 131, 148
Laennec, Christophe (cousin), 15, 16, 21, 91, 94, 100, 103, 104, 105, 110, 111, 127,

218, 243, 255, 256, 282, 328; on Laennec's early practice, 77–79, 82–83; on Marie-Anne, 92–93; marriage of, 93; souvenirs of, 307, 335n.19
Laennec, Désirée de Gennes (uncle's wife), 13, 17, 21, 22, 78, 82, 107, 328
Laennec, Dr. Eric, 307
Laennec, Emerance (infant cousin), 17, 328
Laennec, Emmanuel (cousin), 77–78, 107, 328
Laennec, François, 307
Laennec, Guillaume-François (uncle), 13–23, *14*, 28, 45, 53, 55, 92, 102, 149, 153, 232, 233, 245, 328; appeal for help by, 357n.25; arrest of, 16; on auscultation, 224; on brother's marriage, 91; character of, 107; course on therapeutics, 78; criticism of L's royalism, 103; dismissal of, 105–108, 308; death of, 224–225; early career of, 13–15; letters of, 307; reinstatement of, 223–224; suit with University of, 15; on tartar emetic, 247
Laennec, Julie Lehec (stepmother), 18, 19, 55, 78, 90–91, 336n.36; separation of, 91, 354n.77
Laennec, Marie-Anne (sister), 12, 19, 21, 91, 92–93, 328
Laennec, Mériadec (cousin), 77–78, 93, 110–111, 127, 149, 219, 221, 225, 243, 256, *281*, 281–283, 305, 328; acceptance of criticisms of Laennec, 230, 292; advice on practice of, from Laennec, 251–252; arrival in Paris, 124, 360n.11; error in cardiac diagnosis, 197–199; examination of Laennec, 169; failure to publish lectures, 289–294; hospital work of, 148, 248–249, 251; as literary executor of Laennec, 289, 290; manual of auscultation of, 289; praise of Broussais by, 292; refusal of marriage, 252; thesis on auscultation of, 130, 148, 218, 375n.44
Laennec, Michaud (brother), 12, 19, 22, 23, 30, 79, 90–91, 100, 307, 328; death of, 91; estate of, 91, 354n.76; prizes of, 47
Laennec, Michel (grandfather), 11, 328
Laennec, Michelle Guesdon (mother), 11, 13, 81, 328
Laennec, René-Théophile-Hyacinthe: ambitions of, 17, 18, 350n.7; appointment of to Collège de France, 7, 243; appointment of to faculty, 244; army service of, 18, 21–22; baptism of, 333n.2; birthplace of, 11, *12*, 334n.3; casting of as pathologist, 212,

239, 286; character of, 7–8, 17, 20, 58–60, 82, 83, 166, 210, 260–261, 309; correspondence of, 306–309; criticism of, 7, 64, 85, 160, 174, 200, 201, 202, 209–210, 230, 248, 249–250, 274–279, 291, 294; death of, 283; dogs of, 219, 386n.115; early education of, 13, 17, 18–19, 20, 335n.25, 336n.42; education of in Paris, 30–37, 46–53; family tree of, 328; films about, 333n.5; geology interests of, 17, 19, 20; ghostwriting activities of, 47, 48; health of, 21, 67, 76, 79–80, 82, 149, 154, 162, 169, 196, 250, 252, 279–283, 337n.53; and heart sounds, 174, 189, 192, 370n.98; hunting of, 76, 82, 83, 149, 219, 258, 352n.31; initial publications of, 35–36, 46–47; journalism of, 58–61; lifestyle of, 110; on marriage, 93, 100, 258; marriage of, 255–258, 353n.58; in metaphors, 271; missing papers of, 200, 296–297, 343n.93, 371n.113; musical interests of, 17, 20, 80–82, 252, 380n.6; obituaries of, 288, 289; papers of, 305–310, 348n.85, 389n.51; perceived vitalism of, 274–279; poetry of, 22, 44, 59, 81–82; political opinions of, 17, 85; on politics, 102, 110; praise for, 3, 261, 283–284, 287, 302; prizes of, 30, 47–48, 94, 355n.91; on publishing, 59–60; on Quimper, 59; recording of Bayle's defense by, 340n.42; religious conversion of, 44–46; religious views of, 7, 37, 61, 79, 84–86, 91, 96, 238, 274, 280, 282, 295, 296; reputation of, 254, 284–285, 286, 294; retirement to Brittany of, 147–149, 218–223, 225; reviews by, 58–61; royalism of, 7, 102–108, 233, 270, 274, 296, 353n.66; on social problems, 85; statue of, 291; suppressed ideas of, 7, 71, 279, 291–294, 301, 302; teaching of, 48–49, 110, 229, 251, 260, 270–271; thesis of, 49–53; treatment of himself by, 67, 79, 82, 162, 394n.11; vacations of, 80–82, 100, 254; wills and estate of, 313, 384n.89
—discoveries of: in anatomy, 46, 59, 70; in classification, 49, 61; in parasitology, 56–58; in pathology, 60, 61–64, 62, 63, 70–73, 238
—financial situation of: and early poverty, 19, 21, 22–23, 32, 47, 48, 50, 53, 54, 60, 67, 78; improvement of with practice, 82–84, 255; and sale of treatise, 148–149; and settlement with father, 90–91; summary of, 311

—language interests of: in general, 58; English, 19, 213. *See also* ancient authors, Breton language, Greek language and medicine, Latin
—travels of: to Bordeaux, 254–255; to Brest, 20; to Brittany, 96, 281–282; to Couvrelles, 79–82; to Paris, 23; to Quimper, 19–20; to St. Brieuc, 19, 21; to Soissonais, 258, 352n.31; to Vannes, 22
Laennec, Robert, 309
Laennec, Théophile-Ambroise, 289, 309
Laennec, Théophile-Marie (father), 11–12, 13, 18–21, 32, 37, 45, 48, 53, 54, 55, 67, 82, 83, 149, 222–223, 255, 307–308, 328, 354nn. 76, 77; legal settlement with children of, 90–92; separation from wife of, 91; spying on son by, 55, 255, 282
Lallemand, François, 272
Lammenais, Félicité de, 7, 84–85, 90, 270, 326
Lancisi, Giovanni Maria, 188
Landré-Beauvais, Augustin-Jacob, 139, 305, 326
Larrey, Dominique, 25, 55, 57, 103, 104, 326; on thoracentesis, 218
laryngotomy, 65
Lassus, Pierre, 57, 59, 73
lathe, 129, 258
Latin, 32; at bedside, 132, 254, 361n.49; case records in, 110, 141; essay on angina in, 194; Laennec's uses of, 61, 75, 84, 105, 129, 149, 269, 279; regret for the passing of, 59
Laubrière, Mme de, 32, 80
Laurent, patient, 199
Lavoisier, Antoine-Laurent, 31, 167, 203
Lecadre, Adophe-Aimé, 233; cited, 260
Leclerc, 30
leeches, 88–89, 116, 235, 254; trade in, 229
Lefebvre, patient, 197
Le Floc'h, Canon Jean-Louis, 307
Legallois, Eugène, 55, 261, 266, 326
Legallois, J. J. C., 94, 170, 265, 326
Légion d'honneur, 254
Lehec estate, 18, 19, 21, 83
Léonard, Jacques, 108, 244
leprosy, 271
Lerminier, N. T., 164, 246
Leroux des Tillets, J. J., 33, 35, 36, 48, 60, 139, 326
Lesch, John, 276, 287
lesion, concept of, 202; based on pathological anatomy, 266. *See also* liquid lesion, organic lesions, vital lesion

Levas, M., patient, 142
Lie, Reidar K., 201
Lieutaud, J., 67
life force. *See* vital principle
light, 266
Linnaeus, C., 27
liquid lesion, 266, 267–268, 269, 296;
 concept of based on pathological
 anatomy, 266
Lisfranc, 214
Littré, Emile, 75, 349n.100
liver disease. *See* cirrhosis
Lobstein, J. F., 67
Lorry, A. C., 75
Louis XVI, 15, 16
Louis XVIII, 55, 104, 105, 106, 107, 223,
 241, 243
Louis, P. C. A., 161–162, 214, 247, 292,
 326, 344n.3
Louis-Philippe, 241, 291
Lovejoy, Arthur, 295
Lucas, A., 139
lungs, auscultation of, 132–134, 152–173

MacMahon, Patrice, 139
Magdelain, patient, 199
Magendie, François, 7, 143, 200, 237, 240,
 244, 278, 286, 287, 291, 326, 387n.7,
 391n.81; criticizes Laennec, 275–276;
 Laennec cites experiments of, 265, 267–
 268; politics of, 275; at Société Anatomique, 65
magnets as therapy, 249, 315, 360n.28
Major, Ralph, 278
malaria, 156
Mal de la Baie St. Paul, 271
Malherbe, François, 11
malingering, 116, 298
mania, 269
Marey, Jules, 200
Marion de Procé, Claire, 93
Marion de Procé, P. M., 94, 103, 106, 107,
 326, 355n.94
marsh, 149, 221–222
mass insanity, 389n.47
materialism, 61, 108, 227, 237, 238, 273,
 294, 295, 297, 299, 301; of Bichat criticized by Buisson, 41–42, 45
Matthew Baillie, 211
Maulitz, Russell C., 64, 216
Mazet, A., 148
McKusick, Victor, 177
Medawar, P. B. and J. S., 298
mediator, acoustic, 122–123, 125

Meignen, Le, surgeon, 21
melancholia, 253, 269
melanosis, 62, 63, 70
Mémoire sur l'auscultation (1818), 122, 127,
 128, 132, 136, 137–138, 145
Mémoire sur les vers vésiculaires, 56–57, *57*
Mendel, Gregor, 360n.16
mental illness, 85, 169, 236, 253, 268, 269,
 391n.92
Mérat, F. V., 33, 212, 218
Mercier, L. S., cited, 24
mercury, 115
Mercy, F. C. F. de, 75, 326, 349n.100
Mesmer, F. A., 61
mesmerism, 45
metallic tinkling, 131, 139, 141–142, 254
methodist school, 74
Michel, Antoine, patient. See *cadet Rousseau*
microscope, 58, 129–130, 273, 291, 293,
 345n.14
midwife, patient, 112
military service of doctors, 18, 46, 103, 186,
 226–227, 373n.10
milk, 90, 282
Millet, Jean, patient, 131, 197
Millot, Nicolas, patient, 196, 205, 371n.116
mineral water commission, 254
Miniac, Hervé de, 307, 308
Miniac, Théophile-Anne-F. de (aunt), 19, *20*,
 21, 22, 90, 91, 92, 104, 256, 328
Mitchell, Charles, 261
mitral valve disease, 168, 172. *See also* thrill,
 valves of heart
modesty, 299–300
Moineau, P., patient, 140
Moissenet, patient, 199
Moniteur universel, 280, 358n.28
monomania, 269
Montmorency, Mathieu duc de, 44, 242,
 243, 326
moral causes/therapy, 85, 86, 93, 236 269.
 See also psychic causes of disease
Morgagni, G. B., 28, 49. 61, 65, 67, 70, 75,
 140, 180, 195, 268, 270; Laennec compared to, 213
mortality rates, Broussais and Laennec argue
 over, 233; at Charité, 94, 217, 246, 249; at
 Hôtel Dieu, 358n.31; at Necker, 94, 108–
 109, 214–216; from tuberculosis, 155–
 156; at Val de Grâce, 233
Morton, Richard, 156
Moutard-Martin, L.S., 78
murmurs, 190–194; indicative of valve disease, 190–191, 197–199, 201, 372n.141;

Laennec's rejection of, 192–193, 203, 277; as sensitive but not specific sign, 203; as sign of physiological lesion, 192; as sign of spasm, 191–192, 197
muscle, 191, 287; of bronchioles, 170; experiments on, 185–186; of heart, 182, 184, 185
Musée Laennec (ML), 35, 129, 260, 314, 305–306
music: Laennec's interest in, 17, 20, 80–82, 252, 380n.6; and heart sounds, 174, 189, 192, 370n.98; use in metaphors, 271

N***, Mme, patient 142
Nacquart, J. B., 210
Napoleon Bonaparte, 22, 25, 73, 94, 155, 241; Ambroise's loyalty to, 103, 308; autopsy of, 261; Bayle's disapproval of, 99–100 (Waterloo); and Chateaubriand, 87; and Corvisart, 31, 33, 60; and Fesch, 83, 84; Laennec's disapproval of, 45, 103, 104–105; Laennec *père*'s ode to, 45; One Hundred Days of, 102, 103; and Staël, 126, 308
narcotics, 170, 367n.76
nature: healing power of, 154, 160, 162, 247, 250, 271, 383n.60; Laennec on, 68
Necker hospital, 108–117, 123, 124, 125, 131, 137, 138, 143, 145, 165, 191, 218, 245, 248, 305, 358n.28; impact of auscultation in, 213–216; Laennec's appointment to, 102; mortality in, 94, 108–109, 214–216
Necker, Mme Suzanne C., 108
nemesis, 300
neologisms, 166, 237, 238, 300–301: Laennec on, 59. *See also* words
neuralgia, 196, 249
neurology, 277
Newton, Isaac, 263, 278
Noailles, Comtesse de, 280
nosology, 27, 29, 50, 68–69, 97, 227; Broussais's changing opinion of, 227; criticisms of, 38–40; Laennec retains, 251. *See also* diagnosis: by symptoms
nostalgia, 96–100, 115, 154, 162, 163, 266, 269, 274
Noverre, 148
numerical medicine, 5, 247, 315, 344n.3. *See also* positivism, statistics
nuns, 84, 163, 250, 278, 383n.58
nurses, 142; as patients, 112
nymphomania, 86
Nysten, Pierre, 265

observation: A. L. Bayle on, 121; in G. Bayle's thesis, 38; and discovery, 121, 147; of illness, 271; in Laennec's inaugural lecture, 233, 261; medical emphasis on, 25; of puerile respiration, 171
occupations of patients, 111–113; and disease, 112–113
Olgiati family, 285, 393n.131
Ollivry, George, 219, 256, 282, 326, 375n.49
One Hundred Days, 102, 103–105
Orfila, M. J. B., 254
"organic heart disease," 214, 215, 216. *See also* heart
organicism, 290, 293, 302; Broussais's criticism of, 236–237; failings of as a "discovery," 238; Laennec's criticism of, 206, 236–237, 272–274, 293, 302; product of auscultation, 273, 302
organic lesions: Bayle on, 38; as cause of disease, 151, 207; as cause of stethoscopic sounds, 202; classification of, 62, 181, 267; criteria for recognizing as cause of disease, 274; diagnosis of, 207; falsified as cause of disease, 206; of heart, 176–183; "[in]sufficient," 162, 268, 273; Laennec on, 180–183; Rostan on, 273; as solid lesion, 269, 296; in tuberculosis, 157
Osler, William, 356n.117
ossification: of coronary arteries, 178, 196; of valves, 35, 190–191
oxygen, 166–167, 367nn. 76, 80

Palud du Cosquer marsh, 149, 221–222, *222*
Panckoucke, C. L. F., 75
Paracelsus, 59
parasites, 21, 55–58, 76, 267, 348n.85; Laennec's classification of, 56
Paré, Ambroise, 140, 270
Paris school of medicine, 24–30. *See also* faculty of medicine, Paris
Parry, Caleb, 177, 179
Pasteur, Louis, 147
pathocenosis, 111, 237, 359n.41
pathological anatomy, 5, 6, 39, 25, 28, 40, 46–49, 58, 267, 302; auscultation as contribution to, 151, 209, 273, 280; Broussais's criticism of, 227, 232, 236; compensation for limitations of, 259; courses in, 48; as emerging discipline, 25, 28, 54, 286–287; and Hippocrates, 49, 51; history of, 7, 286; Laennec as hero of, 286, 294; Laennec on, 54, 151, 207, 230–231; Laennec on history of, 68, 69;

448 • INDEX •

pathological anatomy *(cont.)*
Laennec's classification of, 61–65; Laennec's course in, 47, 48–49, 65, 157–158,
271, 297, 306; method in, 33, 46–47, 70,
231; Paris chair in, 28, 293. *See also* Treatise on Pathological Anatomy
pathological anatomy, limitations of, 5, 70,
76, 77, 231; Bayle on, 69, 97; Broussais
on, 227, 232, 236; clinical physiology as
compensation for, 259; compensations for,
101, 173, 259, 273; demonstrated by clinical practice, 76, 77, 101, 154; as a "discovery," 238; invisibility of Laennec's views
on, 287; Laennec on, 207, 236; as unpopular view, 293
patient records, 4, 6; description of, 4,
70, 109–110, 141, 305; as "laboratory
notebooks," 4, 122; samples of, 114–
117
patient records as evidence, 4, 6, 201; in heart
sounds, 197–200; for historians, 6, 111,
214–216; for Laennec, 4, 122, 202, 271,
314; in puerile respiration, 170–171,
172; in research on critical days, 251; in
teaching, 271; in Treatise on Pathological
Anatomy, 71
patients: aristocracy as, 241–242; Breton soldiers as, 94–96, 115, 276; cardinals as, 84;
and charity, 85–86, 252; in family, 78–79;
with heart disease, 197–200; histories of, 5,
141, 162; in hospital, 109–110, 111–116,
214–216; private, 53, 54, 82–90, 240,
241–242, 251–255; with puerile respiration, 170–171, 172. *See also* clergy, nuns,
stories of patients
patients in *Traité de l'auscultation*, 126, 314–
323; additions for second edition, 317,
320–323; full histories of, 316–317; short
histories in first edition, 317–319
pectoriloque: as entry in *Dictionnaire*, 211,
212; as erroneous name for stethoscope,
129, 218, 360n.11
pectoriloquy (or pectoriloquism), 131, 134–
138, 142, 154, 194; and bronchophony,
163–166, 204; discovery of, 134–135,
314; and egophony, 145; threatened specificity of, 204
Pelletan, Philippe, 127
Pelletier, Joseph, 288
pénible carrière, 67, 258
percussion, 97; apparent dismissal of, 46; and
auscultation, 133, 134, 143, 152, 168,
177; in cases, 114, 139; and Corvisart, 32–

33, 46, 60, 177; of dog, 219; inadequacies
of, 132, 142; Laennec's manner of, 241; as
model for diagnosis, 202
Percy, Pierre-François, 55, 127
pericarditis, 193–194
peritonitis, 36, 246, 248, 159
Petit, Antoine, 13
Petit Port, 16, 21, 22, 282
Peyrilhe, Bernard, 30
phrenology, 229
phthisis. *See* tuberculosis
physical diagnosis, 27, 29, 32–33, 39, 60,
116, 152, 167; of Hippocrates, 51, 53; impact of auscultation, 209, 213–217; rapid
rise in, 213–217; triumph of, 302–303; of
tuberculosis, 141, 161. *See also* disease:
without organic lesions
physics, 122, 237, 278
physiological doctrine, 227–230, 260, 287,
292. *See also* Broussais, François-Joseph-
Victor
physiological lesion, 168, 202–203, 204. *See
also* vital lesion
physiology, 5, 25, 69, 267; and auscultation,
151–154, 168, 173, 192, 210, 240, 259,
280, 273, 287; Buisson on Bichat's,
40–43; clinical, 77–101, 141, 294; as
compensation for limitations in pathological anatomy, 259; in disease classification, 166; in disease, 76; as emerging
discipline, 25, 286–288; history of, 7,
286, 294; importance to Laennec of,
280; of Laennec ignored, 7, 212–213,
286–288, 302; Laennec's supposed
ignorance of, 234; suppression of in Laennec's treatise, 212; lesion of modeled on
pathological anatomy, 202–203; and political views, 7, 296–297. *See also* heart,
oxygen, respiration
Pickstone, J. V., 45, 296
Picot, P., 42
Pigeaud, Jackie, 75, 250, 305
Pinel, Philippe, 19, 30, 38, 55, 59, 326; as
alienist, 236, 269; and Broussais, 227, 229,
231; criticisms of, 38, 40, 166, 229, 236,
272; examination of Bayle by, 38–40, 166;
examination of Laennec by, 53; Laennec
on, 48, 49, 69, 132, 263; nosology of, 19,
27, 38, 69; pathological anatomy of, 29,
36, 227
Piorry, P. A., 214, 326
placental murmur, 193, 211
plagiarism, 63, 209, 234, 235, 290

pleural effusion: as admission diagnosis, 214, 215; diagnosis of, 145–147, 152, 216–217; egophony as specific sign of, 205; in tuberculosis, 158–160

pleurisy. *See* pleural effusion

Pliny, 123, 125

Ploucquet, Wilhelm G., 270–271

pneumonia: as admission diagnosis, 214, 215; anatomical pathological anatomy of, 68; and auscultation, 132–133, 134, 152, 172; bronchophony in, 165–166, 204; as disease of respiration or rales, 154, 166, 202; pectoriloquy in, 165–166, 191, 194; Rostan on, 273; stages of, 133; tartar emetic for, 234, 247–248

eumothorax, 140, 142, 172

Poiseille, J. L. M., 185

poisoning, 268

police, 44, 103, 242, 245

political tracts, 104

Pompéry, Charles de, 80

Pompéry, Mme de, 80–82, 94, 96, 107, 256, 327, 328; death of, 257

Ponsard, patient, 197

Pont l'Abbé farms, 96, 149, 221–222, *222*

Pope Pius VII, 45, 87, 342n.73

Popper, Karl, 203, 205

Portal, Antoine, 28, 67, 156, 177, 179, 272, 327; on auscultation, 127; on death of Mme de Staël, 126–127, 361n.30

Porter, Roy, 90

positivism, 5, 25, 68, 173, 227–228, 237–238. *See also* "facts"

postmortem examination. *See* autopsy *and individual cases and diseases*

Potel, abbé, 353n.58

Potel, Marie, patient, 131, 188, 197

Potu, 138–141, 142

Poulpiquet, Bishop, 222

practice: beginning of, by Laennec, 77–101; of Laennec, advice on, 251–252; styles of, 77

precordial lift, 189

"prepared mind," 76, 147

Prevost, patient, 199

priority disputes, 6, 235, 360n.16; with Andral, 164, 278; with Bertin, 180; with Broussais, 235, 238; with Collin, 166; dead predecessors in, 124; with Desportes, 194; with Double 124; with Dupuytren, 63–64; in history of science, 201

Prix Esquirol, 276, 389n.47, 391n.92

Prix Montyon, 280, 288, 313

prizes, of Buisson, 41; of Fizeau, 46; of Laennec, 30, 47–48, 94, 355n.91. *See also* competition

prognosis, 51, 53, 247; in tuberculosis, 97, 99, 283

Propositions sur le doctrine d'Hippocrate, 49–53, 343n.100; facsimile of, 343n.96

Prost, P. A., 29, 59, 61, 227, 230, 277, 376n.84

prostate, 348n.85

psyche and disease, 36

psychiatry, 277

psychic causes of disease, 36, 77, 82, 87, 89, 90–91, 154–155, 163, 178, 250, 256–257, 266, 279, 302; criticized, 278; de-valued, 298; Forbes's suppression of, 212–213; and psychic cures, 77–82, 94–96, 98; of tuberculosis, 115–116

psychology, 43, 298

psychosomatism, 7, 298; of Broussais, 227, 229; of Corvisart, 154; of Laennec, 80, 101, 117, 253

puerile respiration, 132, 151, 152, 166–173, 193, 247, 279, 287, 367n.80; as not indicative of an organic lesion, 168; patients with, 169–171, 172; as sign of asthma, 169; as sign of physiological lesion, 168; as sign of temperament, 167; specificity of, 204

Puget, François, 175, 328, 393n.133

pulmonary edema, 133–134, 152, 168, 192, 216; as admission diagnosis, 214, 215

pulse as sign of heart disease, 188

quartan fever, 116

Quélen, Bishop H. L. de, 44, 83, 243, 327

Quételet, L. A. J., 247

Quimper, 59

quinine, 288

rabies, 97, 253, 258

rales, 131, 132–134, 139; English nomenclature for, 361n.49

Ramée Pierre de la, 269, 389n.47

ramollissement cérébrale. *See* brain softening

Rasori, Giovanni, 248

Rault, René-Marie, 137, 138, 140–141, 148, 164, 219

Récamier, Joseph-Claude-Anthelme, 127, 224, 305, 327; and auscultation, 127, 136, 137, 139; at Collège de France, 275, 291; and Congrégation, 361n.32; Laennec's criticism of, 272; and Mériadec, 218, 219;

Récamier, Joseph-Claude-Anthelme *(cont.)*
as professor, 240, 244, 379n.1; and *Revue médicale*, 394n.19; as witness at Laennec marriage, 256
Récamier, Juliette, 353n.62
reductionism: in Broussais, 229, 230; compared to mania, 273; as excessive self-love, 273; Laennec's opposition to, 61, 230
Reil, J. C., 265
Reill, P., 296
Reiser, Stanley Joel, 303
Reisseissen, David, 170
religion and medicine, 41. *See also* clergy, Laennec, R. T. H.
research: in Hippocratic theory, 240, 247, 250–251; in parasitology, 55–58; in pathological anatomy, 46–49, 61–73; in therapeutics, 240, 247–250. *See also* auscultation, discovery, experiments
respiration: increased "need" for, 167, 169–171; physiology of, 154, 167, 169–171, 367nn. 76, 80
Restoration, 3, 4, 54, 85, 100, 123, 136, 210, 229, 252, 270, 297, 307, 309; and historians, 105, impact on Laennec family, 105–108; Laennec's reaction to, 102–105
retraction of thorax, *161*
revisions for second edition of *Traité*, 137, 151; Broussais's influence on, 233–234; on heart disease, 185, 200; as historical evidence, 202; on lung disease, 155, 158, 169, 171, 269; new patient evidence for, 315, 317, 320–323; research for, 247; summary of, 279
Revolution, 3, 4, 105, 106, 126, 155, 269, 307; as cause of disease, 178, 179; effect on Paris medicine, 24–28, 54, 67; in Nantes, 15–17, 21–22; of 1830, 229, 283, 291. *See also* war
Revue médicale, 210, 229, 394n.19
Rey, Roselyne, 69
rheumatism, 268
Ribes, 139
Richard, professor, 30
Richard, François, patient, 200
Robert, Fernand, 74
Roederer, J. G., 29, 59, 227
Rosenberg, Charles, 303
Rostan, L. L., 55, 168, 225, 254, 272, 291, 293, 299, 327; on cardiac asthma, 134; hostility with Laennec, 276; politics of, 275; review of *Traité* 1819, 210
Rouanet, J., 200, 391n.81

Rousseau, George, 295
Rousseau, Jean-Jacques, 35, 38. *See also* cadet Rousseau
Rouxeau, Alfred, 4, 11, 83–84, 104, 105, 125, 194, 219, 222, 233, 256, 282, 289, 306–309, 333n.2, 336n.36, 354n.80; as physiologist, 297
Royer-Collard, A. A., 149, 248, 289, 357n.25, 382n.46
Rozière de la Chassagne, 32
Ruffo, Cardinal, 84
Rullière, Roger, 371n.107

Sabatier, R. B., 13, 73
Sainte-Beuve, C. A., 252, 327
Saintignon, 342n.73
Salieri, Antonio, 32
Salpêtrière hospital, 94–96, 276, 309
Saunier, Charles, patient, 253, 254, 384n.89
Sauvages, François Boissier de, 27
Savart, Félix, 185
Savary des Brulons, Charles, 44, 94, 263, 327
scabies, 59
Schönlein, Johann Lukas, 155
science: Laennec on, 68, 271; Rostan on, 273. *See also* observation, theory
scientific language, 238, 301, 363n.107. *See also* words
sclerosis, 62, 63, 70
scrofula, 268
Scudamore, Charles, 137, 246, 253, 260, 327
seaweed, 249–250
Sénac, Jean-Baptiste, 177, 178, 187, 195
sensitivity of signs, 202–205
sensualism, 5, 25, 29
Serres, Augustin, 243
servants of Laennec household, 83, 255, 282, 392n.122
signs: auscultatory, 131–147; auscultatory, construction of, 201–206; auscultatory, as diagnosis, 141, 159; in general, 201–206; and medical technology, 302–303; one sign/one lesion priority, 159, 166, 202, 204–205, 234; as theory, 203. *See also* bronchophony, bruit, diagnosis, egophony, friction rub, metallic tinkling, murmurs, pectoriloquy, percussion, puerile respiration, pulse, rales
Signiolle, student, 67
smallpox, 40, 92, 143, 251
Smyth, John C., 36
social healing, 85, 270
Société Anatomique, 28, 48, 60, 64–65, 74,

75, 291; Laennec as president of, 65; papers of, 346n.52

Société de Belles Lettres, Soissons, 81

Société de l'Ecole de Médecine, 54–55, 57–58, 63, 70, 75, 84, 100, 105, 131, 243; emphysema specimen at, 143; essay on angina at, 194; essays on auscultation at, 127, 140, 142; new members of, 344n.4; papers of, 344n.2; publications of, 345n.7

Société d'Instruction Médicale, 32, 35

Société Médicale d'Emulation, 36, 60, 74

Société Médicale de Paris, competition, 194

Société philanthropique, 85–86

Société Royale de Médecine, 55

societies, 25, 54–58, 60, 136

solid lesion. *See* organic lesions

solidism, 266

sophrosyne, 300

Soranus, 74

Spallanzani, Lazzaro, 167

spasm as cause of murmurs, 192, 278

specificity of signs, 202–205; as priority for Laennec, 203, 205

spes phthisica, 79, 351n.17

St. Aignan, L. M. R. de, 107

St. André hospital, Bordeaux, 254

St. Antoine hospital, 193

St. Maur, rue, 258

St. Sulpice church, 45, 256, 353n.58

Staël, Mme de, 44, 108, 136, 327, 353n.62, 361n.30; auscultation of, 126–127

Stafford, Barbara, 28

Stahl, G. 265, 270

statistics, 247, 248, 249

stethoscope, 6, *130*, 85; design of, 129–130; *Dictionnaire* entries on, 211, *212*, 218; first use of, 125–126; made on Laennec's lathe, 129; name of, 129–130; price of, 150; of Wollaston, 125, 186. *See also* auscultation

Stokes, William, 187–188

Stoll, Maximilian, 32, 33, 270

stories of patients, 5, 77, 116, 239, 302; of Bayle, 269; devalued, 298. *See also* patient records

students: "culture" of, 45–46; foreign, 259–260; numbers of, 229, 260, 261, 278, 387n.7; as patients, 112; police surveillance of, 103; theses on auscultation by, 148

succussion, 131, 138–141, 142; on bottle, 219; Hippocrates on, 140, 362n.78

Sue, professor, 53

surgery, 25, 27–28; College of, 25. *See also* thoracentesis

Sydenham, Thomas, 270

Sylvius, F. de la Boe, 156, 157

sympathies of Broussais, 227, 228, 237, 238

symptoms. *See* diagnosis

syphilis, 51, 115, 182, 236, 268, 271, 277

"tact," 33, 38, 60, 148, 180

Taguel, patient, 199

Talaru, Mme de, 251–252, 370n.98

Tardivel, Mr, 149; Institute of, 17

tartar emetic, 85, 148, 234, 240, 246; criticism of Laennec's research on, 288, 293; Laennec's research on, 247–249, 279

telescope, 129

temperament, 114, 116, 167, 358n.34

Tenon, Jacques, 108

Terr, J. L. F., 59

Tesseyre, A. J. P., 44, 327

Testa, Antonio G., 179

tetanus, 97, 185, 268

Théodoridès, Jean, 58

theory, in general, 50, 53, 201; A. L. Bayle on, 121; classification as, 50, 61; coction and crisis as, 234; Laennec on, 50, 61, 67–68; as "scaffolding," 263, 387nn. 20; stethoscopic signs as theory, 147, 203

theory of disease, 77, 97, 239, 258, 259, 287, 298; Broussais on Laennec's, 237; of Laennec, 236, 263–267. *See also* coronary artery theory of angina

therapeutics, 51, 68, 160, 236, 280; of Broussais, 228–229; French indifference toward, 228, 293, 294; heroic, 382n.51; increased in second edition, 315; Laennec accused of neglecting, 218, 224; of Laennec ignored by historians, 235, 302; of Laennec, 271–272; Laennec turns to, 218–219, 234; with tartar emetic, 247–249. *See also* thoracentesis, travel as vital therapy

Thillaye, L. J. S., 53, 58

Thomson, John, 261

Thomson, William, 245, 250, 327

thoracentesis, 28, 139, 218–219; Bouillaud's attack on, 278; as justification for auscultation, 218–219, 234

Thouret, Michel, 50, 73, 75

thrill, 33, 131, 178, 179, 277; Laennec's doubts about, 192

Thucydides, 271

Todd, Robert B., 186

Tommasini, Giacomo, 248

Toulmouche, A., 124, 143, 148, 189, 253, 261, 282, 327, 360n.11

Traité de l'auscultation médiate, 5, 151–206; as contribution to pathological anatomy, 209; as contribution to physiology, 210; income from, 312; patients in, 71, 314–323; printing of, 143; reception of, 209–213, 373n.6, 374n.25

—1819 edition: physiological structure of, 154; price of, 149; release of, 150; sale of, 148; title page of, *153*; writing of, 127

—1826, second edition: cost of, 364n.123; and Prix Montyon, 280, 288

—1831, third French edition, 289, 290, 294

—English editions: first, 211–213; second, 213

—other editions, 213

travel as vital therapy, 82, 87, 99, 250

Treatise on diseases (unpublished), 6, 258, 259, 271; possible suppression of, 291–294; vitalism as reason for suppression of, 293–294. See also Collège de France, lessons at

Treatise on Pathological Anatomy (un-published), 5, 49, 54, 61, 65–73, *66*, *72*, 100, 149; structure of, 71, 343n.92, 348n.85

trismus (lockjaw), 185

Troliguer, 221

Trousseau, Armand, 64

tubercles, 62, 63, 70, 73, 98, 116, 157–158, *159*, 272; inoculation of, 67, 162; latency, falsified as cause of death, 205

tuberculosis, 74, 79, 90, 115, 152; absence of inflammation in, 158–160; as admission diagnosis, 214–215; apparent rise in, 215–216; Bayle on, 96–100; causes of, 161–163, 205, 278, 279; and contagion, 97, 162; cure of, 160, 246, 250, 276; death as diagnostic sign of, 97; diagnosis of, 136–138, 156; as disease of voice, 154, 202; and heredity, 97; incidence of, 193; Laennec on, 155–163; in Laennec family, 13, 18, 162, 250; latency of, 161–162; and liquid lesion, 268; mortality from, 155–156; pectoriloquy as sign of, 136–138; psychic causes of, 115–116; and seaweed therapy, 249–250; specific signs of, 204; treatment of, 160; unification of, 156–158

typhoid, 377n.84

typhus, 94, 276

urinary tract, disease of, 84; calculi in, 243, 267, 268

Usé, Marie-Louise, patient, 248

vaccination, 31, 92

Val de Grâce hospital, 217; mortality in 233

Valentin, Michel, 357n.8, 358n.25

Valsalva, Antonio-Maria: depletive therapy of, 236; maneuver of, 169

valves of heart, 33, 35, 46, 115, 177, 178, 182, 190–194, 372n.141; globular vegeta-tions on, 182, 368n.40

Van Berchem estate, 19

Van Hall, H. C., 260, 327

Varennes, Mme de, 32

Vauquelin, Louis-Nicolas, 254, 267

Vyau de Lagarde, 148

Vicéra, Marianne, patient, 249

Vicq d'Ayzr, Félix, 67

Vieussens, Raymond, 177

Villard, René, 385n.100, 386n.115

Villèle, Joseph, 243

Villemin, Jean A., 155

Villenave, Mathieu G. F., 136, 327, 357n.8

Villeneuve, patient, 197

Villeron, S., patient, 145

Vincenti, Cardinal, 84

vital lesion, 163, 171, 237, 250, 263, 266–267, 268, 269, 278, 289, 296; Bayle on, 69, 96–101; concept of based on pathological anatomy, 266; diagnosed by stetho-scope, 168, 192, 273. See also psychic causes of disease

vital principle, 69, 82, 98, 168, 171, 278, 287, 289, 298; Broussais refutes, 237, 238; Laennec on alteration of, 266–267, 269; Laennec on existence of, 173, 263–266; Rostan denies, 273

vitalism, 6, 7, 227, 228, 273, 289–290; "error" of, 266; as excessive modesty, 299–300; falsification of, 293, 302; Laennec's rejection of, 295–296; perceived in Laen-nec, 274–279, 293–294; as reaction to par-adigm shift, 301; relationship of to politics and religion, 296–297, 299; typologies of, 299; and Wöhler, 293

voice, 147, 154, 166, 202; auscultation of, 134; and physiology of Buisson, 43

Voltaire, 38

Vorogidès, Dr Athanase, patient, 254, 276

Wagler, K. G., 29, 59, 227

Walter, J. G., 65

war: as cause of disease, 155; from 1812 to 1814, 94–96; in Vendée, 16, 21–22, 104, 337n.59

Watson, James D., 299

Weiner, Dora, 28, 85
Weisz, George, 7, 286, 294
Wellington, 102
White Terror, 105–111
Williams, C. J. B., 186, 201, 261, *262*, 327;
   criticism of Laennec by, 202
Williams, Elizabeth, 293, 296, 297
Willis, Thomas, 140
Withering, William, 126, 249
Wöhler, Friedrich, 293
Wollaston, William H., 125, 185, 186
words, 6, 234–235; absence of as "anomie,"

238, 379n.154; Buisson on, 52, 225;
coined by Rostan, 272; and clinical language, 26, 183–184, 216; Condillac on,
346n.33; of decision-making, 202; and differences with Broussais, 238; invented for
stethoscopy, 121, 122, 129–130, 131,
132, 134, 145, 147, 163, 216; Laennec on,
59–60, 70, 104–105, 121; Laennec's uses
of, 287, 294, 382n.51; needed to frame
doubt, 301; and vitalism, 300–301. *See also*
neologisms, scientific language
worms. *See* parasites

ABOUT THE AUTHOR

Jacalyn Duffin earned her M.D. degree at the University of Toronto and her Ph.D. at the Sorbonne. She holds the Hannah Chair of the History of Medicine at Queen's University in Kingston, Ontario, Canada. She is the author of *Langstaff: A Nineteenth-Century Medical Life* and is the cotranslator, with Russell C. Maulitz, of Mirko D. Grmek's *History of AIDS: Emergence and Origin of a Modern Pandemic* (Princeton).